GLAUCOMA—PATIENT
TO PATIENT

GLAUCOMA— PATIENT TO PATIENT

✦

A Coping Guide For You And Your Family

Edith Marks

iUniverse, Inc.
New York   Bloomington

iUniverse books may be ordered through booksellers or by contacting:

iUniverse
1663 Liberty Drive
Bloomington, IN 47403
www.iuniverse.com
1-800-Authors (1-800-288-4677)

Because of the dynamic nature of the Internet, any Web addresses or links contained
in this book may have changed since publication and may no longer be valid. The
views expressed in this work are solely those of the author and do not necessarily
reflect the views of the publisher, and the publisher hereby disclaims any responsibility
for them.

ISBN: 978-1-4401-8320-1 (sc)

Printed in the United States of America

iUniverse rev. date: 3/24/2010

Table of Contents

PART I

1. Windows On The World 3

2. The Many Varieties of Glaucoma 26

3. The Special Child: Primary Congenital (Infantile) and Juvenile Glaucoma 67

4. The Four Horsemen of: Diagnosis 86

5. Medication Treatment—A Drop or Two A Day Keeps The Scalpel Away 118

6. The Remarkable Ability of Light 152

7. The Therapeutic Blade 172

8. Cataract—Clear View Ahead 197

9. The Next Big Thing: Retooling and Protecting The Eye: Neuroprotection, Genetics & Stem Cells 214

PART II

10. Therapies That Complement Medical Treatment 239

11. Nutrition—Its Contents and Discontents 283

12. Take Charge 372

13. How To Make Your Workplace Vision-Friendly 413

14. Graceful Accommodation 419

Glaucoma--Patient-to-Patient is a "must have" book for you.

In it you will find comprehensive information to help you manage your condition. This book takes you on a journey of understanding from definition of the disease to diagnosis-to treatment options and their outcomes. Cataract and macular degeneration and the impact of both are clearly defined.

Part II covers a wide range of activities to help cope with and enhance the treatment options described in Part I—from meditation to herbal treatment to nutrition to supplements to self-help activities to support services and much, much more.

Glaucoma--Patient-to-Patient is a book you will refer to often during your glaucoma journey.

Edith

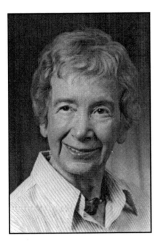

Edith Marks worked for the New York City Board of Education as teacher of emotionally disturbed children, then Supervisor, teacher training. She is co-CEO of the New York Chapter Glaucoma Support and Education Group, of The Glaucoma Foundation and is a founding member of The World Glaucoma Patient Organization. She serves as patient representative on several evaluating committees including the Cochrane Eye and Vision Group, London,England (reviews of eye interventions). She is also an avid gardener and volunteers with an award winning community garden and she has won community achievement awards.

Encomiums

Meeting Edith Marks one can't help feeling that here is someone who really practices what she preaches. Edith is enthusiastic, interested, and involved. She is someone who partners with her doctors to not only obtain the best care she can for herself, but to help her educate others about their own responsibility for their eye care. The theme of "Coping with Glaucoma" is about taking responsibility and partnering with health care professionals to obtain the best possible outcome.

This second edition builds on the successful and informative book that has helped so many to better understand the various aspects of glaucoma, its diagnosis and treatment. Importantly, Edith deals with all aspects of glaucoma including patients' need for support and comfort when dealing with a lifelong, vision-threatening condition.

Those of us in the field of eye care recognize that many of the subjects so masterfully handled by Edith are never discussed in routine doctor visits. Having a book like this as a reference provides answers to many questions and even suggests lists of questions to ask. As a firm believer that each of us has the primary responsibility for our own health care, I appreciate the advice and encouragement Edith provides in her book.

Thomas M. Brunner
President and CEO
Glaucoma Research Foundation
251 Post Street, Suite 600
San Francisco, California 94108

***

Dear Edith,

Your opus is a magnus of the first order. I am bowled over by it - its scope, its depth, its erudition. My only query is whether or not it is just too detailed? It is a vast reference book, almost like a text book. I can't see someone sitting in an armchair and reading through it from go to whoa. I can see plenty of people using it to obtain detailed information about specific topics. I've absolutely nothing to add, subtract, suggest. Go for it! Heartiest congratulations!

Ivan Goldberg, MD
Clinical Associate Professor, University of Sydney
Head, Glaucoma Unit, Sydney Eye Hospital
Director, Eye Associates
President, Australian and New Zealand Glaucoma Interest Group
Immediate Past President, World Glaucoma Association and the South East Asia Glaucoma Interest Group
Past President, Royal Australian and New Zealand College of Ophthalmologists

Writing this volume is clearly a large undertaking but not too overwhelming for Edith Marks, a special and enormously-talented woman who is both dedicated and passionate. As a volunteer, she has worked tirelessly for many years on behalf of a variety of issues and organizations. However, Edith has probably made her greatest impact in the field of glaucoma. With this eye disease, she has been an outspoken advocate, an ardent educator, and a staunch protector of patient rights.

On behalf of the entire family of The Glaucoma Foundation, it is an honor and pleasure to congratulate Edith Marks, a collaborator, partner, and true friend of ours on a monumental achievement. This updated and expanded version of her earlier book is sure to be a gift to the glaucoma community and be enthusiastically used by those who suffer from these insidious diseases we all call glaucoma.

Scott Christenson
CEO
The Glaucoma Foundation
80 Maiden Lane
New York, NY 10038

"As a patient, I usually want to know more about my health conditions, treatment options, and coping skills than what the busy doctor tells me. Edith does just that with her latest book on glaucoma. This book contains a tremendous amount of information in great detail and will be my constant companion as I live with this condition and offer support to other glaucoma patients."

Sherri Holte, owner http://: Glaucoma groups.yahoo.com/group/glaucoma/

Foreword

'It is a great pleasure for me to write the foreword for *Glaucoma - Patient to Patient*, a book which has become the classic reference for glaucoma patients worldwide. Edith is a dynamic and dedicated person, one of the early members of the first glaucoma support group in the United States, founded in 1983 in New York City, an organization which has grown to approximately 3,000 members. She is also one of the founding members of the glaucoma patient Board of Directors and Director of Literature Development of the World Glaucoma Patient Association (WGPA), an umbrella group dedicated to initiating and serving patient glaucoma support groups around the globe.

This work represents the second edition of *Coping with Glaucoma* and has been liberally updated from the first edition of 1997. It is a book which can benefit all glaucoma patients, from those with suspected or early disease to those with advanced visual loss. Glaucoma is a leading cause of blindness worldwide. It is not a single disease, but a specific pattern of optic nerve head and visual field loss which represents the final common pathway of a number of diseases which affect the eye. Most, but not all, of these diseases, are characterized by elevated *intraocular pressure*, which was long equated with the disease itself, but is actually a risk factor (still the most important one known) for visual loss. Primary open-angle glaucoma is the most common glaucoma and leading cause of blindness in persons of African descent, while angle-closure glaucoma is more common in Asia, particularly China. Normal-tension glaucoma accounts for a large majority of the glaucoma in Japan, for unknown reasons, while exfoliative (pseudoexfoliation) glaucoma is the most common recognizable cause of open-angle glaucoma worldwide and is the most common glaucoma in some countries, such as Norway, Ireland, Russia and Greece. Not only has a cure thus far eluded us, but we still lack basic knowledge of the underlying causes of these different diseases. Although significant treatment advances - medications, laser, and surgical - have been made in the last decade, all of these are directed at lowering *intraocular pressure*. We still lack treatment to enhance the blood flow to the eye and to prevent the death of the *retinal* ganglion cells which carry visual impulses to the brain. Nevertheless, we are at the beginning of a major biomedical revolution which will lead to us the eventual goal of nerve regeneration and reversal of blindness, through the promising approaches of gene transfer, stem cell research, nano-medicine, and new methods of drug delivery.

Where does the patient stand in all this? In the United States, it is estimated that half the persons with glaucoma are unaware of it. In developing nations, the number is far greater, while treatment is often minimal or lacking. About 65 million people in the world have glaucoma of one form or another, and about 7 million are blind from it. Most of that blindness could have been prevented with early and adequate detection and treatment. But more is needed than just detection and treatment. Patients take medications, which may have side effects, and are often inconvenient and expensive, for a condition which has no symptoms and no adverse effect on quality of life until it is fairly well advanced. Small wonder that compliance--the patient's ability to adhere to a prescribed regimen--and persistency---continuing to fill prescriptions and staying on a prescribed medication after a period of time are major problems. The more about a disease a patient knows, the more he or she is likely to fare better with treatment. Doctors often don't have the time or ability to answer the many questions which patients have about the nature of glaucoma, how to administer drops correctly, the side effects of medications, and the intricacies and value of the various new visual field and imaging modalities currently being marketed, not to mention the relative potential value of alternative medicine, support groups, and low-vision techniques and sources of assistance for persons with varying degrees of visual loss. For much of this, the patient has to search, but that search can be complicated or derailed by a great deal of misinformation which is readily found in addition to the available information.

Enter *Glaucoma - Patient to Patient*. This valuable, information-filled book is a thorough guide to suit most of the needs of most glaucoma patients. The book begins with a description of the eye and how it functions, an excellent discussion of the optic nerve, often a difficult subject for patients, and also delves into blood flow and the immune system. This is followed by descriptions of the different glaucomas, not only those affecting adults, but infants and children as well. The section on diagnostic testing is one especially valuable for the patient, as it explains the methodology of measuring *intraocular pressure*, visual fields, and the optic disc, including artifacts and limitations. The section on medications contains detailed information on side effects, and that on surgery is similarly detailed. Much space is devoted to alternative medicine, not only vitamins, supplements, and herbal treatments, but also life style and well being. We don't know the effects of these in most cases on glaucoma, but the discussion is well balanced and allows the patient to make his or her own decision. Information is provided on coping with visual limitations, how to start a patient support group, low vision aids, and organizations which provide aid or information to persons with blindness.

All in all, this is a book that every glaucoma patient should own. The information in it is not only a one-time read, but a reference source to which patients can turn over and over again as necessary. Edith Marks has made a superb contribution to the education and well-being of glaucoma patients everywhere.

Robert Ritch, MD
Professor of Clinical Ophthalmology
Chief, Glaucoma Service
Surgeon Director
The New York Eye and Ear Infirmary
310 East 14th Street
New York, NY 10003

Royalties from this book will be donated for research on glaucoma
This book is dedicated to the members of
The Glaucoma Support and Education Group,
without whom it would never have been written.

I also wish to thank Paul Sidoti, MD for his valuable and authoritative assistance in Part I and Dolores Perri, MS, RD, CNS, and Benjamin Lane, FAAO, FCOVD for their insignts on the Nutritional Chapter, Robet Ritch, MD, Ivan Goldberg, MD, and Dan D.Gaton for their invaluable assistance and encouragement, Barbara Friedman and Susan Genis for their insights in body training, and the following medical personnel for supporting our efforts at educating our group with the most recent developments in glaucoma therapy—Christina Alexander, ADBP. Kathy Aquilante, OD, Michael Banitt, MD, Gaetano Barile, Syril K. Dorairaj, MD, Nogs Harizman, MD. Gregory Harmon, MD, Reza Iranmanesh, MD, Mindy Levine, MSW, Richard MacKool, MD, Lorraine Marchi, PhD, Jeffery A. Morrison, MD, Pat-Michael Palmiero, MD, C. Michael Samson, MD, Celso Tello, MD, Gurang J. Trevedi, MD, James Tsai, MD. I also want to thank Sherri Holte and Vivian Werner for their WEB assistance and members of the Support Group, Ann Bially and Linda Flood. And lastly, I want to thank Janice Ewenstein, Sandra Owen for their precise editorial assistance, Kira Zmuda for general assistance and Scott Christensen who has championed my efforts throughout the long process of producing this book.

Preface

Glaucoma has been my constant companion for over thirty years. When my glaucoma was first diagnosed little did I know I would be traveling a long and often arduous path. As with any chronic disease, glaucoma insidiously intrudes into every facet of daily living. Unremitting in its demands if left unattended, glaucoma may lead to severe vision loss. Glaucoma strikes over 65 million people worldwide, 6-to-7 million of whom will be bilaterally blind. It is one of the four major causes of vision loss along with macular degeneration, cataract, and diabetic retinopathy. It is the second leading cause of preventable blindness worldwide.

Glaucoma ranges over the entire population, from babies to seniors. Risk factors increase with age. From age 35, the risk of glaucoma mushrooms with each decade. Although glaucoma is thought of as an aging disease, up to twenty-five percent of those diagnosed are fifty or under. Researchers and doctors believe that, especially in western countries with the increase in longevity, this demographic is on the brink of increased vision problems leading to blindness. By the eighth decade of life, some fourteen percent of Americans will have glaucoma and in patients with diabetes mellitus, glaucoma incidence may be three times as great as in the unaffected population

Untreated, glaucoma can lead to legal blindness defined by the limits of corrected vision to be no more than 20/200 in acuity in both eyes, and/or 20 degrees or less peripherally, or being able to see only the big "E" on the standard eye chart and/or reduced to tunnel vision.

Glaucoma plays no favorites. John Glenn, one of the first astronauts, described the astounding beauty of the universe in his first space flight. Between this and his next flight, thirty years later, Glenn found that he had glaucoma, but with successful treatment, he reported on the later flight, that he could still see these wonders. Over the ages, losing sight has not prevented creative and imaginative people from all walks of life--known and unknown, who have surmounted debilitating eye conditions to produce works of art and literature--political leaders, scientists, explorers who have lived or are living an enviable quality of life.

And it is this quality of life that we seek to retain. Often, however, our tricky vision drives us to distraction. When our visual acuity is compromised, when contrast sensitivity increases our vulnerability to falls-to bumping into things-to requiring more time for reading print, movie titles, or labels in grocery stores-to mistaking a tree for a person--we may despair until we discover we're not alone. Others in support or chat groups on the internet are ready to share experiences and offer advice. Knowledge that help is readily available is one of the gifts available to us.

Early in my glaucoma experience I took advantage of this gift by joining a support group in New York City. Over the years I edited a newsletter based upon the lectures of professionals in the fields of glaucoma treatment, nutrition and the healing arts. These newsletters ultimately formed the basis of my first book, *Coping With Glaucoma.* Writing about glaucoma is a work in progress. The newsletters that I continue to edit for our group report the latest therapies and these, together with the most recent research, has been the basis for *Glaucoma: Patient to Patient,*

Ideally, I hope in the future that such a book will no longer be necessary should a cure be found for glaucoma, but for the present, I believe and hope that this book will empower glaucoma patients together with their medical treatment to embrace self-help and self-determination, and assist in whatever way they can to work towards a cure for this disease.

Edith Marks
New York, New York

PART I

CHAPTER 1

Windows On The World

○ ○

Sight is a hidden gift, apparent only when lost
Edith S. Marks,

"The most pathetic person is someone who has sight, but no vision",
Helen Keller

What is an eye? What is this remarkable organ that lights up our world revealing a universe of color, form and texture? Romantically, the eye might be called the royal road to vision, inspiring odes to its beauty and versatility, or it may be compared to a camera describing how light entering through a shutter (the pupil) stimulates the film (the *retina*) to record images that are sent up to the lab (the brain) for processing. Actually, the eye is an extension of the brain and as such, it is equipped with the necessary tools to provide information to the brain, that grand monarch, governing our entire internal universe. Technically, vision is defined as a process of converting photons (light rays) into electrochemical signals that, via various neurons in the *retina*, a thin body of tissue composed of a number of cell layers, travel to the brain. Through the use of super-speedy spectroscopy, researchers have documented the mechanism for the transformation of the visual pigment rhodopsin. Upon absorption of a photon of light, it is transformed to a different configuration that is then converted into other forms of energy. These biochemical signals, like boxcars on a train with the optic nerve as track, send this information to the visual cortex (about sixty-five percent of the brain is devoted to vision). In a millisecond, you see your dog snatching a cupcake off the table.

Evolutionary development began with the *eukaryote* cells (cells in which the nucleus is surrounded by a membrane—one of the oldest cells on the planet). Throughout time, and in response to newly available oxygen, the eye developed into its present form. Curiously, the lizard still possesses a third eye, which researchers claim, detects time. The eye a teaspoon-sized organ about an inch in diameter, weighs about a quarter of an ounce, and is about one-half cubic inches in volume. An incredible array of specialized cells is packed into this tiny space. The number of cells in the eye is mind-boggling. Consider that the space shuttle has a trifling 52 million parts while the human eye has 137 million photoreceptors alone, along with an additional 2 billion other cells. The *retina* ganglion cells, so vulnerable in glaucoma, number over a million cells.

Basically, the eye is divided into two cavities separated by the lens. The front cavity is further divided by the *iris* into two chambers, *anterior* and *posterior* (front and back.) Both layers are filled with the aqueous fluid. The *anterior* holds about 2 cc (centimeters) of aqueous. Behind the lens, the second cavity contains a gel-like substance called the *vitreous* humor composed primarily of water (90%), hyaluronic acid, collagen fibrils, and *micropolysaccarides* (a form of sugar found in body gels). Three layers surround the entire structure. The outer layer is composed of the *cornea* and *sclera*, a structure that protects the delicate *retina* and provides for the rigidity of the eye. The *cornea* is what you see when you look in the mirror. The *sclera* is the tough white membrane that covers the entire eye. The *uvea*, the middle layer, contains the *choroid* (blood vessels), providing nourishing blood and oxygen to the eye. The Greeks named this part of the eye *uvea* because of its dark color resembling that of a grape. Neurons, essential for transmitting information to the brain, line the innermost *retinal* layer.

Within all species, including humans, eyes have adapted to the needs of the organism. Some animals, the fly for example, have multiple eyes that provide the insect with an extensive view of its environment. The human eye achieves its wide range of vision through its six extra ocular muscles--the *superior* and *inferior, medial* and *lateral rectus muscles* and the *superior oblique* muscle that are cushioned and surrounded by a layer of fat. Movement of the eyes—up, down, side-to-side, and diagonally also allow the eye to register expression. How often have your rolled your eyes at a corny joke?

Scientists have discovered a memory retrieval system linked to eye movement. They have found that to access visual memory right-handed people look up and to the left; left-handed people look to the right. The eyes turn downward to imagine an unusual object; imagining a particular sound causes the eye to look horizontally right. Eye movement, apparently, appears to be essential for activating both sides of the brain—the left for retrieval of information and the right for creative imagining.

The muscles and other structures of the eye also possess interesting features. Properties of the muscles and the *iris* offer several possibilities that affect other diseases. Researchers studying muscular dystrophy are investigating whether properties contained in the eye muscles will lead to therapy that can halt the muscle deterioration of this disease. Diabetics, wearing a series of fluorescent-based glucose lenses, may one day be able to monitor fluctuations of glucose levels by simply looking into the mirror. Their contact lenses would be fitted with disposable plastic fluorescent probes that would change color depending upon glucose level. Diabetics would then be able to match the eye color to colors on a strip indicating safe and unsafe blood glucose levels.

Possible detection of Alzheimer's disease, using a non-invasive optical method that directs an infra-red laser into the lens, has revealed the existence of beta amyloid proteins that form plaques in the brain characteristic of this disease. The method induces a process called quasi-elastic light scattering. In 2003, researchers discovered that these proteins, existing also in the lens of the eye, are capable of creating unusual cataracts specific to the disease.

Mayo Clinic researchers studying 37,786 cases of people in which samples of central nervous system (CNS) fluid were analyzed for various health reasons, found a link among 28 cases with low CNS for glaucoma.

To summarize, the back part of the eye contains the *vitreous body*, the *optic nerve* and the *retina*; the front of the eye, the *cornea, iris, pupil* and *lens*. This part of the eye contains the aqueous humor, the drainage of which is responsible in part for the problems associated with glaucoma. Two pathways for drainage exist: 1) through the *trabecular meshwork* and *Schlemm's Canal* and 2) through the *uveoscleral* pathway accounting for ten-to-twenty percent of outflow. See illustration for drainage image.

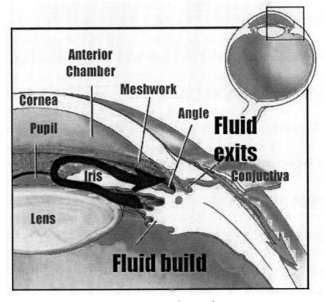

Drainage channel

THE CORNEA

Both the cornea and the lens are transparent, a feature that enables the eye to receive photons of light. Roughly the size of a dime, the transparent tissue in the cornea fuses with the *sclera*. It performs several eye functions, the most important, the production of a clear image, achieved through its focusing powers. Should the normal smooth round curved cornea be football shaped, however, a condition called astigmatism results. Normally, light rays bend equally in all directions. With astigmatism, light rays fall on several points on the *retina* rather than one point, distorting near and distance vision.

The eye is not a perfect sphere for the cornea protrudes slightly in front. Three layers comprise the thin membrane of the cornea. The *epithelium layer* (surface layer of cells) in contact with the tear film and eyelids protects the eye from trauma, bacteria and other invaders. It constantly sloughs off and replaces cells. The *stroma,* the middle and thickest layer consisting of hundreds of thin layers of *collagen* and *kerotocyte cells* is responsible for clarity, transparency, flexibility, and strength. The *endothelium* innermost single cell layer does not grow or reproduce itself. It borders the *stroma* on one side and the aqueous on the other and it helps maintain transparency, hydration and nourishment of the cornea. Injured or lost, these cells cannot be replaced. Some claim that the cornea is the most exquisitely organized connective tissue in the body, and since it is responsible for two-thirds of the refracting power of the eye, this may be a valid claim.

The cornea plays an important role both in the diagnosis of *intraocular pressure* and in the health of the eye. Thin corneas give a false reading of a lower *intraocular pressure* than may actually be the case. Analysis of the cornea is achieved through *pachymetry* (See Chapter 4). If the cornea is thin, doctors may add (to the dismay of patients) an additional four or five points to the *intraocular pressure* reading. *Pachymetry* has proven to be particularly useful in identifying those people with high pressure but who do not progress to glaucoma from those whose glaucomas will progress. In an important study, people in the non-progressive group had thicker corneas. Central corneal thickness has aroused interest in another form of measurement. Corneal resistance as measured by applanation tonometry using just a puff of air (See Chapter 4), provides yet another means to measure *intraocular pressure.*

Cell loss during a surgical procedure is not inevitable, but it does occur. The cornea in my left eye is depleted by half that of my right eye. This is the eye that has been subjected to multiple surgeries. There is a class of eye diseases called the *dystrophies* (See Chapter 2) that involves the *cornea*, and the problems resulting from these eye diseases often lead to the need for *corneal* transplants.

Corneal transplants in existence now for many years are considered one of the most successful of the eye-operations primarily because rejection of the foreign body is avoided for the *cornea* occupies an *immune privileged* site. This site bars the immune system from dispatching its clean-up crew to this foreign body. In addition, because the transplanted cornea is bloodless, it does not become part of the vascular system. Nevertheless, a number of patients still reject the foreign cornea and these patients are candidates for the insertion of a plastic cornea. Whatever type of transplant, human or plastic, careful monitoring is required.

Improvement in corneal transplants continues apace. In use now is a plastic plug pioneered by The Schepens Eye Research Institute, Boston, MA that allows the penetration of light through the opaque corneal surface to the *retina*. The Schepens scientists are also investigating growth factors and other substances to create an artificial cornea that will contain all three layers of the *cornea*. Most challenging is the 500-layer *stroma*.

Other scientists are working on a method to use healthy *corneal* cells as a base to generate a mass of cells in vitro (clones in the lab) that can be transplanted into the eye.

Most contact lens fittings are routine, but in some cases, an abnormal or thin cornea, a condition called *keratoconus,* requires special attention. With the help of computer technology, this condition can be corrected using specific lenses. Special attention is also required for those with glaucoma. To assure the best fit, choose a certified technician.

The Iris

When we speak of beautiful eyes, we usually have the *iris* in mind; this donut shaped gem of multiple hues that has inspired poets throughout the ages to compose odes to their loved ones. But *iris* color, notwithstanding its beauty, is a pragmatic affair, for the color is influenced by the quantity of pigment the *iris* contains. Pigment is an important component for it determines the level of protection present to repel the sun's ultraviolet rays. Dark brown eyes, therefore, containing more pigment are more protective of the sun's rays than blue eyes (Wear sunglasses). But *irises* are not always color compatible. One *iris* may be brown and the other blue or gray. Usually, this anomaly does not indicate a problem, but should this condition occur, check it out with an eye doctor.

Dilating and contraction of the *iris* regulates the amount of light entering the eye. This automatic system governed by the pupil (the black round opening in the center of the eye), enables sight under varying light conditions. Two muscles, the *sphincter* about one millimeter wide contracts the pupil and the *dilator* muscle expands it. The *iris* busily contracts and dilates during your entire waking hours and it has the capacity to dilate wide enough to snare even a tiny bit of light during nighttime. For some glaucoma patients, however, this ability lessens, especially when using drops that constrict the pupil. But age and medical treatment of the eyes also slow down the dilating ability of the *iris*. The sluggish *iris* may require a minute or so to dilate sufficiently to reveal features in a darkened room such as a movie house or theater.

Other more serious problems may involve the *iris*. If subject to inflammation, *iritis* may develop. *Iritis* is a subset of *uveitis* (See Chapter 2) and it is a player in *angle-closure* glaucoma, a condition where fluid behind the *iris* pushes it forward into the drainage channel blocking it.

And lastly, certain forms of glaucoma can be read in the *iris*. *Pigmentary Dispersion Syndrome glaucoma* (See Chapter 2) may be diagnosed simply by observing defects in the *iris* due to loss of pigment. This condition results from the release of pigment granules due to a concave rather than convex *iris*. This conformation presses or rubs up against the *zonules*, (packets of fiber that hold the lens in place) releasing pigment.

THE LENS

The *crystalline lens*, the large and major focusing body of the eye, directs light onto the *retina*. It is a remarkable instrument, for it adjusts to reading fine print to detecting a name on a movie marquee one hundred or more feet away. Biconvex in shape, it is enclosed in a capsule suspended by ligaments called *zonules* just behind the pupil. In addition to its transparency, the *lens* has the capacity to prevent light scatter, the major cause of debilitating glare. Unlike every other tissue in the body containing its full complement of cells, the *lens* contains only a single layer of cells parked alongside its interior edge. At the equatorial sides of the *lens*, the cells transmute into terminal differentiation becoming fibers. Presto, no light-scattering elements! The cell fibers have now has become a bag of protein and have lost their metabolic (physical and chemical change) activity.

Although these *lens* fibers continue to grow throughout life, unlike other cells in the body that are in a constant state of flux (destruction and rebirth), these cells are permanent and contain history. The oldest fibers laid down during fetal growth are at the center of the *lens*; the youngest are at the edges. Like reading tree rings, study of the *lens* reveals past traumas. Say a parathyroid problem occurred that increased calcium concentrations, a condition that produces opaque fibers. Although cured of the disease, the fibers laid down during this period remain opaque. Pre-and post-fibers will be clear. The *lens* and the cornea are the only parts of the body that receive no blood supply! An interesting story told me by an optometrist involved an amateur sailor who piloted his boat across the Atlantic Ocean stopping en route to visit exotic islands. On most days he experienced full sunlight, but he shunned sunglass protection, either because of ignorance or for macho reasons. Examination of his lens revealed a damaged line that corresponded to the year he traveled.

Cataract of the *lens* is the bane of aging and it is often exacerbated by glaucoma drops and surgical interventions. Injury to the lens and exposure to ultraviolet rays also contribute to cataract formation. *Cortical cataracts* form on the periphery of the lens which is softer, and *nuclear cataracts* form in the center of the lens which is harder. *Posterior cataracts* form in the back of the lens.

Inevitable aging of the *lens* in many people causes problems. The *lens* and its surrounding muscles slowly deteriorate over the passage of time, reducing the ability of the eye to accommodate to fine print. This condition is called *presbyopia*. Some doctors claim they can tell the age of the person by his or her ability to read fine print. Actually, the muscles do not weaken but the geometry of *lens* fibers connecting to the muscles shift, and the fibers appear to be less elastic. In some cases, an experimental surgical technique stretches the system out again correcting the problem, but this technique is not widely practiced. *LASIK* surgery, on the other hand, a procedure that reforms the cornea, is widely used to correct near-sightedness and in some cases far-sightedness.

THE LACRIMAL GLANDS

Actors say they need to think of something sad in order to cry on cue. Our tears usually spring forth from emotional and/or physical pain. Although we tend to think of tears as emotional release, their major purpose is to maintain a healthy eye surface. The *lachrymal apparatus* includes glands that secrete tears, and ducts that conduct the fluid from the eye. This fluid flows constantly over the cornea, into the *nasolacrimal* duct and down into the nasal cavity. Discomfort occurs when insufficient fluid is generated. This condition of dry eye affects the *conjunctiva*, a protective tissue that covers the front of the eye and cornea. Deprived of moisture, this tissue causes pain and discomfort. With some people, eye medications are the source, but more likely, dry eye is caused by a number of diseases such as *Sjogren's syndrome*, a disease where white blood cells infiltrate and injure the glands that secrete fluid causing dry mouth and dry eyes. Dry eye can be controlled with a moisturizing drop and in some cases, anti-inflammatory medications.

The naturally-efficient tear ducts discharge only too well as glaucoma patients using eyedrops become aware for a drop of medication instilled into the eye is whisked into the nasal cavity instead of penetrating the cornea. In the nasal passages the medication may cause side-effects such as changes in heart rate from the beta-blockers along with other problems. I experienced cold sweats from the carbacohl drop. Glaucoma patients are, therefore, advised to occlude the passageway into the nasal cavity when instilling a drop of medication. (See Chapter 5).

Some people experience excess tearing, a condition brought about by the eyes' response to irritation such as strong light, high winds and other natural causes. Protective lens and sunglasses may solve this problem. Other cases may be due to obstructed lacriminal drainage problems requiring medical attention.

THE VITREOUS BODY

The *vitreous body*, located in the back of the eye between the *retina* and the lens, is a jellylike mass composed of water (90%). plus hyaluronic acid and collagen fibrils. It fills the eyeball to help keep it rigid. Mainly inactive, the *vitreous*, with age, breaks down a bit often causing the release of floaters-- small bits of proteins or cells floating in the *vitreous*. As light passes through the *vitreous*, the floaters cast annoying shadows on the *retina*. Usually these floaters are benign, but should a shower of black floaters appear, it may indicate that the *retina* may be detached or in process of detachment. Laser treatment most often corrects a number of these *retinal* problems. Less common, but more harmful, another type of floater involves specs or goblets of blood that result from *retinal* bleeding, usually caused by diabetes. At times, removal of the *vitreous* (vitrectomy) may become necessary. The cavity is then filled with a sterile physiological saline solution. Unfortunately, this solution robs the lens of the protection of the *vitreous* gel from toxic oxygen. That floaters are distracting and as some patients complain "driving me crazy" cannot be denied, but when they are not sight-threatening, the general advice appears to be to leave them alone. Only when the lens has been removed in a cataract operation, can the *vitreous* gel be tampered with to rid the eye of the floaters.

THE CILIARY BODY

A glaucoma patient sometimes becomes painfully aware of the existence of the *ciliary body*. In healthy eyes, the *ciliary body* bathes the front of the eye with the nourishing *aqueous humor*. When glaucoma strikes, the *ciliary* body continues to produce this fluid but its outflow apparatus may become blocked. The ciliary body then becomes one of the targets of glaucoma therapy.

Several classes of glaucoma medications, among them the *beta-blockers* and the *carbonic anhydrase inhibitors,* lower *intraocular pressure* by interfering with the *ciliary* body's production of fluid. (See Chapter 5).

The ring-shaped structure of the *ciliary body* is joined at one end to the *iris* sitting directly behind it and at the other end to the *retina.* The *ciliary body* is composed of layers of cells forming seventy folds quite like a lineup of tiny sausages served at cocktail parties. These cells are covered by two layers of *pigmented* and *non-pigmented epithelium.* The *pigmented* cells produce the fluid and export it via three methods—diffusion, active transport and osmosis. The *non-pigmented* cells contain two important enzymes, *carbonic anhydrase* and *adenosine triphosphatase (ATPase).* These cells are targeted by the *carbonic anhydrase* inhibitors found in the glaucoma medications, *Azopt* and *Trusopt.* The muscle attached to the *ciliary body* is another feature of this structure. The contraction of this muscle decreases the diameter of the ring, releasing tension on the *zonular* fibers thereby allowing the lens to accommodate for near vision.

Ideally, the *aqueous* humor circulates naturally through both chambers in the front of the eye, nourishing the lens and cornea with a concentration of vitamin C and minerals. It drains through the *trabecular meshwork* into the *Schlemm's canal* continuing to further drain into the general circulatory system via the *episcleral* veins. About a teaspoon averages the daily fluid production. Should this system fail, fluid builds quite like a river behind a dam. This trapped fluid presses against the *scleral* walls. In adults the *sclera* is quite rigid and the effect of the damned fluid cannot be observed, but in infants whose *sclera* is still elastic, the eye bulges outward resulting in a *cow's eye* appearance, most often a diagnosis of glaucoma in this age group. This build-up of fluid can have disastrous consequences on the eye's ability to maintain its visual properties. Trapped fluid presses against the delicate *axons* of the *ganglion* cells injuring and eventually destroying them.

Given the eye's size (tiny), the efficiency of the system is remarkable; for the fluid to circulate, it must squeeze through a very narrow space between the *lens* and the *iris.* If this space narrows even further or closes altogether (the eye leaves little margin for error), the trapped fluid pushes the *iris* into the angle blocking the fluid from reaching the trabecular meshwork, leading to *angle closure glaucoma* (See Chapter 2). A second possibility is that debris floats into the *trabecular meshwork* and clogs up its pores.

Why the eye's apparatus fails to function raises important questions, one of which involves the role of proteins, vitamins and other substances in the delivery and excretory systems of the aqueous fluid. Some researchers have found evidence of differences between glaucoma patients and those without glaucoma for various substances, but further investigation is needed to determine whether these differences are artifacts of glaucoma or are involved in the development of glaucoma. Scientists are also questioning whether the *ciliary* muscle cells, in addition to their role in regulating tension of the *iris* for near and far vision, possess an additional role in regulating the flow of aqueous humor. These and other questions are still being sorted out.

THE TRABECULAR MESHWORK AND SCHLEMM'S CANAL

A *trabecula*, derived from the Latin word for beam, designates a framework. In the eye, the framework composes an anatomic supporting structure of strands of connective tissue. Viewed under a microscope, the appearance of the *trabecular meshwork* resembles a natural sponge. Responsible for the outflow of fluid, this porous structure, if blocked, prevents the fluid from exiting the eye. Dammed up fluid creates ocular pressure damaging *retinal* fibers, the optic nerve, and surrounding tissues. Like all structures in the eye, the *trabecular meshwork* is tiny, only about one-eighth inch at the juncture of the *cornea* and *iris*. This space is called the angle (See Illustration above). Should the aqueous fluid be prevented from exiting through to the *Schlemm's Canal* (a ring-shaped porous network of passages and giant *vacuoles* (fluid filled cavities), *intraocular pressure* rises. There is evidence in the literature that high pressure changes the shape of the cells rendering them less effective.

Researchers continue to explore this bit of tissue and investigate its molecular structure. The trabecula beams among other elements contain a core of collagen, cells, a growth factor, and enzymes. The enzyme, *metalloproteinase (MMPs,)* regulates the outflow, transport of *electrolytes*, *steroids*, environmental chemicals, oxidative substances, and *cytokines*. *Cytokines* have the ability to change and alter cells. They are important for controlling inflammation and other substances and when unavailable may affect the *trabecular meshwork's* ability to do its job. One major factor may lie in the loss of the cells' ability to rid the *trabecular meshwork* of the secretions of an extracellular ground substance along with the cells' debris, the weight of which forming a plaque-like substance, collapses the meshwork. Specifically, the syndromes of *exfoliation* and *pigmentary dispersion glaucoma*, both of which produce debris, are believed to clog up the meshwork. An examination of enucleated eyes (eyes removed from the body), revealed the presence of debris in the *Schlemm's Canal*, on tissues within the system, and in the *trabecular meshwork*. (See Chapter 2 for more information on these conditions.)

Oh, for a click of the mouse on your computer to clean up the meshwork. The amino acid tyrosine plays a positive role in the functioning of the trabecular meshwork by relaxing the trabecular meshwork allowing a freer flow of fluid.

Understanding just how the *trabecular meshwork* and the *Schlemm's Canal* function to move the liquid out of the eye is becoming increasingly clear through the use of powerful electron microscopes. The outflow system appears to be operated by a mechanical pump action powered by the *elastin* properties of the *trabecular meshwork* and the *Schlemm's Canal*. As scientists study this system, they will, no doubt, develop new therapies to engineer the pump's capability.

Apparently, each system of the body can go awry and cause problems. If there is too much *collagen,* the trabecular cells deteriorate. Also, with advancing age as with other parts of the body, a portion of cells die off. This natural process exerts a toll on the *trabecula meshwork.* In normal eyes, loss of cells appears to be insignificant, but in the presence of glaucoma, loss of cells may cause serious problems. Furthermore, according to some studies those with glaucoma may begin to lose cells by middle-age. Age-related issues are not encouraging. Studies have also indicated that the giant vacuoles, pores and canal width of the *Schlemm's* Canal narrows. Other age-related factors include stiffening of *sclerotic trabecular meshwork* or one that is too flaccid, both conditions impacting on the outflow of fluid.

Damage by a high IOP is not exclusive to the *ganglion* cells for high pressure can also apparently reduce the effectiveness of cells in the outflow system.

With the discovery of the *TIGR* gene expressed in the *trabecular meshwork*, there appears to be, in some cases of open-angle glaucoma, of genetic influence on the *trabecular meshwork*. More glaucoma genes are being identified. One gene alone has been established as being responsible for *exfoliation* glaucoma. (See Chapter 9)

THE RETINA

"The *retina* is the most accessible part of the central nervous system for genetic and surgical manipulations. In fact, because of its similar organization, of development and signaling, the *retina* has been considered a model system for study of the brain's pathways. Many neurotransmitters and hormones signal their target cells through cascades comparable to those of *retinal* and *cone* receptors." This concise description by Stephen Tsang, M.D., Ph.D., a clinician-scientist trained in clinical ophthalmology and molecular biological research, stresses the central position of the *retina* both in eye health and its relevance to the entire body. Recall the simple comparison of the *retina* to the film in a camera, although in our digital age, this comparison begs the question. In the digital camera, the image is captured on a photo-sensitive silicon computer chip and stored as digital data. In the eye, the *retina* sends light image data captured from the superbly designed photo-sensitive cells onto the brain where the image is reconstituted to sight and is also stored as visual memory. Technology and body processes have amazing similarities.

This vital innermost layer of the eye looks and feels like wet tissue paper, but it is a large, light-sensitive structure completely lining the back of the eye right up to where the cornea and *sclera* meet. It is an extremely active body, for it contains millions of cells. Perhaps the action of microchips might clarify to some degree the *retina's* capacity for capturing light-sensitive information and sending these packets to be decoded by the brain's visual cortex. The *retina* consists of ten interconnected layers containing neurosensory cells. It consists of three parts: one, the sensory or nervous structure extending from the optic disc forward; two, a part immediately behind the *ciliary processes*, and three, a part forming the back structure of the *iris*. The rods and cones, two basic cell types, occupy the sensory structure. About seven million cones (neurons) grouped in the central area of the *retina* handle detail and color. They snap to attention at the flick of a switch. In less than perfect light, one-hundred twenty-five million rods leisurely take up the challenge. This lag (only a few seconds), nevertheless delays instant play, usually not a problem, except for glaucoma patients whose rods may need longer time to suck up the available light, especially at twilight and in darkened rooms. An additional set of cells called the *bi-polar* cells are connected to each of the rods and cones. They, too, are divided into two types: the more numerous *parvo* cells comprise ninety percent of the total; the smaller number but equally important ten percent, are *magno* cells. These neurons refine the information that the rods and cones deliver. The system resembles an assembly line in a factory. Many parts are needed to complete the product. *Magno* cells detect fine detail--outlines of letters, edges of objects and deliver in dim light, separating figure from ground, such as observing a rock on a dirt path or distinguishing navy blue from black. The *parvo* cells fill in the rest. The cones respond also to certain wavelengths, the range of which is determined by *opsin*, a pigment protein found in the cones. The capacity for the cells' mutability continues to amaze. Pacific salmon contain a maximum absorbency of light in the ultraviolet range allowing the small fry to swim and eat near the water's surface, but as the fish grow and descend into deeper waters, the cones stop producing that particular chemical and begin producing another type with maximum sensitivity in the blue range, enabling the fish to navigate deeper waters.

Whatever is sent the brain's way mimics the processing that began with the light-gathering information in the *retina*. These bits of information (think millions of computer chips)—color, contrast, shape, contours, etc. sent onto the brain spread all over the cortex, which is organized into columns corresponding to one element of the image. The brain binds these together to produce a complete image. This stream of sensory data travels first to the thalamus where it is synchronized and coordinated into a rhythm of electrical activity and then moves onto the cerebral cortex, the thin pleated layers of cells that coat the outer surface of the brain. Each sense has its own relay station and claims an area of the brain. How the brain coordinates all the senses, sight, sound, taste, and touch for a comprehensive image is still being explored, but there now seems to be evidence that the cerebral cortex masterminds the whole process.

Empirically, we do understand that it happens and that if our *retinas* keep sending the messages off to the cerebral cortex, we have sight. Instantaneous sight is truly all the more remarkable for there is an actual inverted image of the object on the *retina* appearing continuously and incorporating any changes in position of the eyes or objects. Should light be dimmer, or fixation a problem, the image slows down to allow additional time to sufficiently evaluate details of an object in imperfect light. As you whiz by in a car objects may blur or elude sight registration altogether. For the visually imperfect, subtitles at the bottom of foreign films lacking contrast sensitivity also may cause reading problems. Even a menu in a dimly lit restaurant will become a reading challenge. But many of these problems not only affect glaucoma patients, but also aging eyes. Baby boomers are up in arms about some of the poor lighting conditions.

What happens in the *retina,* such as loss of cells, is reflected in the brain. Corresponding cells in the part of the brain called the *lateral geniculate nucleus* and *visual cortex* disappear as well. It's a two-way street. In animal studies, the presence of elevated pressure indicates loss in the visual pathways (the *ganglion* cells), as *metabolic* and other visual changes impact on the brain. Investigation into this function has revealed that neurons constantly sample the microenvironment of connection to the brain by way of axons seeking the delivery of *neurotrophins* (food). Loss of this food transport occurs in the brain early in the disease process, before the neuron cells in the *retina* begin to die. Further investigation will, of course, reveal in greater detail the mechanics of this minuet, but we do know that loss in any part of the visual system diminishes the brain's ability to provide the needed growth factors and nutritional elements necessary for a healthy *retina.*

While the *ganglion* cell loss is considered the main reason for vision loss in glaucoma, there is some evidence found in genetic studies that cones may also play a role and researchers are busy exploring other reasons for neuron vulnerability. The possibility exists that the blood-brain barrier may be disrupted and thus render the neurons in the *retina* vulnerable to blood-borne toxic substances. Cells that surround the *retinal* cells influence how the *ganglion cells* maintain function. A complex relationship exists between the *ganglion* cells and the *Muller* cells which, when healthy, act to maintain proper *glutamate* (an amino acid transmitter) levels but when damaged, lose this ability and glutamate builds up becoming *toxic glutamate*. Another type of cell, the *astrocytes,* also supports the *ganglion* cells, and if these are dysfunctional, *ganglion* cells die. A great deal of research is directed at exploring the death of *retinal ganglion* cells. A research team investigating *glial* cells that provide structure and nutritional support to the eye and brain found that these cells may secrete harmful agents such as *nitric oxide* and *TNF-alpha* (tumor necrosis factor) following exposure to stressful conditions. The researchers found they could inhibit *retinal* ganglion cell death by eliminating the effects of these agents. Researchers have found that *glial* cells appear to be the earliest event signaling the progression of glaucoma, well before neuronal loss is detected and before vision declines. Scientists are exploring the impact of these different classes of cells and methods for intervening before they become dysfunctional.

High-level imaging systems continually reveal intricate mechanisms in the eye and, of course, the *retina* is no exception to exploration. A study conducted by researchers at Vollum Institute at Oregon Health and Science University, Portland, revealed that synapses in the *retina* become strengthened or remodeled in the presence of a sudden change of ambient light. This means that the *retina* is capable of rewiring itself.

You would think that with the millions of neurons in the eye and brain that we could afford to lose a few and still retain our sight, and you would not be wrong, for before noticing visual loss, a sizeable number of neurons may have already disappeared (See Chapter 4). The *ganglion* neurons are fewer in number than the rods and cones, unfortunately for glaucoma patients, and cell loss adds to the vulnerability of this structure. These neurons are also prone to damage from *intraocular pressure*, for their axons extending to form the *optic nerve* are fragile and they are also unique, for each ganglion neuron serves as a collection depot for several hundred rods and cones that form a field around it. Loss of even one *ganglion* neuron, therefore, disorders that field of rods and cones affecting quality of vision. When quality of vision declines, patients may assume that their vision is permanently deteriorating, but this may not be entirely the case. Some people, including myself, who believed that glaucoma had taken a heavy toll especially in color sensitivity, found sight restored to near normal capacity following a cataract operation.

There may be another class of cells in the *retina* that enables the resetting of the biological clock each morning and night. The *circadian* clock is present in all living systems from bacteria to humans. While the *circadian* clock works independently, it requires daily resetting based on available light. We think of our biological clock as our wake-sleep cycle, the maintenance of which if interrupted can cause many problems. What is particularly interesting about the discovery of these particular cells is that they may be responsible for a blind person's *circadian* rhythm. Researchers found that blind mice deprived of rod and cones still demonstrated *circadian* rhythms. Only when their eyes were removed did the mice lose that ability.

There are also other similar rhythms in the body leading to homeostasis such as temperature, immune system activity, gastrointestinal activity, and drug metabolism. You may have noticed that you see better or feel better at certain times of the day. Chances are it's not your imagination, for feeling good may indicate a synchronicity of bodily functions.

Special molecules also play a role. Those mechanical receptors located throughout the brain and *retina* that, although their function is still unclear, when disordered, appear to be a cofactor in *intraocular pressure*.

Research on animals provides important information that may at a later date be applied to improve the human condition. Scientists attempting to fathom how a particular bee, the nocturnal South American sweat bee, manages to see in almost total darkness, found that the bees had neurons twice as wide as honey bees. This feature allows the South African sweat bee greater access to the smallest possible photon of light. Scientists speculate that this information may be translated into processing simpler ways of digital image sequences gathered in dim light.

We hear a lot about *macular degeneration* these days. As people live longer, there is a build-up of stressors from pollution, poor diet and excessive sunlight that affects the functioning of the *macula*. The *macula* is a tiny bit of tissue in the center of the *retina* packed with millions of *photoreceptor* cells that transfer images through a series of cell exchanges—*bipolar* to *ganglion* cells-to optic nerve-to *visual cortex*. The *macula* is your locus of central vision providing fixation (focus) for both near and distance vision. Should you lose cells in this area, except for the peripheral neurons that are unaffected, central vision is severely affected. *Macular degeneration* is the exact opposite of glaucoma. Patients with glaucoma lose peripheral neurons first; the *macula* is affected only in late stages of glaucoma. Fixation, however, may be a problem, for many glaucoma patients, me included. I discovered this problem when taking the visual field test (See Chapter 4). There are some people, like Cynthia, who have the double whammy of glaucoma and *macular degeneration*. Cynthia doesn't know which condition to worry about first. As people age, unfortunately, it is not uncommon for both of these diseases to be present.

Many of the diseases such as *cataract* formation and *macular degeneration* are now believed to be at least partially caused by ultraviolet and blue light rays. But not all light rays are harmful. Researchers in Milwaukee have found that red light heals diabetic skin ulcers, burns, mouth ulcers and blindness caused by an overdose of *methanol*. Just one shot glass of neat *methanol* can blind a human permanently and every year there are over 5,000 accidental overdoses in the United States. Researchers shone red light into the eyes of rats intoxicated with *methanol* and were able to prevent blindness in these animals. Human trial studies have yet to be done. Other environmental factors involve being in the vicinity of a lightning strike. This intense flare of light, under some conditions, may injure the eyes, causing macula holes and/or cataracts in both eyes, both conditions which can be corrected with surgery.

Truly precise seeing is accomplished by the *fovea,* an even smaller body of neurons located in the center of the *macula.* This is such an important area that each neuron is connected to its own *ganglion* neuron. The *fovea* is your pathway to the stars. On a clear night in the country (or where light pollution is at a minimum), you can gaze at the tiniest star. In daylight, your *fovea* enables you to detect animal statues atop high buildings, a bird's nest high in a tree, or see the struts of a bridge. Often wonder how a bird of prey can swoop down from a pinnacle to snare dinner from the height of 9-to-13,000 feet? Its *fovea* provides that ability. In fact, the eagle has double *foveas*, an evolutional development probably to assure survival.

Along with the *retinal* functions described above, examination of the *retina* provides insight into the physical conditions of the body as well as diagnostic evidence for some diseases. For example, a doctor with the aid of an ophthalmoscope can detect substances called cotton wool spots in some patients. These are actually diseased nerve fibers present in people with *diabetes mellitus.* Other vascular *retinal* diseases such as *macula edema* (swelling), tiny *hemorrhages*, blood flow disorders, occlusions in the blood vessels, infections, radiation-induced toxicity, infectious diseases (*HIV, Rocky Mountain Spotted Fever, cat-scratch fever*, etc.), and diseases that result from bacterial and fungal infections may also be indicated. Obviously, since many diseases or anomalies may be detected in the *retina*, examination should be included in a comprehensive eye examination and, for that matter, a comprehensive physical as well.

Members of our Group often ask if high blood pressure is related to a high *intraocular pressure.* While not directly implicated, elevated blood pressure may indeed affect the *retina*, for elevated blood pressure may compress the openings of tiny arteries at the juncture of the veins and arteries. *Optic disk* swelling may also result from extremely high blood pressure.

Some diseases of the *macula* may or may not be associated with glaucoma. *Macular Pucker* results from a membrane that wrinkles the *macula.* Surgeons can remove the membrane, although on occasion the *macula* spontaneously flattens out and the symptoms improve. Uncommon complications include infection, bleeding, and *retinal detachment.* This condition may mildly blur vision but if it does not interfere with daily activities, surgeons do not recommend treatment.

A *macula hole* is another matter particularly if vision is dramatically affected. Treatment, however, requires removal of the *vitreous* gel (*vitrectomy*). The gel is replaced with a special gas bubble that slowly dissolves, creating a post-surgical dilemma for the patient, who must maintain a face-downward position for one or two weeks to keep the gas bubble in contact with the *macula.* If well positioned, the *macular* hole closes and some or all of the lost vision may be restored. Until the gas bubble is gone, air flight is ruled out. If you have normal vision in one eye and are not troubled by the *macula hole* in your other eye, you can forego surgery.

Cystoid Macula Edema (CME) is a condition where clear fluid fills multiple cyst-like formations in the *macula* creating swelling. It may occur after cataract surgery or may be part and parcel of *retinal* diseases such as *retinal vein occlusion, uveitis* or *diabetic retinopathy.* This condition causes blurred central vision and may be present even when there is no visual loss. If inflammation occurs, treatment consists of steroid and non-steroidal drops, and in recalcitrant cases, a steroid injection that delivers the medicine for about three months. Diuretics to reduce swelling, laser surgery, and a *vitrectomy* are also part of the treatment. Persons having this condition may develop glaucoma because of increased pressure in the eye.

And lastly, scanning of the *retina* is taking the place of fingerprints as an identify tool.

THE OPTIC NERVE

Glaucoma is an *optic nerve* disease. The *optic nerve* head, 1.5 mm in vertical diameter, has three important regions: the margin; the nerve fibers, and the cup. While high *intraocular pressure* is a major consideration in the diagnosis and treatment of glaucoma, it is now understood that along with its damaging effects on the *optic nerve,* non-pressure factors may also play a major role. The *optic nerve* head or *disc* has been described as looking like a donut. Nerve fibers form the donut and the donut hole is the cup, a space where the fibers fan off from the *retina.* The cup is the area to which doctors refer when they describe cupping of the *optic nerve.* The size of the cup varies from patient to patient. On average it occupies thirty percent of the optic disk surface. The size can vary from zero-to-seventy percent. Size alone, however, does not necessarily indicate a glaucomatous condition. An individual may possess no cup or an abnormally large cup but still be unaffected by glaucoma; larger than seventy percent, however, suggests the presence of glaucoma. A cup-to-disc ratio of 1.0 represents total loss of optic nerve fibers. Also, if there is a difference of the cup-to-disk ratio between both eyes, glaucoma is suspected. But with every form of glaucoma, the enlargement of the cup size indicates loss of nerve fibers, a clear indication that progression of glaucoma is occurring.

In a healthy eye, the cells in the eye talk to the cells in the brain continually through electrical and chemical signals. This communication is made possible by a little over a million *axonal* neurons originating in the *ganglion nerve fiber layer* located in the *retina,* which comprise the *nerve head.* These *axons,* bundled into packages of two thousand each, form the *optic nerve head* by winding round and round. But this formation of the *optic nerve* requires the bending of its axons at a ninety-degree angle, possibly weakening the structure and contributing to one of the factors leading to glaucoma.

Evaluation of the state of the rim or margin of the optic nerve head can be measured through the use of various imaging systems--optical coherence tomography (OCT), scanning laser polarimetry (GDx), and confocal scanning laser ophthalmoscopy (Heidelberg Retinal Tomography or HRT II), (See Chapter 4). The areas indicating glaucoma's presence include the rim of the optic disc, defects in the nerve fiber layer, and hemorrhage, where there is no other cause such as vitreous detachment. Assessment of the nerve fiber layer is an important diagnostic measure, for although IOP may be measured in the normal range, the nerve fiber layer may still register thickness loss. Doctors focus also on the condition of the lamina cribosa. This is a multilayered mechanical support structure at the base of the optic nerve head that can affect the health of the axons. Some researchers speculate that increased intraocular pressure deforms the lamina cribosa by compressing bundles of axons that then impedes axonal transport. An exposed lamina cribosa (it is white), is an indication of more nerve fiber loss.

Traditionally, doctors, upon examining the *optic nerve* and measuring the width of the cup, draw a picture to establish a parameter for future reference. In lieu of sophisticated instruments described in *Chapter 4,* this practice serves patients and doctors well. Also, usually, during the initial workup, doctors photograph the *disc.* Depending upon the glaucoma condition, your doctor may take additional photos yearly to chart changes in the *optic nerve head. Stereo* photography consisting of three-dimensional images is a more sophisticated approach that doctors may choose to use.

Optic disc pallor, a blanching of *retinal nerve fibers* and of the *neural rim* is atypical for glaucoma, but it still may occur. The *ciliary* and *retinal* arteries and the *retinal veins* carry the blood supply to the eyes. Where a condition in the eye interferes with the blood supply, pallor may be observed. *Pallor of* the *optic nerve* is an indication that not enough blood is circulating within the eyes.

Other considerations that impact on the eye causing glaucoma include congenital anomalies, hemorrhage, tilted and in some cases, myopic disks. Racial differences also need to be taken into account. Studies indicate that Latinos and blacks have smaller discs, cups and neural rim areas but glaucoma patients, whatever the race, also have this effect. As well, patients with symptoms of glaucoma whatever the race may not all have the configurations.

Glaucoma patients tend to think of the *optic nerve* in terms of their own disease. But a number of other diseases may cause *optic nerve* problems. One is called *optic neuritis.* Both ophthalmologists and neurologists figure in the diagnosis of this disease, for it is often the first indication of *multiple sclerosis,* a debilitating disease affecting young adults. Patients experiencing blurring vision that progresses over several days accompanied by eye pain that worsens with eye movements are candidates for this syndrome. Early intervention is advised.

That undue pressure, chemical imbalances, genetic abnormalities and reduced blood flow affect the cells' activity is well known. Nevertheless, the formation of new *dendrite* connections continues throughout life. *Dendrites* are projections from neurons that form synaptic connections to other neurons. Although the dying off of cells called *apoptosis* is serious business, the knowledge that those cells still remaining are capable of making new connections is comforting. These exceptional multi-taskers have the ability to perform subtle changes at their synapses in response to a barrage of input information, and a plasticity that paves the way for incorporating and retaining information. Scientists theorize that neurons, by delegating management skills to the synapses, require protein synthesis (manufacture of suitable proteins) in addition to the protein synthesis that occurs in the cell. To keep the synapses at the ready, the neuron sends *RNA* nuggets ready to be used as needed. Scientists are exploring *RNA* as a possible application for treating glaucoma and other eye diseases. For example, researchers have identified an Inhibitor of *axon* regeneration. (The *ganglion nerve* has a long *axon* that is easily damaged). If a drug is developed from *RNA* blocking this inhibitor, *axons* may then be allowed to regenerate when injured.

THE LAMINA CRIBOSA

This is a thin, sieve-like section of the *sclera* lies at the base of the *optic disc.* *Ganglion* fibers leave the eye through this structure in the process of forming the *optic nerve.* In myopic eyes, the *lamina cribosa* has been found to be thinner than in normal eyes.

THE BRAIN

The eye is an extension of the brain. All neuronal activity in the eye becomes part of the visual information transported to the brain. Sight is possible, however, only when these electrical-chemical impulses reach the *visual cortex* unimpeded. Our sensory organs are designed to constantly feed the brain information. Our busy brain is the ultimate multi-tasker, but it can hold only seven items at a time. Nevertheless, it forms internal maps of the space surrounding us, providing clues for navigation such as knowing exactly the height to lift each foot when mounting stairs, or when to duck under a low doorway. The brain is also superbly equipped to recognize objects. Given a bit of stimuli, it fills in the rest of the object. Should the senses become unable to feed much of anything to the brain, imagination takes over. But alas, the results in this case may be less than perfect and perhaps embarrassing—like greeting someone with open arms and then discovering you've erred, as did a friend of mine who thought she saw an old friend. She opened her arms to him and much to her consternation, the gentleman wanted to develop a relationship. The brain craves patterns, necessary to establish pathways for ordering the world, the design of the universe. This system of cranial pathway development begins at birth and continues throughout life.

Technology increases our understanding of how the brain processes the jumble of biochemical-electrical impulses. *Functional Magnetic Resonance Imagery (FMRI)* measures the oxygen levels in the blood throughout the brain and identifies which neurons are at work processing these impulses. The brain, like other natural systems, abhors complexity. Scientists studying brain chemistry speculate that vision is accounted for by two or three super maps with many sub maps nestled inside--sort of like a set of Russian dolls. The super map is formed, scientists believe, by the activity of the *retina* that, through a biochemical reaction, distributes a point of information to a corresponding point in the visual cortex.

Those valuable neurons, when lost in the *retina* are also lost in the brain, altering the spatial map. This loss may add to problems with depth vision, a condition occurring with some glaucoma patients who have what they refer to as a good and a bad eye. When sight worsens, information is no longer fed to the brain that in turn loses the ability to create or alter the spatial maps. Like all neurons when damaged or destroyed, regeneration is, as yet, not possible. Loss, unfortunately, leads to more loss, for not only do vital cells die, but in their demise, take with them surrounding cells succumbing to the toxic environment formed by the dying cells.

THE CHOROID AND BLOOD FLOW:

The *choroid* contains a major blood supply for the eye and is also responsible for supplying nutrition to the outer *retina* as well as removing waste products. Other functions include temperature and IOP homeostasis. In birds and to a somewhat lesser degree in mammals, the thinning and thickening of the *choroid* helps to focus images on the *retina*.

The *choroid* and *retinal* circulation processes are distinct with different regulatory mechanisms although both flow from the *ophthalmic* artery. Age brings a decrease in blood flow that reduces the supply of nutrition to the *retina*. With certain forms of *macular degeneration*, blood flow may be decreased by as much as thirty percent. A study from Australia indicated that both *open-angle* and *ocular hypertension* patients had decreased blood flow. Increasing age also weakens the body's ability to regulate blood pressure. While not comparable to a rise in IOP, blood pressure elevation can impede blood flow to the capillary system of the eye causing *ischemia* (deficiency of blood supply). Lack of nourishment from the blood supply is considered one of the causes of cupping. Increased cup size may also result from the stretching of the capillaries, possibly responding to diminished blood flow weakening the capillary capacity and allowing *disc hemorrhages* (bleeding) to occur. While the pathology for *optic disc hemorrhage* needs further refinement and is present in other diseases of the eye, doctors consider disc hemorrhage to be serious. Researchers have reported that sixty percent of the eyes diagnosed with *disc hemorrhages* will progress in glaucoma patients over a period of sixteen months.

Systemic diseases, too, play a role. *Cardiovascular disease, arteriosclerosis* or *arterial hypotension* (too low blood pressure), *diabetic neuropathy*, and sleeping patterns are cited. Glaucoma patients may be affected by reduced blood flow to the eye by a dip in blood pressure during a phase in the *circadian rhythm*. Hemoglobin may be one of the control mechanisms determining how much blood is delivered to the body's tissues. Hemoglobin picks up and sheds *nitric oxide*, the molecule that signals the arteries to dilate or contract. As the blood flows through the lungs, hemoglobin loads up on oxygen that promotes a change of shape allowing it to add a specific form of *nitric oxide*. When tissue oxygen is low, hemoglobin causes arteries in that area to open wider; when high, hemoglobin narrows arteries. Studies comparing blood flow velocity between normal healthy subjects and glaucoma patients reveal that glaucoma patients experience a weaker blood flow velocity.

Inadequate blood flow apparently is implicated in a number of other conditions such as *myopia* and *contrast sensitivity*. But its most pernicious effect is the linkage of reduced blood flow to *normal tension* and possibly *open-angle glaucoma.* A study of patients with *normal tension* glaucoma indicated prolonged *retinal* circulation that was related to *vasospasm* (reversible constriction or insufficient dilation of a blood vessel) or arteriosclerosis in the *retina* along with *nerve fiber* loss. A small protein, *endothelin-1 (ET-1)* that constricts blood vessels is another factor affecting blood flow. Higher levels of this factor are present in patients with glaucoma.

That all parts of the body are intricately connected is corroborated once again by findings that *retinal* images may help predict risk of stroke. Researchers following patients for seven years found that damage to the tiny blood vessels in the eye were seventy percent more likely to have a stroke during the term of the study those than those without damage.

Medications to promote greater blood flow have been mixed. In a study comparing normal subjects with glaucoma patients, researchers found that while beta-blockers did help with the vasospasms, when compared with normal subjects, they had no effect on vasoconstriction. Ginkgo biloba extract (See Chapter 11) may improve blood flow to the eye and brain.

THE IMMUNE SYSTEM

What does the immune system have to do with glaucoma? Lots, for apparently the immune system is involved in the life and death struggle of neurons. Some neurons die naturally, but some neurons subject to toxic substances or pressures create a problem for healthy neurons surrounding their dying buddy. In the process of demise, toxic environmental factors spread to neurons in the surrounding field. Small studies have indicated that cells may be rescued if the immune response is boosted by neutralizing the toxic environment, thus slowing the degeneration of the *optic nerve.* Based on the work of the Michel Schwartz group in Israel, the possibility exists that a vaccination they have developed will protect "bystander" damage to *axons* adjacent to dying neurons. This immunization consists of *copolymer-1 (Copaxone),* which cross-reacts with many different self-reacting *T cells.* That, along with a form of *retinoid,* has successfully protected *retinal* fibers from damage in animal studies. Trials on human subjects are underway.

Inflammation, the immune response to injury and the invasion of bacteria and viruses, is not necessarily a negative factor, for inflammation is one of the body's attempts to heal. If inflammation goes awry, however, it leads to a chronic, low-level condition, a major risk factor for a multitude of diseases. Chronic *uveitis* is an example of inflammation affecting the eyes, resulting in secondary glaucoma. Other chronic diseases such as *arthritis, gum disease, bronchitis, sinusitis, urinary tract infections, asthma* or allergies and even cancer are rooted in the inflammatory processes. Glaucoma patients appear to have one or more of the above conditions. A marker for chronic inflammation is *C-reactive protein* that can be measured in a blood test. Levels less than 1 mg are considered low risk, from 1-to-3, average risk and greater than 3, high risk. Therapeutic medical strategies include aspirin, statin drugs, and *COX-2* inhibitors which have, unfortunately, been implicated as possibly causing heart attacks. Inflammation has also been linked to raising *intraocular pressure*. Researchers have found that by blocking a type of inflammatory molecule tumor, *necrosis-alpha (TNF-alpha)* that the neurons may be protected.

The use of steroid medication is one of the most common remedies to combat inflammation, although with some people, steroids can worsen or even cause glaucoma. Steroid products have been found to cause changes of cells in the *trabecular meshwork* inhibiting the movement of *aqueous humor*. Even the use of topical steroids as in medications and creams that contain *dexamethasone* may, in some instances, be a causative factor in *open-angle glaucoma*.

Life style changes described in Part II of this book provide a non-medical approach to bolstering the immune system and lowering inflammatory responses.

Obviously, there is more to an eye than simply a sight organ. It is one of the most complicated structures in the body and scientists are still unraveling its mysteries. Glaucoma, our major interest in this book, is also far from simple. It, too, especially since there are many forms of the disease, poses both universal and unique problems that are in the process of resolution. In the next chapter, we will take a look at the many forms of this disease.

CHAPTER 2

The Many Varieties of Glaucoma

○ ○

"It is best to do things systematically, since we are only human, and disorder is our worst enemy,"

Hesiod, 8th century BC, 471

Like so many words in our vocabulary, the term glaucoma has an ancient derivation. Several Greek words suggest its source; (*glaux*) for owl, (*glauco*), a Greek prefix meaning bright, shining, sparkling, (*glaukos)* identified by Guthrie in 1823 as coming from the Greek word describing a dull, grayish green or blue covered with a powdery bloom as in grapes. Obviously glaucoma is an old disease, probably extending beyond recorded history. The ancient Greeks described all eye diseases leading to blindness as glaucoma. Arabic manuscripts from the tenth and fourteenth centuries correlated vision loss with the hardness of the eyeball. The separation of glaucoma from cataract dates from early AD and the linkage of glaucoma to eye pressure is attributed to an English oculist and author, Richard Banister, who wrote the first book on glaucoma in 1622.

Primary open-angle glaucoma (POAG) is the most prevalent form in Western countries of the more than forty diagnosed eye conditions that are grouped under this condition. Once believed to be a disease characterized only by *high intraocular pressure*, it is now known as an *optic nerve disease* often, but not always, associated with elevated pressure. As with all diseases, genetic markers are present. While a number of markers have already been identified for glaucoma, the total genetic picture is still elusive. Glaucoma occurs throughout the world and while it strikes most individuals over the age of forty, it does have a toehold in all age groups, including babies, but it is most prevalent in those over sixty-five. Family history most often sets the stage for the possibility of acquiring the disease. When I was first diagnosed with glaucoma I was told that two forms of glaucoma existed—*primary-open angle* and *closed angle*. This cleavage into the two forms occurred in the 1930's. Of the two, *open-angle* was considered less dangerous, primarily because it did not set the stage for an acute *angle-closure attack* associated with *closed angle glaucoma*. Since living with this disease for many years, while not being subject to *angle-closure*, I have found that *POAG* is hardly a benign condition.

Some forms of *POAG* are called secondary for the the glaucoma is caused by a primary condition. Many members in our group possess secondary glaucoma from such conditions as *uveitis, pigmentary dispersion,* and *exfoliation*. At present writing, the combination of IOP pressure (mmHg) and optic nerve disease is labeled *POAG* although this definition may change as more genes causing glaucomatous conditions are identified. Since my initial diagnosis, I subsequently learned that my glaucoma was probably linked to *exfoliation*, for which a single mutated gene has been identified. There are a number of risk factors associated with glaucoma. Being female is apparently one. A Canadian study found glaucoma in women occurred twice as likely as in men. The authors speculated that the condition might be related to hormonal changes. *Intraocular pressure* is a telling sign (although there are those with high pressures who do not necessarily develop glaucoma), ethnic origin, family history, age (considered one of the *degenerative* diseases associated with age), *myopia* (epidemiological studies indicate that *myopic* subjects compared with *hyperoptic* subjects have a statistically significantly higher risk), reduced blood flow to the *optic nerve*, hypertension, systemic and vascular diseases such as *diabetes, thrombosis, autoimmune disease,* and *occlusive* (blood flow blockages) *diseases* of the eyes. And sedentary life style, obesity, smoking, and ingestion of a higher ratio of polyunsaturated fats, (the omega 6's to the omega 3's (See Chapter 11), may also play a part. Unquestionably, glaucoma is now considered a mutlifactorial disease and is a far cry from what I learned when I was first diagnosed.

There are studies on *myopia* suggesting that the *retina* determines the length of the eye. This finding further suggests that there is a direct correlation between the *retina* and the *sclera*. Elongation of the eye affects the *retina* Myopia commonly believed to develop from early reading experiences may be more of an inherited factor. Furthermore, it may also be worsened by the use of pressure controlling eyedrops as happened in my case.

Certain populations are more at risk. In the *Baltimore Eye Survey*, African-Americans were four times more likely to have glaucoma than white people, and first degree relatives had two-to-nine times the odds of having glaucoma than non-relatives. A study of one large family in Rotterdam found that siblings and offspring had a two-to-nine time higher risk. White people and

African-Americans seventy years and older are three-to-five times more likely to have glaucoma as compared with a younger group of forty-to-fifty year-olds. The same odds are apparently true for Latinos according to a study in Los Angeles. Newer medications such as the prostaglandins (See Chapter 5) narrow the gap between African-Americans and whites. African-Americans, however, while doing better with laser surgery in certain cases, may fare less well with incisional surgery because their incisions scar over more quickly.

Although glaucoma is known as a progressive disease that can and does lead to blindness in some cases, most glaucoma patients who comply with treatment do quite well. In some patients the rate of progression is relatively slow. In the *Early Manifest Glaucoma Trial (EMGT)* two hundred fifty people were randomized to receive *argon laser trabeculoplasy* (See Chapter 4) plus *beta-blocker* drops or no immediate treatment. The results, after six years, showed a fifty-three percent progression, but in the group treated, progression was halved. Factors leading to progression included higher baseline IOP's, *exfoliative* glaucoma, both eyes affected, and *disc hemorrhages*. This study, admittedly small, given the large number of glaucoma patients, does raise questions concerning the remaining forty-seven percent who did not progress. The "why" still needs to be further studied.

Researchers at Johns Hopkins University in Maryland suggest that patients whose glaucoma progresses slowly do lose some cells each year, but at a reduced rate enabling them to retain decent vision throughout life. According to an analysis from the team at Johns Hopkins, the majority of glaucoma patients especially those whose glaucoma occurred later in life, die before they go blind from the disease. Data gleaned from several studies below found a thirteen-year period for white individuals and a sixteen- year period for African-Americans to go blind from glaucoma. The *Baltimore Eye Study*, the *Beaver Dam Eye Study* and the *Framingham Eye Study* found only four percent of white individuals and eight percent of black individuals became legally blind from glaucoma. Furthermore, the *Ocular Hypertension Study* revealed that only a small percentage of people with pressures above 21 mmHg lost sight. An analysis of the data from the *Baltimore Eye Survey* and the *Barbados Eye Study*, found that up to ten percent of blacks seventy years and older had glaucoma. These studies also found little evidence for those with moderate glaucoma field damage to have an effect on health-related quality of life, but when central vision was affected, the situation changed. All told, these studies have had an impact on treatment of glaucoma. Some doctors now weigh prognosis with effects of treatment on life style, and base their recommendations for intervention accordingly, taking into account such factors as age of onset, severity of loss when first diagnosed, skin color, and the availability of medical care in rural areas and poor countries.

These studies also help us, as patients, to better understand the intricacies of differential treatment and depending upon the diagnosis, whether treatment is even necessary, especially for those of us who have high pressures but no field loss. The *Ocular Hypertension Study (OHT)* revealed that only 4.4% of the treated patients compared with 9.5% of the untreated developed glaucoma. This study has provided evidence based on the individual's medical history of whether it is necessary to medically treat such high-intensive individuals or simply follow them yearly and medicate only when signs of damage are detected. With the sophisticated *imaging systems* now available (See Chapter 4) subtle changes in the *nerve fiber layer* can be detected before damage occurs. Patients whose IOPs were higher than 25 mmHg and had corneal thickness less than 555um and who did not have treatment had a 36% chance of developing glaucoma in a five-year follow-up. Conversely, 64% of these high risk patients did not develop damage over the same period.

For those of us whose glaucoma continues to eat away at our optic nerve cells, controlling *intraocular pressure* is a key factor in preserving vision. Cure through genetic intervention or medical protection of the nerve cells is close to fulfillment, but for the moment, the control of *intraocular pressure* is the Gibraltar for slowing down the ravages of glaucoma. While doctors stress that each case is different, in general, when glaucoma patients' pressures climb above 14-to-15 mmHg, risk of vision loss increases. One study found a 35% risk in patients with an IOP over 30 mmHg. Many doctors now feel that the cutoff point of 21 mmHg should be reduced to between 12-to-16 mmHg or even lower. When we patients compare our IOPs, we envy those whose pressures are no more than 9 mmHg.

Blood flow plays a fundamental role, for blood nourishes the eye. Diagnosis using the *Doppler flow meter* that measures blood flow has found evidence that blood flow is decreased in some patients with glaucoma. As glaucoma advances, blood flow decreases. Areas receiving the least amount of blood flow may show the greatest defects.

High systemic blood pressure, not to be confused with blood flow, is tricky for glaucoma patients. High blood pressure may starve the capillaries by reducing the flow of blood to the eye. But, if blood pressure is drastically lowered, the *optic nerve* may be deprived of blood. It's a thorny problem for, as people age, blood pressure often increases as does the incidence of glaucoma. It's important, therefore, for both the patient's general practitioner and glaucoma specialist to review the protocols for reducing both forms of pressure and try to achieve a balanced therapy for these conditions. As stated above, glaucoma can possibly be linked to various forms of vascular diseases, or at the very least, a co-factor. In the best of circumstances, your auto regulation of blood flow at the capillary level in the *optic nerve* and the *retina* should be unimpeded, but the fine tuning of this system is constantly threatened as you age.

Genetics is playing a more and more significant role in determining the etiology of glaucoma for genes can alter normal protein production (See Chapter 9). Other conditions may also be causative factors. Researchers at Tulane University in New Orleans have found a significant level of antibodies to *Chlamydia pneumoniae* (a parasitic disease). In a group of thirty-nine patients, nineteen demonstrated antibodies to this infection, but this finding requires further investigation.

Secondary glaucoma may occur following other eye conditions such as *uveitis, exfoliative syndrome, pigmentary dispersion syndrome,* extreme near-sightedness, previous eye surgery, corneal and *iris* diseases as well as low blood pressure (possibly a result of hypertension medications).

There is evidence that *hypothyroidism* (low thyroid) may be linked to the development of glaucoma. In the presence of *hypothyroidism, hyaluronic acid* (a gelatinous substance acting as a lubricant and shock absorber) may build up causing blockage of the *trabecular meshwork.* Other disorders include *lukemia* and *sickle cell anemia.*

There is some epidemiological evidence from the *Beaver Dam Eye Study* that glaucoma is largely undiagnosed. In this study of roughly six thousand people, 83% of the residents between the ages of 43 and 86 were given visual field tests. Researchers found 119 cases of undiagnosed glaucoma. Mass screenings are important, for glaucoma is a preventable blinding disease. One organization, the Lion's Club, provides for mass screenings throughout the world. Awareness, fortunately, has grown especially in developed countries where a standard eye examination includes a check for eye pressure, but in the undeveloped and outlying districts, glaucoma assessment is still woefully scarce.

Aside from all these possible complicating factors, as we alluded previously, glaucoma comes in many forms, the most common, *primary open-angle glaucoma (POAG).* What follows are short descriptions of the more common glaucoma forms.

PRIMARY OPEN-ANGLE GLAUCOMA (POAG)

When most people think about glaucoma, *POAG* comes to mind for indeed, this is the most prevalent form of glaucoma in western countries, affecting about one percent of the over-forty population in the United States. Originally, it was termed primary because doctors could not detect an underlying cause and, although for years this form of glaucoma was thought possibly to be of genetic origin, not until1997, with the discovery of a mutation on the TIGR gene located on chromosome 1, did that premise prove true. Subsequently, with the identification of five other possible gene mutations, scientists are beginning to unravel the complexity of *POAG*. Wherever a mutation occurs a wrong signal is given to the *RNA* molecule to manufacture a faulty protein. The TIGR gene was found to manufacture the protein, *myocilin* a mutation found in most of the forms of juvenile glaucoma and about three-to-five percent of adult-onset POAG. This number represents about 100,000 people in United States alone. Worldwide, the figure expands exponentially. Yet undoubtedly, there are millions of people for whom genetic linkage has not yet been made. Obviously, other factors contribute to this disease that damages neurons in the eye.

When I received a diagnosis of glaucoma, every one of my colleagues at work visited his or her eye doctor for a checkup. At that time, optometrists and some ophthalmologists did not routinely check eye pressures. Examination of the eyes for detection of glaucoma, while certainly improved in western societies, is still not a routine medical procedure in a large segment of the world-population, and therefore, many people remain undiagnosed. Glaucoma is a manageable disease for the most part and sight could be saved if facilities were available.

Like other chronic diseases such as high blood pressure and diabetes, for example, medical care and life style changes are important for healthy maintenance of vision.

The risk factors of age, genetic heritage, family member, African-American, hypertension characterize most glaucoma patients. Most of the members of our glaucoma group do have one or more of these risks. Both Bess' and Judy's fathers became blind from glaucoma, and both were diagnosed with glaucoma before the age of 35. *Myopia*, not the form that can easily be corrected with eye glasses or contacts, but severe *myopia* requiring thick eyeglasses may also lead to glaucoma. Although African-Americans are at greater risk, the introduction of prostaglandins, especially *Travatan* combined with a more aggressive treatment has narrowed the gap between the white and black populations, but blacks still remain at greater risk. African-Americans have thinner corneas increasing their risk factor. In our Group, two African American members are virtually blind, and another is slowly losing sight. Nevertheless, in my acquaintance, two other African-Americans are doing fine with medical and surgical treatment.

Each of us reacts differently when receiving a diagnosis of glaucoma. Nancy cried and then went into a research mode, reading all the information she could access on the Internet. I denied the diagnosis, although I faithfully took my mediation. But within six months from the time of diagnosis, I experienced early signs of central vision loss in my left eye. Friends much wiser than me insisted that I visit a glaucoma specialist.

Intraocular pressure is intricately tied to all glaucoma conditions. *POAG* patients often wonder how low their pressures should be to stem progression. When my glaucoma was diagnosed, pressure below 21 mm Hg. was believed to be safe. We have since learned that the safety valve for each individual is determined not by numbers but when a series of visual fields appears stable and no nerve loss is detected. Your friend John, diagnosed with glaucoma, may be able to sustain pressures of 21 mmHg, without loss of vision, while you may need to have your IOP lowered to a single digit (six-to-nine mmHg) to protect your eye. Some people have pressures above twenty-five mmHg and lose little or no sight throughout life. These lucky people are called *ocular hypertensives.* The *(Ocular Hypertension Study {OHT}* sponsored by the National Eye Institute found that persons with high IOPs and thin corneas were likely to experience glaucoma damage. With some patients, the condition remains unclear and these people become glaucoma "suspects." They still must be vigilant, however, and visit their doctors regularly for periodic eye examinations.

A high IOP results from a buildup of fluid in the eye because of impaired egress through the trabecular meshwork, the outflow channel of the eye. This buildup damages the optic nerve, the organ that sends messages to the brain that in turn, interprets these signals into sight. Although the wish for genetic therapy to correct unruly pressures is not yet a reality, the medical, laser (trabeculoplasty) and incisional therapies for stemming the ravages of the disease that have been developed over the years are quite effective in the majority of cases,

Patients often wonder whether systemic hypertension is related to a high *intraocular pressure.* Systolic and diastolic blood pressures have been shown to have a modest association with *POAG*, and those patients with visual field deterioration have been found to have significantly lower nighttime diastolic pressure possibly corresponding to reduction of blood flow to the eye. Blood flow velocity to the eye has been studied extensively, since reduced or restricted blood flow can lead to capillary damage. Many studies confirm that lowered cerebral blood flow is one of the factors leading both to many forms of glaucoma.

Can *POAG* be related to an ulcer? A study of bacterium *Helicobacter pylori (H. pylori)* was implicated as a possible cause for ulcers. This bacterium may also play a role in a number of ischemic diseases, (starved of blood) such as heart disease, vascular disorders, *Raynaud's* Disease (peripheral vascular disorder), migraine, and most recently, open-angle glaucoma. Infection with *H. pylori* may cause clumping of the platelets, a condition rendering the blood flow more sluggish resulting in reduced nutrition to the optic nerve. It also produces inflammation and an uptick in nitric oxide, a condition that can induce the blood vessels to constrict blood supply to the optic nerve. Researchers in Greece found *H. pylori* present in 88% of patients with *POAG* or *exfoliation* as against 47% in an anemic control group. In a subgroup of patients who underwent antibiotic treatment, visual fields and *intraocular pressure* improved. This study has met with some skepticism in the general ophthalmic community. While the rationale makes sense, more studies need to be conducted before *H-pylori* is linked to glaucoma.

Diagnosis of any form of glaucoma requires scheduled periodic visits to your doctor or clinic. Timing of these visits depends upon the severity of the condition. Most often the glaucoma condition can be followed with a yearly visual field test along with a thorough eye examination. Should your condition require further analysis, more sophisticated imaging instruments may be used (See Chapter 4).

NORMAL-TENSION GLAUCOMA (NTG)

The discovery that Jenny still lost vision even though her IOP was determined normal terrified her. How could this be? She discovered that she had *NTG*. Diminished blood flow and poor blood circulation are considered to be primary causes of this form, but other undiagnosed factors may still be undiscovered for some patients do not fit in with the above syndromes.

Treatment of the disease before the *Collaborative Normal Tension Glaucoma Treatment Study (CNTGTS)* was largely intuitive, but the result of this study indicated that the IOP should be lowered to low double digits or even single digits in some cases. Caught in time, damage to the optic nerve may be slowed. Doctors, therefore, advise reduction of pressure by at least thirty percent.

Women, particularly, are more susceptible than men to *NTG*. Migraine, but not the common-run of-the-mill headaches, disc hemorrhages, possibly other vascular disorders affect women more frequently than men and low blood pressure is also associated with *NTG* according to a study that detected trends but could not identity one single cause among those participating. What the study did reveal, however, is that the natural progression of glaucoma is more rapid in women, those with disc hemorrhages, vasospasms (like *Raynaud's Disease*), and possibly other vascular disorders.

How vascular disorders affect *NTG* depends on the autoregulation of the circulatory system. Should a spasm in a blood vessel occur, it impairs the blood supply. . Other factors negatively acting on blood supply include a rise in IOP or a decrease in blood pressure or both. There is also evidence that the blood vessels fill more slowly in *NTG*. Some systemic problems such as breathing problems during sleep (*apnea*) and possibly hearing loss have been associated with *NTG*. Disc hemorrhages often indicate ongoing damage as does a thinning of nerve fiber thickness. A comprehensive study from Japan that followed *NTG* patients for a mean of 5.6 years revealed that disc hemorrhage, age, systolic blood pressure and pulse rate significantly influenced visual field defects. The authors concluded that disc hemorrhages may be a sign of progressive damage to the optic nerve eventually showing up as deterioration of the visual field.

Apparently, people with *NTG* have thinner corneas. Using the ultrasound *pachymetry* researchers compared *NTG* eyes with *POAG*, ocular hypertension and normal eyes. The *NTGs* were the thinnest. Doctors may, therefore, be undertreating *NTGs* if this finding is not taken into account. Not everybody with *NTG* loses visual field progressively. In some people, especially with older patients, loss is so slow that doctors may elect not to treat.

Although the *CNTGTS* had only a few black patients in its cohort, the rate of progression of this population was more rapid. With Asians the rate was less. While reducing IOP by thirty percent became the golden rule based on this study, researchers have found that in a subset of cases, despite lowering of IOP, visual loss progressed. This finding raised the question of whether in certain patients the disease is not pressure-related or if further IOP reduction is necessary.

At times an avocation may contribute to vision loss. People with *NTG* who play a high resistance wind instrument may produce a transient rise in IOP. Blowing hard produces *uveal* engorgement (the *uvea* section of the eye is distended with fluid). This reaction, in susceptible individuals, can lead to glaucoma damage. Some doctors, however, disagree with this assessment.

OCULAR HYPTERTENSION (OHT)

A considerable group of people possess high *intraocular pressures* but do not, in some cases, appear to lose visual field. Until the *Ocular Hypertension Treatment Study, (OHS)* doctors were puzzled about whether to medicate these individuals or just simply follow them. If visual field loss became evident, they would then medicate. An important finding to emerge from this study revealed that persons with thin corneas, less than a measurement of 555um of corneal thickness had higher rates of progression than those with thicker corneas. This finding took precedence over other physical conditions such as *myopia*, high blood pressure, and race with respect to the onset of *POAG*, for a thinner central cornea measures lower than the actual IOP reading. This insight gave rise to a simple measurement device, *pachymetry,* now a routine procedure. Other risk factors for identifying *OHT* patients include larger cup-to-disc ratio, age and an IOP above 25 mmHg. Regardless of other parameters such as the visual field test, patients with IOPs of 30 mmHg or above, are at risk for visual field loss. The medical community generally concurs that these patients should receive medical treatment. Should the patient's central cornea measurement be 555um or better, have no visual field defects, and with an IOP less than 30 mmHg, depending upon the circumstances, some doctors simply follow the patient. Should medication be indicated, usually only one drop is prescribed. On the whole, and despite the small number of people who do progress into glaucoma as the study indicated, doctors are a cautious lot, and many of them prefer to treat patients even when visual loss is not evident assuming that at a later date loss may occur.

CONFIGURATION OF THE EYE LEADING TO GLAUCOMA

Narrow-Angle /Primary Angle-closure Glaucoma (PACG)

A narrow angle may be considered a structural problem of the eye. This can lead to several different eye conditions--*Narrow angle* and *Primary Angle Closure glaucoma* that can develop into *Acute* and/or *Chronic Angle Closure*. Considerably fewer people in the United States have this problem with the exception of Alaskan natives, but worldwide, in countries such as China, Japan and India, *PACG* is the most prevalent form. Glaucoma screening should begin at age thirty for this group, especially East Asians who experience the highest rate of blindness in the world from *angle closure*. Chinese and Intuit Eskimos are also highly vulnerable. As with *POAG*, relatives of those afflicted are more at risk. With older patients the most common cause for *angle-closure* is *pupillary block*.

Fortunately, not all people with narrow angles develop glaucoma. As with any organ, a width range varies and doctors consider this variation when diagnosing this syndrome. The angle in question is formed by the meeting of the *iris* and the wall of the eye. Generally, doctors use four grades to assess the angle width. Numbers 1 (10 degrees) and II (20 degrees) are considered *narrow-angle*; numbers III (30 degrees) and IV (40 degrees) are termed *open-angle*, although, in truth, the angle width is more of a continuum pattern than a strict cut-off point. Doctors maintain a watchful eye on patients with narrow angle problems. Everybody's angles, however, are routinely examined for signs of possible blockage.

Several diagnostic techniques help to determine the extent of the angle closure. The first test simply involves observing the reaction of the pupil in both light and dark conditions. The pupil will normally widen or dilate in a dark condition--this normal reaction allows the eye to capture all available light. In susceptible people, dilation of the pupil may cause blockage of an already narrowed angle.

There are four parameters that doctors use to determine etiology of the narrowed angle condition. The first is caused by an excessively narrow space (narrow *iridocorneal angle*) in the outlet channel. Any pressure on this space such as dilation of the *iris* can block the egress of fluid. The second type is caused by an enlarged ciliary body. This gland can cause blockage of the angle if it is anteriorly placed. The third cause of *angle closure* is an abnormally large lens that pushes the *iris* up against the outflow space, blocking it. The fourth type is caused by an anteriorly positioned ciliary body. Known as malignant glaucoma, this condition pushes the *iris* and ciliary body into the outflow space. It is often found in patients who undergo trabeculectomy.

According to the American Academy of Ophthalmology, the gold standard at the present writing for diagnosing *angle-closure glaucoma* is *gonioscopy*. A *gonio* lens is placed on the eye and through the mirrored magnification, the doctor is able to clearly see the angle. Some doctors assert that best results are obtained if this examination is performed in a completely dark room and this finding was evident with a small cohort of patients, where it was determined that fifty percent of the patients were more likely to be identified with *narrow angle glaucoma*. Since gonioscopy is uncomfortable for the patient, a group of researchers conducted an alternative *gonioscopy* using the slit-lamp adapted *Optical Coherence Tomography (SL-OCT)*. During this procedure the patient sits upright and a non-contact laser snaps pictures of the eye. In this small study results were quantitatively and qualitatively compared with *gonioscopy* in total darkness. More patients were identified as having *angle-closure* using the above method.

Should you be diagnosed with a narrow angle but with no evidence of glaucoma or optic disc damage, you still should be followed periodically. Although you may be one of the lucky ones to escape eye damage or glaucoma, you will probably still become a "glaucoma suspect." Your doctor in this case monitors your angle closely for should there be any changes in the various configurations as stated above the doctor might recommend a prophylactic procedure. A group of scientists researching this condition found upon examining a volunteer with so-called perfectly healthy eyes to be on the brink of *angle-closure*. His *iris* was poised to move into the angle blocking the outflow channel. This is the dreaded sequence of events that can lead to a precipitous rise in IOP resulting in significant nerve damage and visual field loss. The subject had an *iridotomy* within the next few days.

Dilation of the pupil is a fact of nature. Sitting in a darkened theater, certain drugs, stress, fatigue, anxiety or excitement, intensive close work, upper respiratory problems—all cause dilation. In most people this normal reaction is inconsequential but for *narrow angle* patients, any of the aforementioned conditions poses a real threat. A narrow angle event can occur in the doctor's office during a *retinal* examination or by taking medications such as anti-anxiety agents, antidepressants, anti-Parkinson drugs, antispasmodics, atropine agents, general anesthetics, ophthalmic vasoconstrictors (dilating drops), psychotropic agents, and stimulants that dilate the pupil. To avoid problems, advise your general practitioner that you have this condition, or when buying over-the-counter medicines, read labels carefully for contraindications for glaucoma. Be sure to check with your pharmacist if you are in doubt and if you are filling a prescription for the first time.

In all other cases glaucoma stealthily plucks off cells one by one until the loss mounts up to where it is finally noticed, but in an *acute-narrow angle attack,* the patient realizes that the eye is in deep trouble. There is a critical point where the *iris* moves into the blockage position, but it is hard to identify when that point will occur. This is the major reason that doctors treating certain patients who have *narrow angle* advise *iridotomy* as a prophylactic operation. An attack can cause a grim scenario—a fifty percent chance of severe optic nerve damage and a twenty percent chance of blindness in the affected eye.

Do not take *PACG* lightly. An attack can shoot your IOP up as high as 80 mmHg. Permanent damage to the optic nerve may occur. Scars can form on the angle and instant cataracts may form. Immediate treatment is vital to avoid damage to the optic nerve. To paraphrase Hamlet, *Get thee to an ophthalmologist or eye clinic immediately.* Be aware. An eye that has had an acute-angle glaucoma attack is at risk of another attack as is the contralateral eye. While nobody likes the idea of a prophylactic procedure, sight retention may hinge on the kind of treatment you receive.

What really frightens people about *PACG* is the almost instant loss of sight coming from out of nowhere as it did with Roger who developed a severe headache and noticed halos around lights. He was knowledgeable enough to see an ophthalmologist the next day and discovered his pressure to be 90 mmHg. Treatment was immediately instituted and while the pressure was reduced within a few hours, a sizeable chunk of damage had already occurred. In retrospect he ruefully admits, that although vaguely aware of the potential for dire consequences, instead of waiting until morning to call his ophthalmologist, he should have immediately gone to the emergency room of a hospital nearby.

In African-Americans and Asians, narrow angle follows a different pattern. Their thicker and more rigid *irises* usually result in a category called *chronic angle-closure glaucoma (CACG)*. This pattern slows the movement of the *iris* into the angle when the eye is dilated. But patients with *PACG* do not go scot-free, for although the situation may not be as dire as described above, severe problems can still occur.

People under fifty who are diagnosed with *PACG* may actually have *plateau iris syndrome*. This is a condition where the ciliary body in a more forward position pushes against the *iris* driving it into the angle and causing blockage. This condition also requires careful monitoring. Doctors usually recommend treatment of an *iridotomy* or *iridoplasty* for patients with *plateau iris*.

SECONDARY GLAUCOMAS

Glaucomas that arise as a result of systemic diseases or genetic factors are called secondary glaucomas. Some of these diseases are readily identifiable. *Pigmentary-Dispersion* Syndrome *(PDS)* and *Exfoliation Glaucoma (XFS)* are two such diseases that create blockage of the trabecular meshwork.

PIGMENTARY DISPERSION SYNDROME (PDS)

PDS usually affects people in their mid-twenties and is most prevalent in *myopic* males below the age of forty. Both men and women are equally affected, but men develop glaucoma about three times as often as women and at a younger age. It is an inherited structural condition of the eye. In the mid-age group doctors can readily diagnose this disease through the observation of a characteristic appearance called *Krukenberg's spindle* in the cornea; transillumination (defects) and dense pigmentation in the *trabecular meshwork*. The *iris* color may darken as the pigment particles accumulate. Along with the *Krukenberg's spindle*, the *iris* becomes more concave as it is brought in closer to the *zonules* (packets of fiber that hold the lens in place). Movement of the *iris* rubs against the *zonules* causing release of pigment. Certain forms of cataract surgery, implantation of an intraocular lens in the posterior chamber may result in pigment release because of the abnormal position of the lens. Examination requiring pupillary dilation may also cause a release of pigment. Whatever the reason, once released, these granules float in the fluid in the eye and end up in the *trabecular meshwork*, where they become trapped blocking the pores and slowing down the outflow of fluid.

They are also deposited on the *zonules*, the cornea, and on the lens capsule. The flakes of pigmentary from the *iris* may gradually block off the *trabecular meshwork*, resulting in glaucoma. It occurs in both eyes. According to one study, its prevalence is greater than previously suspected and some 2.45% of the Caucasian population may have this syndrome. Apparently with older patients, when the presence of *PDS* has not been diagnosed at a younger age, the signs are more subtle and it is often designated as *normal-tension glaucoma* or *POAG*.

Accommodation (eyes focusing on near-and far-objects) may also cause release of pigment granules. The pupil constricts for reading and other close activities; conversely it expands when looking at more distant objects. This action of the pupil may cause release of pigment. In eyes free of *PDS,* accommodation does not result in this problem.

As with other glaucoma conditions, mutated genes may be in part responsible for this condition. Researchers have identified a gene affecting the development of the middle third of the eye early in the third trimester of fetal development. It is reported at chromosome *7q35-36* and *18q*. This is the same gene implicated in juvenile *POAG*. Robert Ritch, MD suggested that either the serotonin or dopamine pathways are involved in the genesis of *PDS*. Animal studies indicate that *tyrosinase* (an enzyme that acts on the amino acid *tyrosine* that produces melanin) may correct the deficiency.

About sixty-to-eighty percent of patients are *myopic* and there is evidence that the greater the *myopia*, the earlier the onset of glaucoma. *Myopic* patients also experience a higher incidence of *retinal* detachment. Also, this disease may be mistaken for *juvenile glaucoma*. Doctors unfamiliar with this syndrome, even in the presence of the *Krukenberg's spindle* may misdiagnose the syndrome. In some patients, it's possible to have a double whammy with *pigmentary dispersion* in one eye and *exfoliation syndrome the other eye*. More optimistically, one eye might have a much less severe case of the disorder.

Reverse pupillary block is a mechanism of *pigmentary dispersion* that occurs when the *iris* is in a concave position. This causes the eye pressure to be greater in the front of the eye than in the back. In this case, the increased pressure in the front of the eye pushes the *iris* up against the lens. Because of the unequal pressures, the *iris* is forced into a concave position promoting release of pigment and possibly scarring. Not comparable to *narrow-angle glaucoma* this condition can be relieved through a procedure called a laser *iridotomy*. Blinking, yes, blinking may also cause concavity of the *iris*. Apparently a blink deforms the cornea for a split second, innocuous except for *PDS*. Researchers using animal models demonstrated that the *iris* would flatten out if blinking were prevented. But this is obviously not an option for blinking bathes the eye in protective fluids.

PDS does not always lead to glaucoma. A number of retrospective studies found a ten percent occurrence over a period of five years, and fifteen percent at fifteen years. It has also been reported in the literature that fewer than half will develop glaucoma. They may be blessed with a more aaccommodating *trabecular meshwork* or an immune system capable of clearing away the pigment granules. There is evidence of the white blood cell clean-up crew scrubbing down the *trabecular meshwork*. Nevertheless, when patients are diagnosed with this syndrome they are generally considered "glaucoma suspects" This syndrome can, in later life, morph into *exfoliation syndrome*.

Treatment of the disease where glaucoma is present requires lowering the *intraocular pressure*. First line medications now include the *prostaglandins* (*Xalatan, Lumigan*, and *Travatan*). *Miotics (Pilocarpine, carbacohl)* that constrict the pupil is another option. *Miotics,* however, are difficult to take, especially for young patients because of pupil constriction preventing accommodation that in turn limits or constrains work-related and recreational activities, such as driving and sports. In older patients, *miotics* reduce vision. Nevertheless constricting the pupil rebalances the distribution of fluids between the back and the front of the eye releasing the *iris* to return to its convex shape and also preventing the *iris* from rubbing against the zonules. Beta blockers are no longer recommended, for by reducing fluid, removal of debris from the trabecular meshwork may be compromised. A *laser iridotomy* may be recommended in some cases. A *trabeculoplasty* might be the better choice for younger patients. Some doctors prefer to treat the problem medically and then move into surgery if an elevated IOP no longer responds to medical treatment. Aerobic activity is especially contraindicated since jogging loosens up the particles.

There is good news associated with *PDS*. Unlike other glaucomas, regression of the disease has been documented. Loss of accommodation because of thickening of the lens, that pesky bit where you suddenly find that you need glasses for reading, alleviates the problem of pigment release. IOP may return to normal and some patients who have been treated for a number of years with *miotic* therapy may be able to reduce or to do away with their drops altogether. Remission of glaucoma has also been recorded following glaucoma surgery. Ben, whom we discussed in our earlier book, *Coping with Glaucoma*, happily states that he is in remission. Now in his mid-fifties, he has carefully monitored the progress of his disease. His IOP pressure is no longer threatening his sight and he, along with many older patients with *PDS,* are in the blessed state of glaucoma remission. Ben's diligence did help him to avoid serious damage from the disease, for being aware of the consequences of *PDS* he developed a doctor-patient relationship that served him well. He recalls how in the early stages of his condition, he alerted his doctor to the possibility that he might have a problem and asked to have a visual field test The test did show a defect and Ben switched doctors for one more knowledgeable about *PDS*.

EXFOLIATION GLAUCOMA (XFS)

This syndrome characterized by the production and progressive accumulation of whitish material or microfibular deposits is an apt description of this secondary glaucoma condition. The material loads onto many ocular tissues causing in about twenty-five percent of those affected elevated IOP, cataract and angle-closure. It is believed that environmental factors such as impaired blood flow, oxidative stress, and low grade inflammation may set the stage of those with *XFS* to develop glaucoma. Nevertheless, if you have *exfoliation,* chance of developing glaucoma are six times higher than average.

The flaking resulting from this condition affects more areas than the lens. Since it is a systemic disease, it may also affect the skin, heart, lungs, liver, kidney, spinal chord, brain membranes, gallbladder, and possibly lead to transient ischemic attacks, stroke, angina, myocardial infarction, hypertension, *retinal vein occlusion, Alzheimer's,* abdominal aortic aneurysm, and elevated *homocystinuria* (increased risk of atherosclerosis).

While this syndrome has not captured the general practitioner's interest to the extent that it has within the ophthalmologic community, it may well reveal upon research, that *XFS,* as scientists have observed, affects connective tissues and muscle cells as well as the eye. Furthermore, in an observation of patients undergoing stomach aneurysm surgery (abnormal dilation of a blood vessel), over half the patients had *XFS*.

Typically *XFS,* resulting in impairment of the blood-aqueous barrier that in turn results in *pupillary block*.

The prevalence of the disease increases with age and it is more commonly found in certain ethnic populations such as in South Asia, Sweden, Norway, Iceland and Russia. Since medical and surgical procedures will be affected by the presence of *XFS,* eye doctors should be encouraged to check for *XFS* at the initial examination of people from the above countries. Several members in my family have been identified with the syndrome but not all of them have glaucoma.

In August of 2007, scientists using a new device, DNA scanning chips, have identified two variant sites on the same gene that pose a risk for *exfoliative* glaucoma. Both sites lie on the gene known as the *Lysyl oxidase-like 1* gene, or *LOXL1,* responsible for the formation and maintenance of elastin tissue. Defects in one gene can account for essentially ninety-nine percent of the cases of *exfoliative* glaucoma. The effects of the genetic variant of the gene seem to lower the production rate of protein it specifies. The protein appears to play a role in the accumulation of microfibular deposits causing *XFS*. The protein built by the *LOXL1* gene is produced in many tissues of the body. It helps build the network of fibers and elastin that looms the body's tissues together. This would possibly account for the prevalence of this syndrome throughout the body.

Management of the disease requires special consideration. Cataract extraction, in particular, raises a red flag in the presence of *XFS*. My sister, although developing glaucoma much later in life than I, sadly discovered the reality of complications during a cataract operation. She lost of over fifty percent of her vision in her eye. Evidently her doctor was unfamiliar with the destructive effects of *XFS*. The main problem lies with the *zonules*. The lens sits in a capsule, like a pillow in a pillowcase, and it is held in place by *zonules,* bundles of fibers (like a rope). The *XFS* material coats these fibers, Imagine snow coating bare tree branches in winter. If the branches become heavily laden, they may break under the weight. The same is true for *zonular-laden fibers.* These delicate fibers weaken, stretch, and may even break or detach from their moorings dislocating the capsule.

Intraocular pressure is much harder to control when *XFS* is present. The material loads on to what is called the *juxtacanalicular* (a type of tissue) that is adjacent to the *Schlemm's Canal*. Deposits of *XFS* material swell this tissue and because of its proximity to the *Schlemm's Canal* it disorganizes that body causing greater susceptibility to blockage. Other problems involve pupils that are asymmetrical, a condition possibly decreasing rigidity, leading to scarring affecting the outer cells of the *iris* and lens capsule. This condition occurs when cells coated with sticky *XFS* material adhere together. Degeneration of the *iris* may weaken the structure. The *trabecular meshwork* may become clogged up with melanin granules from the affected *iris* and the cornea may also be affected. This, in turn, may lead to *corneal decompensation* (failure to maintain structure). A possibility also exists of retinal detachment and *pseudouveitis.* The above is a most impressive and scary list of problems associated with *XFS* syndrome. I have and have had some of them--retinal detachment and a difficult-to-control IOP, but one of my eyes still possesses decent vision after some thirty-odd years with this syndrome.

This confluence of events complicates treatment. Diagnosed, however, treatment follows the same sequence as in *POAG*--medication, laser, filtering surgery. Of the greatest importance is control of the *intraocular pressure* that may require maximum glaucoma therapy. Although out of favor given the many new IOP medications now available, the *miotic* drugs once widely used have taken a back seat. Yet these drugs, despite their serious side effects may still be useful for some patients. Researchers studying *XFS* have not yet documented a clear biochemical composition of this invasive material but they do possess good information on its effects on the various structures of the eye. Some scientists speculate that the fibers might not even be biochemical in nature.

People who have *XFS* or *PDS* do not necessarily get glaucoma. In my family, my sister and brother, as well as I, have glaucoma but a third sister does not, nor does my niece, diagnosed with *exfoliation syndrome*.

In Ben's family, his sister has *PDS*, but no sign of glaucoma. Is it life style, stress or some other not yet undiagnosed factor or it just the luck of the draw? Impossible to answer these questions at the present writing. What does matter, however, is that should you be diagnosed with either syndrome, even without the presence of glaucoma, be sure to have at least a yearly eye examination with a doctor experienced in *XFS* or *PDS*.

UVEITIC GLAUCOMA

Why should two apparently healthy individuals such as Sally and Mary develop inflammation (any disease ending in "itis" is an inflammatory disease) in their eyes? The *uvea* as we have learned is the pigmented middle layer of the eye. It incorporates the *iris*, the fluid manufacturing *ciliary body* and the *choroid* responsible for carrying nourishing blood into the eye. *Uveitis* is a generic term describing inflammation inside the eye. It occurs in 115 out of 100,000 people. Inflammation may be confined to only one of the bodies in the eye, such as the *iris* or the *choroid*. If so, it is called *iritis* or *choroiditis* respectively. When inflammation occurs in the front of the eye *(anterior uveitis),* it tends to be the most symptomatic, causing pain, redness, decreased vision and sensitivity to bright light. Affecting twenty-eight of all *uveitis* cases, it is associated with eye trauma and cataract surgery. *Intermediate uveitis* occurs in the center of the eye just behind the *iris* and lens and *posterior uveitis* can be found in the *retina*, the optic nerve, and other parts located in the back of the eye. Both *intermediate* and *posterior uveitis* are usually pain free, but floaters and decreased vision may occur. Often, inflammation affects only one eye causing that eye to be particularly vulnerable and giving rise to what many of us call the good-eye/bad-eye syndrome. It is estimated that over 300,000 people in the United States are affected by intraocular inflammation.

Neither Sally nor Mary fit the clinical picture of a *uveitis*-prone individual. They are in mid-life and are actively engaged in their respective careers. So then what causes this dread disease? To probe the source of *uveitis,* ophthalmologists and researchers are delving into past medical histories of patients with the syndrome. About forty percent of people suffering from *uveitis* have or have had another inflammatory disease. C. Stephen Foster, MD, Harvard Medical School, asks patients to fill out a comprehensive survey of the patient's medical history that includes family members as well. Apparently any past or present illness and diseases such as cancer, *diabetes*, allergies, *sickle cell anemia, hepatitis, pleurisy, pneumonia*, ulcers, *herpes* (cold sores, etc.), *AIDS* or *chicken pox* may be causative. Other causes include *HLA-B27* (*ankylosing spondylitis*—inflammation of the spine and large joints), *sarcoidosis* (granular lesions that may affects any organ or tissue of the body), *Fuch's syndrome, Behcet's Syndrome* (inflammatory condition that can affect the eyes, blood vessels, nervous system and digestive tract,), *Vogt-Koyanagi Harada Syndrome (*rare, may result in *uveitis* or *retinal* abnormalities*),* and collagen vascular disorders such as *systemic lupus erythematosus* (chronic rashes). In older people, diseases such as *serpiginous chorioretinopathy* (may result in artery occlusion), *birdshot retinochoroidopathy* (inflammation of the *retina*), *acute retinal necrosis* (death of *retinal* tissues), *Sjogren's syndrome* (dryness of the mucous membranes), and *tuberculosis,* and *syphilis* may also be responsble. Water from an untreated stream, raw meat, uncooked sausage, unpasteurized milk or cheese, intravenous drugs, cat or dog possession, bisexual or homosexual relationships all may induce parasitic or bacterial infections such as *toxoplasmosis, toxocanasis, endogenous endophthalmitis, histoplasmosis* (fungal infection), *cystercicosis* (parasitic infection), *Whipple's disease,* (infection), *Lyme* disease, *cat-scratch disease, Brucellosis,* or *nephritis.* Some clinical studies have shown a higher incidence of this syndrome in women but other studies deflate this finding. A poor visual prognosis may result from a condition called *granulomatous uveitis* (accumulation of inflammatory products—the white blood cells and macrophages) and adhesions in the eye.

Auto-immune diseases--*lupus, arthritis, rheumatism,* fungal infections and *coccidiodomycosis* are not exempt. Children can also be affected but more rarely except for those exposed to unsanitary conditions and are infected with parasites. More common is *juvenile rheumatoid arthritis* that affects youngsters in their teens. *Toxoplasmosis, retinochoroiditis* (inflammation of the *retina* and choroid) caused by a pathogen may also be involved in this syndrome. Testing of all these diseases is obviously unwieldy. The following tests recommended by Ernest L. Bowling. OD, MS, FAAO and Daryl F. Mann, OD include *juvenile rheumatoid arthritis, sarcoidosis, ankylosis spondylitis, Lyme disease, syphilis, tuberculosis.* Your doctor, of course, may want to order additional tests. Do the tests reveal a connection? One study found in a group of some 200 patients that forty percent had a systemic disease.

So what does this all mean? Some studies indicate that secondary glaucoma resulting from *uveitis* mainly affects nearly ten percent of the patients with *open-angle glaucoma.*

How do you know if you have *uveitis*? If it is mild, only your doctor can tell, but if it is severe, you may experience pain, redness of the conjunctiva, photophobia (sensitivity to bright light) and lowered vision. Your doctor can detect the presence of *uveitis* by checking for tell-tale white blood cells seen floating in the fluid in the front part of the eye or deposits of white blood cells on the inside surface of the *cornea* or in the *vitreous*. You might see floaters (those pesky black spots) if the *uveitis* is in the back of the eye. *Retinal* detachment may also occur. *Uveitis* can also cause swelling of the *macula* leading to *macular edema* and cataract formation. Uveitis is graded from 0-4, depending upon both the leakage of serum from diseased vessels into the aqueous portion of the eye and the numbert of white blood cells.

How does *uveitis* cause glaucoma? At first, the diagnosis of *uveitis* appears non-problematical, for the disease might, with some patients, reduce the production of aqueous fluid thus lowering IOP, but if this situation becomes chronic, the *retina* can become damaged. When the aqueous normalizes, however, the trabecular meshwork may become blocked, causing a rise of pressure. Inflammation can scar tissues at the border between the *iris* and surface of the lens. If scarring is extensive, fluid may be prevented from flowing through the pupil raising pressure in the back of the eye. This syndrome pushes the *iris* forward into a bowed position precipitating *secondary angle-closure glaucoma*. *Uveitis* is not considered an optic nerve disease, but one that affects the *retina*.

Yet with all the diseases and medical conditions that can contribute to *uveitis*, researchers have found that in about half the patients the syndrome is idiopathic (unable to determine origin). About ten percent of seniors with glaucoma have uveitis. A retrospective study of patients with glaucoma from the Royal Aberdeen Infirmary in Scotland suggests that glaucoma is a major complication of *uveitis*. Although not all persons with *uveitis* develop glaucoma, this statistic places greater emphasis for those diagnosed with *uveitis* to have frequent check-ups.

Treatment involves control of both the inflammation and of the IOP. Inflammation can respond to corticosteroid or non-steroid drops. Should drops be ineffective, systemic steroids in pill form or by an intraocular injection right into the eye or periocular (around the eye) may be recommended. The injected material affords protection for about three months. A drug *infliximab* in trials has been found to be effective with some people but it also causes side-effects. Glaucoma treatment follows the *POAG* guidelines—pressure-reducing drops and possibly filtering surgery bypassing laser treatment because of the possibility of increased inflammation, and lastly, a glaucoma drainage implant (See Chapter 7). Most important is reduction of inflammation before surgery. Both Sally and Mary have had surgery. Sally has done well with one eye, but not with the other. Mary did not do well with laser surgery and had to have a filtering operation.

Research continues to establish the most effective protocols for managing *uveitis*. The Casey Eye Institute in Oregon is studying cells and tissue as well as genetic factors to determine treatments, both standard and experimental that will eliminate the ravages of this disease. The drug *Kenelog* (*triamcinolone acetonide*—a corticosteroid) has been used with a small number of patients. Researchers have found it to be effective, but more research on this drug is needed.

There has been some indication that a higher level of *arachidonic acid* (an unsaturated fatty acid) that is a precursor of *prostaglandins, thromboxane* (constrictor of blood vessels) and *leukotrienes* (mediators of inflammation) may affect *uveitis* adversely. Taking medications other then eye drops that contain *arachidonic* acid may load up more of this substance than the body can tolerate. Some practitioners advise taking an aspirin which blocks synthesis of *prostaglandins* to clear up this problem.

Loss of sight need not occur with *uveitis* if it is treated and caught in time. Both Sally and Mary have lost some sight, mostly in one eye (the good eye/ bad eye syndrome) but both of these women developed the condition in their early thirties. Some twenty-odd years later, they are still functioning well.

The Neovascular Glaucomas

Several of the diseases that cause secondary glaucomas fall into this category. The term *neovascular* is defined as new blood vessels, which instead of beneficial, create problems, for these new products are weak, leaky, rupture easily and hemorrhage. Furthermore, they proliferate over the eye causing blockage.

The most common diseases associated with the *neovascular syndrome* include *diabetic retinopathy, central vein occlusion (CRVO),* and *carotid artery occlusive disease (CRAO)*. They are associated with systemic problems that block the flow of blood to either the central vein or the *carotid* arteries. What causes these runaway blood vessels? One of the theories submits that blockage starves the vessels of oxygen, which is crucial to circulation and nourishment. Stimulated, the blood vessels release substances that promote growth of new blood vessels. And, indeed, researchers have found a high level of *VEGF (vascular endothelia growth factor)* in the aqueous humor of eyes with neovascular glaucoma, as compared with patients who have cataracts or *POAG*. The body does attempt to counterbalance blood vessel growth. A protein *PEDF (pigment epithelium derived factor)* inhibits *VEGF*, although in the *neovascular* glaucomas, this protein may be in short supply.

A substance, *C-reactive protein* that has been linked to *rheumatoid arthritis* and cardiovascular disease, may also be a risk factor. While these studies are illuminating, additional research is necessary to nail down a cure for this syndrome.

Fortunately, not all patients who have the above diseases develop glaucoma, but when runaway blood vessels proliferate over the *retina, iris, optic nerve*, and *trabecular meshwork*, blockage of the outflow channels promotes a glaucomatous condition requiring treatment. It is of utmost importance, therefore, that scheduled visits to the doctor for both the glaucoma and the *neovascular* conditions be instituted.

DIABETIC RETINOPATHY

I belong to a community garden. One of our most stalwart members was Charles, a diabetic. Charles joined the garden about five years after I did, and he immediately assumed a leadership role. Not many of us knew that Charles had *diabetes*, but, as the years marched on, we noticed that Charles was slowing down. Being a man of pride, Charles kept his failing eyesight to himself. When I learned that Charles was diabetic, I asked if his eyes were routinely checked for signs of disease. Charles assured me that this was so. In teaching hospitals and clinics, such an examination is usually routine, but world-wide, checking for *proliferative diabetic retinopathy* may not be so. Unfortunately, although Charles did have treatment, the disease exacted a toll on his eyesight. Charles finally succumbed from his *diabetic* condition, almost blind. His case is a stark example of the dire consequences of that deadly disease.

Genetic susceptibility is known to play a role in *diabetes*. When this disease affects the eyes, the condition is called *diabetic retinopathy*, which can be either *nonproliferative* or *proliferative*. *Diabetic retinopathy* affects almost half of all Americans diagnosed with *diabetes*. Statistics about loss of vision are alarming. Yearly, about 40,000 *diabetics* will lose their sight to *diabetes* as incidences of *diabetes* increases due to poor diet, excessive weight gain and lack of exercise. With the rise of *diabetes* nationwide, blindness from *Diabetic Retinopathy* has become a front-burner issue.

The eyes are not the only organs associated with this condition. *Diabetes* also causes poor circulation, heart disease, stroke, gangrene of feet and hands due to poor wound healing, impotence, infections, kidney failure, nerve damage, poor digestion, erratic blood pressure, and increased susceptibility to urinary tract infection, skin problems, and *Carpal tunnel syndrome*.

There are two classifications of *diabetes mellitus*. Type I, accounting for ten percent of the *diabetics*, occurs in young patients who produce little or no insulin resulting from the destruction of ninety percent of the insulin producing cells in the pancreas. These are the patients who require daily injections of insulin when first diagnosed.

Type 2 diabetes most often called *Adult* or *Maturity Onset Diabetes* is not necessarily insulin-dependent. This syndrome is believed to be caused by excessive carbohydrate intake that is stored as fat when not used up entirely for energy. It is possible that when patients carefully heed their food intake and maintain blood sugar levels within the normal range of 90-to-120 mg/dl of blood, medication is unnecessary. Charles feasted on bread, cookies, cake and fast food low in nutrition but high in fats and sugars. Overweight people require a larger amount of insulin to meet their dietary needs to counter insulin-resistance. It is estimated that eighty-to-ninety percent of obese people have Type 2 *Diabetes*. Fat cells secrete hormones such as *leptin, adinonectin* and *resistin* that help tissues communicate. These hormones apparently work differently than other hormones in Type II diabetics. Only a few types of tissues are susceptible to the negative effects of these hormones and of these the *photoreceptor* cells of the *retina* and the *vascular* cells are especially sensitive. High intra-cell sugar in these cells causes the *mitochondrial* cells to burn more fuel resulting in excessive oxygen free radicals.

In the *nonproliferative* form, small blood vessels in the *retina* weaken and develop bulges (micro-*aneurysms*) that can leak and possibly swell. If swelling occurs, the *retinal* cells may be damaged, resulting in loss or blurring of vision - especially if the *macular* region is affected. High blood pressure, often accompanying *diabetes*, puts patients at greater risk. High levels of blood sugar are directly related to the weakening of blood vessels. In the *proliferative* stage, impaired circulation, caused by narrowed and damaged blood vessels, deprives the *retina* of oxygen. The eye tries to redress the problem of oxygen deprivation by growing new blood vessels that extend all over the eye. These vessels are fragile and when they rupture, they release blood into the interior of the eye leading to blurred vision and temporary blindness, forming scar tissue that eventually pulls the *retina* away from the back of the eye (retinal detachment) and leads to permanent vision loss. Therapeutic laser treatment (See Chapter 6) can help alleviate this situation.

Your doctor can diagnose the type of *diabetic retinopathy* that you possess by visually examining the *retinal* or by using a test called *fluoroscein angiography* that takes a picture of your blood vessels. Guidelines exist for determining the severity of the condition.

Treatment of the ravages of *diabetic retinopathy* involve *ablating* (destroying) the peripheral *retinal* cells in an effort to halt the progression of these wayward blood vessels. When these blood vessels stray into the *trabecular meshwork*, glaucoma occurs. Traditionally, laser treatment is the therapeutic approach, but it is known to fail. Some of the same drugs in use with macular degeneration may relieve the ravages of *diabetic retinopathy*. New drugs are constantly being evaluated and these may become more effective. A *vitrectomy* (removal of the vitreous) is another method for controlling this problem.

Control of early stages of the disease is possible through careful diet considerations. A study that followed four thousand diabetics over twenty-five years documented that *diabetics* who controlled their blood sugar levels did not develop *diabetic retinopathy* as frequently as those with poor sugar control. Nevertheless, there is robust research ongoing to determine some of *angiogenic* (development of blood vessels), factors involved in *diabetic retinopathy*. As researchers learn more about growth factors and forms of enzymes, new drugs for treating the disease will inevitably follow. This research covers a large field, for both *macular degeneration* and *diabetic retinopathy* share some of the same problems, and as a result, many of the strategies being explored for one of the diseases will find applicability to the other. Controlling the *vascular endothelial growth factor (VEGF),* implanting steroids capable of delivering medication to the eye for up to three years, and developing medications that can reach down to the cell level are some of the strategies already in use. One of these new medications under study, taken orally, is hoped to prove effective enough to eliminate the drastic treatment of destroying peripheral vision in order to preserve central vision.

Diabetes mellitus can also lead to *neovascular glaucoma,* the proliferation of blood vessels that may clog up the outflow passage. Studies have revealed that two percent of the *diabetic* population and twenty-one percent of those who have *proliferative diabetic retinopathy* will also experience a form of *neovascular glaucoma.*

One of the persistent effects of *diabetic retinopathy* is *macula edema* (swelling of the macula). A novel therapy involving five patients consisting of delivering four liters of oxygen per minute into their noses for three months reduced the thickened macula by an average forty-three percent. Visual acuity increased by two lines and macular thickness by half. Although pregnancy tends to lower eye pressure, possibly because of hormonal changes, women who are pregnant and also have *diabetes,* need extra medical attention to assure a healthy delivery.

Traditionally, the level of glucose control for *diabetics* requires a blood sample, but the time may be ripe when the *diabetic* can simply look in the mirror and check on his/her condition. This information can be obtained by wearing specially prepared contact lenses that are outfitted with a particular kind of crystal that detects glucose levels.

CENTRAL RETINAL ARTERY OCCLUSION (CRAO)

With no history of eye disease, Raymond, a fifty-five year old black man, discovered that he could no longer see out of his right eye. He did not suffer a headache, see flashing lights or floaters, nor did he have or recall trauma to that eye. Yet within hours of reporting to the emergency room and being referred to Ophthalmology, he discovered he had experienced an occlusion of the *central retinal artery*, described to Raymond as a stroke in the eye. This is a rare disease affecting one in ten thousand patients in the United States, and of these only one-to-two percent have a bilateral episode. The disease affects men more frequently than women but women are not entirely exempt. The sixties is the mean age when the event occurs. Life expectancy, unfortunately, is shortened in patients diagnosed with *CRAO*.

Blood supply to the *retina* derives from the *carotid* artery, the principle source of blood supply to the brain. This artery branches into the *ophthalmic artery* that then branches into the *retinal and ciliary arteries*. Each eye is served by a separate branch. The inner layers of the *retina* are supplied by the *retinal artery* while the *ciliary artery* supplies blood to the outer layer of the *retina* as well as to the *choroid*. Blood flow may be impeded by blockage at any point within this system. Should blockage occur in the *ophthalmic artery*, blood flow to the entire system fails, producing a sudden painless loss of vision in the eye. In some patients, severe loss renders the eye capable of seeing fingers held only a foot or so away. Within hours, the *retina* becomes pale, except for the *fovea* that retains its reddish hue.

Patients at greater risk for *CRAO* include those with hypertension. About two-thirds fall into this category, one-fourth with plaque in the *carotid* artery. Other risk factors include *atherosclerosis*, cardiac problems, chronic inflammation of the *ophthalmic artery*, vascular diseases, traumatic insults that include X-ray irradiation, *retrobulbar* injection, migraine, lesions that may appear on the *optic nerve*, swelling of the *optic nerve*, *Central Retinal Vein Occlusion*, abnormal tissue growth, *sickle cell* disease, or just simply a spontaneous incident.

When blockage is remediated, in most cases, vision, except for some ten percent of the lucky ones who retain central acuity, remains very poor even though blood supply is normalized. This is a true emergency. If the patient is able to receive treatment within the first ninety minutes of the event, vision may be saved. Restoration may still be possible in the first twenty-four hours. Treatment consists of lowering the IOP, dilating the blood vessels and medically attempting to improve the flow of blood, breathing in five percent carbon dioxide gas, massaging the eye, removing a small amount of fluid from the eye to further lower the pressure, and possibly dissolving the *fibrin* in the blood. Although this disease is rare, doctors are investigating preventive measures such as *neuroprotection* and *fibrin* reduction in the blood. Steroid medication is recommended should inflammation occur and your doctor will usually suggest this treatment to protect an inflamed fellow eye.

CENTRAL RETINAL VEIN OCCLUSION (CRVO)

This syndrome is complicated, for it may manifest in a mild (*non-ischemic*) or a severe (*ischemic*) form. This syndrome as, with others affected by blood flow, is the result of an obstruction. When the drainage system turns sluggish, it becomes occluded, a condition similar to the *aqueous fluid* attempting to drain through a clogged *trabecular meshwork*. With *CRVO,* it is a clogged venous channel. Blood vessels feeding the *central retinal vein* become engorged and swell. As pressure builds, blood begins to seep out leading to hemorrhages in the *retina*.

In the mild form, swelling and hemorrhage, while occurring, are generally minimal, and while the sluggishness is still evident, some practitioners opt not to treat, considering this condition to be relatively benign. *Cystoid macular edema* (swelling caused by fluid in the macula) is a major complication and a permanent *scotoma* (gap in the visual field) may form. According to one study, however, sixty-five percent of the patients retained good vision.

A severe condition involves a backup of blood that impedes *(ischemia)* the flow of fresh blood from the arteries, starving the cells of oxygen. With extreme *ischemia*, the starved *retina* dies off, resulting in vision loss. During this event, the eye attempts to self-protect by growing new blood vessels *(neovascularization)* which is, unfortunately, a destructive solution. If the *neovascularization* grows over the *anterior chamber, angle* and *trabecular meshwork*, glaucoma develops. This glaucomatous condition responds poorly to medication and may lead to blindness in the affected eye. According to Sohan Singh Hayre, MD, who was honored for his work by The *Association for Research in Vision and Ophthalmology,* risk of severity develops in the first seven-to-eight months of the disease. 45% of these patients develop *neovascular* glaucoma. In the study that Dr. Hayre mentioned, 12.6% of the eyes progressed from *non-ischemic* to *ischemic* within eighteen months. Dr. Hayre also found that both aspects of this disease were self-limiting, notwithstanding the severe damage to the eye in the *ischemic* phase.

Systemic anticoagulants may contribute to the formation of this disease, leading to an increase in *retinal* hemorrhages that in turn, may promote a benign *CRVO* into a severe form. Patients on antiplatelet agents such as aspirin are not immune from this effect. Dr. Hayre suggested that based on a review of the literature for treatment of *CRVO* over the past three decades, anticoagulants and antiplatelet therapies are of no therapeutic value.

Scientists are, of course, seeking better treatments. One such, *hemodylution,* an attempt to thin the thickness of the blood, is according to Dr. Hayre of little value. Some patients may respond to high dose systemic corticosteroid treatment for *macular edema* resulting in improved vision, but when the steroid dose is lowered, the condition reverts to its former parameters. It is possible to inject the steroid directly into the eye packaged in a drug called *triamcinolone acetonide (Kenelog)* that lasts for three months. The injection leaves a little bump in the area where the needle was introduced. Patients willing to tolerate side effects from high doses of steroids may be rewarded with vision retention. But steroid use may be of no value when the form is severe.

Diamox, one of the drugs used to control severe forms of glaucoma, may help. *Diamox* is a very difficult drug for it may produce systemic effects in some vulnerable people. Although some patients may be able to tolerate *Diamox sequels,* Dr. Hayre has found that if a patient doesn't respond within two weeks, the treatment should be discontinued.

Internally, high IOP is not a problem associated with *CRVO*; for some unexplained reason, pressure is actually lowered. If a high IOP registers in the fellow eye, however, and is free of *CRVO,* pressure should certainly be lowered.

Vascular endothial growth factor (VEGF) has gained prominence as a central cause for *neovascular disease.* A *retina* starved of blood will attempt to remedy this problem by creating new blood vessels that are weak, given to bleeding, and proliferate mercilessly. The growth factor *VEGF* sets this scenario in motion. Inhibiting *VEGF* is, therefore, one of the therapeutic goals for neovascular control. Progress is being made with several drugs designed to inhibit the production of *VEGF.*

CORNEAL IRIDOCORNEAL ENDOTHELIAL (ICE) SYNDROME

The *ICE Syndrome* characterizes a group of diseases affecting the *iris.* These include; **Progressive Iris Atrophy, Cogan Reese Syndrome, Chandler's Syndrome, Iris Nevus Syndrome,** along with various *iris* abnormalities. In some cases, a membrane, called *Descemet's membrane,* is also affected. These syndromes are rare, but if present can lead to glaucoma. Regarded as a single disease with multiple features, each is distinguished by a group of related syndromes affecting the *cornea* and *iris*. Abnormalities of the endothelial layer of corneal cells, notable for "beaten metal" appearance, *corneal edema* (varying degrees of swelling,) wasting away of the *iris*, formation of holes in the *iris*, abnormalities of the interior chamber, and *secondary angle-closure glaucoma* that occurs when an opaque membrane from the inner layers of the peripheral corneal lining spreads over the angle and onto the surface of the *iris*, are common to each. The diseased lining grows over the *iris* shrinking it. This shrinkage pulls the *iris* back up towards the cornea blocking the angle that then elevates the IOP. The *iris* in this form unfortunately, does not heal. While the *iris* transformations sound grim, they are generally not visible to the naked eye. Most often only one eye is affected. Onset of the disease usually occurs in early or middle adulthood.

Treatment of all of the syndromes is focused on reducing the swelling of the *cornea*. Control may be possible with the use of hypertonic saline drops or ointment (e.g., five percent sodium chloride.) Simply using a hair dryer to blow warm air onto the face may also relieve the swelling that is usually greater in the morning. Some patients do find that as the day progresses, swelling subsides somewhat.

Should glaucoma develop your doctor will usually recommend eye drops to reduce pressure and if drops cease to be effective, either *laser* and/or a *trabeculectomy*--although the *trabeculectomy* may fail within a few months. Some people, however, consider themselves lucky as Lily did whose *trabeculectomy* served her for ten years. Shunts are known to work somewhat better but present a problem should a *corneal* transplant be necessary. Nevertheless, doctors do not advise a prophylactic transplant, for the post-operative procedure requires a year of taking drops and the special care of a corneal specialist.

This syndrome is believed to be a developmental disorder occurring during the final differentiation of the *cornea* lining when cells are prevented from completing their normal growth. Although it is believed that this abnormality affects only a small portion of the lining, it does cause proliferation. There is a possibility, observationally-based, of a high percentage of *herpes simplex virus* found in corneal graft specimens, which were taken from *ICE* patients undergoing *corneal* transplants. It is speculated that the infection from this virus may have occurred during fetal development. Females are more affected than males. Lily discovered she had the disease while at college. Noticing that she didn't see well, she visited her eye doctor and discovered she had *ICE Syndrome* in one eye along with high IOP pressure. Therein, for the next five years she battled progressive loss of vision in the eye, which finally stabilized at the count fingers" stage. Despite this loss, her glaucoma free 20/20 vision fellow eye enables Lily to bicycle all about New York City, through varying degrees of traffic, weather conditions and what have you with absolute confidence. This exercise helps to both keep her IOP low in her affected eye and to maintain good blood sugar levels.

PROGRESSIVE IRIS ATROPHY

This syndrome is characterized by severe thinning of the *iris* that results in *corectopia*—an abnormal position of the pupil. The thinning produces holes in the *iris* called either "stretch holes" or "melting holes" along with pupil deformation.

COGAN-REESE SYNDROME

This is one of the rarer eye disorders that is fortunately unilateral. It is characterized by abnormal proliferation of the *corneal* cells over the *cornea* and the angle where the *cornea* and *iris* meet. The surface of the *iris* appears matted or smudged. Multiple *Iris nevi* (small colored lumps or nodules) cover parts of the *iris*. Portions of the *iris* adhere to the *cornea* and may be wasting away. As well, the *Descemet's Membrane*, the only barrier between the interior chamber and the surface of the eye is abnormal.

CHANDLER'S SYNDROME

This syndrome is somewhat milder than the others and is characterized by a fluid filling the anterior chamber even under normal eye pressure. This condition results in swelling of the *cornea* (edema). Mild *iris* atrophy may also occur.

DYSTROPHIES MAINLY INVOLVING THE CORNEA

This group of corneal dystrophies includes: *Fuch's Corneal Dystrophy, and several other rare dystrophies—Anterior Polymorphous Dystrophy, Map-dot-fingerprint Epithelial Dystrophy, Central Crystalline Dystrophy and Central Cloudy Dystrophy of Francois.*

FUCH'S CORNEAL ENDOTHELIAL DYSTROPHY

Unlike the *ICE Syndrome* this disease affects both eyes. Signs and symptoms are attributable to a primary malfunction of the inner lining of the *corneal endothelial* cells. Three stages characterize this disease. The first covers a span of ten-to-twenty years. In the beginning the patient is asymptomatic until an abnormal *Descemet's Membrane* occurs and *guttata* (warts) appear on the surface of the *cornea*. The second stage is characterized by *corneal edema* (swelling) and cloudy vision. Increasing edema promotes folds in the *Descemet's Membrane* worsening vision. In the third phase, tissue arising from the central *cornea*, an irregular, dense gray, swirling sheet of scar tissue consisting of active fibroblasts (connective tissue) and collagen fibrils, decreases vision further. One positive feature at this stage is the possible lessening of the edema heightening the comfort zone. Mild changes in the *iris* occur, but corneal edema is the predominant sign. A corneal replacement corrects this condition. If glaucoma occurs, the high IOP further exacerbates the high fluid condition in the eye. Cataract extraction may be problematic.

Posterior Polymorphous Dystrophy

In our glaucoma group, although these dystrophies are not common, we have found several members with one or other of these syndromes. The member with *polymorphous dystrophy* has had it from her early thirties and has lost one eye to the disease and barely manages to retain vision in the other. She has had two failed *corneal* transplants and now has a plastic *corneal* implant that has been successful. We are all rooting for her.

Map-Dot-Fingerprint-Epithelial Dystrophy

Shapes in the lining of the external surface of the *cornea* resemble map lines, dots, microcysts or fingerprints. Otherwise the symptoms follow the pattern of the dystrophies

Central Crystalline Dystrophy

Multiple white crystals appear in the center of the *cornea* although the surface of the cornea is not involved.

Central Cloudy Dystrophy Of Francois

Like a cloud formation, nebulous grayish opacities form on the *cornea*, mostly in the center and the back of the *cornea*. These are separated by clear zones.

GLAUCOMA ASSOCIATED WITH ELEVATED VENOUS PRESSURE

Elevated Episcleral Venous Pressure may be induced by blowing on a brass wind instrument such as a trumpet or from conditions in the eye that include abnormal sinus cavities, involvement of the *carotid artery,* tumors, thyroid function or may be idiopathic should no secondary cause be present. The flow of aqueous humor is impeded by the elevated venous pressure resulting in a rise in the *intraocular pressure* that is then characterized as secondary glaucoma. Normally, the aqueous pathway flows through the *trabecular meshwork*, to the *Schlemm's canal* to the aqueous veins to the anterior ciliary veins to epi*scleral* veins to superior and inferior ophthalmic veins to cavernous sinus to inferior petrosal sinus to jugular veins. Whew! What a roadmap the flow of aqueous follows! Anywhere along the line, a stop sign blocking the free flow of traffic can occur. As mentioned above, musicians run a risk of creating *episcleral* pressure through exertive efforts on their brass instruments akin to string players running a risk of *Carpal Tunnel Syndrome* from repetitive motions.

When the glaucoma is caused by one or more of the conditions listed above, it may occur in only one eye. At first this symptom may be diagnosed as *uveitis* or *acute angle-closure glaucoma*, but further investigation may reveal the syndrome of *low-flow carotid cavernous sinus fistula*, i.e. *episcleral glaucoma*. With the exception of *Xalatan*, and possibly *Travatan* and *Lumigan*, other antiglaucoma medications do not work for this condition and the patient may need a *trabeculectomy*.

ANGLE RECESSION GLAUCOMA

Recall being hit by a baseball when you were ten, or falling and banging your head when you were fifteen, or surviving an automobile accident when you were thirty-five? Any of these and countless other traumas may resurface down the road as *angle-recession glaucoma*, a type of *secondary open-angle glaucoma*. This condition is often under-diagnosed due to delayed onset of a distant history of eye injury. First reported on examination of an enucleated (from a cadaver) eye in 1892, angle recession with or without glaucoma is characterized by a separation of the circular and longitudinal fibers of the *ciliary body*. In 1944, a physician observed unilateral (in one eye) glaucoma associated with ocular trauma, but it was not until 1962 that the relationship was firmly established.

The sequence of *angle-recession glaucoma* may start with a sock in the eye or any blunt force. *Angle-recession,* according to several reports, occurs in more than seventy-five percent of the eyes experiencing injury. It is estimated that over one million Americans are hit in the eye. Work-related injuries may account for some eighteen percent, home injuries twenty-to-thirty percent, assault eleven-to-thirty percent, recreation twenty-three percent, travel five percent. A 1987 study of boxers found nineteen percent in one eye and eight percent in both eyes. Generally, ocular trauma occurs most frequently with young adults and declines steeply with advancing age, although falls in the elderly may lead to the condition. Reports from other countries found people in Nigeria to also have the above rate of injuries; Israel in l988 reported that home injuries were most frequent for this syndrome.

The incidence of glaucoma with such injuries is relatively mild, with reported zero to twenty-percent cases. The onset of glaucoma may occur directly after the trauma or may be latent for many years. The risk of *angle recession* causing glaucoma appears to be a matter of the depth of the front of the eye. A blow initiates compression in one part of eye and expansion in another. Sudden indentation (think of what boxers do to each other's eyes) of the *cornea* may force the aqueous fluid into a position that deepens the front of the eye while increasing the *corneoscleral* structure. Although this deformity is transient, it results in a shearing force to the angle structures, disrupting, if the force is very strong, the weakest points of the tissues. The ciliary body is most affected by *angle-recession glaucoma* where front-to-back compression of the eye leads to equatorial expansion, like squeezing a rubber ball. Expansion beyond the elastic properties of the eye results in a tearing of the ciliary muscle between the circular and longitudinal inside layers. Associated contusion damage such as scarring of the *trabecular meshwork* leads to impaired aqueous drainage and thence, elevated IOP. Also, as a result of this trauma, the arteries in the ciliary body may disrupt, leading to bleeding. And, of course, the rest inevitably follows. Elevated IOP leads to cupping of the *optic nerve* accompanied by visual field loss. Doctors can identify this condition using *gonioscopy* or through microscopically examining tissues although they still don't quite know the sequence of events that lead to late-developing glaucoma in people who have experienced a blunt force to the eye, but they suspect that these patients have a predisposition to glaucoma. Formation of cataract in only one eye provides another clue to *angle recession.*

Retinal Disorders That May Lead To Glaucoma

Recently I met a woman, my age, with somewhat the same history as mine. She was highly *myopic*, had a tear in her *retina* that developed into a detached *retina*, and subsequently developed glaucoma. Although my condition was not as serious as hers, the doctors had difficulty in reattaching the *retina*. The outcome for both us was similar. When *myopia* develops in early childhood, a deformation of the eye may ensue. As the eyeball transforms from basketball to football shape, the *retina* thins and stretches raising the risk of *retinal* problems and possible detachment. Visualize this process by the stretching a rubber band to the breaking point. Early on, of course, *myopic* vision is easily corrected by the use of contact lenses, Lasik treatment or eye glasses. For the majority of patients these remedies suffice, but for those persons with severe *myopi*a, regular visits to an eye doctor are necessary.

Retinal treatment for holes or detachment may lead to glaucoma. I am certainly one who falls into this category. Perhaps my form resulted from the use of steroids following laser treatment to repair *retinal* holes in both of my eyes or the laser treatment itself, which can damage cells. Steroidal anti-inflammatory medication may cause a rise in *intraocular pressure*, although this is generally transient and resolves with cessation of the steroid medication. Not everybody experiences glaucoma following *retinal* repair, and as with many other syndromes such as *exfoliation syndrome* or *pigmentary dispersion syndrome,* some people are more susceptible,

Retinal detachment, a serious condition, requires a device called a *scleral buckle* that puts pressure on the large veins that drain through the *sclera*. Unfortunately, this may cause congestion of the *ciliary body* that may push the *iris* against the *trabecular meshwork*, blocking it and causing scarring and secondary *angle-closure glaucoma* in some cases. When detachment is not corrected, a condition called *Schwartz's Syndrome* may result. Outflow of fluid is reduced, possibly by trapped photoreceptor cells outer segments (possibly damaged areas in the *retina*) in the *trabecular meshwork*. Usually this situation resolves following successful *retinal* realignment.

Tumors

As if having a tumor, whether benign or malignant wasn't bad enough, tumors in the front of the eye may lead to *open-angle glaucoma*. Blockage occurs in the *trabecular meshwork* that may clog up from blood, blood products, inflamed cells, dead cells from the tumor or pigments released by the tumor.

If the tumor occurs in the back of the eye, *angle-closure glaucoma* may result. The treatment itself may cause glaucoma. Radiation therapy can lead to *neovascular glaucoma* for the irradiation may damage the *retina* or *ciliary body*, and steroid therapy can produce *steroid-induced glaucoma.*

MEDICALLY INDUCED GLAUCOMAS

When your doctor tells you there are complications after an operation, just what does that mean? Is it *iatrogenic,* a term not implying incompetence but that treatment of the problem was unsuccessful or misjudged; or was the procedure actually caused by incompetence on the part of the physician or surgeon; or was there an unsuspected anomaly that screwed up the procedure; or was the procedure not suited to your particular problem? Unfortunately, for the patient, cause, other than a subject for litigation, is not as much an issue as correcting the side effects of the procedure. Below are some but not all of the consequences of medical injury.

POST-CATARACT GLAUCOMA

Advances in cataract extraction have made this form of induced glaucoma a rare occurrence, but glaucoma may still occur after a cataract extraction. In the immediate aftermath, a slight increase in pressure may occur. Usually it resolves within a short time. When glaucoma does manifest, it may not be for lack of skill on the part of the doctor, but rather that tiny bits of the pulverized cataract or even trapped air released into the aqueous fluid are transported into the *trabecular meshwork.* A healthy meshwork will discharge these particles but an aging meshwork may no longer be equipped to manage this event and debris then clogs it up.. Also, a slight shifting of the parts of the eye, the pupil, etc. can lead to *angle-closure glaucoma,* usually with a mal-positioned lens or if the procedure was performed with an iridotomy.

Glaucoma patients, undergoing cataract extraction, however, may find their conditions worsened by the operation. Some glaucoma patients, both within and outside our group, speak of having lost most of their sight to cataract operations. In one case, the doctor had not considered that the patient had *exfoliation syndrome* and for the operation to succeed, should have taken into account that the *zonules,* the ligaments holding the lens in place might be compromised. In another case, a newly-minted doctor dropped the lens into the eye and its retrieval damaged the tissues. In a third case, the reason was unclear. In all three cases, the doctors were not glaucoma specialists. The possibility that the cataract surgery will undo former filtering surgery is another problem glaucoma patients may face. For this reason some glaucomatologists opt to perform both operations at the same time using the same site of entry and thus sparing the patient additional scarring, although this procedure has not been proven to be better than two separate sites or two separate procedures.

GHOST CELL GLAUCOMA

THERES A GHOST IN MY EYE! Not actually, but there is a phenomena where degenerated cells inhabit the eye. These cells result most often from an operation on the *vitreous body* intended to stop hemorrhaging. The released blood, if not cleared by the eye in three or four weeks, breaks down, forming khaki-colored cells. *Ghost cells* can also be present after a cataract operation should hemorrhage occur. These cells migrate into the front of eye and are carried by the fluid into the drainage passages. An active *trabecular meshwork* may be capable of cleaning itself of these cells.

Sometimes this syndrome is misdiagnosed as *neovascular glaucoma, hemosiderotic, hemolytic* or *uveitic glaucoma*. But when, upon examination, ghost cells are present in the aqueous only, the diagnosis reverts to *ghost cell glaucoma*. There may be ocular pain associated with this syndrome. If glaucoma develops, your doctor will probably try medication first and if that doesn't lower the pressure, surgically wash out the cells from the anterior chamber and vitreous cavity, and if not resolved, implantation of a shunt.

POST-CORNEAL-TRANSPLANT GLAUCOMA (PENETRATING KERATOPLASTY)

So, you've lived with this difficult *cornea* for a number of years and at last you've decided to go for a *corneal transplant*, especially, since you are aware that there is a waiting list for donor *corneas*. Consider, however, the complicating factor of glaucoma. If you have had a number of surgical procedures, a history of eye inflammation and a failed *corneal* transplant, your risk of a successful *corneal transplant* is compromised. Furthermore, with each surgical procedure, *corneal* cells are most probably lost, reducing the resiliency of the eye and possibly increasing the formation of scar tissue. Following the transplant, a dangerous dialogue occurs between the transplant and the IOP. The transplant surgery may cause severe IOP fluctuation requiring glaucoma medication that in turn, imperils the transplant.

In a non-glaucomatous eye, glaucoma may develop immediately following or months or years later. The *trabecular meshwork* may collapse, or may be blocked up by either debris from inflammation or blood released into the *uvea*. Both *steroid-induced* and *angle-closure glaucoma* may occur.

While a *corneal* transplant is often considered to be a relatively safe operation, complications may occur when glaucoma enters the picture. Subsequent inflammation along with an elevated IOP may follow the procedure. Control of IOP even with filtration surgery and shunt procedures may not be successful. Furthermore, the transplant may be rejected. One patient in our group, after two *corneal* transplant rejections, was fitted with a plastic implant that requires constant steroid medications to tame the inflammatory processes. Her IOP has been controlled with *cyclophotocoangulation* (See Chapter 6).

STEROID-INDUCED GLAUCOMA

Cortisol produced by the adrenal glands is a key player in the body's chemistry. One of its major effects is to reduce inflammation. Other effects maintain blood-sugar levels, blood pressure, help control the balance of salt and water, and play a part in maintenance of muscle strength. That's the positive side of its regulatory functions necessary to keep the body humming along. The negative side is the readiness of the *adrenal gland* to pump *cortisol* into the body at the least hint of danger—yes, the fight or flight response. The *adrenal gland* is responsible for the surge of *cortisol* that floods the body when a dangerous situation is perceived. It provides a surge of energy for either fighting or fleeing. In the Stone Age when the enemy happened to be a predatory beast, adrenalin saved the day. But deep into our present-day civilization—although sometimes one wonders if we have merely substituted the tiger for deadly tribal conflicts—*cortisol* continues to play its role. With any stressful event--impossible work habits, substance abuse, war, illness, loss of loved ones, etc. a flood of *cortisol* is released. Excess *cortisol* negatively affects the body in various ways. Weight gain, slower recovery from injury following exercise, and possibly a rise in IOP are a few of the more common effects. Should a tumor be located in one of the *adrenal glands* causing excess release of *cortisol,* elevated IOP may result, but when the tumor is removed, IOP has been known to return to normal.

Steroids, however, are major players in the treatment of a host of inflammatory diseases such as *asthma, arthritis* and autoimmune syndromes. Eye doctors rely on steroid treatment to quell inflammatory conditions that include relieving tear duct obstruction, easing contact lens discomfort, healing *blepharitis* (eyelid inflammation), and reducing inflammation of the conjunctiva (*conjunctival hyperemia*). Steroids are also indispensable for treating inflammation following any invasive therapy and for control of *uveitis.*

Steroid sensitivity is primarily found in individuals who may be genetically predisposed and who may respond to steroids by producing an excessive amount of cellular ground substance in the *trabecular meshwork* (the TIGR gene product *myocilin*) that clogs up the drainage channels. They may also not be able to metabolize a complex carbohydrate known as the *glycosaminoglycans* that if not broken down, causes blockage in the outflow channels. If a person lacks the full action of an enzyme found in tears, steroid drops may lower the functioning of healthy eyes. Also steroids may alter the drain itself by acting on the tissues, collagen and fibronectin that form them. How do you know that you may be steroid-sensitive? The usual risk factors apply, but perhaps for the genetically susceptible individual, delivery, strength of the medication and duration may be an important factor. One of the members of the group was on systemic steroid therapy for *asthma* as a child, and she believes that all her consequent eye problems resulted from that extended therapy.

People who are susceptible to *steroid-induced glaucoma* may not be aware that a hand cream or ointment containing even a minute amount of *cortisol* can trigger a rise in pressure if contact with the eye is made. Systemic absorption is not the problem, but touching the eyes may be. It is rare that a person will wash hands after applying cream or lotion. We inadvertently touch our eyes all the time, and because so many of us, especially over fifty, suffer from aches and pains, we use more of these steroid-laced topical creams and lotions.

Chronic use of nasal steroids can raise IOP according to a small study from Vanderbilt University. None of the patients in the study realized that their nasal sprays contained steroids. If you have a stuffy nose, be sure to check for steroids should you use nasal spray.

MACULAR DEGENERATION/AGE-RELATED MACULAR DEGENERATION (ARMD)

Age Related Macular Degeneration leads the eye diseases causing low vision and blindness in the United States, eclipsing persons affected with glaucoma. The *macula,* located in the center of the *retina,* is a small, more deeply colored area dense with cone cells and containing the *fovea,* an even smaller area. With age, in certain susceptible individuals, cells in the *macula* degenerate. *ARMD* is considered one of the degenerative diseases, a characterization of which is hardening of the arteries. In the case of some forms of *macular degeneration,* the arteries feeding nourishing blood to the *retina* harden, depriving the *retina* of sustenance.

The disease is divided into two forms, the wet (*exudative*) which is the most serious, affecting ten percent of the patients, and the dry (*non-exudative*) affecting ninety percent. Four independent studies defined strong association of specific *Complement Factor H,* and/or haplotypes on an *Y402H* variant with fifty percent of the *ARMD* cases. The association is the same in patients with all (early and late) forms of *ARMD*. A variation in *Factor H* strengthens the immune response, a good thing for serious infections, but when unchecked causes chronic inflammation, a factor in both *macular degeneration* and a rare kidney disease called *MPGN II*. Researchers speculate that other organs in the body may also be affected.

Non-exudative, the dry form resulting from genetic disposition and environmental influences is characterized by deposits of *drusen,* an accumulation of material which may be seen beneath the *retina*. It may or may not devolve into the wet form.

Exudative (the wet form) develops when blood vessels invade *Bruck's Membrane*. This condition is called *choroidal neovascularization*. These new blood vessels also invade the dense network of photoreceptors. As well, diskiform scars can form in untreated *neovascularization*. The pathways to these destructive effects are triggered by inflammation that then leads to oxidative stress, damage to the *Bruch's Membrane*, etc. When deposits of *drusen* become large, a first sign, they lodge in the interface of the *retinal ganglion layer* and *Bruch's Membrane*. Central vision loss can be devastating although in many cases peripheral vision is spared. Therapies, therefore, have been primarily directed to treatment of the wet form. In the wet form, the *retina* has to be relatively dry for it to function and capture light signals for, if wet, images get wavy and distorted.

Ordinarily, the *choroid,* (blood vessels beneath the *retina*, the region that has the highest blood flow in the body), nourishes the eye. But with the wet form, an angiogenic signal is triggered and new blood vessels sprout. This signal causes capillaries on the blood vessels to form. Normally, this reaction is necessary for healing, during pregnancy and maintenance of the menstrual cycle, but when uncontrolled new blood vessels proliferate, this function becomes pathological, for these sprouts, (*endothelial cells*) may penetrate and migrate through the wall of the blood vessel from which new blood vessels form. While the delivery of blood is important for the health of the eye, these new blood vessels are fragile and subject to fluid leakage and bleeding causing destruction of the overlying *retina*.

The problem area of this syndrome is with the *retinal pigmentary epithelium cells* (*RPE*) that separate the *choroidal* layer (the blood supply) from the photoreceptor cells. Scientists have not yet identified why these particular cells lose function, nor do they fully understand if waste products from cells that accumulate in the *retina* are more than an age-related phenomenon. The various *retinal* analyzers are shedding more light on this very important question.

Possibly, these new blood vessels are formed during the time that the *RPE* is sending out distress signals that tell cells to manufacture new blood vessels. This syndrome results in *choroidal neovascularization* as described above. The *neovascularization* may be classic where the damaging blood vessels are well defined or occult where they are less evident. Two other forms may occur—*bulb-like,* often found near the optic disc and also in the central vision, and *angiogenic proliferation*, blood vessels emanating from the *retinal* blood supply.

As if having glaucoma were not enough, some patients are also stricken with *ARMD*, and while the disease attacks different parts of the eye, people with glaucoma may find that they need to enlist both *retinal* and glaucoma specialists for management of the two diseases. These conditions affect vision differently. In glaucoma the peripheral vision and then at late stages, the central vision is affected; in exudative macular degeneration, the central vision is affected but the peripheral vision is spared. Scientists, however, in a large retrospective comparative study, closely observing the *optic neuropathy* of *macular degeneration,* have found signs of glaucomatous damage as well. Even if you do not have overt signs of glaucoma, it is wise, therefore, to have a glaucoma specialist examine your eyes.

Exposure to ultra violet light may be one of the causative factors in this disease. Ultra violet light refers to three types: UV-A, UV-B, and UV-C, (which is a milder form and is normally screened out by the ozone layer). UV-A rays, the more powerful, are of longer wavelength. Exposure to these rays cause skin tanning and premature skin aging. They can also reach the *retina* and long-term exposure can lead to *macular degeneration.* The UV-B rays are shorter wave lengths and these can lead to blistering sunburn and skin cancer. A report from the *Beaver Dam Eye Study* found that people, who in their teens had more than five hours daily of sun exposure, had a higher risk of developing early *macular degeneration.* In contrast, more than ten sunburns did not raise the risk. Ultra violet UV-B exposure was not linked to *ARMD*, but those who wore sunglasses and hats during their teen years had significantly lower rates of early *ARMD* compared to those who rarely took this precaution.

Obesity has also been associated with an increased risk of *macular degeneration.* Researchers studying the results of the *Physicians Health Study* that followed twenty-one thousand men found that obese men had more than double the risk as compared with men of normal weight. Watch your waistline. A spare tire can speed up the progression of *age-related macular degeneration.* A waistline of more than forty inches for men and thirty-four and a half inches for women doubles the risk of *macular degeneration.* The wrong kind of fat (excess omega 6 and saturated fats) may possibly promote inflammation or oxidative stress. A smaller study of roughly two hundred and sixty people who had intermediate *macular degeneration,* found risk of progression to an advanced form doubled for the overweight individuals. Being too lean may also be a risk factor according to a study at *Brigham and Women's Hospital,* Boston, but the researchers were at a loss to come up with a plausible explanation of this finding. Is it possible that skinnies have a deficiency in the essential fatty acids?

Certain diets may promote the onset of *macular degeneration.* A diet low in fruits and vegetables, especially deep green vegetables such as kale and spinach may stage the eye to be more susceptible to the disease. Low antioxidants may also be a factor. Vegetables, fruits and supplements are high in antioxidants. (See Chapter 11).

Smoking is another risk factor. Nitrite (a smoking by-product) may be the cause. Smoking reacts harmfully with three types of proteins in the body—collagen, elastin and *alpha-crystallin* that make up the connective tissues in the skin, bones, tendons, arteries and organs such as the lungs and eyes. Collagen provides the scaffolding of body parts, and for this reason, it is the most abundant protein in the body. *Alpha crystallin* is found in the lens of the eye; collagen and elastin in the membranes beneath the *retinal.* Nitrites may cause damage to the structural integrity of these proteins through a chemical process that is called non-enzymatic nitration. Exposed to nitrites, collagen becomes rigid, elastin cracks and fragments, and *alpha crystallin* clumps and scatters light. Exercise is a given--subjects who exercised had a less severe form.

Certain medications may possibly be a factor. *Beta-blockers* may promote a slight increased risk. A decreased risk was found in patients who used hormone replacement therapy or *trycyclic antidepressants.* This data came from three pooled population studies, but the authors suggest further study. Diagnosis of the source of the problem includes an *angiogram* using either the drug *fluoroscein* or *ICG (Indocyanine green).* Images are taken of different sections of the *retinal.*

EXAMINE YOUR DIET

Diet may be a factor in the development of ARMD. For more information consult the chapter on nutrition. (11).

IN SUMMARY

Although doctors have referred to more than forty types of glaucoma as a collection of eye diseases causing optic nerve degeneration, we have listed only those that are most prevalent. Systemic diseases may also be at the root of some syndromes, such as endocrine disorders, *Herpes Zoster* infection, and *sickle cell* disease. As genetic studies provide greater understanding, glaucoma, in all of its variations, may one day be recognized as mainly genetically-based. Yet this explanation may also be fraught with doubt, for why does one patient with an obvious syndrome develop glaucoma while another having a like syndrome escape the disease entirely? The interdisciplinary approaches now common among research models promise to throw more light on the etiology of glaucoma. Although glaucoma is an old disease recognized in ancient Greece and probably even earlier than recorded history, we have yet to determine if it is, in part, an environmental disease, a viral or solely a genetic disease.

Neurodegeneration underlies a variety of diseases such as *Alzheimer's*, *Parkinson's*, *Huntington's*, *multiple sclerosis*, *Mad Cow disease*, and glaucoma. Studies worldwide on the etiology of these diseases may one day lead to a unified theory of the cause or causes of *neurodegeneration*. Most important for the glaucoma patient is that such studies will positively impact on future treatment of glaucoma. There is a normal death rate of neurons in the eye called programmed cell death or *apoptosis*. In glaucoma, this rate of programmed cell death may accelerate.

Dry Eye Syndrome

Many glaucoma patients complain about "dry eye" syndrome. *HRT (hormone replacement therapy)* may be the culprit behind the condition. An article published in *JAMA (Journal of the American Medical Association*--November 7, 2001 *286* 2114-9) established a relationship of dry eye syndrome using data compiled on nearly forty thousand female health professionals. About seventy percent of the respondents had passed through menopause, and the odds of having dry eye syndrome increased in women taking estrogen alone by about seventy percent and by about thirty percent for women taking estrogen combined with progesterone/progestin; the higher the duration of *HRT therapy*, the higher the risk of dry eye. Although *HRT therapy* is no longer routinely prescribed, it is still available for remission of menopausal symptoms. Some eyedrop medications to treat glaucoma, especially *Alphagan P* may also contribute to dry eye problems. A number of over-the-counter medications exist that relieve dry eye symptoms. New medications also become available from time to time. One of the more recent medications, *Cevimeline* appears safe according to a double-blind study and patients did report improvement. Dr. Jeffrey Morrison, who practices nutritional therapy, has reported that Vitamin A drops that are non-toxic to be effective.

CHAPTER 3

The Special Child: Primary Congenital (Infantile) and Juvenile Glaucoma

∘ ∘

"One always hopes that the children—that things will turn out better for them…"
　　　　　　　　　　　　Ugo Betti, Goat Island (1946)3.2 Ed, Gino Rozzo

Most feared by a prospective parent is the specialness of a child born with a defect or abnormality. Defects may result from genetic disorders, environmental factors ranging from carcinogens in the water and soil, herbicide, pesticide and fungicide use, and mercury poisoning. The fetus may also be affected by the mother's smoking, use of alcohol, or drugs, both legal and illegal. Factored in as well are complications during delivery. Is it any wonder then that parents delight in the birth of a healthy infant and despair when informed that their infant will need immediate surgical intervention and special attention to his or her eyes for the rest of life?

Jerry is a member of our group. When he first joined, he told us that his glaucoma had been diagnosed when he was three months old. At that time, a protocol had not yet been established for treating congenital glaucoma. His parents consulted with various doctors, and finally one of them performed an operation, an iridectomy—partially removing the *iris* when Jerry was seven months old. The doctor's intention was to use that opening to reach the trabecular meshwork but when the doctor detected the movement of fluid, he closed the eye hoping for the best, although he informed Jerry's parents that their child would probably not see. Surprisingly, this procedure worked for one eye providing Jerry with sight still maintained at this writing. His present doctors cannot satisfactorily explain why this operation succeeded. Perhaps his stem cells were still functioning at that tender age and repaired the damage; perhaps the faith of his parents that a miracle would occur or perhaps an unknown factor that will one day be revealed took place. Whatever the reason, sight, however tenuous, has provided Jerry with the means of living a normal boy's life, participating in sports even at the risk of injuring his good eye. Since three months of age, Jerry's doctors, and there have been several of them, have carefully monitored his eye condition, and recently he called me to tell me that since his IOP had risen to just below 50 mmHg., his doctors decided to perform a *trabeculectomy* (See Chapter 7) along with a *vitrectomy* (removing the *vitreous* gel and replacing it with a sterile fluid) plus a cataract extraction. Yet, after that very involved procedure, he still has sufficient sight to adequately perform his everyday activities, and when his eye heals, he will be fitted with either a contact lens or a special pair of glasses and his vision should be considerably improved. Jerry is thankful that he still has sight despite the incredible odds that he faced. He is grateful to the teams of dedicated doctors who worked to save his sight.

Although glaucoma in infants occurs much less frequently than adult-onset glaucoma, there still are a sizeable number of babies (1 in 10,000 in Western countries and 1 in 2,500 in the Middle Eastern countries) who are born with *Primary Congenital Glaucoma*.

Infantile glaucoma is divided into three categories. The first, *primary congenital or infantile glaucoma* (accounting for tenty-two percent of the cases) is present at birth or appears shortly thereafter, but it is not necessarily inherited. The second category, (forty-six percent of the cases), *secondary glaucomas*, called *anomalies* result from a group of congenital diseases such *as Sturge-Weber syndrome, aniridia, Axenfeld's syndrome, congenital rubella, and Lowe's syndrome* plus other genetic disorders. These diseases may affect the heart, the skeletal system, blood vessels, cause multiple birth disorders, and mental incapacity. The third category, another form of *secondary glaucoma*, stems from conditions such as tumors, trauma, cataract or inflammation of the eye.

At birth, the infant's eyes are still developing. Normally, the eye is beautifully clear. Its cornea is 10 mm and its IOP is 16 mmHg. The collagen fibers are soft and elastic from infancy to about four years of age. The *iris* and the trabecular meshwork undergo changes that occur in the first six months. If elevated pressure occurs during this period, especially in the first six months when the collagen fibers are softest, the infant's eye will bulge out, a condition commonly called "cow's eye." One clear sign of disease is a cloudy cornea. A number of conditions may be present as well. These include cupping of the *optic nerve*, an enlarged globe, *myopia*, IOP greater than 20 mmHg, problems with the inner structures of the eye, and aversion to light (*photophobia*). Some infant eye diseases are readily apparent while others may not manifest immediately: one, two or three years may elapse before the parents realize that their infant's eye or eyes are not functioning normally.

In general, both your obstetrician and pediatrician are alert to signs of eye disease. But in some cases, glaucoma may be present in an eye diagnosed with *conjunctivitis*, an inflammation of the membrane covering the eye. Such an eye should be examined for possible glaucoma by checking the eye pressure. The drawback to this simple procedure is that the infant must be anesthetized. Should glaucoma be present, anesthetization will be necessary until the child is ready to accept the routine eye examination. But children are adaptable little creatures and most often they will be cooperative once they understand procedures, provided their roles are carefully explained to them. Some children profit from practicing eye care on their favorite toys.

Basically all eye therapy is to prevent blindness. Babies diagnosed with *primary* or *secondary glaucoma* run the risk of becoming blind if treatment is not instituted within a short period of time, often within days of birth. If light is blocked from reaching the *retina*, impaired vision results (*amblyopia*), for the *retina* cannot export important information to the visual center of the brain. This vital information allows the brain to interpret as sight every photon of light that travels from the *retina*.

Should the presence of glaucoma not be evident at birth, as a parent, you may notice that your infant or toddler displays sensitivity to light such as tearing or turning away from a light source. You may also notice a slight haziness or cloudiness of the cornea. Myopia may also be present. Should any problems be evident, the child should be seen by a doctor.

PRIMARY CONGENITAL (INFANTILE) GLAUCOMA

When the pediatrician observed a problem with one of Joe's eyes at birth, she told Joe's parents that this condition was an operation waiting to happen. *Primary Congenital Glaucoma* affects between sixty-to-sixty-five percent of boys--(a problem consistent with other diseases affecting more boys than girls, including hyperactivity). Most often bilateral, it is more likely to be present at birth or to be diagnosed within the first year. Up to eighty-five percent of *Primary Congenital Glaucoma* is attributed to a mutation in a gene known as *CYPIBI*, located on chromosome 2. It has also been associated with thin central *corneas*. *Primary Congenital Glaucoma* is a condition where the anatomical structure of the eye is abnormal, that is, the drainage system is dysfunctional. Doctors need to provide an alternative method for fluid to exit the eye. Joe's parents at first could not comprehend that their beautiful baby needed immediate surgery. Both mother and father had no eye problems except that mother wore glasses to correct her nearsightedness.

Yes, the tiniest of us may undergo surgery when it is *congenital glaucoma*. Two procedures correct the situation. One is a *goniotomy* where the doctor passes a knife through the *cornea* into the anterior chamber and severs 120 degrees of the *trabecular meshwork*: the other consists of a *trabeculotomy*. In this procedure, a probe is introduced into the *Schlemm's Canal* and rotated into the anterior chamber rupturing the *trabecular meshwork*. These surgeries may be considered a first-line treatment for *infantile* and *juvenile glaucoma*. While a pediatric ophthalmologist may prefer one or the other, which procedure to use may depend upon the *cornea's* clarity. Should the *cornea* be cloudy, a *goniotomy* cannot be performed for the doctor cannot see the interior of the eye. A *trabeculotomy* performed on the surface of the eye does not require visualization.

Timing is essential. Apparently, as little as several days delay can consign the child to a lifetime of severely impaired vision or even blindness. The vulnerability during this period, along with the natural elasticity of the *sclera*, renders the baby's eye most receptive at this stage to an operation. Should an operation be delayed, fluid build-up can lead to scarring of the inner structures of the eye along with other problems possibly resulting in poor image quality, cloudy *cornea*, and *astigmatism*.

Although the methods differ slightly, the end result of freeing the flow of *aqueous* fluid is the end game. Attempts to spare the knife such as *cyclocryotherapy*, the destruction of part of the *ciliary body* by freezing, have afforded only modest success. The good news is that surgery performed in a timely fashion results in a ninety percent cure rate, and unlike in the adult, where, although surgery may correct the outflow of fluid, cupping before and after the operation remains the same; in the infant, the *optic nerve* reverses to normal. Also, unlike adults, the child's eye is more likely to retain the rim margin of the *optic nerve*.

GLAUCOMAS ASSOCIATED WITH OTHER CONGENITAL DISEASES.

Aside from mutation of the gene *CYBIBI*, a number of other congenital conditions may cause a child's glaucoma. These conditions are not necessarily inherited but they are present at birth or appear shortly thereafter, and are usually part of a larger syndrome that affects other organs of the body. Incomplete development of various organs usually underlies the conditions exhibited in the eye. Although rarer than those of *Primary Infantile Glaucoma*, they do occur and are worth examining. Treatment follows the same protocols as described for *Primary Congenital Glaucoma*. Should your baby's eyes look suspicious, be sure to have your neonate evaluated by a pediatric ophthalmologist.

Actually, if there is anything abnormal about the condition of your infant's eyes that are attributed to conjunctivitis or inflammation, get a second opinion. This is one case when confirming a diagnosis is of utmost urgency. *Congenital glaucoma* is believed to be caused by maldevelopment of the *trabecular meshwork* where the *iris* is inserted into the drainage passages. The *iris* may also be mislocated in front or not fully developed. Blood vessel irregularities and a *cornea* that is either too small or too large may also be associated with *Primary Infant Glaucoma*. This syndrome occurs in only about one in thirty thousand babies.

Congenital glaucoma is divided into three areas differentiated by the position of the problem. *Trabeculodygenisis* is an isolated maldevelopment of the *trabecular meshwork*. Its cure rate is ninety percent using surgical procedures. *Iridodysgenisis* is a condition where abnormalities of the *iris* are present at birth. This condition has a poor medical prognosis. The third is *Corneadysgenisis* where the *cornea* is either tiny or too large, possesses lesions, a thinning of the supporting foundation, swelling, and elevated pressure. Prognosis is also poor in this case.

With the conditions described above, the sooner the treatment is instituted, the better the prospects are for a more positive outcome. The operations are comparable to those described in *Primary Congenital Glaucoma*.

Other surgical options for children whose glaucoma develops during later stages of growth and whose glaucoma presents problems, reduction of the aqueous fluid can be achieved by destroying or in medical terms, ablating part of the ciliary body, either by freezing (*cyclocryotherapy* or by *laser cyclophotocoagulation*) (See Chapter 6). Although this procedure is drastic, it may save the child's sight. Another option is a tube implant or shunt that redirects the aqueous fluid to a reservoir concealed in the outer surface of the eye.

ASSOCIATED SYNDROMES

There are several syndromes under the rubric Iridocorneal Dysgenisis that are grouped together because they involve the cornea and iris. These are Axenfeld's Syndrome, Rieger's Anomaly, Axenfeld-Rieger's Anomaly and Peter's Anomaly.

AXENFELD-RIEGER'S SYNDROME

Half of the babies with this syndrome develop glaucoma. Both the *iris* and the *cornea* are affected. *Iris* strands adhere to the peripheral *cornea* causing blockage. Some of the symptoms include abnormal development of the anterior chamber, the *iris*, dislocation of the *lens*, and thinning of the eye's structure. *Iris* problems account for fifty percent of the glaucoma cases. Myra, born with *myopia*, more serious in one of her eyes, was not diagnosed until she visited an ophthalmologist as a teenager complaining of not seeing well. She was told she had *Axenfeld-Rieger's syndrome*. To her dismay, she found that she had already lost seventy-five percent of her sight in one eye, a common occurrence with this disease. With 20/20 in her good eye, Myra is thankful that she has perfect sight in her one good eye. As with many of the congenital diseases *Axenfeld-Rieger's syndrome* may vary in intensity. Some children may be mentally retarded. Myra, fortunately, has only glaucoma in one eye and none of the other debilitating effects.

RIEGER'S ANOMALY

This syndrome is sometimes referred to as *Axenfeld-Rieger's Anomaly* for both share many of the same symptoms and may be an expression of the same gene. This genetic disease strikes the fetus in the third trimester and developmentally, may affect other parts of the body such as the brain, causing mental deficiency, abnormalities in the fingers and toes (shortened or long and spidery), the absence of some teeth, distorted facial features such as a flat nose, and wide-spaced eyes. The child may also be short of stature. When the eye is involved, the *cornea* is immaturely developed leading to adhesion between the *iris* and the *cornea*. Scarring results and blocks the *aqueous* fluid movement resulting in a rise in pressure. Control includes medical treatment and/or surgery.

PETER'S ANOMALY

Three days after Billy was born, he was diagnosed with *Peter's Anomaly*, a rare disease affecting the anterior segment of the eye that resulted in maldevelopment of the *cornea, iris, anterior chamber* and *lens*. Because the central portion of the *cornea* is often very thin, it is extremely vulnerable. Possibly it can be opaque, and portions of the *iris* may become attached to the periphery of the cornea. Upon the advice of doctors, ten days after his birth, Billy had a *corneal* transplant on one eye and a month later on his other eye. In the process he lost both of his *lenses*. Three months later glaucoma developed requiring medical therapy. Although Billy was fitted with contact lenses, his sight is still precarious.

Not all cases are as severe as Billy's. Doctors usually recommend a *corneal* transplant before the age of six to prevent *amblyopia*, especially if *Peter's Anomaly* strikes only one eye. Glaucoma results when the condition flattens the *anterior chamber* (front of the eye) giving rise to the sticking together of the *iris* and *cornea* that subsequently blocks the drainage areas.

Associated disorders that have similar syndromes include *aniridia* and *familial iris hyperplasia*.

ANIRIDIA

While *aniridia* means absence of the *iris* affecting both eyes, in some cases a bit of *iris,* little more than a margin, is still present. It appears to have no color and the pupil is larger than normal. The *cornea* and the *lens* of the eye may also be affected, both becoming cloudy, and possibly requiring either or both a *corneal* transplant and an intraocular *lens*. This rare genetic condition occurs during the twelfth week of pregnancy, and it affects one in fifty thousand to one in one million children.

Glaucoma develops when the vestigial *iris* stump moves forward and adheres to the wall of the angle where it obstructs the movement of fluid through the *trabecular meshwork*. Some patients with *Aniridia* have associated *open-angle glaucoma*. If medical treatment fails to control the IOP, either *goniotomy* or *trabeculotomy* is performed, (See Chapter 7) depending upon the condition of the eye. Since the eye is extremely vulnerable, any surgery including *cornea*l and cataract extractions as well as the above, may cause more harm than good. Long term prognosis is guarded.

While some babies do have normal vision, the visual acuity in the majority of cases settles around 20/200, a definition of legal blindness. *Aniridia* may be associated with or related to a number of other syndromes that include underdevelopment of either or both the *retina* and *optic nerve*, *amblyopia* (loss of vision in the non-dominant eye), *microcornea* (abnormally small *cornea*), and *strabismus* (eye misalignment). Its effects on the brain include *anosmia* (impaired sense of smell), problems in recalling individual words or understanding meanings of words, glucose intolerance (a precursor to *diabetes*), absence of the *pineal gland* resulting in a lack of *melatonin* (the sleep inducing hormone), and malformation of the cerebral cortex. When severe, the baby may be born with absent eyes, a misshapen brain, and a disconnection between the nose and the mouth.

This syndrome has been identified with the gene *pax6* that is located on band One on the short arm of the 11ᵗʰ chromosome *11P13*. Genetic counseling is generally advised.

Phacomatosis Diseases

This group of genetic diseases involves tumors and the neurological system. For the most part glaucoma is a secondary manifestation. These diseases include (*von Recklinghausen's disease, neurofibromatosis), Sturge-Weber syndrome, Wyburn-Mason syndrome (Racemose angioma), tuberous sclerosis (Bourneville disease), von Hippel-Landau disease, incontinentia pigmenit, Bloch-Sulzberger syndrome, ataxia, and Louis-Bar syndrome.*

Neurofibromatosis

This particular syndrome formerly known as *von Reckinghausen's disease* affects one in four thousand babies. Pigmented areas appear shortly after birth (*café au lait spots*) and by late childhood, multiple tumors on or underneath the skin ranging from just a few to thousands appear. About two-fifths of the tumors are malignant. These tumors may appear on any part of the body and may lead to congenital deformities. In addition, the patient may have high blood pressure or be subject to leukemia. When the eyes are affected, as occurs with ninety percent of the patients, tumors appear as nodules on the *iris* surface; and in fifty percent on the *optic nerve*. About one-third to one-half of the adults with this syndrome have lesions on the *choroid*. Glaucoma may be one of the secondary problems associated with this disease. Since this disease affects the entire body, coordination among ophthalmologists, orthopedists and cardiologists is recommended.

Glial Cell Lesions

This particular syndrome is divided into at least three kinds of *neurofibromas* classified as N-1 and N-2. The N-1's are more numerous and typically begin in the first two years of life, but may be delayed until adolescence. The N-2's are less common and usually are seen at teenage and early adulthood placing them in the *juvenile glaucoma* category. Symptoms sending patients to their doctors include *tinnitus* (ringing in the ears), decreased hearing, early cataracts and self-limiting tumors.

Glaucoma, usually affecting one eye, may be present in infants and is identified by enlargement of the *cornea* (cow's eye). Associated high pressure can leave in its wake *corneal edema* (swelling) and severe *myopia*. A number of glaucoma abnormalities can result from N-1 and N-3. These include an abnormal *trabecular meshwork*, scarring of the angle, or a tumor blocking the angle. The glaucoma is difficult to treat but should definitely be followed, for should any of the tumors become malignant, the eye will need to be removed. Other physical characteristics of this disease include skeletal defects, elevated blood pressure, central system abnormalities that include *macrocephaly* (enlargement of the head), seizures and mild retardation.

These lesions are classified into three forms: first, nodular, typically begins to appear in late childhood increasing in number in some cases to one-hundred in adolescence and adulthood. When there are a large number, disfigurement may be a problem. One eye is usually affected. Second, *plexiform* (network of tissues), less common than the *nodular*, develops earlier becoming evident in infancy or early childhood and the nodules over time can enlarge and become disfiguring. When the face is involved (about ten percent of the cases), the upper eyelid thickens and eventually droops over the eye causing considerable discomfort. Although the eyelid can be thinned to restore binocular vision, this correction is a temporary fix, for the bulk grows back again. The third, *optic glioma* is the most potentially serious, for the *optic nerve* is affected and unlike the other two, often affects both eyes. This form is found in about fifteen percent of the cases, almost always in patients younger than ten years. Many other abnormalities may occur that include *hydrocephalus* (enlargement of the head), *hypothalamic dysfunction* leading to precocious puberty. A malignant tumor alarmingly predisposes death in fifty percent of the cases, although chemotherapy treatment may lower this figure. Surgery to remove the tumors sacrifices vision.

STURGE-WEBER SYNDROME

Not a genetically-transmitted disorder but present at birth, this syndrome is believed to be caused by an insult to the fetus during the first four to eight weeks of embryonic development when primitive facial structures are developing. A birth mark called a "port wine stain" on the face is indicative, but not always a sign of glaucoma, but when this birthmark covers the lid or conjunctiva, it is responsible for fifty percent of the cases. The stain is the result of a collection of capillaries just underneath the skin. Primarily the disease involves blood vessels that proliferate on the lid, the epi*scleral*, conjunctiva, ciliary body, and *iris* along with a maldevelopment of the angle. Mental deficiency can vary, and seizures can occur, but there are those who escape retardation altogether. Children with this syndrome may have tumors on the *meninges*, (three membranes that surround the brain), disfiguring skin lesions on the forehead and upper eyelid, scalp, trunk, arms, and legs. Laser treatment (See Chapter 6) may reduce some of these symptoms.

The eye becomes involved when the skin lesion affects the eyelid. The blood vessels in the *choroid* multiply and during adolescence or adulthood may thicken leading to degeneration or detachment of the *retina*, possibly resulting in severe visual loss. Glaucoma is the most common and serious complication however, for it occurs in approximately half of the cases. It is believed that elevated pressure in the *episcleral* (outermost layer of the *sclera*) veins, *ciliary body*, or an *interior chamber* anomaly causes blockage of fluid outflow. Glaucoma can be present at birth or may develop later in childhood.

When this syndrome is detected in infants, doctors generally treat immediately for the *trabecular meshwork* is abnormal and signals severe problems in the future. Treatment follows much the same pattern established in general for treatment of glaucoma—medication first and then the intervention strategies of either *goniotomy* or a *trabeculotomy* (See Chapter 7). Complications from surgery include choroidal detachment and hemorrhage. In children four years or older, a *trabeculectomy* is the surgery of choice. When the condition becomes intractable, shunts may be used. Should these fail, freezing or using a laser to destroy part of the *ciliary body* may be attempted to reduce the flow of fluid.

WYBURN-MASON SYNDROME (RACEMOSE ANGIOMA)

This syndrome is a non-hereditary malformation of the eye and the brain involving the *optic disc*, *retina* and/or the midbrain. Central nervous system lesions, seizures, mental changes, paralysis on one side of the body, and swelling and inflammation of the *optic nerve* may develop. Usually only one eye is affected. Vision can range from normal to low. Glaucoma may occur from *neovascularization*—weakened blood vessels proliferating over the affected eye.

TUBEROUS SCLEROSIS (BOURNEVILLE DISEASE)

This disease rarely strikes. (1:6000 or 1:100,000.) Two distinct genetic mutations give rise to a variety of abnormalities involving the skin, eye, central nervous system and other abnormalities leading to mental retardation, facial tumors and seizures. Present at birth, a white spot located on the skin is one of the first indications that the disease is present. Two types of tumors affect the *retina* and other bodies in the eye. The first, not easily visible, is defined as flat and translucent, the second more readily seen has been compared to a cluster of tapioca grains or fish eggs. But they have also been called giant *drusen* and coincidentally, these *drusen* are also found in the *macula* of patients with *macular degeneration*. These conditions, however, are unrelated. Eighty percent of the cases involve one eye.

VON HIPPEL-LINDAU DISEASE (RETINAL ANGIOMATOSIS)

In this disease, tumors affect the central nervous system and the *retinal* blood vessels. While these tumors on the blood vessels are generally non-proliferative, they do weaken structures in the eye and may produce an accumulation of fluid causing *retinal detachment* and loss of vision. Secondary results involve degenerative changes leading to glaucoma and cataracts. Lesions can usually be seen between the ages of ten and thirty-five, with onset typically at age twenty-five, ten years before effects on the brain are identified. Both eyes may be affected. Laser treatment or freezing can zap the errant blood vessels. Patients with this syndrome need to be carefully monitored. The Cambridge Screening Protocol recommends an annual complete physical examination and dilated eye examinations, renal ultrasonography, a 24-hour urine collection; neuro-imaging every three years to age forty and every five years thereafter. Relatives should also undergo thorough annual screening.

INCONTINENTIA PIGMENTI (BLOCH-SULZBERGER SYNDROME)

Nearly all babies affected with this genetic syndrome are female. The first characteristics may be seen on the skin that appears normal at birth but within a few days, redness and blistering may develop. Although this condition subsides after a few months, a more troubling syndrome may occur--one-third of the babies may develop *microcephaly* (abnormally small head) *hydrocephalus* (fluid on the brain), seizures and varying degrees of retardation. About two-thirds of the patients have dental abnormalities and less common findings include *scoliosis*, skull deformities, *cleft palate* and *dwarfism*. One-quarter to one-third of the cases have ocular problems mainly found in the *retinal* blood vessels. Glaucoma can result when the blood vessels proliferate blocking the *trabecular meshwork*. Remediation of the blood vessel problem using laser therapy has had mixed success.

ATAXIA: (LOUIS-BAR SYNDROME)

This is a rare genetic disease located on *chromosome 11*. It occurs in one-to-forty thousand births and can cause severe problems. In the second year of life, speech impairment and jerky muscles may appear. By the age of ten, this syndrome can lead to deterioration of muscle movements. Retardation if it occurs is usually mild. Effects of this disease may first be seen in ocular motor abnormalities that include difficulty in involuntary eye movements (*saccadic*), ability to follow a target, misalignment of the eyes (*strabismus*), and rapid involuntary movements of the eyeball (*nystagmus*). Although glaucoma is not one of the main problems associated with *Ataxia*, the presence of the disease can cause considerable difficulty in processing visual material especially reading.

MARFAN SYNDROME

Caused by a dominant gene, *Marfan syndrome* is an inherited connective tissue disorder affecting the musculoskeletal and cardiovascular systems of the body. People with this syndrome are unusually tall and thin, flat-footed, have long fingers and toes and because of their stretchy tissues, may have flexible joints enabling them to perform contortionist exercises. Symptoms can range from mild to severe. The mild form is often not apparent until adulthood when a physical structure, a deformed breastbone or humpback, becomes prominent. Although life span is shortened to about sixty years because of an adverse effect on the heart, intellect and creativity are often unaffected and unusual flexibility of joints enables and enhances such endeavors as gymnastics and/or musicianship. Believed to have *Marfan's* disease, Nicola Paginini, favored with unusually long fingers, who lived in the early 1800's, excelled as a violinist, Although not documented, Abraham Lincoln, the tenth president of the United States, has been suspected of having this disorder.

In the eyes, *exfoliation* may be present. As well, because of the aberrant connective tissue, weakness may affect one or both of the eyes; the *lens* may become displaced and the *retina* detached. Glaucoma can result from the dislocation of the *lens*, which may obstruct the pupil and push the *iris* into the *trabecular meshwork* (the outflow channel), blocking the aqueous fluid from leaving the eye. Other syndromes include *uveitis* and astigmatism. Medical and surgical intervention can often save vision. A retinologist may be enlisted to repair *retina* problems. Since this syndrome affects the entire body, it is often fruitful to initiate a correspondence between the orthopedist, cardiologist, and ophthalmologist. Cardiac arrhythmia and spontaneous pneumonia may occur.

WEILL-MARCHESANI SYNDROME OR MIRCO SPEROPHAKIA

Considered to be inherited, this syndrome is a rare form of glaucoma. It is usually identified by a *lens* that is spherical in shape and smaller than average. From early childhood on, the *lens* may become dislocated and move to the front of the eye where it obstructs the pupil resulting in a forward movement of the *iris* which blocks the drainage pathways causing a rise in the IOP. *Myopia* may sometimes occur, as does occasional blindness. Other physical symptoms include malformed and misaligned teeth and a cardiac condition. Genetically, this disease has been found most frequently in American Amish communities where second cousins often wed.

Glaucoma appears at about three years of age when the *lens* in the eye may dislocate and cause *pupillary block,* a condition that occurs when the aqueous fluid is blocked from squeezing between the *lens* and *iris* in its passage from the back to the front of the eye. The fluid builds up behind the *iris* and pushes the *iris* into the drainage channel.

MORE CONGENITAL DISEASES

A group of genetic diseases, in addition to causing severe physical handicaps, may also cause a high *intraocular pressure*: *Trisomy 18* (an extra copy of chromosome 18), causes severe deformity and mental retardation; children born with this anomaly usually do not survive beyond the first year. *Trisomy 21,* commonly known as *Down's syndrome,* is associated with varying degrees of mental retardation. Features of all these children are quite similar and are easily visually identified. With medication these children can live into midlife. They have various levels of mental capacity including the ability to read and do mathematics. *Trisomy 13,* (located on an extra copy of chromosome 13) causes severe congenital deformation and mental retardation. These children usually do not survive beyond the first year of life. *Congenital mircrocoria* (tiny pupil) has been linked in a study to *myopia* (near-sightedness) and glaucoma.

HOMOCYSTINURIA

The outward appearance of this syndrome is somewhat like that of *Marfan's Syndrome,* with skeletal abnormalities. These babies are born normal but lack the enzyme to metabolize (break down) the amino acid *homocysteine* causing toxic byproducts, building to a variety of mild to severe symptoms. Behavioral disorders and mental retardation are common, but most devastating is the condition of *homocystinuria* that is likely to promote blood clots resulting in strokes and high blood pressure. Also, the child may suffer from *osteoporosis*. A nutritionist can help the parent select foods that do not exacerbate this condition, and it has been noted that some children improve with the addition of vitamins B6 and B12.

Glaucoma appears at about three years of age when the *lens* in the eye may dislocate and cause *pupillary block,* a condition that occurs when the aqueous fluid is blocked from squeezing between the *lens* and *iris* in its passage from the back to the front of the eye. The fluid builds up behind the *iris* and pushes the *iris* into the drainage channel.

RETINOPATHY OF PREMATURITY (ROP)

Premature infants are prone to a number of diseases that affect various organs in their bodies and the eyes are no exception. Because of increased *in vitro* fertilization, there are more multiple births that place babies at risk for premature delivery. In the twelve year period from 1984 to 1996, the number of preemies increased from nine and four tenths percent to eleven percent—about 400,000 babies in the U.S. alone. The visual system affected by prematurity involves a *retinal* condition called *retinopathy of prematurity (ROP).* This is a condition where new blood vessels grow over the immature avascular (lacking in blood) *retina* which, if not treated, leads to blindness. The treatment as with *diabetic retinopathy* sacrifices side vision to preserve the central area. These babies may also develop lazy eye *(amblyopia)* and will probably be quite near-sighted requiring strong correction with glasses. The condition may advance, but this circumstance is now rare, for greater awareness and improved screening identifies and treats at earlier stages, thereby preserving vision. In the past, the use of high O2 (oxygen) to treat premature infants led to blindness in some cases, because the oxygen constricted blood vessels depriving nourishment to the developing *retina.*

CONGENITAL RUBELLA (GERMAN MEASELS)

Before routine vaccination in developed countries, the *rubella* virus was able to cross the *placenta* during pregnancy. If the fetus is infected during the first trimester of pregnancy, *rubella* infection can be severe. The virus may damage the tissues of the inner ear, *lens* of the eye (cataracts), *retina*, heart, brain, liver and/or spleen, lymph nodes, and disrupt dentition formation and also promote skin lesions and easy bruising.

Infection of the eyes resembles *infantile glaucoma* with maldevelopment and poor function of the drainage channels. Surgery effectively opens these channels. The condition may cause cataracts but not glaucoma. Should this occur, the cataract is removed and a *lens* implanted which should last a lifetime. Inflammation (a *uveitis*-like condition) may also occur. Medication usually relieves this problem.

Although the rate of infection has dropped dramatically in the United States due the availability of a vaccine, in countries where the vaccine is difficult to come by or where parents refuse it, newborns are at risk of developing the disease.

SECONDARY INFANTILE GLAUCOMAS

This category differs from those already described, for the problems associated with secondary infantile glaucoma result not necessarily from a birth defect or genetic anomaly, but are caused by conditions stemming from a preceding eye problem. These include inflammation, tumors and trauma. In some cases, tumors and traumas can be treated and the glaucoma reversed when the baby's eyes are stabilized. Trauma, however, often causes irreversible damage to the *trabecular meshwork* resulting in persistent glaucoma. Inflammation, if not treated early, can lead to glaucoma.

Inflammation of the baby's eyes does not differ greatly from *uveitis*. Why *uveitis* occurs in babies has given rise to a number of inconclusive theories. When inflammation cannot be associated with a particular disease, it is termed *idiopathic* (no known cause), or *endogenous* (arising from within the body). Prostaglandins, a large group of unsaturated fatty acids that act as regulators of many bodily functions, or an autoimmune response may be possibly responsible. Inflammation causes damage when the inflammatory debris clogs the trabecular meshwork leading to a diagnosis of *open-angle glaucoma*. Inflammation may also cause *pupillary block,* a condition that occurs when the aqueous fluid is blocked from squeezing between the lens and *iris* in its passage from the back to the front of the eye. The fluid builds up behind the *iris* and pushes the *iris* into the drainage channel. Effective treatment consists of a *trabeculectomy* or a *goniotomy.*

TUMORS

In the first year of life, a skin tumor, *Xanthogranuloma*, produces skin lesions on the scalp, face, and upper trunk; these tumors may also invade the *iris* and other parts of the baby's eyes. Although spontaneous regression does occur during the period that these tumors are present, bleeding may occur driving up the IOP in the baby's eyes. If not resolved, the *trabecular meshwork* becomes blocked. Elevated pressure is treated with topical medication and steroids.

TRAUMA

An outside force that impacts the eye causes trauma. Many different kinds of trauma can damage an infant's eyes. During birth delivery, trauma may result from the use of forceps. When glaucoma is detected, it may be difficult to differentiate whether the condition is caused by trauma or the consequences of *primary infantile glaucoma*, but a careful inspection of the infant's forehead and possibly cheeks may reveal trauma as the underlying cause. If over a period of weeks or months the condition resolves, doctors assume the cause to be trauma, but continue to carefully monitor the baby's eyes to exclude the diagnose of *primary infantile glaucoma* where quick action is needed to preserve the infant's sight.

CATARACT

Cataracts can be removed early in babies born with the condition but the operation often results in glaucoma developing somewhere down the line. More recent information about the procedures suggests that surgery be delayed until the infant is at least four weeks old, rather than proceeding with surgery during the first few weeks of life. It is not yet clear as to whether waiting longer or removal at birth is the most preferable option.

JUVENILE GLAUCOMA

Aaryn was diagnosed as a glaucoma suspect at the tender age of thirteen and then graduated at the advanced age of fifteen into *juvenile open-angle glaucoma*. Like many glaucoma patients when first diagnosed, Aaryn took the news in stride and faithfully followed her doctor's medical recommendations. Her experience with medications has been similar to those of adult patients. At one period in her life, her IOP rose dramatically and her doctor, with varying results, tried a number of different medications. *Alphagan* produced a reaction that mimicked *meningitis* and it was Aaryn who observed the condition was due to the medication. *Pilocarpine* caused severe migraines which lasted for a week. *Trabeculectomy* surgery, because of the possibility of scarring, was not recommended due to Aaryn's age. (Youth confers a more rapid healing response).

Aaryn's diagnosis of glaucoma surprised her family, for she had a healthy infancy and glaucoma had not surfaced in her immediate relatives. Since her diagnosis, however, her material grandfather has developed the disease and her mother and brother are glaucoma suspects. Genetics appear to play a role here.

While friends and family supported her, Aaryn needed to connect with other young glaucoma patients and to spread the word that glaucoma can occur at any age. She launched an interactive web site called YUP (Young Under Pressure) that links together those young people who have juvenile glaucoma. Aaryn is now married, a mother and continues to support glaucoma awareness.

Yes, glaucoma does strike teenagers. Juvenile glaucoma brackets the period from early childhood through adolescence. The same susceptibilities—greater frequency found in African-Americans and those with *myopia* occur as with adult *POAG*. The problem appears to lie in a thickened *trabecular meshwork* formation that signals immature development of the meshwork, impairing the flow of aqueous. In the United States, *juvenile glaucoma* is considered rare, occurring in one out of fifty thousand persons. As with glaucoma in general, it favors no specific nationality occurring in people who are Japanese, French, French Canadian, American, Panamanian, German, English, *Iris*h, Danish, Italian, and Spanish. Males may be more frequently affected. Onset of the disease may occur between five-to-ten years especially if there is a history of glaucoma in the family, although with Aaryn, she rolled the ball first. But if glaucoma is present in the family constellation, it is wise to have young children's' eyes monitored for elevated pressure.

Juvenile glaucoma has also been associated with systemic anomalies that are present at birth. These include *Sturge-Weber syndrome, Neurofibromatosis, Stickler syndrome, Oculocerebrorenal (Lowe) syndrome* (a genetically transmitted disease), *Rieger's syndrome, SHORT syndrome, Hepatocerebroretinal syndrome, Marfan's syndrome, Rubinstein-Taybi syndrome, infantile glaucoma* associated with mental retardation and paralysis, *Oculodentodigital dysplasia, open-angle glaucoma* associated with *microcornea* and absence of frontal sinuses, *Mucopolysaccaridosis* (an enzyme deficiency), *Trisomy 13, Trisomy 21 (Down's syndrome)* skeletal dysplasia, *Michel syndrome, non progressive hemiatrophy (impaired nutrition), PHACE syndrome, Sotos syndrome, Linear scleroderma syndrome (*a binding of tissues in the skin and visceral organs*), Duplication 3q syndrome, Cutis marmorata telangiectasia congenita, Warburg syndrome, Kniest GAPO syndrome, and Roberts pseudothalidomide syndrome.* It has also been associated with abnormalities of the eye that include: *congenital glaucoma with iris and pupillary abnormalities, Aniridia, congenital ocular melanosis, sclerocornea, iridotrabecular disgenesis, Peters syndrome, and ectropian uveae,* *posterior polymorphous dystrophy, idiopathic or familial elevated episcleral venues pressure, anterior corneal staphyloma (a protrusion on the cornea), congenital microcoria (tiny pupil) with myopia, congenital hereditary endothelial dystrophy, congenital hereditary iris stromal hyperplasia (*underdevelopment of tissues*), and Rieger's anomaly.*

Secondary glaucoma may result from trauma such as a blunt injury to the eye, or acute glaucoma caused by concussion, blood in the eye or *ghost cell glaucoma* (degenerated red blood cells).

Secondary glaucoma may also result from tumors in the *retina, xanthogranuloma* (a skin disease present at birth), hemorrhaging in the eye after an operation, *leukemia, melanoma* of the *ciliary body, melanocytoma,* a benign tumor on the *optic disc,* and a tumor or tiny tumors on the *iris* that become aggressive.

A dislocated *lens* found in some syndromes such as *Marfan's Syndrome, homocystinuria,* or *Weill-Marchesani syndrome,* or *lens* material after surgery may obstruct the *trabecular meshwork* if inadvertently retained, resulting in secondary glaucoma. *Rubeosis,* a condition of runaway blood vessels like that found in *diabetic retinopathy* may be caused by a variety of *retinal* problems. Infection with the *rubella* virus may continue to reoccur, affecting the *iris.*

The above list is amazing. It's as if researchers have thrown everything in the barrel to account for the presence of *juvenile glaucoma* that in the United States accounts for one in fifty thousand persons. What is evident, however, from the list of diseases is that glaucoma can derive from a number of different physical conditions. We do know that in a small proportion of patients with *primary open-angle glaucoma* that the *TIGR* gene (*myocilin*) is responsible. Whatever the source, the pathology remains fundamentally the same. Filtration of fluid is blocked. Examination of the *trabecular meshwork* reveals thickened tissue and abnormal deposits of tissue in the drainage passages. These mutations are linked to the *TIGR* gene now called the *myocilin* gene that codes for the *glycoprotein myocilin* found in the *trabecular meshwork* and other tissues in the eye. It was the first gene to be identified in connection with glaucoma and caused great excitement when the discovery was announced.

We are now increasingly aware that obesity in developed countries promotes *diabetes* in young people, a condition that may lead to *diabetic retinopathy* characterized by poor blood flow to the *retina.* This condition results in *angiogenesis,* a stimulation of new blood vessel growth that proliferates over the entire eye and eventually blocks the *trabecular meshwork.* Over the age of twenty-five, *diabetic retinopathy* is one of the leading causes of blindness in the United States. Genetic problems such as *exfoliation* and *pigmentary dispersion syndrome* in otherwise healthy individuals may affect the eyes in juveniles. In both *pigmentary dispersion syndrome* and *exfoliation*, debris from these conditions clogs the *trabecular meshwork*, as does inflammation associated with *juvenile arthritis*.

Although the history of maintaining the sight of children and juveniles was once a dismal prospect, treatment with both medication and surgery has improved the prospects of these young patients. For the littlest ones, medication is titrated taking into consideration the age and weight of the child. When the anomaly affects the structures of the eyes as it does with some serious infant diseases, the outcome may be less promising. In the evolving brave new world, it may one day be possible to medically disarm the genetic flaw while the baby is still in the womb.

Diagnosis is essential. Take a look at the following chapter that delineates the many steps leading to a complete diagnosis of glaucoma conditions.

CHAPTER 4
The Four Horsemen of: Diagnosis

o o o o o o o o o o o o o o o o o o o o o o o o o o o o o o o o o o o o o o o o o o

"A disease known is half cured."
Thomas Fuller, MD, Gnomologia (1732), 75

A diagnosis determining an existing disease shocks one to the very roots of being. You visit your doctor for a nagging little something, an itch, a sore that won't go away, stomach distress, loss of energy, or a change of glasses, and wham, you're hit with a full-fledged disease. Or you may discover during a routine procedure a heretofore hidden and more serious problem, as it did in my case. After successfully sealing up a *retinal* tear, my doctor diagnosed early stages of glaucoma in my left eye. Joseph discovered he had glaucoma upon on a visit to his optometrist for his yearly check-up. To his dismay, he had lost the sight of one eye to glaucoma. At whatever stage diagnosis confirms this unwelcome news, glaucoma is a disease that, up to the present, because no cure yet exists, will be a lifetime companion. I recall overhearing a woman reiterating again and again that she could not understand how SHE came to be diagnosed with glaucoma. How indeed—for those of us with no family or as yet undiscovered family history, glaucoma arrives, an uninvited guest, permanently establishing itself into our households.

Diagnosis of glaucoma can range from simple to sophisticated. Measuring your *intraocular pressure*, examining the condition of your *optic nerve*, measuring corneal thickness and visual field testing are part of the examination. Equally important is examining the angle formed by the meeting of *iris* and *cornea*. If necessary, your doctor may also use the more sophisticated imaging instruments.

Fortunately, due to awareness in developed countries and increasingly in developing nations, screening for glaucoma is becoming routine. Yet despite this greater awareness, the sad fact remains that countless individuals still lose sight because screening still has not achieved the level of awareness given to blood pressure, *diabetes,* and cholesterol. At the very least, all routine eye exams should include glaucoma screening.

Recently I spoke with a woman who was in a dither about her mother, age eight-five scheduled for a glaucoma operation. I asked this woman if she, too, had been evaluated for glaucoma. She hesitated, and then said no, but hastened to add that her sister, ten years older, fearful of learning an unwanted truth, had also shunned visiting her eye doctor. The one taking her mother to the eye doctor rationalized that looking after her mother ate up all of her free time, while the older sister flat out said that she preferred to remain oblivious. Diagnosis is at the heart for detecting glaucoma. Screening for glaucoma is not a diagnosis. A routine screening checks *intraocular pressure,* which if high, suggests that glaucoma may be present. The patient is then referred to a doctor who can complete a comprehensive evaluation.

THE ROUTINE EYE EXAMINATION—WHAT'S YOUR ACUITY?

The routine eye exam, depending on your age, eye condition, and need, is generally performed yearly. Basically, the exam determines your near and distance vision (how well you see at a standard distance of twenty feet). For near distance, reading newsprint is the key. To measure your acuity, your doctor will ask you to read letters or numbers on the *Snellen Eye Chart* that is placed twenty feet away or flashed on a screen in the doctor's office. This chart is a marvelously simple instrument. It displays rows of letters, numbers or symbols that decrease in size. A person registering 20/20 can read at 100 feet what a person with 20/100 can only read at 20 feet. Alternatively, the *Snellen chart* may be replaced by a completely objective instrument that automatically records your refraction error and provides a read-out of your prescription.

Often there is a variation between your eyes. Patients noting the discrepancy between their eyes often refer to their good and bad eye.

A card bearing a graduated line of words or numbers, each line becoming tinier than the one preceding it checks for print readability. Those with good near vision but uncorrected distance vision (*myopia*) usually experience little difficulty during this section of the exam. Those with excellent distance vision, but who whip out glasses to read fine print (*presbyopia*) have the opposite experience. Progressive lenses, however, often provide excellent distance-and-near vision.

While the *Snellen* chart appears to be unsophisticated, it is a well-designed instrument that provides your doctor with baseline information on your ability to process the elements that comprise an object. Each object possesses a number of elements of varying complexity. Letters and numbers are structures built from disparate elements. The greater the number of elements in a figure, the more complicated it appears. With less than perfect vision, look-alike letters baffle. For example, "P" and "B" have one upright bar, plus one or two semi-circles. The circles raise problems with limited visual acuity. "G" and "O" may present similar difficulty, for both letters may be perceived as having closed circles. Or the "B" may be indistinguishable from either of these letters. "T" and "P" may stump you, since both letters have the similar configurations.

Some visual problems may simply be an artifact of age. With age, even those with perfect vision may need reading glasses. This situation is a result of the loss of flexibility of the accommodating *ciliary* muscle, which is part of the *ciliary body*. When it contracts for near vision, it pulls the *choroid* forward, reducing the tension on the *zonules* (ligaments holding the *lens* capsule) allowing the *lens* to assume a more spherical shape for near vision accommodation. Cataracts also reduce acuity. When I had my cataract removed I was amazed at the brightness, clarity and color that I thought I had lost forever.

"Seeing is believing," but that premise loses its impact for glaucoma patients who complain that they do just fine on the *Snellen* but in the real world, they no longer see competently. Several possibilities exist for this discrepancy. Glare, or light scattered from sunlight, overhead lights, or fluorescent lights can decrease visual acuity. Competing light situations create visual noise that disturbs the act of seeing. Even fully-functioning eyes are affected by twilight that diminishes acuity. If the quality of light interferes with your contrast sensitivity, discuss this situation with your doctor who may be able to recommend colored *lens* that will lessen glare and improve contrast sensitivity.

MAGNIFICATION OF YOUR EYE
THE DIRECT OPHTHALMOSCOPE

This instrument is the oldest but perhaps the most widely used method for evaluating the *optic disc*. It is a hand-held instrument providing for a magnification by 15x of the *optic disc*. It is useful for screening and taking a look at the *disc* when the patient has small pupils. It is limited, however, in that regard, for it does not provide a three-dimensional view. A newer development, a hand-held laser *ophthalmoscope*, however, is rivaling the use of the slit lamp for taking *intraocular pressure*.

The Workhorse Of The Doctor's Office-- The Slit Lamp

The slit lamp is the instrument that your doctor uses to examine the inner structures of your eye. Following your reading of the *Snellen* chart, your doctor may either examine you with an *ophthalmoscope* or a *slit lamp.* You will be asked to place your chin on a chin rest and lean your forehead against a forehead rest.

The lamp itself is part of an instrument that both magnifies and lights up the front portion of your eye, the first part of the eye that your doctor will examine. He or she will evaluate the health of the *conjunctiva, sclera, cornea, iris, lens* and a portion of the *vitreous.* In this position your doctor will anesthetize your eye and measure your IOP.

To ascertain the angle width, your doctor will do a *gonioscopy,* using one of a variety of contact lenses or *goniolens,* (a *gonioprism*). During this part of the examination, your angles, the drainage ports for the fluid discharge, will be measured. The width of the angle determines the type of glaucoma you possess--*open-or narrow-angle,* an important distinction that determines the method of treatment.

In the course of the examination, your doctor will examine the *optic disc* or *optic nerve head.* This may be viewed in a number of ways--looking through the center of a convex lens, dilating the eye for greater visual access, and/or using a high-powered convex lens attached to the slit lamp. Whatever method, examination of the *optic nerve* head or *disc* is vital for evaluation of the condition of your eyes. Another method that is possible through the use of advanced software elimiminates touching the eye.

While the eye is dilated your doctor may choose to examine your *retina.* For this test, you will be asked to look up, down, right and left. This is an important examination for those with vulnerable *retinas,* for *retinal* holes or *detachment* can lead to loss of vision. Problems can most often be repaired with laser treatment.

A photograph of the *optic nerve* provides the doctor with a baseline of the condition of your eyes. This test may be performed yearly or at greater intervals and is now a routine part of the initial examination.

Each section of your eye will be assessed. The *cornea* should be smooth, clear and free of irregularities. Cause for concern includes a bloodshot eye, ground-glass appearance (possibly *corneal edema*—swelling due to fluid retention), or cloudiness. In a child, the *cornea* should not exceed eleven millimeters, for, if larger or bulbous, *congenital glaucoma* may be present. An accurate reading of your IOP is impacted by the thickness of your *cornea.*

A thin *cornea* gives a false lower reading of your IOP. Doctors now perform *pachymetry*, an ultrasound measurement that assesses central *corneal* thickness (*CCT*). (More on cornea problems in Chapter 2)

Your doctor, in examining your pupil, checks for a nice round orb and its response to light stimuli--expanding in dim light and contracting in bright light. This simple mechanism regulates the quantity of light falling on the *retina* and provides for decent vision. Prior to the wide selection of medications now available for managing *intraocular pressure*, miotic drops (*pilocarpine* and *carbacohl*) narrowed the pupil reducing visual acuity. Although these medications are still available, given the alternatives, fewer people need to use them. If the pupil's shape is distorted, disease may be present. Certain conditions waste away the *iris* corrupting the pupil's integrity. An inflammatory condition of the *iris* can cause it to adhere to the *lens*, distorting the pupil. Radial slit-like defects in the *iris* may indicate the presence of *pigmentary-dispersion syndrome*, a secondary form of glaucoma where loss of pigment results in a spindle shaped pigment on the *cornea* (*Krukenberg's spindles*), resembling somewhat the framework of a bicycle wheel. Diagnosis is achieved using the slit lamp light (*transillumination*) that, shining onto the pupil, bounces light back out of the eye through the abnormal slits.

The *lens* is examined for transparency. A cloudy *lens* indicates the formation of a cataract. Cloudiness also obscures the amount of light falling on the *retina* affecting vision. Grayness or opaqueness of the lens indicates advanced cases of cataract.

THE IOP--PRESSURE, PRESSURE--WHAT'S RIGHT FOR YOU--BUT NOT FOR ME

Once the hallmark of glaucoma diagnosis, the IOP measurement now comprises one leg of the total eye examination. Measurement of eye pressure is most often performed with a Goldmann tonometer attached to the slit lamp apparatus. There is no magic number. What might be high for me will be just fine for a person with no sign of glaucoma. What might be great for Mary at 16 mmHg, who has lost minimum sight and over time maintained stability on one drop, is detrimental for Eleanor who has *normal tension glaucoma* and whose pressures are ideally in the low teens or single digits. On the other hand, Elliot, who has not yet shown any signs of damage with pressures in the mid-twenties range (an *ocular hypertensive*), can apparently tolerate elevated pressure. Although glaucoma is regarded as an optic nerve disease, the level of *intraocular pressure* still ranks high for controlling vision loss, for research has linked pressure control to management. *The Advanced Glaucoma Intervention*

Study and the *Normal Tension Glaucoma Study* both concluded that pressures in the low teens were most protective of field loss.

That the IOP is intricately associated with a number of factors that comprise the glaucoma diagnosis is certainly not controversial. But the effect of elevated pressure on parts of the eye other than on the sensitive *ganglion* nerves continues to unfold. Researchers have found that elevated pressure swells the *cones* in the eye causing subsequent vision loss.

THE GOLD STANDARD OF A PRESSURE CHECK-- GOLDMANN TONOMETER

In treatment of a disease, certain tools, medications, and protocols are termed "gold standard." This is the standard used as a measurement of quality and reliability. The *Goldmann Applanation Tonometer* is designated as the gold standard for measuring *intraocular pressure* and examining the eye. Standards change, however, as continuing research reveals new findings. One such finding derived from the *Ocular Hypertension Treatment Study (OHTS),* revealed that the thickness of the central cornea had a direct impact on an accurate measurement of the *intraocular pressure*. The study discovered that people with *ocular hypertension* had not lost vision as was projected. These subjects possessed thicker *corneas* that masked lower IOPs. Ophthalmologists proposed that thicker *corneas* may account for the health of the subjects' *optic nerves*.

A flurry of measurement followed this revelation. The researchers discovered that eyes with thin central *corneas* registered four-to-five points less than eyes with thicker *central corneas*. This finding added another dimension in the evaluation of the IOP prompting eye specialists to routinely perform *pachymetry* that with a zip across the center of the *cornea* provides a reading of *corneal* thickness that may impact on a true IOP reading. Thin *corneas* may give a false lower reading requiring that an adjustment be made in glaucoma management.

Scientists established a possible norm of 550 micrometers (um) as normal central *corneal* thickness. Additional studies, however, may further refine this figure. Nevertheless, deviations from this value are considered important, for studies have indicated that either an over-or-under estimation of IOP by as much as 7 mmHg exists. Thin *corneas* were underestimated by as much as 4.9 mmHg, while thick *corneas* were overestimated by as much as 6-to-8 mmHg. There are also racial differences. Mongolians and African-Americans apparently have thinner corneas, with Latinos falling somewhere in the middle of Africans and whites. Age of whites did not show any difference in most studies, but with various ethnic groups, differences may be revealed for in some studies, Japanese and African-Americans were found to have greater corneal thinning with age.

Pachymetry has also proven to be essential for performing *LASIK* (laser correction of the *cornea* for either near-or far-sightedness). When performing *LASIK* surgery, the doctor must evaluate the central *cornea* thickness to determine if the tissue is thick enough for the procedure; if the tissue is too thin, the operation might cause an abnormal bowing of the *cornea*.

When you are having your IOP checked, be sure to loosen tight clothing (neckties, belts, etc.). These items may restrict natural breathing and possibly cause a temporary rise in IOP. Place your chin in the chin rest and lean your forehead against the forehead rest. The use of the *Goldmann* tonometer to measure the IOP is a deceptively simple procedure. Your doctor or practitioner administers an anesthetic drop to numb the eye for a very short period. A drop of fluoroscein is then added. When illuminated with the cobalt blue light the fluoroscein appears yellow. Some people have trouble opening their eyes wide enough and doctors can assist by gently raising the eyelid. Initially, you will note a blue spot of light. When the instrument touches the *cornea* a fluorescent ring is formatted at which point the examiner presses the tonometer against the *cornea* flattening it and causing the two halves of the fluorescent ring to form a half-circle. This procedure registers the IOP reading. Contact lens users need to remove their contacts before this procedure for the fluorescent drops will stain the lenses.

A Puff Of Air—The Pneumotonometer (Pneumatic Tonometer)

Some people have such sensitive *corneas* that even the lightest touch of the probe causes irritation; also young children may not be cooperative. An alternative system using a puff of air may solve the problem but it may not provide as accurate a reading as the *Goldmann*. This instrument includes a built-in evaluation of the central *corneal* thickness and adjusts the IOP measurement accordingly. It is unlikely that this instrument will be found in an ophthalmologist's office, although there will probably be one in the ophthalmologic department of a training hospital. It is cheaper than the *Goldmann* tonometer and it is portable, features that make it attractive for mass screenings or in rural and outlying areas where access to an eye doctor is limited.

This test does not require anesthesia, is performed in seconds and aside from the air puff, is a completely benign procedure. The puff of warm air into the eye equals a blink. Of course, there are those sensitive people who object to even a puff of air directed to the eye and these individuals may tense up and distort the readings. It's a good idea, if possible, to compare the reading of both systems and with your eye doctor determine if they are in sync. I found that with the pneumotonometer, my IOP was several points below what I normally register on the *Goldmann*. As with the *Goldmann*, use of the pneunomotometer requires removal of contact lenses.

SELF-EVALUATION

Want to take your own pressure? It's possible with a device called the Proview manufactured by Bausch & Lomb. This device does not need anesthetizing drops, for only the eyelid is touched lightly with a probe. When you view the phosphene (like a flash of light) you remove the probe and read your pressure. I'm not able to use this instrument for I've lost too many peripheral cells and I can't locate the phosphene. Those with *trabeculectomies* may find interference with the *bleb* since the probe is placed over that area. People recently diagnosed and who have not lost much peripheral vision are able to use this device. Researchers feel that this instrument is a good indicator for detecting large changes but not for small ones.

MASS SCREENINGS

The knowledge that visual field loss is routinely found in newly-diagnosed glaucoma patients underscores the importance of glaucoma mass screenings. Many of the affiliates of Prevent Blindness America provide vision screening as do chapters of the Lion's Club. Mass screening is facilitated using the *FDT Visual Field Instrument.* This is a noninvasive machine that registers information by targeting the activity of a particular group of cells in the eye. The screening takes no more than several minutes. It accurately determines glaucoma damage in the moderate-to-severe range. Ideally, when these screenings take place, there will be a trained assistant to measure *intraocular pressure* using a hand-held tonometer.

Another instrument, the *Damato Campimeter*, is sometimes used for mass screenings. Deceptively simple, it consists only of a rectangular chart containing a diagram of fixation points. An occluder (cover) is provided for the eye not being tested. You hold the chart at a reading distance from your eyes with one hand, and with the other place the occluder over the eye not being tested. You are instructed to locate a center dot on the chart and then to focus on an asterisk and tell the examiner if you can see the center dot. Initially, you will fail at this exercise for the examiner is checking your blind spot (the area of your *retina* where your *optic nerve* exits your eye to connect with your brain). As you shift focus from one numbered fixation point to another, the examiner registers what you are able to see.

VARIABLES THAT MAY AFFECT A GLAUCOMA READING

There are many variables that may affect the pressure reading--tight clothing, neckties, hip-hugging pants that constrict stomach breathing, inability to get close to the instrument because of obesity, pillow pressure (a small study out of Brazil found that sleeping on one side might cause asymmetrical glaucoma. Patients had more severe glaucoma in the eye that rested on the pillow.) Pillow pressure, however, should not affect IOP measurement in your doctor's office. But your mental state, as well the time of day, may impact on your pressure reading. If you're feeling low you may discover that your pressure is somewhat elevated. Diurnally, pressures rise and fall according to the time of day. Pressures are lower in the morning and tend to rise as the day progresses. In some people, the difference can be as large as five or six points.

OPTIC NERVE EVALUATION-
HOLDING ONTO THE RIM

Careful observation of the optic nerve is a given upon a diagnosis of glaucoma. Evaluation consists of visually examining the optic nerve and/or using one of the diagnostic instruments (see below) that electronically produces a reading of fiber thickness. To view the *optic nerve* the doctor will dilate your eye, a process that requires thirty minutes or so for the eyedrop to widen the *pupil*. The dilating drops commonly used include *Mydramide (Tropicamide 0.5 %,)*, sometimes in combination with *Phenyl phone HCI 10%, Scopolamine,* or *Cyclopentolate Hydrochloride*. The most often side-effect complaint is the length of time involved (sometimes as long as eight hours before the *pupil* resumes its normal shape.) Other side effects are infrequent, but may include an elevation of IOP, an allergic reaction, photophobia, hallucinations, convulsions, and blurred vision. Even death may occur with *Atropine*. Most frequently, however, patients experience discomfort, especially on bright, sunny days for the wide-open pupil absorbs an oversupply of light affecting the neurons in the *retina*. This effect is simply uncomfortable, not dangerous. If you are severely disoriented when having this examination, for heaven's sake bring somebody along to assist you, or at the very least, wear sun glasses to block the light pouring into your eye.

While it is preferable to dilate the eye for the *optic nerve* examination, patients who have had a cataract operation that required the stretching of a bound *pupil* (because of the use of *miotic* drops), a condition I have experienced, in certain situations the stretched *pupil* provides sufficient access to view the *optic nerve*.

Dilation of the pupil in patients who have *angle-closure glaucoma* is risky, for widening the *pupil* may move the *iris* into the smaller angle space and block the flow of fluid. Dilating drops are also contraindicated for people with brain damage, Down's syndrome, or spastic paralysis. In some of these cases more sophisticated imaging instruments for *optic nerve* assessment may be used.

A squirmy two-year old can present an examination problem, which is solved by using a hand-held laser ophthalmoscope. This instrument is capable of diagnosing *nystagmus, photophobia, eccentric fixation*, and problems with the cone receptors.

WHAT YOUR DOCTOR LOOKS FOR

Formed from the *ganglion nerve fibers* originating in the *retina*, the *optic nerve* carries visual information to the brain. In the eye, the nerve fibers form a cup-like shape before exiting to the brain. This cup or *disc* is surrounded by a pink rim. Imagine a white teacup on a pink saucer. Thinning of the nerve fibers around the *disc* signals loss of vision, for these fibers are pathways to the brain. Pallor of the nerve fibers may signal inadequate blood supply, for although potentially serious, nerve color does vary among individuals. Cup size is one of the most potent indicators of glaucoma damage. A large cup most often is associated with fiber loss. But again, cup size may vary. Near-sighted people possess larger cups due to the elongated shape of their eyes. African-Americans also tend to have larger cups. The *Blue Mountain Study* that enrolled 3,654 elderly people found cup ratios ranging from 0.66 mm-to-1.5 mm. Cup-disc ratios may range from .55- to-2.00 mm in the population at large. A study conducted by the University of California, Los Angeles documented that Latinos forty years plus had smaller discs, cups and neural rim areas as compared to blacks and whites. A small study found that glaucoma patients appear to differ from those without the disease.

Pressures, diurnal (during the day) and nocturnal (during the night), appear to be higher in newly-diagnosed patients than in those who do not have glaucoma. Of greater concern for normal pressure glaucoma patients is the systolic pressure (the top number) dropping at night possibly reducing nourishing blood flow to the optic nerve.

CONTRAST SENSIVITY

A decline in visual acuity is often accompanied with a decline in contrast sensitivity, not to be confused with contrast diminishment because of a cataract. Glaucoma patients lose contrast because specific cells die. Loss of contrast sensitivity hampers just about every task—reading labels, computer work, colored print on colored paper, distinguishing color variables in vegetables, fruit and flowers, dark garments, grease or dirt spots on clothing and even observing traffic signals. Books, magazines, journals and newspapers printed in various font sizes and/or tight spacing between lines may confound. Fortunately, computers provide users with a choice of both screen and font size. Objects designed for young eyes challenge glaucoma patients. Cell phones, IPods and the like, for example, provide information on a distressingly tiny screen. Any technological product (fax machines, copiers, cash registers, ATM's etc.) provides consumer information located on tiny black rectangles with barely visible print. Often, one simply ignores or fails to see the message and resorts to calling the manufacturer to complain of a faulty product (something I've done) and then sheepishly admitting that I hadn't read a simple message, for example, that the machine merely needed to clean itself and was politely asking me to "please wait." In another instance, when my printer gave me trouble, I called for "support." A technician guided me through a series of steps, during which process I discovered a feature previously invisible to me unless viewed in a strong light. People over fifty and those who are visually disadvantaged are challenging the technological industry to provide better visual and /or auditory access. If you are one of those who are challenged, complain to the company.

Contrast screening is important for glaucoma patients who continue to drive. Depending upon the speed of the car, you may have just a few seconds to apply the brake or veer to avoid hitting an object. The threshold at which you see the target when taking a *visual field test* is an indication of your threshold sensitivity. Another means, the Sine-wave (a wave form that is graphically expressed as a sign curve), assesses threshold levels by assessing your ability to distinguish forms.

Many organizations working with people who have vision problems suggest filling out a questionnaire assessing Daily Living Tasks. Depending upon the state of your vision, such a questionnaire is helpful in determining how contrast sensitivity affects your daily life. Other tests of contrast sensitivity include the *Reading Index Test* that checks your reading speed (loss of vision reduces reading speed) and/or a *Computer Task Analysis Test* that correlates closely with the *visual acuity test, contrast sensitivity test,* and *color vision defects.*

THE MARVELS OF TECHNOLOGY

The secrets of the body are unveiled through the use of powerful electron instruments. Scientists can now view a living cell in process, such as determining cell movement. The cell does a two-step sort of walk. As scientists produce useful applications, better therapies for protecting the eyes from the ravages of glaucoma may follow. George I. Cioffi, MD at an *ARVO* conference (*Association of Research and Vision Ophthalmology*) gave as an example of acid-sensing ion channels that when exposed to mechanical or ischemic (lack of blood) stressors, allow the influx of substances into the cell that can ultimately destroy it. When *retinal ganglion* cells are lost, unfortunately, corresponding cells in the brain follow suit. Another example involves the *free radical, singlet oxygen* molecule, which is very toxic. With digital infrared microscopy scientists have been able to detect this culprit.

THE NERVE FIBER LAYER

Thickness of the *nerve fiber layer* is of grave concern for glaucoma patients. A thick *nerve fiber layer* indicates a healthy eye. Thin, it most often signals a diseased condition. Anatomical changes in the *nerve fiber layer* can lead to loss of vision. Different diseases affect the *nerve fiber layer* in specific ways. With glaucoma, the *nerve fiber layer* thins; with *diabetes* it swells. Other diseases may cause distortions such as holes, cavities and *retinal detachment*. Structural damage precedes functional loss and therefore, assessment of nerve damage is essential. Fortunately, non-invasive imaging instruments exist today capable of objectively evaluating the *optic nerve*. These include the *scanning laser tomography, scanning laser polarimetry* and *optical coherence tomography* among others.

DEEP INTO THE EYE--IMAGAGING INSTRUMENTS

Laser Tomography Ophthalmoscope

The development of the *laser ophthalmoscope* has improved the ability to determine the scope of glaucomatous field loss. The *Heidelberg Retinal Tomography Analyzer* (*HRT*) and other similar machines are the instruments of choice for this delicate analysis. These devices measure across the spectrum of loss. They create an image of the *optic nerve* and the *retinal nerve fiber layer,* providing an analysis of the life and death of *retinal* cells.

The information gathered comprises a 3-D color-coded topographic map of the *optic nerve* including a contour outline of the optic cup. The instrument performs this task by detecting reflected laser light. The nerve fiber layer contains a property called *birefringence* that reflects polarized light. Within the nerve fibers are microtubules that compose the *birefringent* area. The greater the amount of reflected light, the greater number of microtubules present. The more the better. Measurements include the surface contour of the optic nerve head and nerve fiber layer thickness, disc area, cup-to-disc ratios, cup shape, height variation contour, rim area, rim volume, maximum cup depth, cup area, cup volume, *retinal nerve fiber layer (RNFL)* cross-section area, and mean *RNFL* thickness. It measures the thickness of ten *retinal fiber layers*. In other words, it provides a detailed picture of the *optic nerve head*.

As with all imaging systems, information of your visual field is compared statistically to other patients in your age range. Findings are especially useful for evaluating those people labeled high ocular intensives where no detected vision loss is apparent through the use of other evaluative tools. Early glaucoma detection is one of *HRT's* strengths for it can possibly detect minute changes in the *nerve fiber layer* possibly signaling glaucoma progression. Testing can be performed on either dilated or non-dilated eyes if the pupil measures a 6-mm area and fixation is no problem. An image takes 2 seconds. Astigmatism apparently does not distort the results.

The *HRT* is usually recommended when patients can't take the *Visual Field Test*, for children who have a short attention span, and when a physician needs to assess the extent of glaucoma damage. Although the *Visual Field Test* (see below) and the *HRT* are used diagnostically, each test provides a different aspect of glaucomatous damage. The *Visual Field Test* evaluates the extent of vision remaining; the *HRT*, the *optic nerve* condition. Together they complement each other.

SCANNING LASER POLARIMETRY

The *GDx* is one example. This technology assesses the condition of the *retina* and *optic nerve*. It does not image the nerve, but rather utilizes a nerve fiber analyzer consisting of a diode laser and a computer. It is basically used to examine the integrity of the intercellular structures of the *retinal nerve fiber layer*. In this system, it is the amount of reflected light that provides this reading. It works this way: a single source of light hitting the eye splits in two directions and then travels in two optical paths. One path travels into and back out; the other travels to and from a reflecting surface. By moving the reflector, researchers can examine tissue. This double pass (polarized light) penetrates the *retinal fiber layer* providing the examiner with a measurable degree of change. This degree of change is proportional to the thickness of the *retinal fiber layer.* This process is computerized and a printout provides the examiner with graphic information about the condition of the *nerve fiber layer.* A thin layer indicates that cells have been lost. These instruments can work with non-dilated pupils and see through lens opacity. An age and racial database provides a comparative scale that helps determine if cell loss is comparable to those in the age and race range. The test is easy on the patient since it may or may not require dilation. Corneal contact and a bright light flash are minimal. Some studies indicate that African-Americans may have thinner *retinal* fiber layers which may account for the greater preponderance of glaucoma in this group. This is a highly portable instrument.

Imaging instruments continue to evolve. Researchers at Aberdeen University in the UK have developed a true color *scanning laser ophthalmoscope.* This instrument employing low light intensity and is more comfortable for the patient, but one of the drawbacks consists of only single color images, thus possibly obscuring important diagnostic information. New instrumentation to study the effect of diabetes on the blood vessels may soon become routine. *Diabetic Retinopathy* causes blood vessels to proliferate all over the eye. But this process may be stopped cold if doctors can detect the tiniest breaks and hemorrhages. To reveal these blood vessels, scientists need to overcome the obscuring effect of melanin (brown pigment). In the UK, scientists are developing software that can be attached to an *ophthalmoscope.* This technology should be especially useful for patients who have dark *iris*es.

Doctors caution, however, that these instruments alone do not make a case for glaucoma, since the variation in the normal population must be taken into account. Nevertheless, because the tests are objective, less error should occur albeit obbjective interpretation of the data may still present a problem. Studies have documented differences among technicians analyzing the results of a scan. Furthermore, since there is so much variation in the appearance of the structures of the eye, the instruments may denote false positives or false negatives. An experienced clinician certainly takes these considerations into account.

The instruments may prove to be most productive for evaluation of younger patients with little visual field loss. Taking into account longer life expectancy, a fraction of *nerve fiber* loss may, over time, incrementally add up to significant vision loss if treatment is not instituted early. These instruments also help determine whether glaucoma is progressive. There are some patients who do just fine using only drops with no need of further interventions, while others (me included), must be closely monitored. You may be a patient who on the first go-round has little evidence of damage but over the course of several years, may benefit from being followed with an imaging system.

The term for these follow-up measures is called *serial analysis* and is especially important to determine whether a "suspect" patient needs treatment.

These imaging instruments are also useful for analyzing *macular holes, diabetic retinopathy*, and other optic nerve conditions.

Optical Coherence Tomography (OCT) or Confocal Scanning Laser Ophthalmoscope (CSLO)

The *OCT* provides a cross-section evaluation of the *retina*, assessing the *retinal* layers affected by disease. The *OCT* is the instrument of choice by many physicians for it offers an in-depth look at the *retina* (axial resolution). Laser light travels along two pathways--one branch to the *retina* and the other to a reference mirror. Light from the mirror along with backscatter of light reflected from the *retinal* structures combine on the return pathway. Interference pathways are then detected.

The *OCT* is a neat, noninvasive little unit. Compact, powered by a confocal scanning diode laser, it is relatively low in cost and can be mounted on the slit lamp. It measures all ten layers of the *retina* and creates a contour map of the *optic nerve*, optic cup and *retinal nerve fiber layer* thickness. Unlike instruments that use sound waves, the OCT employs light waves that provide a higher resolution than sound waves. Simply, reflected light from your *retina* and *optic nerve* is displayed by means of a video camera providing viewing access to these structures. The ultra-high resolution enables clinicians to observe subtle disease processes affecting the *retina*. The instrument is also used to check for *macular holes* and *macular* changes, analyzing for non-organic vision loss in patients who complain of poor vision. The test requires good fixation, for the instrument constructs the composite image from nine individual scans. Your eyes must remain fixated throughout the process.

An advanced optical coherence device *(OCT3)* is capable of measuring the central *corneal* thickness, an important feature for evaluating *intraocular pressure*. It uses cross- sectional images of the *retina* and computes the incident light reflected for a given tissue. With this instrument, the *retinal* layers can be analyzed for a more detailed diagnosis of a number of different eye conditions. Also using an adaptation of *Doppler* technology that provides for lower power, the velocity and pattern of distribution of the blood flow can be measured. Other advances include reduction in scanning time.

Technology moves so quickly that it's hard to keep abreast of all the developments. *HIGH-DEFINITION OCT* provides higher resolution, resulting in more precise diagnosis of various conditions. Accuracy not previously attained is possible with this instrument. Known about in theory, histological images of the layers of the *retina* have finally been viewed. The first white layer is clearly defined as is the *retinal nerve fiber layer* which is the most superficial layer in the *retina*. This layer if damaged is responsible for glaucoma. It is possible also with this imaging device to locate the damaged and the healthy segments and to measure the normal thickness. Imaging of the *retina*, the *fovea* and the *macula* add to the analysis of *retinal* health preempting what eventually appears on a visual field. Puzzling cases become clearer with an *OCT* scan as in the case of a patient who complained of a blue haze over one eye. All the findings were normal and the case was not solved until the scan revealed a condition called *central retinopathy*, in which fluid accumulates underneath the *retina* and causes visual distortions and even vision loss.

In Hanover, Germany, scientists have developed an *OCT* guided laser instrument capable of cutting or ablating tissue. In addition, the confocal scanning lasers have other applications. Researchers at Rockefeller University in New York have discovered that migrating proteins move in a two-step stroke motion. This particular type of imaging still at the exploratory stage but may one day give scientists insight on how structures in the brain are built, how nerve cells migrate and eventually reveal underlying factors driving genetic malfunctions that cause glaucoma. The newer instruments combine speed with accuracy and higher definition.

A large study of high IOP individuals revealed differences in the *optic* nerves of African-Americans who possess significantly larger *optic discs*, *neuroretinal rims*, optic cups, and cup-to-disc ratios than other groups. This information calls for a different set of standards for this ethnic group. Although hypertension has been associated with the African-American's greater susceptibility to glaucoma, a study did not confirm this finding.

ULTRASOUND BIOMICROPOSY (UBM)

We are all familiar with ultrasound used routinely to view the developing fetus. *UBM* follows some of the same principles. It is calibrated to detect a structure as tiny as fifty microns (a micron is half the width of a human hair). The reflected sound waves provide important information on the internal anatomy of the eye--*iris, lens*, especially the *ciliary body* and most importantly, the angle where the *cornea* and *iris* converge. This instrument is particularly useful in diagnosing *narrow-angle* glaucoma, for it provides a clear picture of the angle and surgical effects on the angle. There are two forms--the A-scan provides pre-op evaluation prior to cataract surgery and the B-scan for examination of the interior of the eye. The B-form distinguishes between cysts (water based) and tumors (solid). To take this test, the eye is anesthetized and a transducer (liquid in an eyecup) is placed on the eye. The transducer receives the reflected beams. The instrument is helpful in diagnosing *plateau iris, pigmentary dispersion syndrome, nanophthalmos* and possibly suspected *ciliary body* tumors. Measurement of the thickness of the *cornea* equals the *pachymetry* measurement. To take this test, you lie on a table. The technician applies a pen-sized instrument to your anesthetized eye close to the surface of the *cornea* for a few minutes and that's it.

DARC (Detection of Apotosing Retinal Cells)

This non-invasive imaging istrument allows your doctor to visualize a single *retinal* nerve cell's death. This imaging technique detects early glaucomatous changes enabling doctors to make rapid and objective assessment of potential neuroprotective sight-saving strategies as well as response to treatment. Furthermore, it should dramatically shorten the length of glaucoma clinical studies.

Digital Stereo Disc Imaging

This method is an update of *Stereo Disc Photography* still in use in a number of settings. *Optic disc photography* can document glaucoma progress. Unfortunately, individuals reading the photographs tend to be subjective and this may pose long-term evaluative problems. This updated version may correct the problem, for its black and white stereo images can be viewed in stereo and stored on the hard drive. The images provide cup-to-disc ratios at all orientations. The examiner can monitor changes in the *optic nerve* through comparison of new data with that already on file. The system can also be modified for examining the *macula*. This updated version, thankfully, reduces to minutes the time involved in the painstaking series of evaluating stereophotographs. Good dilation and fixation are necessary for taking this test. For those who qualify, according to some clinicians, the test is invaluable, for it provides an excellent tracking record of the *optic nerve head*, despite problems associated with technicians' subjective interpretation of the results.

Measuring Blood Flow

Blood flow is one of the paramount considerations in treating certain forms of glaucoma, especially *normal tension glaucoma.* The *optic nerve* requires a steady blood supply as does every tissue in the body. Pressure inside the eye plays against the pressure inside the blood vessels and this physiological mechanism acts on the blood supply that reaches the optic nerve. When equilibrium exists between these two pressures, blood flow to the *optic nerve* is unimpeded. But should high pressure exist in the eye, blood flow will be affected. On the other hand, should the pressure in the eye be normal but the systemic blood pressure abnormally low, blood supply to the optic nerve is also affected. When the supply is such that it starves the *optic nerve* of blood, the condition often leads to *normal-tension glaucoma.*

The rate of blood flow is also apparently affected by factors other than blood flow dynamics. Second-hand smoke can lead to decreased blood flow, cold air may increase blood flow, decreased estrogen in older patients may affect blood flow, and decreased blood flow may affect different parts of the eye. Rate and volume of blood flow may also differ in each eye. Systemic, environmental, medical treatment for other problems and age are additional factors. Obviously this is a complicated issue. There is, however, a group of glaucoma patients who fall into the category of what is called "vasculopathic." These people have a history of *Raynaud's Disease,* systemic hypertension, migraine, *normal-tension glaucoma,* vascular damage, diabetes, tumor, sleep apnea, or even suffer from nutritional damage. Blood flow in this group may affect the course of their glaucoma. *Optic disc pallor* is one of the telling signs.

When doctors observe a pale *optic nerve,* they enlist a number of instruments designed to assess the rate and volume of blood flow. The instruments listed below assess whether the *optic nerve* receives its complement of nutrition ported by the blood. While a number of instruments ostensibly measure blood flow in the eye, accuracy may be difficult to determine, although in animal studies, scientists are coming closer to this goal. Nevertheless, should the *optic disc* be pale, the clinician may want to attempt to establish a baseline at the very least. Below are some of the instruments used for that purpose.

FLUORESCEIN ANGIOGRAPHY (EXAMINATION OF THE DISC AND RETINAL VESSELS)

This most commonly-used instrument requires an injection of fluorescein *sodium,* a red dye, into a vein in the arm. Some people experience a reaction to intravenous *fluorescein.* I did. I felt nauseous but the condition subsided within a few minutes. The dye circulates through the veins and when it reaches the blood pathways of the eye, the rate of flow is computer analyzed. The printout is then compared against a standard.

Indocyanine Green Angiography— (Examines The Choroidal Vessels)

This procedure follows the same process as above, except the dye is *Indocyanine green.*

Infrared Scanning Laser Tomography

This instrument combines infrared imaging and a *scanning laser ophthalmoscope.* Fluorescein is also injected. Lesions and new blood vessels not always visible with standard fluorescein angiography are easier to see, since the instrument's light penetrates more deeply into the eye. Use of the instrument may increase the understanding of underlying causes of *macular* problems and provide serial analysis (follow-up) to determine whether a "suspect" patient has moved into the glaucoma category.

Scanning Laser Ophthalmoscopic Flowmetry (measures retinal blood flow)

This system uses an infrared diode laser to scan the eye. It assesses the rate of blood flows into the arteries, veins and capillaries. The image can be viewed on a monitor or a printout either in black and white or in color. Another technique uses computerized polarization imaging to illuminate the tissue. This device is attached to a video camera providing a view of the blood flow. It is especially attractive, for the probe is surrounded by a stabilization device, designed to eliminate image distortion by steadying the examiner's hand, a problem inherent in involuntary hand movements. The quality of pallor is assessed using a digital color image of the *optic disc.*

COLOR DOPPLER FLOWMETRY (Limited resolution of larger nerve, *retinal* and orbital vessels) Prints out color images.

Tracking Laser Ophalmoscope

This adaptation of the *ophthalmoscope* overcomes the fixation problem that older patients often experience. Researchers at Physical Sciences Inc. and Schepens Eye Research Institute and *Retinal* Specialists developed this instrument. It is capable of observing blood flow in the *retina* and underlying *choroids* in real time. Combined with fluorescein imaging technology, the tracker adjusts for eye movements allowing researchers to precisely view blood flow. At this writing, this device has yet to reach the marketing stage.

The search continues to develop instruments that provide even greater precision for assessing blood flow dynamics. Many glaucoma patients remark about the good-bad eye syndrome. A recent report about an experimental two-photon imaging system that captures information on capillary blood flow may provide some insight into this disparity between the two eyes. Researchers found that blood cell velocity and density vary independently of each other but both systems contribute to vascular signals.

ELECTROPHYSIOLOGY

Two tests--*the eclectroretinogram (ERG) and the visual-evoked potential (VEP)* measure the *retinal ganglion cells.* The *ERG* registers the electrical response of the *retina* to a brief pulse of light that illuminates the entire *retina.* People with glaucoma register less light. Some studies have indicated that this test is useful for identifying patients at risk for *neovascularization* (proliferation of blood vessels), especially those patients who have had *central retinal vein occlusion..*

OBJECTIVE VISUAL FIELD TESTING--MULTIFOCAL VISUAL EVOKED POTENTIAL (MFVEP)

A visual field test can be either objective or subjective. The subjective test most commonly used is the *Humphrey Visual Field Analyzer* (see below). The objective field test requires no patient input. Currently, two objective field tests exist--the *Multifocal Visual Evoked Potential (mfvep)* and the *Magnetic Encephalogram (MEG).* The *mfvep* (many flashing lights) records the potential or electrical activity in the brain when lights are seen. The *MEG* evaluates damage from glaucoma. Through electrical stimulation, the *VEP* test probes the primary occipital visual areas located in the lower back of the brain. It measures the brain's activity as the *EKG (electrocardiogram)* measures that of the heart. Different pathologies such as *retinitis pigmentosa* or glaucoma will produce characteristic variations in electrical responses. Studies on the effectiveness of the test for detecting glaucoma are generally favorable and despite the required length of time, the patient is relieved of action and may actually prefer the experience. Since this is an objective test, the patient is only required to look at a series of images. The setup involves placing electrodes on the back the head to record responses.

The *mfvep* reveals information about the visual pathway. Studies indicate that assessment on the *mfvep* is comparable to the *Humphrey Visual Field Test Analyzer* (see below) although each test assesses different pathways. These instruments are especially sensitive for detecting changes in the *magno* cell pathways and they also have the potential to signal *retinal* damage before it is visible on the *visual field test*. A study of fifty glaucoma patients compared the *mfvep* results with the *Humphrey Visual Field Analyzer* and found a favorable comparison in detecting visual field loss. Each instrument, however, did detect abnormalities not found in the other. What sets apart the *multifocal mfvep* as a favorable assessment instrument is its objectivity. Its chief drawback is the time required (about 20 minutes each eye) to fully display the geometric images. It is also not foolproof. While "patient subjectivity" no longer presents a problem, other factors such as the greater time involved, poor electrode contact and patient movement are.

LOW VISION EVALUATOR

This instrument measures the light perception in patients who have very low visual function. Light is graded into nine different intensities and delivered randomly. Each eye takes four minutes for testing.

SPIRAL COMPUTED TOMOGRAPHY

There is some evidence that various sophisticated instruments can detect other diseases as well as glaucoma. German researchers found that the use of *spiral computed tomography* revealed a tumor in some *normal tension* patients, the *optic nerve* sitting unusually close to the *carotid artery* and atherosclerosis the *ophthalmic arteries*. This is essentially a CAT scan of the eye.

LASER TREATMENT FOR MACULAR DEGENERATION (ARMD)

`The *Thermal Laser*, one of the earlier developments, is practical only if lesions are outside the *foveal* center (extrafoveal). It photocoagulates (destroys) the *neovascular membrane*, but its application is limited because of the fifty percent rate of reoccurrence and few cases of *extrafoveal ARMD*.

Photodynamic Therapy (PDT is Another *ARMD* treatment. It does stabilize acuity (as compared to natural history) and it is somewhat more successful. The procedure involves injecting a photosensitizing dye *Visudyne (verteporfin)* into the arm of the patient. The dye travels through the body and is taken up by proliferating blood vessels. It is then directed at these vessels destroying them. Both used only with the wet form of *ARMD*.

RAMAN SPECTROSCOPE

Is it possible to measure the level of carotenoids in the eye? Well, yes it might be. Researchers at the Moran Eye Center, University of Utah, Salt Lake City, using a device called the *Raman Spectroscope,* ostensibly measured the level of *carotenoids* and other compounds in the human eye. A small experiment revealed that levels of *carotenoids* were fifty percent lower in the average fifty-five-year-old compared to the typical twenty-six-year-old. Early studies indicated that *carotenoids* in the *macula* were a third lower in the *macular degeneration* group than in an age-matched control group.

From the range of instruments listed above, it is increasingly evident that scientists are searching for a deeper understanding of the physiology of the eye and are amassing a body of information that may one day lead to better treatment and possibly a cure. The instruments detecting loss before it is observed in the visual field posit the question of whether earlier intervention will prevent visual loss further down the line. Loss of *nerve fiber* in the *optic nerve* is a clear indication of glaucoma damage. The greater the loss of fiber accompanied by increasing cup size foretells greater visual field damage. As more knowledge accumulates from present and future imaging instruments, it is hoped that the ravages of glaucoma will be stemmed.

Nevertheless, one size does not fit all. There are a range of physical structures found in the general population in the body and the *optic nerve* is no exception. Different structural characteristics between African-Americans and Caucasians, for example, call for individual approaches. A study of these two groups found the rim area of the African-Americans was independently predictive of field loss. Age also plays a part. Treatment varies depending upon the age of the individual. Obviously, what is right for you may not be right for me.

Whether your eye doctor subscribes to some of the newer methods of detecting nerve-tissue damage or relies on visual observation, the goal is to closely observe changes in the *optic nerve*. Should damage be detected, steps will be taken to stop, or at least slow *nerve-fiber loss*. At present, unfortunately, expense may be an issue, for using sophisticated instruments for monitoring may not be covered by insurance. Some doctors claim that these instruments provide no more information than a series of *visual field tests.* This routine test is commonly administered once or twice a year. The majority of glaucoma patients, as well as others with varying eye diseases, will probably have experienced it. Below is a description of the test along with tips for understanding it and for doing better at it.

THE VISUAL FIELD ANALYZERS

You can get a rough idea of your visual field by simply fixating on a spot or picture on the wall in front of you. Now note whether you can see the left and right walls without turning your head or your eyes. The amount of wall you can see on either side of you crudely represents the perimeter of your visual field. Naturally, the instruments used to test your actual visual field are far more sensitive than this little experiment. If your vision is normal, you see up to 109 degrees on the temporal side (away from the nose), 65 degrees toward the nose, 60 degrees above the nose and 75 degrees below the nose. If you train your eyes on a fixed point, you can still see from side to side and up and down. A graphic illustration of the visual field is depicted as a hill or island. The largest cluster of cells representing cones in the macula is at the top or center of the hill. The tippy tip, incredibly just a speck of tissue provides clear, focused vision for seeing both distant and near objects. Along the sides of the hill the collection of cells diminishes. These are the peripheral cells that work at dusk into night. They also are the detectors of motion. School teachers are well aware of the action of their peripheral cells when cut-ups in their classes accuse teacher of having eyes in the back of the head. It's catching a movement response—that corner of your eye phenomenon that puts the kid back in his or her seat. Actually, your eye can see a complete circle except for the natural blind spot where the *optic nerve* exits on its way to brain. The eye also performs saccadic movements when reading or watching a moving object. To comprehend the object, the eye must also fixate rapidly and this function is often slowed down in patients with glaucoma. A study confirmed what glaucoma patients know—it takes longer to perform a visual search task than it does for persons with normal vision.

The *Humphrey Visual Field Analyzer* is a quick, easy, and accurate test for examining the status of your visual field. It also provides information about patients with high *intraocular pressure*, glaucoma suspects or *ocular hypertensives* (patients with higher than average IOP), who do not show field defects. It has the advantage of being compact, portable, and easy for patients to use, although some patients complain that it is tedious and scary. The *visual field test* detects nerve cell loss after a percentage of loss has already occurred. This drawback lies with the non-specific nature of the test and it is less capable of detecting early glaucoma loss than the electronic instruments described above. The test relies on three *retinal ganglion* cell subtypes that send information to the brain. When glaucoma begins to damage these cells, some of which may be non-functioning, other intact cell types will respond but the sensitivity of the test is reduced.

Since there are over one million nerve cells forming the *optic nerve*, loss of a few cells shouldn't make much of a difference, and it doesn't, for as we age, we continually lose cells. But with glaucoma, cell loss is endemic and when die-off accelerates, your doctor takes steps to stem this destruction—primarily taking steps to lower your IOP. I notice my loss of peripheral cells most acutely when walking in the street and someone unexpectedly materializes at my side. Or if I'm walking with a person and unpredictably that person moves to my other side, I start looking about wondering what happened to my companion. When preparing meals, I often miss seeing an object at elbow range and end up—oops another spill to clean up. My experiences are shared with other members of the group who have lost vision.

Since glaucoma typically damages those peripheral cells first and there are fewer of them, loss of these cells primarily determines the read-out of your visual field. While loss of central vision is not as common, some people with severe glaucoma damage may be reduced to tunnel vision (an extremely narrow visual window) or no central vision at all, comparable to, but not, *macular degeneration*. Rules don't always apply. Some of us, me included, have experienced early central vision loss. When this loss occurs, fixation (your ability to focus on a single point) is compromised. Furthermore, this situation places you in the serious risk category. Usually, your doctor will try every method available to lower your IOP. There are some patients, however, who show *optic nerve* changes, but still retain a perfectly good visual field. These people fall into what is called the "preperimetric" group. They have lost nerve fiber and when identified, they too, need to be followed and treated accordingly.

The results of a field test provide your doctor comprehensive information for interpreting generalized field depression, local depression, short-and long-term fluctuations, individual attentiveness and comparison between fields. Furthermore, your doctor may be able to determine if you require careful follow-up or if you're a lucky low-risk candidate.

There is a learning curve to taking a visual field. Studies indicate you may need to take up to four visual field tests before you reach a comfortable plateau. The learning curve, however, begins to diminish in six months. If this is your first shot at taking a visual field test and you feel you haven't done your best, ask to take another before a baseline is established.

Points of Light

Although the *Goldmann* and the *Humphrey Visual Field Analyzers* are both valid *visual field tests*, the two instruments differ in the form of presentation of the target or stimulus. The *Goldmann* uses a kinetic system; the Humphrey uses a system called static perimetry. They both use a white on white screen. The manually-driven *Goldmann* may soon be mothballed, for it requires the full-time services of a technician, but for some patients, especially those older, and those who also have lost a lot of sight and become rattled by the pace of the *Humphrey*, the *Goldmann* is a more comfortable experience. Although there is some evidence that fixation is easier with a kinetic target rather than the static target, this information has not deterred the general use of the Humphrey. If you do need a technician, however, to nudge you awake and question whether you actually see the target, you may still have the option of taking the Goldmann provided one is available in the facility you use. Both of these instruments are computerized and chart the status of your visual field.

The setup is similar. You are positioned with your forehead resting against the headrest and your chin settling into the chin rest. One eye is occluded (covered) and you are handed a buzzer. The examiner adjusts the instrument and instructs you to focus on the center dot. You may find it easy at first, but because of its length, you may experience difficulties, often resulting in searching for the pulse of light. When you see a spot of light (target) you press the buzzer. Apart from the anxiety of taking a visual field test, and this can be considerable, the actual process couldn't be simpler.

Kinetic Perimetry

As discussed above, although the *Goldmann* has been mainly replaced by the *Humphrey*, you may be more comfortable with this form of visual field testing. For many years I happily, if I can use that word together with low-level anxiety, took my visual fields on the *Goldmann*. The technician in that office made sure that I saw the target. Alas, my ophthalmologist retired. My present ophthalmologist uses only the Humphrey and while I'm still uncomfortable with this instrument, I grit my teeth and buzz away. With the *Goldmann* the target light moves from the periphery to the center. As peripheral loss occurs, your field of vision becomes narrower. These losses are indicated on a chart containing concentric lines that indicate the status of your visual field.

STATIC PERIMETRY

Light stimulus remains fixed but brightness is increased until it becomes apparent. The *Humphrey* relies on automated computer programming to probe the threshold of light--that is, the very dimmest pinprick of light that you can see. To do this, a point of light is presented at its dimmest and progressively increased in brightness and size until you see it. If you have lost cells in a particular area, whatever the size or brightness, you will be unable to see the light in that area. Two programs are available, differing in the number of targeted points: the 30-2 program evaluates seventy-four individual points within the central 30 degrees of the visual field; the 24-2 program evaluates fifty-eight points. The 24-2 program eliminates some of the points where patients make the most errors, and is generally preferred by ophthalmologists. It also takes less time. The *Humphrey* is designed to prevent random buzzing through intermittent flashing of the target. People who have lost little vision can tolerate the system unlike those who have lost a sizeable amount that affects their ability to fixate. Not seeing anything even for a second or two increases tension. In the desperate search for the stimulus fixation becomes uneven. Some technicians will gently chide you into refocusing. If you're anxious and fearful that you won't be able to take the test, request that your technician remain at your side.

Humphrey has also produced technology using *short wave-length automated perimentry* (*SWAP*). The background is bright yellow, the stimulus blue. The yellow background adapts to the rods and the red and green cones. The blue target on a yellow background isolates the blue pathways found in the periphery, which may be the first to be affected by glaucoma. This test has been found to be particularly useful for detecting early glaucoma field loss. It appears to be an excellent tool for evaluating possible field damage in persons with high IOP readings but show no visible field loss on other instruments. Although the time span is shorter, veteran glaucoma patients usually find *SWAP* difficult to take. Some studies, however, still claim that the white on white using a #1 stimulus (tiny light) format is superior in detecting early losses in the perimeter.

The main problem with the *Humphrey* is the time involved. Each eye can take as long as 15-to-20 minutes for a full scan. In some cases, your doctor may elect to use another system that is gaining in popularity and is part of the standard equipment of late model *Humphrey Field Analyzers*. It is called the *Swedish Interactive Threshold Algorithm* (*SITA*). Although a brief test, this instrument has been found to correlate highly with the standard *Humphrey*, for it can track down a defect in the *nerve fiber* bundle. The program is correlated to concentrate on visual field defects bypassing for the most part healthy tissue. If you find yourself in a busy clinic, you may well be tested on *SITA*.

COMMON PITFALLS

- You start to search for the target light.
- You buzz too soon or not often enough.
- Your attention wanders or you drowse off or even in the worst scenario you drift off to sleep.
- Your head slips off the chin rest and drifts off the forehead bar-rest reducing your ability to view the targets.
- You are physically uncomfortable. Your back hurts.
- If you are amply endowed, you may not be able to get close enough to the instrument.

Test anxiety may cause a stressful reaction such as tightening up your muscles.

AVOIDANCE OF PITFALLS:

- Be aware that you are not supposed to see all of the targets. The computer determines the state of your vision and delivers a program according to your capability.
- Be sure you're seated comfortably. The technician can adjust both the chair and the headrest to your needs.
- Get a good night's sleep.
- Don't be intimidated. Ask the technician to explain a procedure.
- Should you become fatigued during the test, simply hold down the button on your buzzer and the program will automatically pause to give you a rest. Lifting your thumb from the button tells the computer to resume.
- If troubled by excess light in the room, background noise, or whatever else may disturb your concentration, discuss this situation with the technician.

ERRORS

That dreaded word has reverberations of school days. Well, you're not in class. Unless you're legally blind, you *cannot fail* the test. If you're asked to repeat the test, however, it's not because you've messed up, but because your doctor wants to verify its accuracy. To avoid the fatigue factor, do not repeat on the same day. Should the computerized model be too difficult for you, it's possible to still be tested on the *Goldmann Perimentry* if one is available.

HOW TO READ THE PRINTOUT:

Depending upon your condition, the printout will show a mixture of black and white areas. These indicate how much functional vision remains. The black areas indicate where cells have died off. The top three numbers in the right hand corner indicate fixation losses, false positive and negative errors. The bottom schematic is the pattern of deviation that corrects for age-matched controls. For example, your assessment may appear worse than it is if it were not based on people in your age bracket.

Fixation error

This reading reflects your search for the target. If you make twenty percent fixation errors, the test is unreliable. This does not mean that you are unreliable, but that there is something hampering your performance. A technician can assess and correct the problem.

False Negative Errors

The computer knows what you can and cannot see. If you miss a bright light, the computer assesses that you're not paying attention and this constitutes a false negative error. More than a third false negative errors render the test unreliable.

False Positive Errors

You respond to lights that you should not be able to see. Here again if you produce a third of false positive errors, the test becomes unreliable and needs to be repeated.

How often should the test be repeated? This depends upon each individual case. Where glaucoma progression is suspected or if the test you've taken is considered unreliable, more often; when there appears to be stability, yearly. Remember, there is a learning curve. If you have to repeat the test it's not the end of the world.

Many times the technician wanders in and out of the room while you're taking the visual field test. For experienced confident people, this spotty oversight may not affect your performance but if your test registers both false negative and false positive errors, the technician should be on hand to help you through the process.

OTHER PROBLEMS YOU MAY EXPERIENCE

You may be sensitive to the lighting. When there is considerable loss, it is important that the room is dark or dim to eliminate any light competing with the screen illumination. Your clothing, skin, or hair may absorb or reflect light depending on color and style. Eye conditions other than glaucoma, such as cataracts, may thwart your efforts to do the best you can. You may have a constricted pupil, a result of either having taken *carbacohl* or *pilocarpine*. Other possible physical problems may occur with your reaction time. You have been advised to buzz almost simultaneously when you see the stimulus light. But let's face it, the *Humphrey* test is long and boring especially if you see fewer stimuli. Your mind may wander or just close down.

Most importantly is your state of mind. If you are depressed, upset, worrying not only about the test but about other life situations, you may not do well. Distracted by the death of her husband, Jane could not keep her grief in check during a routine visual field test. Although glaucoma was in her family, previous visual fields had not indicated signs of glaucoma until that particular test. Her ophthalmologist, aware of her loss, scheduled a repeat in three months. This time Jane's field test, reflecting her more positive frame of mind, was more in keeping with the previous tests. Medication for other physical problems may reduce your alertness. Some medications cause sleepiness, others affect reaction time. Discuss these possibilities with both your doctor and the technician and see if adjustments can be made.

Other reasons to question the accuracy of a field test lie with the physics of the eye. Researchers have found that the *retina* needs a bit of a rest, two seconds worth, after it has responded to the dimmest light, and that as the threshold of light advances, it needs greater light. These crucial seconds may produce less accurate visual fields. Additionally, if you are mature, your *retina* no longer has the capacity of its younger days and if you're *myopic* to boot, your field of vision is decreased (even in people who do not have glaucoma). If these conditions apply to you, discuss them with the technician. A high IOP may also give a misreading of a test and that's another reason for keeping your pressure within the prescribed range.

Be aware that if you're a smoker, your visual field may be compromised. The effects of smoking in healthy people taking *visual field tests* revealed a decrease in *retinal* sensitivity. A small study in Sweden matched normal visual acuities with smokers and non-smokers. Although there was no *optic neuropathy* with either group and central vision was unaffected, there was loss of *retinal* sensitivity in the smokers.

FREQUENCY DOUBLING TECHNOLOGY (FDT)

This is an appealing test for mass screenings for it is easily transported and the test takes only minutes. This instrument is also part of the *Humphrey* family. It isolates a small section of *retinal ganglion cells*--the magno cellular pathways, that researchers believe indicate early signs of glaucoma. Interestingly, loss of these cells is also noted in dyslexia (inability to interpret written language). *Magno* cells respond to movement and contrast and loss of motion sensitivity is a predictor of glaucomatous loss. The test consists of sixteen flickering patterns of black and white bars that create the illusion through rapid counter-phase flicker that there are twice as many bars (hence the term frequency doubling). Strain-free on the patient, the test can be taken in ambient lighting. Patients can wear their glasses; are relieved of the chin rest because the test is fast. Taking this test is simplicity itself. You gaze into a viewer and press a button each time the target flashes. An occluder built into the machine blocks the eye not being tested. One pattern is projected at a time. You receive a printed form immediately upon completing the test indicating whether you are within normal limits or have a mild, moderate or severe vision loss. The *FDT* takes forty-five seconds for each eye. I tried it out and of course, it indicated that I had glaucoma.

Possible is an expanded version of the *FDT* that compares favorably with the *Humphrey*. This version takes 4-to-5 minutes in each eye. Some researchers claim that results are comparable to the standard *Humphrey*, for because the eye is sensitive to flicker and contrast, the instrument has the capability of detecting glaucomatous loss especially in the early stages, providing in a few minutes information that equals the standard *Humphrey*, albeit that different sets of cells are targeted. People with cataracts can still be tested accurately with the *FDT*. Some studies claim that detecting visual loss in persons with *normal-tension* glaucoma is equal to if not better than with the standard Humphrey.

Should you ask your doctor to administer the *FDT* and save you time? You can, provided that your doctor agrees and has access to the instrument. What usually happens in real time is that your doctor has his or her own preferences for a particular instrument, one that is readily available and which in concert with the technician, offers a substantially accurate reading of the *optic nerve*. For children under the age of eight, however, given their limited attention span, the *FDT* is ideal.

Corneal Cell Count

The *cornea*, so crucial for sight, may lose cells. There is a likelihood that cells will be lost each time an invasive procedure is performed on the eye. Various eye diseases, especially those affecting the *cornea* as described in Chapter 2 can affect the cell count of the *cornea* dramatically. Before any invasive procedure surgeons now routinely perform a preoperative *corneal* cell count. The instrument that makes this possible is called a *specular microscope* combined with an *automated cell counter*. Light is reflected from the cell layer allowing for visualization of the individual cells.

Color Vision Test

Color vision defects are usually inherited and are more common in males. My husband has the common color blindness that confuses the red-green spectrum. Acquired color vision defects, however, are caused by diseases that affect the *cone cells*, inner *retinal layers*, optic nerve fibers or *visual cortex*. *Macula* lesions cause a defect in the *cones* concentrated around the edge of the *fovea*. Cloudiness of the *cornea, lens* or *vitreous* will distort color vision. While the color vision test is not routine (I was tested only once), faulty color vision may have a profound impact on the quality of life.

The Retina and Glaucoma

Should a *retinal* problem be suspected, your doctor may refer you to a retinologist. This is a good idea, especially for people with severe *myopia*, for the stretching of the *retina* due to the elongation of the eye may result in *retinal* tears or *retinal detachment*. That's how all my eye problems began, and I now have a yearly check on my *retina*. A retinologist will also evaluate the health of the *macula* to rule out *macular degeneration*.

Systemic Diseases Affecting Glaucoma

Blood pressure rhythms during sleep may be a central or a peripheral reason that glaucoma worsens. A study by the Scheie Eye Institute, University of Pennsylvia,   monitored a group of glaucoma suspects against a group of normals throughout the night. Results of the study indicated reduced blood flow in the glaucoma suspects. To add insult to injury, the IOP also rises at this crucial time. This raises the question of the delicate balance again. Patients on blood pressure medication may experience a reduction in blood flow that will impact on the *optic nerve*. If you are taking such medication, ask your eye doctor to work with your general practitioner to calibrate a safe dosage. Overnight monitoring of your blood pressure is possible using *Laser Doppler flowmetry.*

In the years to come, systemic problems may well enter into the diagnostic evaluation. Scientists exploring the acid-sensing ion channels in a rat model of glaucoma found that a subtype of one of these channels is increased in *retinal ganglion* cells, suggesting that this effect is related to mechanical and ischemic (lack of blood) injury.

Now that you've been diagnosed as a glaucoma patient, you will be under your doctor's care for treatment of this chronic disease. In most cases, such treatment begins with medication. The types, uses and side-effects of the drugs are explored in the next chapter.

CHAPTER 5

Medication Treatment—
A Drop or Two A Day Keeps The
Scalpel Away

○ ○

Good Medicine Is Bitter To The Taste

Chinese Proverb

Treatment for glaucoma traditionally begins with drops that lower elevated *intraocular pressure*. In some cases, laser treatment is initially recommended, for findings from a number of collaborative studies, some of which are still ongoing, has equalized this playing field. With double-blind data collection (neither doctor nor patient know whether treatment or a placebo is being administered) or field studies using strategies for protecting the *optic nerve*, treatment of glaucoma may be leading to new directions. While long-term glaucoma patients may not yet fully benefit from innovative applications, newly-diagnosed patients may find their eye doctors suggesting treatment that does not have a familiar ring. Below is a brief summary of some of the more important studies that will most likely infuse treatment of glaucoma.

THE EARLY MANIFEST GLAUCOMA TRIAL (EMGT)

This is the first randomized trial to determine the effectiveness of treatment vs. no treatment for moderate *open-angle, normal-tension*, and *exfoliative* glaucoma in the presence of IOPs of 20 mmHg or less. This landmark trial has illuminated whether treatment for glaucoma is effective in stemming visual field loss. The multicenter trial conducted in Sweden lasted six years and followed 225 patients, aged fifty-five-through- eighty diagnosed with early stage glaucoma. Those patients treated with a *trabeculoplasty* plus *betaxolol* had lesser field loss than those who were not treated. While some of the patients not receiving treatment did fine, the *exfoliative* patients did not. The worse outcomes included a higher baseline IOP, *exfoliation, bilateral disease*, more severe visual field loss, older age and disc hemorrhages. One-third of the non-treatment group had no field loss after five years. There was a trend towards higher death rate and cataract formation in the treated group. Nevertheless, while the results of the study indicate that some low-risk patients (glaucoma suspects) may be followed closely, elevated IOP does constitute a real threat of vision loss in susceptible individuals and overall, reviewing the data, evidence confirms that treatment, regardless of the condition of the *optic nerve*, is beneficial towards protecting the visual field. An interesting and important finding from this study suggested that lowering IOP by as little as one mmHg improved the risk for developing glaucoma by about ten percent.

The option of whether to use medical therapy vs. laser *trabeculoplasty* as a first line treatment may rest with the doctor's bias, but this study did indicate that blacks and whites respond differently. Blacks did better with laser treatment first, and whites did better when laser treatment followed medication within four years.

THE COLLABORATIVE NORMAL-TENSION GLAUCOMA STUDY (CNTG)

This study conducted on a white North American population, may not impact other races. Nearly half the *normal-tension* glaucoma patients in India and Japan have IOPs in low teens in contrast to a white population whose IOP at baseline is generally higher. The study addressed and confirmed that lowering pressure slowed visual loss, but did not investigate the problems of the autoregulation of blood flow believed to be one the root causes of *normal-tension* glaucoma. Patients with this syndrome experiencing steady visual loss also display evidence of poor blood circulation, migraines, and disc hemorrhages.

THE OCULAR HYPERTENSION TREATMENT STUDY (OHTS)

This study evaluating 1,636 individuals aged forty through eighty was divided into two groups--medicated and non-medicated. The study posed one of the thorniest questions facing eye doctors—whether or not to treat persons with *ocular hypertension* (defined as IOPs above 24 mmHg), a majority of whom have no visual field loss. The study found that about one percent of the OH patients will develop glaucoma and visual field loss. Eighty percent of OH patients did not develop glaucoma during the length of the trial. To read this data another way, 4.4% of those taking medication, compared with the non-medicated, 9.5%, did not develop glaucoma within five years. Statistically, this difference makes a case for treating high-intensives. But wait a minute. What about all those others who showed no signs of glaucoma? A good diagnostic work-up will usually untangle this problem. At risk of developing glaucoma are those with IOPs over 25 mmHg, and those with higher IOPs and larger cup-to-disk ratios. Measurement of central *corneal* thickness factors in, for a thin *cornea* reflects an erroneously low reading of the IOP. Other long-term trials found that 34 percent of the study group developed field loss after twenty years. Generally, the findings indicated that older patients may be more vulnerable, but then some doctors claim that vision loss is so gradual that these patients may be better off not medicated because of their shortened life span, and also because they may already be on a number of different medications. Even so, the results of this study raise questions about treatment for younger patients, who did not lose vision, but who may not be scott free over time. Many doctors still prefer the time-tested approach of medication first and following all patients with high *intraocular pressures*. The *American Academy of Ophthalmology* recommends a reduction of *intraocular pressure* of twenty percent for mild damage, thirty percent for moderate damage, and thirty-to-forty percent for severe damage.

THE ADVANCED GLAUCOMA INTERVENTION STUDY (AGIS)

What is the best approach for treating patients who already have glaucoma? This study evaluated the outcomes of different surgical treatments when medications failed to halt the progression of glaucoma. This randomly controlled trial followed 591 patients ranging in age from thirty-five-through-eighty for seven years. One group received laser treatment first, followed by a *trabeculectomy* if the laser failed, and a second *trabeculectomy* if the first one failed. The second group received a *trabeculectomy* first and if that failed, laser, and if the laser treatment failed, a second *trabeculectomy*. Blacks did better than whites with laser first. None of the eyes received the *antimetabolite* medications that serve to keep the wound from healing (see Chapter 7). Outcomes for both blacks and whites may reflect a better picture with *antimetabolites*. Probably the most important finding from this study was the IOP level. Patients did better when their IOPs were below 14 or 15 mmHg. Members of our support group cheer when their IOPs drop as low as 8-to-10 mmHg.

Los Angeles Latino Eye Study (LALES)

This study found that Latinos equaled Blacks in the prevalence rate of glaucoma. During the course of the study one in five individuals was newly diagnosed with *diabetes mellitus* and twenty-five were found to have *diabetic retinopathy*. These grim statistics, given that the Latino population is one of the fastest-growing in the United States, suggest that efforts to reach this population should be accelerated.

Smaller studies also offer new insight on medical therapy. Researchers have found that each eye possesses individual needs. What works in one eye may not work in the other. Many of us already have experienced this phenomenon, having lost some or most of the sight in one eye, while using the same therapeutic approaches in both eyes.

Other studies that shed light on pressure control include diurnal variations. In untreated *POAG* with IOP's of less 21 mmHG, twenty percent had pressures higher than 21 mmHG while sleeping. Risk for glaucoma for high intensives apparently increases during sleeping.

Medication

When I was first treated for glaucoma some thirty-odd years ago, only a limited number of medications were available. Not so today. The medical pantry provides a selection of more than twenty different drugs plus the convenience of taking some that have been combined. The medication choices now available have benefited many patients increasing the possibility that glaucoma can be adequately controlled with medical therapy. Furthermore, the success of some of the newer drugs may actually delay laser and/or *infiltration* therapy. As medical therapy continues to be the first treatment option in many countries, pharmaceutical companies are inspired to develop new classes of drugs from a possible 1,000 unique combinations. Even considering the results of the *Early Manifest Glaucoma Study*, suggesting that laser treatment first may be as effective as medication first, it appears from informal conversations that eye doctors and patients may still prefer to start with medical treatment. Both the *American Academy of Ophthalmology* and *The European Glaucoma Society* recommend that a diagnosis of glaucoma requires immediate therapy to lower *intraocular pressure* most often in the form of eyedrops.

Shock and dismay are often a patient's first reaction when told about the need to be on medication for possibly a lifetime. Bill complained about this inconvenience, reminding me of my own reaction when I learned that glaucoma would be my constant companion.

Taking a medication, however, is not a benign activity. What seems be an innocuous drop may produce unpleasant, and at times, serious side effects. A randomized study of 295 patients found that sixty-four percent suffered from drug intolerances and/or ineffectiveness of the drug. Of this group forty-one percent had adverse reactions. I certainly fall into the adverse reactions for although there are a larger number of medications available since my diagnosis, I am still limited to only a few. Andrea, a member of our group is allergic to the preservatives in drops, one of which, *Benzalkonium* is possibly toxic to the *trabecular* cells. Andrea has had laser but now needs to consider a *trabeculectomy.* A study involving 310 patients found that twelve percent were allergic to *Benzalkonium.* Unfortunately, medical side effects are common among glaucoma patients. Most often, however, patients do tolerate some of the effects if the medication sufficiently lowers IOP.

We who have lived with glaucoma over a period of time have developed a hate-love relationship with our medication. We understand that medication while necessary can also produce uncomfortable side effects, and in some cases, related eye problems, but, nevertheless, we are also aware that careful use of medication may stave off more serious interventions and help to preserve vision. That said, it is helpful in assessing the effects of a medication to recognize that not all will work for you. Our body chemistries are as variable as the color of our hair or the shape of our noses. When you are diagnosed with glaucoma, you may find that your doctor needs to evaluate the effectiveness of a series of drops before settling on the formula that consistently lowers your IOP. Piling on a variety of drops to lower pressure may also not be advisable. According to a study published in *The Journal of Glaucoma,* a third or fourth anti-glaucoma medication produced a clinically significant reduction in IOP in about forty-to-sixty percent of the patients, but the cumulative effect, at six months to a year, however, including safety outcomes, was relatively poor.

Stop and Go—
the Action of Pharmaceuticals

Medications must target the programmed actions of particular cells to produce an effect. Basically, the production of a medicine requires the union of two disciplines--biology and chemistry. In the laboratory, scientists study the mode of action, the effect that by stimulating or inhibiting a group of cell receptors a positive outcome results. Take the case of the amino acid *glutamate* (*glutamate* is the only amino acid metabolized in the brain and is responsible for neuronal transmission.) When there is an excess it may excite neurons too drastically possibly killing them. Development of a medicine to inhibit just enough *glutamate* to maintain transmission of messages at a healthy level and still not murder neurons challenges research scientists. Such a medication, if developed, would fall under the rubric of *neuroprotection.* Medications are divided into classes and within each class a number of medications are available. The *beta-blockers*, for example, are either *selective* or *non-selective. Selective* medications target only certain cell receptors; *non-selectives* take on the whole crew. Some medications are taken systemically and others in drop form. Medications also play double roles. The *beta-blockers*, taken for heart problems, block the action of the hormones *adrenaline* and *norepinephrine*, powerful stimulants released by the body during stress or exercise that raise blood pressure; in the eye, *beta-blockers* target the *ciliary body* cells blocking the secretion of aqueous humor, a strategy for lowering *intraocular pressure.* Less fluid in the eye protects the eye in some cases from a pressure build-up. The *prostaglandins* loosen the intracellular spaces on the *ciliary body* allowing increased *uveoscleral* outflow. The *miotics* contract the *ciliary muscles*, an action that widens the pores in the *trabecular meshwork* thus increasing egress of fluid from the eye. All drugs interact with receptors, the specialized cells or molecular structures that are located on the surfaces of the cells. This interaction is a complicated process, for substances such as hormones and neurotransmitters also get into the act. By linking up with one or more receptors in the body, like a key fitting into a lock, the drug's chemical structure then modifies the cell's activity.

Fortunately, with a large number of medications for glaucoma, your doctor can choose the most effective treatment for you, given your age and the condition of your eyes. Even so, doctors tend to favor those medications they have found to be most successful with their patients. Should you hear of a medication that someone is using successfully, you are certainly free to suggest that this might work for you. Your doctor is primarily interested in keeping your IOP at the level where your visual field remains stable.

Although the effectiveness of a medication when launched is documented, scientists still continue to study them with various groups of glaucoma patients. Partly, this continuing observation is driven by the fierce competition among the pharmaceutical companies and partly, continuing studies bolster the eye doctor's confidence in prescribing a particular drug. Many of the studies are funded by pharmaceutical companies but that may not necessarily influence your treatment. For example, although a single-center study found that 0.03% of *Lumigan* reduced IOP to a greater extent than *timolol,* a *beta-*

blocker, given individual differences, you may still be more comfortable with the *beta-blocker*.

Loss of effectiveness over time is another problem that glaucoma patients experience. This situation requires the need to re-establish a new set of protocols. Some patients find that if they discontinue a medication for several months, returning to it at a later period of time, the medication will again produce effective results. The bottom line is, of course, use the medication that works best to preserve your vision. Below is a description of the various classes of medications and their side effects. Keep in mind, however, that your ophthalmologist has the prerogative to determine which medication is best suited for your condition.

Variability in eye pressure may occur throughout the day, and if your doctor suspects this, he or she may suggest a diurnal curve check. This involves having your pressure checked throughout the day beginning as early as seven in the morning and as late as five in the afternoon.

Most drops are viable at room temperature and for one year with the exception of *Xalatan* that requires refrigeration after the bottle is opened, which limits it shelf life, although the company, given the competition, is attempting to remove these restrictions. Although two medications, the *prostaglandins* and *Timoptic XE,* require only one instillation per day, other medications require two-to-three instillations. When using these drops, take them at regular intervals—twice a day, twelve hours apart, three a day, eight hours apart, etc.

FIIRST LINE MEDICATIONS

THE BETA-BLOCKERS: TIMOLOL (TIMOPTIC, TIMOPTIC XE, BETIMOL), ISTALOL, (BETAXON) LEVOBUNOLOL (BETAGAN), CARTEOLOL (OCUPRES), METIPRANOLOL (OPTIPRANOLOL) BETAXOLOL (BETOPTIC, BETOPTIC S)

Two forms: *selective* and *non-selective,* comprise the *beta-blockers* that hook up to beta receptors found in the heart, lungs and eyes; beta one receptors are present in the heart, beta two in the lungs and both one and two are in the eyes. *Selective beta-blockers* connect with a particular site, the *non-selective* to more than one site, thus increasing the range of possible therapeutic effects but also of side effects. *Timoptic, Timoptic XE, Betimol, Betaxon, Betagan, Ocupress, Optipranolol* comprise drugs in the *non-selective antagonist* family that bond to the *beta-adrenergic receptors* that act on both forms of the *beta-blockers* in the eye. *Betoptic, Beptopic S.* (beta one) are *selective* and these drugs are usually easier to take for patients with pulmonary and cardiovascular problems. These medications, however, are only eighty-five percent as effective as the *beta two* in lowering IOP, although there is a possibility that they may facilitate blood flow by reducing the level of calcium flowing into the blood vessels. An animal study also suggested that *Betoptic* may act as a *neuroprotectant*. A Japanese study suggested that *carteolol* and *betaxolol* increased blood flow to the eye.

Pressure is reduced twenty-to-thirty percent with these medications. If you are on systemic *beta-blockers* for other conditions, the drops will be less effective.

It is preferable to take *Timoptic* in the morning, as the flow of aqueous humor decreases naturally during the night. Glaucoma patients, however, according to some evidence in the literature, do not experience as much decrease as those who are disease free, and it has been noted that at 3 A.M. there is a pressure rise.

The only *beta-blocker* that has been established as safe for infants is *carteolol HCI (Cartrol, Ocupres)*. Safety for use during pregnancy has not been established in any of the *beta-blockers*. And for the most part, they are contraindicated in breast feeding.

Although the mechanism by which *beta-blockers* in general lower IOP is not completely understood, the indiscriminate receptor-connections affords a first-line defense for a great number of glaucoma patients. Different bottle cap colors refer to the strength of the drug. There are some studies that claim that the dosage of .25% concentration of a *non-selective beta-blocker* is as effective as 5% *beta-blocker*. Speak to your doctor about this especially if you're on multiple medication therapy.

Side Effects

Medical students say in studying various diseases that they experience periods where they believe they have contracted a particular disease. As you read about the many possible side effects, resist believing they all apply to you. The effects of medication either by swallowing a pill or putting a drop into your eye are often idiosyncratic, that is, you react in a particular way that may not be reflected in the literature. At times, you need to bear with the medication as the body incorporates this new substance. If the medication lowers your IOP sufficiently, you may find yourself weighing the advantages and disadvantages of this particular drug. Glaucoma patients, in general, according to a study conducted by the Glaucoma Research Foundation found, will put up with discomfort and redness of the eyes if vision is protected.

That said, the most widely used *beta-blockers Timoptic* and *Timoptic XE,* while highly effective in controlling *intraocular pressure*, do have significant topical and systemic side-effects. Some of these are vague such as reduced vision, for this effect is known to disappear with continued use. For susceptible patients, the most severe side effects include hypersensitivity, worsening of asthma by decreasing airway resistance in people who already have heart and bronchial problems, congestive heart failure and/or reduction of cardiac output. It is advisable for patients in this category to check-out their respiratory function before using the *beta-blockers*. This effect is also true for healthy individuals who, as they age, may find they are acquiring the symptoms of asthma or chronic obstructive pulmonary disease. In rare cases, reduced blood flow can be mistaken for clogged arteries and it is wise, if you are diagnosed with this condition, to advise your cardiologist to consult with your eye doctor before undergoing any invasive heart procedure. In addition to the heart and pulmonary problems, *beta-blockers* may also affect blood circulation such as claudication (inadequate blood supply to the limbs) and *Raynaud's Disease* (inadequate blood supply to the extremities), as well as decreased blood pressure, lowered pulse rate, fatigue, fainting, or lethargy.

Other problems include slowing of sinus rhythms, muscle weakness, stomach distress, nausea, diarrhea, and impotence (men generally report this effect). The nervous system may also be affected. *Myasthenia gravis* may worsen. If you have trouble falling asleep, *beta-blockers* may aggravate this condition, or if you finally do sleep, you may be beset by nightmares. There have been reports of confusion, hallucinations, anxiety, disorientation, nervousness, and memory loss. People who are subject to skin conditions may find a worsening of *psoriasis*, rashes and loss of hair. *Diabetic* patients need to be especially careful for *beta-blockers* can mask symptoms of *hypoglycemia*. After filtration surgery, *choroidal detachment* may occur. Depression is also experienced by some patients either in mild or severe form. Symptoms of *hypoglycemia* (low blood sugar) may be masked in some patients.

Cholesterol can also be affected by decreasing the good HDL and increasing the triglycerides. Falling appears to be more prevalent in those with glaucoma than in the general population, and some patients attribute their tumbles to dizziness caused by *Timoptic XE*, a formulation that is taken once daily, a preferable routine for many patients. Extending the action of *Timoptic* over twenty-four hours is made possible by the addition of a gel (Gel rite).

An additive effect may occur should you be using prescription medicines to lower high blood pressure. The *beta-blockers propranolol (Inderal), atenolol (Tenormin),* or *nadolol (Corgard)* and the *calcium-channel blockers* especially may require that your general practitioner and eye doctor confer in order to adjust the dosages between the two prescriptions and so prevent over-medication. In older women the *beta-blocker carteolol* may be a better choice of drug, for it does not affect the plasma lipid structure as much as *Timoptic*.

The *beta-blockers* may also possess sulfites possibly causing allergic reactions in people hypersensitive to the preservative. *Timoptic XE* may be less allergenic, for it is formulated with the preservative, *benzododecinium bromide,* found to be better tolerated. Should you, however, be unable to tolerate any preservative, be heartened that *Timoptic* is available preservative-free. The cost, of course, is increased. There are both single and multiple versions of preservative-free *Timoptic.* Possibly the preservative in *timolol* and *carteolol* promotes *free radical* damage especially with long-term use.

Another problem associated with long term use of a *beta-blocker* is that the drug becomes less effective over time. Should this occur your doctor will probably switch you to other medications and after a period of time should these medications be less effective, resume *beta-blockers.* Often the *beta-blocker* will again be effective.

Topically, *beta-blockers* may cause irritation of the eye, inflammation at the roots of the eyelashes, dry eyes, decreased corneal sensitivity, *macular* swelling, and visual disturbances.

Members of our group cite their own litany of complaints. Yvette claims she can no longer sing operatic arias. Denise had unexplained crying jags. Lillian and Sally cite forgetfulness. Betty had to discontinue *Timoptic* for it made her depressed. I find that even using *Timoptic XE* in one eye and faithfully occluding for 5 minutes, walking pace is considerably slowed. Taking *beta-blockers* makes it impossible to reach an aerobic level.

This long list of side effects does not mean that everybody experiences them. Patients may complain of many symptoms that they attribute to *beta-lockers* that upon examination may be caused by other substances. Be sure to discuss your complaints with your doctor before *kicking the dog.*

THE PROSTAGLANDINS—

ANOTHER WAY FOR FLUID TO EXIT THE EYE

Latanoprost (Xalatan), bimatoprost, (Lumigan), travoprost (Travatan, Travatan z), unoprostone (Rescula)

These drugs have changed the medication therapy radically gaining first or second place in the pantheon of drugs prescribed for glaucoma. While the *prostaglandins* have not toppled the *beta-blockers* as a first-line defense completely, they do provide an excellent alternative. Depending upon your glaucomatous condition, the *prostaglandins* may be what your eye doctor prescribes. Often, the *prostaglandins* are added to the *beta-blocker* routine. An Israeli study cited an astonishing effect with *Xalatan*. The researchers found that newly-diagnosed glaucoma patients needed to only dose once a week to maintain their target IOP. Another study with *normal-tension* patients found that some patients with non-fixation-threatening glaucoma were able to maintain low pressures using only *Xalatan*.

The *prostaglandins* provide an additional route (*uveoscleral*) for the fluid discharge. *Xalatan,* the first drug in this class to reach the market lowers pressure by 25%-to-32%, *Travatan* and *Lumigan,* by 27%-to-33% and *Rescula,* 13%-to-8%. *Travatan Z* is a formulation of *Travatan* which has a different preservative and it may be easier for some patients to use.

Prostaglandins occur naturally in the body. They are chemical mediators and have a variety of biologic effects that react with the cellular receptors found throughout the body including the eye. They are synthesized from fatty acids and regulate many physiological processes including the flow of *aqueous fluid* across the *ueoscleral* route, Blood flow to the eye increases with *Xalatan* use. The *prostaglandin* involved in *Rescula* is *docosahexaenoic acid (DHA—an omega 3-fatty acid)*—essential for development and functioning of photoreceptor cells. DHA is endogenous to the central nervous system, including the *retina*. It is neuroproctective, but there is, as yet, not a great deal of evidence that *Rescula* meets neuroproctectant criteria. A review of the research suggests that the four *prostaglandin* formulas produce more or less equal effects on IOP management. Subtle differences however, do exist, and as with any medication, one of the *prostaglandins* may be better for your condition. *Travatan,* for example, has been found to be more effective with African-Americans.

Side effects

Although *prostaglandins* are involved in a myriad of bodily functions, their activity is not always benign. Most susceptible are people with a medical history of kidney or liver diseases, allergies,) high blood pressure, swollen or itching eyes, *macular edema* (excessive fluid in the macula. Nevertheless, lesser side effects occur than with other eye medications. Systemically, some people may get colds and flu more often than previously. The flu-like symptoms noted in patients using *Xalatan* may be averted with antioxidant therapy. I have this side effect and I find I can handle it by taking a combination of *echinacea* and *goldenseal*. Chest pain, muscle, back and joint pain and allergic skin reactions have also been reported. Although some patients have multiple health problems, the *prostaglandins* should not induce central nervous system side effects, uterine bleeding, or be contraindicated for persons with prostate cancer. You may be advised by your doctor if you use contact lens that *prostaglandins* are not for you.

Reversible side effects include redness, burning, itching or stinging of the eyes, foreign body sensation, dry eye, tearing, eye pain, blurred vision, crusting, uncomfortable eyelids, light sensitivity, hyperpigmentation of the eyelashes (or lashes growing where they should not), two or three rows of lashes, longer lashes and/or abnormal growth of hair, *uveitis* (usually contraindication for those with *uveitis* and *iritis*), inflammation, and worsening or development of herpetic eye disease.

Xalatan is the least likely to cause *hyperemia* (redness) but there still might be a mild *hyperemia* present. *Lumigan* is more likely to cause redness of the eye. I couldn't handle it, but Gloria, a group member, does quite well with it. Browning of the *iris*, a condition that may be related to an increase in the enzyme *tyrosinase* may occur. This effect occurs mainly in people who have hazel eyes. It increases melanin (brown pigment) which in of itself protects against UV rays. A problem may arise if only one eye needs treatment, possibly resulting in differently colored *iris*es, or conversely of the unaffected eye also becoming darker because of a crossover of the medication.

In addition to the general side effects mentioned above, *Lumigan* may also cause abnormal liver function; *Rescula*, corneal inflammation, cataract, back pain, *rhinitis* and *sinusitis*.and there is some indication that *Rescula* may bind with *free radicals*. Should you be using it, be sure to maintain an antioxidant routine. *Travatan* may decrease visual acuity, provoke abnormal vision; systemically, it may promote an inclination to accidental injury, *angina pectoris*, anxiety, arthritis, back pain, *brachycardia* (slowed heartbeat), and chest pain.

Manufacturers of *prostaglandin*s stimulated by the effects of hair growth produced by these substances have produced a cosmetic version as an eyelash thickener and growth factor and a cure for baldness is in the works using this drug.. Control your IOP and grow and thicken your hair and eyelashes. Now there's a thought.

SECOND LINE MEDICATIONS

Alpha Receptor Agonists. Apraclonidine (Iopidine), brimonidine (Alphagan, Alphagan P)

This class of drugs inhibits aqueous production and increases uveo*scleral* outflow by targeting the *ciliary body*, the structure of the eye responsible for secreting the *aqueous humor*. *Iopidine* is the mother of *Alphagan* and *Alphagan*

P. These drugs are *highly selective alpha 2 agonists* with fewer side affects and allergic reactions. As well, the medication is effective for a longer period of time. *Alphagan P* is gentler due to the use of *Purite* as a preservative and it improves absorption. This enables the company to put less of the medication into the bottle but still retain the same efficacy as a generic of higher concentration. Generic brimonidine is cheaper. Dosage is 0.2% brimonidine, whereas *Alphagan P* can be had at 0.1.55% or 0.1%.

These medications both increase outflow of fluid inside the eye, while at the same time, decrease production of fluid. Although they may not be prescribed as frequently as the first line medications described above, they are often used as an additive medication. One of the disadvantages of these drops is that they need to be taken two-to-three times a day, unlike the *prostaglandins* that require only a drop at bedtime.

Apraclonidine

Iopidine was approved for reducing temporary spikes in IOP that often occur after *trabeculoplasty* (See Chapter 6). In 1995 it was approved by the FDA (*U.S. Federal Food and Drug Administration*) for general management of glaucoma, but because of side effects experienced by over thirty percent of the users, it fell out of favor and was replaced by *Alphagan*. Intolerance to *Alphagan* as with *Iopidine* affects a fairly sizeable group of patients. To overcome this handicap, *Alphagan P* was developed. This formula lowers the concentration and substitutes the preservative *Purite* matching the pH factor found in our bodies. Some patients are better able to tolerate *Alphagan P*. that coincidentally, works equally well to reduce temporary spikes following laser treatment.

Some ophthalmologists feel that *Alphagan*, if not for the need to instill it two-to-three times a day, could be used as a first-line medication. Its multiple actions include reducing IOP by 20%-to-30% peaking two hours after instillation, an increased perfusion of blood to the eye adding protection to the optic nerve, and possibly increasing *uveoscleral outflow*, a pathway more commonly associated with the *prostaglandin* drugs. A randomized clinical trial comparing *Alphagan* with *argon trabeculoplasty* found that patients after a year on *Alphagan* had less visual field progression than those who received the laser treatment.

Patients using *Alphagan P* and *Timoptic* may welcome the combination drug that combines both of these medications in one drop.

Side Effects

Alphagan P, although considerably less allergenic than *apraclonidine*, still causes side effects. Only about thirteen percent of those taking the drug suffer reactions and it is, therefore, considered a safe drug for the majority of users. Systemic side effects include fatigue, low blood pressure, sedation, abnormal taste, dry mouth and depression. The drug causes allergic topical reactions such as red eye, eye discomfort, corneal staining, burning, stinging, lid crusting, *contact dermatitis, conjunctivitis*, dry eye, dry mouth, swelling of the eyelids, slight dilation of the pupils, movement up of the eyelids, and photophobia. Less common are fatigue, drowsiness, headache, insomnia, depression, anxiety, and fainting. Hypersensitivity may occur in patients taking *MAOis (monoamine oxidase inhibitors* (drugs used to counteract depression). If you are taking *trycyclic anti-depressants*, the effectiveness of *Alphagan* may be lowered. Barbiturates, opiates and sedatives may increase *Alphagan's* side effects. The drug is usually considered when pregnant, but preferably this decision should rest with a consultation between your obstetrician and your eye doctor. The medication is contraindicated for infants and children (causes central nervous system side effects.)

ADRENERGIC AGONISTS

Epinephrine & Dipivefrin, Propine

While *epinephrine (Epifren)* is in the grouping of second-line medications, it is seldom used because of its many side effects and, because at least one-third of the patients do not respond to this medication. It acts on the *alpha* and *beta* receptors in the eye, increasing the outflow of fluid while at the same time reducing the production of *aqueous humor*. Old time glaucoma patients may recall various versions of the drug that went by the trade names of *Epifrin, Epinal, Epitrate,* and *Glaucon. Epinephrine* is chemically identical to the hormone *adrenaline*, which is secreted by the *adrenal gland* and which has an effect of controlling IOP. Because of its severe side effects, pharmacists combined it with the drug *dipivefrin*, naming it *Propine*, which as a pro-drug does not begin to work until it is instilled in the eye, thus preventing some of the side effects.

This drug has some possibly positive side effects for it dilates the pupil tending to counteract the pupil-constricting properties of drugs such as *pilocarpine* and *carbacohl*. Also, since it constricts the blood vessels on the surface of the eye, the whiteness of the *sclera* is improved enhancing the eye's appearance, although the eye reddens as the medication wears off. Long-term use of *Propine*, however, may cause some of the same allergic problems as *epinephrine* eye drops.

Side Effects

About twenty percent of those taking these medications report allergies. The dilation of the pupil may lead to *angle closure* in susceptible people. The eyelids can move up, a bothersome event, and black spots on the surface of the eye and on contact lenses may occur. Systemic side effects include increased heart rate or *arrhythmia* and high blood pressure, dry mouth, headaches, nervousness, and drowsiness. Contact lenses and *epinephrine* are contraindicated.

Generally considered safe for pregnant patients, but it is advisable to have your obstetrician and eye doctor concur in its use. The pediatric dose has not been established.

CARBONIC ANHYDRASE INHIBITORS

Acetazolamide (Diamox), methazolamide (Neptazane), brinzolamide (Asopt), dichlorphenamide (Daranide, Oratrol), and dorzolamide HCI (Trusopt)

These drugs work by reducing the secretion of the *aqueous humor* by inhibiting the *carbonic anhydrase* enzyme in the *ciliary body*. Its action splits the carbon dioxide molecule into bicarbonate and hydroxide. Sodium then steps in and neutralizes the bicarbonate to form *aqueous humor*. *Carbonic anhydrase inhibitors* thus slow down the production of fluid. The drugs are sulfonamides (sulfur) medications possibly causing allergic reactions in some people. They act on the kidney and increase urination which can cause a side effect that of changing the electrolyte balance leading to systemic acidosis in some people and, which is possibly a serious condition.

The oral medications *Diamox* and *Neptazane* are most often prescribed when drops no longer manage pressure, or given intravenously in cases where the patient is hospitalized for extremely high pressures.

The drop forms of these medications include *dorzolamide (Trusopt)* and *brinzolamide (Asopt)*. With the availability of the drop form, these medications moved into second tier. They perform as do the systemic medications, but with fewer systemic side effects, although these may still occur. The mode of action is similar to diuretics. Some small studies indicate blood flow increase to the optic nerve brought about by the release of additional oxygen, an effect known as the *Bohr Effect* named after Neils Bohr (Danish physicist—Nobel Prize, 1922). Simply stated, hemoglobin packs highly concentrated oxygen and as it rides the blood stream, oxygen is deposited where needed. To do this job, hemoglobin must come into contact with carbon dioxide that has been generated by cell metabolism. Carbon dioxide distorts the hemoglobin molecule enhancing its release of oxygen. *Trusopt* and *Asopt* are inhibitors of *carbonic anhydrase*, and in the blocking of this enzyme, carbon dioxide builds up, shedding the pH factor, resulting in dilation of the blood vessels.

Side Effects

Systemically, most side effects are caused by *Diamox* or *Neptazane*. *Diamox Sequels* and *Neptazane* are better tolerated, but common side effects include malaise, fatigue, weight loss, depression, agitation, confusion, decreased libido, overgrowth or loss of hair, urinary stones (*urolithiasis*), anorexia, nausea, heartburn, cramps, diarrhea, tingling, prickling, carbonated drinks taste flat, urinary frequency, kidney stones (calcium in the kidneys—less with *Neptazane*), or *Stevens-Johnson syndrome* (severe form of allergy which can cause scarring of the surface of the eye—rare). People who take *digoxin* for heart disease should mention this to the doctor because severe electrolyte imbalance, specifically with potassium, can occur. Low potassium can cause heart *arrhythmias* which can be fatal. The pill form rarely causes the side effects in the eyes.

Dorzolamide reduces the hydrogen ion secretion in the kidney which then increases the kidney's secretion of sodium, potassium bicarbonate and water. This is the action in the eye that is responsible for lower fluid generation but when this same reaction occurs in susceptible kidneys, stones may develop. Decreased formation of red blood cells leading to anemia may develop into *aplastic anemia*, a serious condition. Usually this condition appears within the first two months of therapy and in most cases is reversible provided the medication is discontinued at its first sign. Persons who are susceptible to sulfur or who have liver or kidney disease should not take these drugs, although sulfur reactions have been questioned. According to a University of Iowa study self-reported reactions often stem from a patient's perception unrelated to evidence. Based on this study, reaction to a sulfur-containing drug should be considered in documented cases.

Diamox causes more side effects than *Neptazane*. Should you need to take the systemic form of these drugs, do establish a base-line of white blood cells and an electrolyte balance (sodium, chloride and potassium). Headaches and loss of chloride and potassium may occur when taking these medications.

In general, the systemic drugs increase the acidity in the body, a condition called *acidosis*, which can cause muscle weakness, deadened reflexes and at its most extreme, paralysis. Side effects occur less frequently with the drop form but drops may still cause side-effects. *Dorzolamide* 2% (Trusopt) and *brinzolamide* 1% (Azopt) are the drop forms of these medications. The pH factor of *Azopt* is closer to natural pH factor and so is better tolerated unlike that of *Trusopt*, which is lower and burns more upon instillation. *Azopt* stings less and may produce fewer side-effects, but both medications are equally effective. Other side effects include burning, stinging and blurring of vision due to corneal swelling which reverses upon cessation of use. Less frequent complaints include a bitter or sour taste, tearing, dryness and photophobia (intolerance to strong light), fatigue, skin rash, *blepharitis* (inflammation at the root of the eyelashes), and foreign body sensation. On rare occasions, urinary stones or inflammation of the *ciliary body* may occur. Interactions may also occur should you be taking high-dose *salicylates* (aspirin and other products) and sodium.

These medications peak at approximately two-to-three hours after instillation and wash out in about two days—much quicker than other medications. They pair well with *beta-blockers* as evidence by the drop, *Cosopt*, a combination of *Trusopt* and *timolol*. They are considered equally effective and are well tolerated.

Known to cause birth defects in animals eliminates these medications during pregnancy and pediatric use has not been established. *Trusopt* is contraindicated for breast feeding.

THE PARASYMPATHOMIMETICS

Miotics—Direct-Acting And Indirect-Acting (Pilocarpine And Carbachol

These drugs act on the *pupillary sphincter* constricting the pupil. The direct-acting includes *acetylcholine (Miochol)* (used in the operating room for rapid pupil constriction to blunt post-operative IOP spikes), *pilocarpine (Isopto Carpine, Pilocar, Pilopine Gel)* and *Carbacohl*, a synthetic compound with both direct and indirect action. These drugs reduce the pressure by 15%-to-25% by increasing the *trabecular meshwork* pores allowing more fluid to exit the eye. *Carbacohl* doesn't penetrate the cornea as well as *pilocarpine*, but it is more potent.

These medications were once the mainstay of glaucoma therapy, but they have taken a back seat to newer forms of medication described above. Nevertheless, they do work well, although side effects are more severe than with the other medications. Some patients, including me, still use them. The mode of action is comparable to *acetylcholine*, a derivative of the amino acid *choline* that plays a role in transmitting nerve impulses. The *cholinergic* agents work on the autonomic system causing the ciliary muscle to contract, increasing egress of the aqueous fluid. This action expands the *trabecular meshwork* pores, quite like tugging the rim of a flexible perforated disk to widen the perforations.

Side Effects

Constriction of the pupil is a serious side effect, a condition that may become permanent after long use. This narrowing of the pupil affects vision especially in low light. While these drugs are effective in lowering *intraocular pressure*, they do present a number of problems. In some cases they are contraindicated for people with *exfoliation* They aggravate the blood-aqueous barrier and decrease the mobility of the sphincter muscle raising the risk of scarring and cataract formation. In the extreme, use of miotics may lead to *angle-closure* glaucoma. Yet, even though I have exfoliation, I have used miotics for years (since I'm allergic to many of the other drops) and although I did get cataracts, I seem to have escaped the other problems.

The journey of *pilocarpine* from a medicinal plant to an eye drop is one of the more interesting stories in glaucoma therapy. Discovered by a Brazilian physician who noted that natives used the plant *pilocarpus microphylus* to induce sweating and salivation, the physician brought it to Paris where both the French and Germans experimentally found that it reduced ocular pressure. Used in the eye, *pilocarpine* acts on the *ciliary muscle* and the *sphincter muscle* as described above, both widening and constricting the pupil in response to light stimulation. Concentrations of *pilocarpus* range from 0.25%-to-10%. In general doctors start with the lowest dose and increase if necessary. Patients with dark *irises*, an indication of heavy pigmentation, often require a heavier solution to penetrate the eye. A gel form used at night reduces the need for the four-times-a-day routine. Its longevity of action is increased by the gel creeping up and into the eye attracted by the tear film; because it is sticky, it remains on the eye throughout the night. There is divided opinion from those using this form as to its tolerability.

Side Effects

Decreased vision is the most troubling side effect. The problem is aggravated in dim or dark areas when the pupil cannot respond to lower light levels. Driving at night may become hazardous especially in unfamiliar territory. People with *myopia* are particularly plagued by a constricted pupil for they may already have some reduced vision. Other side effects include brow ache, or ache around the eyes and forehead, itchiness of the eyelids and conjunctiva. While less common, side effects may occur such as *retinal tears* or *detachment*, inflammation after surgery (but that happens, no matter what), cloudiness of the lens, a jump-start on cataracts, cysts on the *iris* and the possibility of *angle closure* Like all topical drugs, systemic side effects are not absent although the frequency is definitely lessened. These side effects may include nausea, vomiting, diarrhea, sweating, bronchial spasm, pulmonary edema and a slower heartbeat.

CARBACHOL

First synthesized in 1932, it has become a back-burner drug trotted out when the newer drugs fail to adequately control pressure. Doctors are reluctant to prescribe it because of its many and sometimes serious side effects. Like *pilocarpine* it is a miotic, and its pupil constricting effects are similar.

Side effects

The transient symptoms of stinging, burning and brow ache when first instilled are minor in comparison to the systemic side effects that may occur. It may produce the symptoms of a *cholinesterase inhibitor*. When I instilled the drop without occluding the tear duct, I experienced cold sweats. This was a most disconcerting development since I needed the drug to control my eye pressure. Other side effects include salivation, fainting, cardiac *arrhythmia*, gastrointestinal cramping, vomiting, asthma, hypotension, diarrhea, frequent urge to urinate, increased sweating, and irritation of the eyes. The drug should not be used if the eye is inflamed for it readily permeates the blood vessels. It is contraindicated for people with *narrow-angle* glaucoma. It should definitely not be used by people who have severe respiratory, cardiovascular or gastrointestinal tract disease. Fortunately, fewer people resort to it and in the future, it may no longer be on the market. When I told a retinologist that I was using the drug, he expressed surprise that it still was available. Incidentally, it is one of the least expensive of the eye medications.

Safety for pregnancy, pediatrics and breast feeding has not been established.

INDIRECT ACTING MIOTICS

Demecarium (Humorsol), physotigmine (Eserine) and *echothiophate (Phospholine Iodide)* are used less frequently. They are in the *anti cholinesterase* family and are very potent. This class of drug was originally used in chemical warfare and as insecticides.

Side effects

These include dim vision (especially at night because of small pupil), brow ache, redness, irritation, *myopia*, cataracts (better used in eyes where the lens has been removed), and disruption of blood-aqueous barrier which causes inflammation (especially in those with a history of *uveitis* or *iritis*.) Inflammation can lead to scarring on the surface of the eye, *conjunctivitis*, scarring of tear ducts and increased tear production. The *lens* can shift forward causing *angle-closure* in those with narrow angles. At risk also is *retinal detachment* in myopic eyes. Possible systemic side effects include nausea, vomiting, diarrhea, sweating, breathing problems, slow heart rate, and increased urination.

MEDICATIONS USED FOR VERY HIGH PRESSURE

Used only for emergency situations when pressure is very high, the following medications may be contraindicated in patients who have heart, kidney or liver disease and who are elderly.

Glycerin administered either intravenously or orally, is a very sweet-tasting liquid. It rapidly decreases the pressure by reducing the fluid out of the eye by shrinking the *vitreous* gel. It is of short duration and is contraindicated for people with lung or kidney disease, and *diabetics* because it is highly caloric. The oral form has fewer side effects than when given intravenously, in which case vomiting and nausea may occur.

Regular *ethyl alcohol*, 80-to-100 proof given orally, will also reduce pressure, but it too, is highly caloric and can cause nausea, vomiting and central nervous system depression. It penetrates the eye rapidly lessening its effectiveness and it promotes frequent urination.

Mannitol, given intravenously, works in as little as ten minutes and lasts six hours. It is a hyper osmotic agent that rids the body of fluid, thus lowering (sometimes dramatically), pressure in the eyes.

PREGNANCY

It is important for your gynecologist to consult with your eye doctor. Generally, the minimum amount of medication if possible should be prescribed during the first trimester. Glaucoma suspects or patients with limited optic nerve damage may be able to dispense with medications during the first twelve weeks, but frequent monitoring is required. Recent research, however, indicates the dangers of discontinuing medications. Advances in diagnostic tools have revealed that, although pressure typically drops during pregnancy, visual fields worsened in sixty percent of the pregnant women in a study. Those continuing with medication should religiously practice punctal occlusion (see below). Laser trabeculoplasty may also be an option and that can be performed anytime during pregnancy. *Trabeculectomy*, for the most part, is now performed with local anesthesia and should not be harmful. General anesthesia is rarely used, but if necessary, should be used in the second trimester. *Brimonidine* is a Class B pregnancy drug which means that animal studies show no harm to the fetus, but there are no well-controlled human studies. All other glaucoma medications are Class C which means that animal studies showed adverse fetal effects, but no controlled human studies have been conducted. The *carbonic anhydrate inhibitors* cause birth defects in animals. The *prostaglandins* increase uterine contractility.

Concern does not end with delivery of the baby. Should you decide to nurse, have your pediatrician consult with your eye doctor about your protocol. Just as medication may enter the bloodstream of the fetus, it may also be secreted in mother's breast milk. Most likely *beta-blockers* will not be recommended for they concentrate five-fold in breast milk, nor will *Humorsol* or the oral form of the *carbonic anhydrase inhibitors.* Chances are you will be on eyedrops and while few of them have been subjected to long-term study of possible harmful effects from nursing, you should discuss with your eye doctor the most appropriate form of drop for you and your baby. Of course, the concentration of other noxious chemicals are also present in breast milk, and pediatricians attempt to weigh the protective benefits of nursing against the toxic environmental substances such as *dioxin* that, unfortunately, has been detected in breast milk. Unquestionably, to nurse or not to nurse is a difficult decision. Consult the nutritional chapter in this book for healthy choices. Be sure to practice punctal nasal occlusion to minimize the amount of medication entering your system.

CHILDREN

The miotics are less effective in children than in adults. *Alpha agonists* are contraindicated in young children due to somnolence and fatigue, presumably due to central nervous system depression. A single drop of 0.5% timolol (*beta-blockers*) can reach cardiac *beta-blocker* levels in infants under two years of age. The *prostaglandins* and *carbonic anhydrate inhibitors* in oral liquid form for pediatric dosing are well tolerated.

MEDICAL THERAPY FOR MACULAR DEGENERATION

A promising treatment for the wet form of macular degeneration considered to both stabilize acuity and actually improve vision has had a profound effect on management of the disease. The treatment focuses on the vascular *endothelial growth factor (VEGF),* an endogenous (produced within the body) protein. This is a growth factor, but too much of it stimulates *neovascularization* (runaway blood vessels)--another example of a natural order running amuck causing damage to vital organs; in this case, to the *retina* resulting in diseases such as *ARMD* and *diabetic retinopathy.* Three medications have been developed that can be delivered directly into the eye by *intravitreal* injection. *Macugen (pegaptanib)* administered every six weeks was the first compound shown to specifically inhibit *intraocular VEGF.* The drugs, *Lucentis (ranibizumab),* which has gained FDA approval, and *Avastin (bevacizumab),* which at this writing has not, but which is much cheaper and essentially works the same, are the line of drugs under intense study.

Intravitreally injected they penetrate the *retinal* layers. The smaller antibody fragment developed by *Lucentis* clears more quickly, 48 days as opposed to *Avastin's* 149 days, but *Avastin* has a higher binding affinity. *Lucentis,* therefore, systemically eliminates the medication 100 times faster. Clinicians, however, have found the results of both of these drugs pretty much the same. Two trials demonstrated mean visual improvement in neovascular *ARMD* at one year for *Lucentis* with a seven letter gain vs. a ten letter loss for the controls. A trial using intravenous *Avastin,* demonstrated anatomic and visual efficacy in *ARMD,* but there was a mean increase in blood pressure, risk of heart attack and strokes, so its use may be limited. *Lucentis* has been studied more extensively (randomized clinical trials) than *Avastin,* but similar results have been achieved based on published case histories. Injected in the eye where *macular degeneration* occurs, it forms a depot delivery system that is comparable to the implants. The National Institutes of Health is engaged in a head-to-head analysis of these two therapies.

ARMD treatment has advanced from the goal of stabilization of acuity to improvements in acuity. Scientists are engaged in developing long-term sustainable delivery systems to decrease the need for frequent *intravitreal* injections. They are also actively seeking treatments to decrease transformation of dry to wet forms of *macular degeneration.*

Possibly a combination therapy (*anti-VEGF* agent with the above therapies and *photodynamic therapy* or steroids will be more effective in stemming the changes brought about by *ARMD.* None of these systems is as yet perfected but they all offer promise. The downside of any of these drug delivery systems is that for protection of the *macula*, additional medication will need to be instilled within a matter of months.

Treatment with *anti-VEGF* agents for other eye diseases that stimulate *angiogenesis* due to *endothelial* cell injury is now possible, for excess *VEGF* is implicated in the diseases of *Choroidal Neovascularization, Diabetic Retinopathy, Edema, Central Retinal Vein Occlusion, (CRVO), Branch Retinal Vein, Occlusion,(BRVO, Retinopathy of Prematurity, Corneal Neovascularization, and Iris Neovascularization.*

Other growth factors being explored such as pigment epithelial cell derived factor (PEDF), Gial cell line derived neurotropic factor (GDNf) and lens epithelial cell derived growth factor (LEDGF) also show promise for stemming the ravages from ARMD. Scientists at the Cole Eye Institute (Cleveland Clinic) and Case Western Reserve have found a greater amount of a substance called carboxyethylpyrrole (CEP) in the blood of ARMD patients than in controls. The presence of CEP may be a valuable biomarker that can be isolated in blood tests.

Photodynamic therapy (PDT) that combines medication and laser treatment is not ruled out as a therapy in some cases. A drug, *Visudyne (verteporfin,)* is injected into the arm where it accumulates preferentially in the fast growing blood vessels and attaches to molecules called *lipoproteins.* Cells which are rapidly proliferating require more *lipoproteins* than non-dividing cells. After ten minutes, a non-thermal laser is shone into the eye activating the *Visudyne* that then destroys these fast-growing blood vessels.

Combining *photodynamic therapy* with *photocoagulation* is another option. Small studies indicate that the combined therapy saves vision. Some patients suffer severe backache when injected with the drug *Visudyne* spurring clinicians to study lower doses and slower infusion. But other medications are in the pipeline and this problem may be overcome.

Side Effects

Drug breakthroughs, however, although initially hailed as cure, may turn out to be too toxic for use. An example is the drug *Accutane* that suppresses the toxic accumulation of chemicals called *lipofuscin* that promote the death of *retinal pigmentary epithelial* cells. While *Accutane* does halt the build-up of *lipofuscin,* the use of this drug might seriously affect the liver, induce severe depression, and cause birth defects. *Intravitreal* injections risk infection and cataract stimulation. Side effects of *PDT* therapy include temporary sensitivity to bright light, and the need to avoid exposure to sunlight and bright indoor light for the first five days after treatment. Protective clothing and sunglasses are advised during this period.

While most attention has been focused on the wet form of *macular degeneration,* an oral treatment for the dry form is poised to begin trials. Named at present SIR-1047, this potent medication is contraindicated for women of child-bearing age. Another drug, *Fenretinide* is also being tested for dry *ARMD.* This drug reduces the accumulation of *lipofuscin,* toxic copmpounds known to cause *retinal* damage and vision loss.

PRESERVATIVES IN OPHTHALMIC PREPARATIONS

In nature, the microbial action that breaks down and recycles organic material is a necessary cycle of regeneration. Simply, it is a natural process that refertilizers the soil. Yet this cycle built into every organism has stimulated humans for thousands of years to tinker with this conversion of foodstuffs by salting, drying, brining, pickling, smoking, marinating with herbs and to lacing with synthetic preservatives. The latter, the synthetics have found their way not only into our food supply but into just about every product we use. Medicines are no exception. The chemicals used are not benign, and while they do preserve the medicine from spoilage and contamination, they may also cause allergic reactions that for some of us may make certain drug preparations intolerable. Furthermore, some of the chemicals may worsen the glaucoma condition. Most eyedrops, both over-the-counter and prescribed, contain preservatives, important to protect against possible sight-threatening, dangerous infections. But the chemicals used may set up a different set of toxic reactions such as inflammation and *corneal,* tear-film and *conjunctiva* changes. Persons with dry eye, a problem often following *LASIK* Surgery (the thinning of the cornea to correct near-or-far-sightedness), or who use multiple glaucoma drops, are usually most adversely affected.

The preservatives fall into two main categories—detergent and oxidative. *Benzalkonium (BAK),* a detergent commonly used in glaucoma medications, zaps microorganisms effectively but because mammalian cells are incapable of neutralizing chemical preservatives, it causes cellular damage by incorporation into the cell.

Oxidative preservatives are smaller but they, too, interfere with cell function but usually to a lesser degree. They have an advantage over detergents by providing sufficient clout against the microorganism and because the cells in this case, equipped to deal with oxidation, become neutralized. *Stabilized Oxychloro Complex (SOC)* is an oxidative preservative that is one of the gentlest. While its use is newer for ophthalmics, its key component, sodium chloride, has been used since 1944 in such products as toothpaste, mouthwash and antacids.

Only one medication, *Timoptic*, can be purchased preservative free, but it comes in one or several-dose forms and needs to be refrigerated. It is inconvenient and expensive. Until manufacturers begin to use less toxic preservatives, it is a good idea, if possible, especially when using multiple medications, to choose those with the least amount of preservative.

Manufacturers of ophthalmic drops use varying percentage levels of preservatives in their preparations. See below.

Alphagan	0.005	BAK
Alphagan P	0.005	SOC
Azopt	0.01	BAK
Betagan`	0.005	BAK
Betimol	0.01	BAK
Betoptic S	0.01	BAK
Cosopt	0.0075	BAK
Lumigan	0.05	BAK
Rescula	0.015	BAK
Timoptic	0.01	BAK
Timoptic XE	0.012	BDD*
Trusopt	0.0075	BAK
Xalatan	0.02	BAK

Over the Counter

Gen Teal	Sodium Perborate	
Hypo Tears	0.01	BAK
Refresh Tears	0.0005	SOC
Tears NaturelleII	0.001	polyquaternium-1**

* BDD benzododecimnium bromide—a product similar to BAK

**studies indicate polyquaternium-1 moderate to extensive superficial eye surface erosion

MEDICAL INTERACTIONS

In this age of a pill for everything, we may find that we are taking multiple medications in addition to our eyedrops. Here are some of the interactions to bear in mind when you swallow a pill and put a drop in your eye. But, please, don't stop what you're doing until you consult with your ophthalmologist and general physician.

The *beta-blockers* may interact with a number of other medications. Note the possible interactions.

Timoptic or Ocupress

--Hypertension after abrupt withdrawal from *Catapres*

--Hypertension when taking *Adrenalin*

--Hypotension with *Cordarone*

--Peripheral ischemia (lack of blood flow) with *Ergostat, Cafergot, Bellerga-S*

--Migraine; hypotension, congestive heart failure with *Procardia*

--Airway resistance with *Theo-Dur*

Timoptic, Betagan, Ocupress

--Hypotension and b*rachycardia* with *Luvox*

Timoptic, Betoptic

--Exaggerated hypertension response

--Arrhythmias with *Aldomet*

Ocupress

--Hypotensive response to first dose of *Minipress*

Timoptic, Ocupress, Betoptic

--May affect d*iabetic* patients with loss of glucose controls

The Alpha Agonists Alphagan, Iopidine

--May result in hypertensive emergency when taking *monoamine oxidase inhibitors—Parnate, Eldepry.*

It is important for both your primary physician and your ophthalmologist have information on all the medications you are taking. A side-effect believed to be a result of an eye medication may, in fact, be caused by an interaction between medications. An excellent source of this information can be fund on The Glaucoma Research Foundation website *http://www.glaucoma.net. nygri/glaucoma/topics/guide.asp.* This material is a practical guide to ocular side effects, which has been reprinted from a Review of Ophtalmology.

The statins and other cholesterol lowering medications, according to a study of clinical data bases maintained at the *Veterans Affairs Medical Center* in Birmingham, Alabama, may be associated with a reduced risk of *open-angle* glaucoma, particularly among patients with cardiovascular and lipid diseases. Even the non-statins were associated with a reduced risk. Another study found that men over fifty who had used cholesterol-lowering medications for five years had a lower risk of developing glaucoma. Scientists are investigating whether this class of drugs might be an additional therapeutic option for glaucoma.

THE DELICATE BALANCE

Taking a drug is in no way a benign activity. Unfortunately, once you are diagnosed with glaucoma, there is very little alternative choice, since neglecting your eye disease may lead to blindness. Despite our own experiences with the difficulties of medicine and the evidence in the literature that this is universal (one study cited four percent experiencing adverse effects and sixty-four percent general intolerance), medications for glaucoma patients are a fact of life. Nevertheless, you may feel that you are being overmedicated, especially when your schedule requires that you instill multiple drops. And there is merit to your discontent. Some studies suggest that piling on more medications will do little to affect the IOP level. After a certain point there is no gain. The adverse affect of multiple medications has the potential to increase side effects.

Drops do increase *free radical* damage and you may experience subtle changes in your vision. Long term use of *beta-blockers* has been shown to affect visual sensitivity. Glaucoma patients complain they have difficulty detecting subtle contrasts between colors and low-contrast print materials. *Pilocarpine* and *epinephrine* have been found to cause distinct changes in the cells of the *cornea*. How these changes affect sight is not clearly understood, but those of us who have been on drops for many years speculate that the drops might have something to do with reduced vision. As glaucoma patients we can only report what we experience. It is up to the researchers to document glaucoma-related changes and weigh these effects against the therapeutic value of glaucoma medications. In the face of this quandary, the majority of glaucoma patents would be reluctant to part with their medications if these are doing some good, and would instead, hope that the pharmaceutical companies would be able to produce less toxic drugs with fewer side effects.

Cataract formation tosses another ingredient in the mix of visual sensitivity. I was amazed at the improvement in my vision when my cataracts were removed, Suddenly, I could read newspapers, street signs and effortlessly detect discoloring in my vegetables. Muscle mobility may also be linked to visual sensitivity. With age, muscles lose their elasticity--even the tiny ciliary muscles in the eye. And to boot, medication may quicken this degenerative process. Animal studies suggest that chronic use of the miotics (*pilocarpine* & *carbacohl*) may irritate the *conjunctiva*. When cells are irritated, inflammation occurs, damaging cells and possibily leading to *closed-angle glaucoma*. Fortunately, for most users of glaucoma drops, newer medications do not affect the ciliary muscle.

Why take drops at all since glaucoma is an optic nerve disease? The fact is that there is ample evidence in the literature recommending that the IOP, especially with vulnerable patients, should be in the lower teens or single digits. If drops can do the job, we're spared the scalpel to lower IOP to the level where vision remains stable. So at this juncture, most of us would rather use multiple medications, if necessary, than risk irrevocable damage to our eyes.

OUTSIDE THE BOX

The drug arsenal for fighting glaucoma is constantly expanding and a number of promising drugs, still in the experimental stage, may soon reach the marketplace. In a two-center clinical trial, a two-percent solution of a *carbonic anhydrase inhibitor* called *MK-926* with decreased IOP by an average of 24.6% and 23.7% after six and eight hours, respectively. Two agonist drugs, called *UK-14303-18* and *B-Ht-920,* respectively, have reduced IOP up to forty percent in animal studies. Researchers believe these drugs work by decreasing aqueous production. Scientists are also working on a number of drugs that will directly address the *trabecular meshwork* for even with the aqueous suppressant drugs, if the *trabecular meshwork* drainage dterioates further, the IOP is more difficult to manage. Very promising is a drug *Anecortave Acetate.* A medication, *Latrunculin,* is under study and has shown promising results. It acts on a completely different mechanism on the outflow system of the eye and it is long acting, possibly as long as a month. What doesn't work for one disease may very well work for another one. *Anecortave Acetate* originally developed to control wet macular degeneration was found to be ineffective for that disease but was serendipitously observed to reduce the high pressure in patients who had glaucoma since the drug possesses an anti-inflammatory action. The method of application is also novel for glaucoma patients. A supply of the drug (a liquid containing a white powder) Is injected into the *juxtascleral* section of the eye. This injection does not penetrate the eye. The FDA has cleared an investigatory glaucoma drug, INS117548 Ophthalmic Solution for early stage clinical trials. This treatment targets the *trabecular meshwork.*

Basic science is the bedrock girdling many of the substances in various exploratory stages and there is no end to new findings. One such involves the action of a *neurotransmitter.* Commonly believed to be a one-one synaptic transfer (the junction point between two neurons), researchers have discovered that release of *neurotransmitters* can be multiple. A study of the *amino acid glutamate* revealed multiple release sites. As mentioned previously, the release of excess *glutamate* is implicated in the death of neurons. The thrust for more effective medications to curb the destructive elements in the cells is found in some of the *neuroproctective* agents currently being assessed as possible treatment for glaucoma. The potential to regulate body fluids impacts on glaucoma therapy and a new class of drugs called *vasplans* may eventually join forces with other glaucoma medications to regulate *intraocular pressure.*

It takes years, however, to bring a new drug to the market, but advanced technology may soon transform this situation, for with imaging systems now available and also in development, scientists can view the action of the medication in vivo and evaluate whether or not it works. Whether this will eliminate human trials of 4-to-5 years duration remains to be seen. Making the cells stronger has also stimulated some interesting research. Cells and tissues adapt to stress. In the laboratory, mice exposed to a low-oxygen environment forced the mouse cells to adapt. If this treatment proves successful, possibly a medication could be developed to mimic controlled stressful situations forcing cells and tissues to adapt for survival.

Furthermore, a low oxygen level implies that carbon dioxide is elevated offering some interesting insights as to the effects of this gas on glaucoma. Once formed, carbon dioxide rapidly reacts with water to form *carbonic acid*, a reaction catabolically assisted by the enzyme *carbonic anhydrase*. This is a powerful enzyme inhibitor that provokes a rise in acidity. The *carbonic anhydrase inhibitors* (*Trusopt, Asopt*) work on this system to reduce production of aqueous. Now, if circulation in the brain is inadequate to keep up with metabolic needs, carbon dioxide tends to build up and cerebral blood flow correspondingly increases. At high levels of carbon dioxide, both blood flow and oxygen transfer to central brain tissues. At low levels of carbon, dioxide the opposite occurs. Since *carbonic anhydrase* is abundantly spread throughout pigmented tissues of the eye, including the *retinal pigmentary layer* which is adjacent to both *retinal* and *choroidal* blood vessels, high carbon dioxide should increase blood flow and oxygen to the tissues.

There is a great deal of attention directed towards rehabilitating *central nervous system* injuries. Since the *retina* and *optic nerve* are part of the central *nervous system*, development in this field will certainly migrate into rehabilitating the *optic* nerve.

Many glaucoma patients long for a medication to rehabilitate the trabecular *meshwork* by washing out debris clogging it. Researchers focusing on *ethacrynic acid*, a diuretic, may answer this need. This compound appears to increase the *trabecular meshwork's* permeability by temporarily causing the cells in the meshwork to separate, possibly promoting a flushing of abnormal material from the meshwork, restoring its normal fluid outflow.

Hypertension medication—lowering blood pressure, may have a deleterious effect on some glaucoma patients. While healthy eyes are not affected, studies indicate that lowering blood pressure in glaucoma patients may deprive the cells of needed blood flow. What a dilemma this poses for both patient and doctor. Many seniors find their blood pressures rising along with their years. People who have normal-or-low-pressure glaucoma may suffer from insufficient blood flow to the eye's vascular system. Here is a situation that calls for a dialog between your ophthalmologist and cardiologist to determine the best medical approach for your condition.

CHANGES AFOOT FOR GETTING EYEDROPS INTO YOUR EYES

Do you find it a chore to put drops in your eyes? Well, who doesn't? Help may be on its way. Scientists have realized that eyedrops are not the most efficient delivery system to direct medicine to the *choroid* or *retina* because of the long diffusional pathway drops must travel. Also, since the *cornea* is somewhat impermeable, large molecules have difficulty squeezing through to the inner eye. Add on tearing when a foreign substance is introduced. All these factors along with patient compliance reduce the amount of medication reaching the inner eye. Systemic, oral, or intravenous medications do have a better chance of reaching the *retina* and *choroid*, but this approach is hazardous for the drug will most probably act on other organs as well.

In developing non-eyedrop systems of drug delivery, scientists need to consider duration length of the drug, patient or in-office administration, nature of drug, location, form and materials used to carry the drug to the eye. While relief from instilling eyedrops may be welcomed, periodic injections, for the life of the injected or an implanted drug, is limited, and may give rise to patient resistance. On the other hand, for patients who are chronic non-compliers, drug delivery systems may save these patients from considerable loss of vision.

Here are some of the methods under investigation and which have reached study status that may soon be adopted in medication delivery systems. Through *nanotechnology* (tiny structures), scientists have developed a class of self-assembling *peptides* that form *nanopores* capable of carrying a wide variety of drugs (biomedicine). The structure of the *nanopore* allows the drug to diffuse slowly into the eye's environment, but getting the medicine to enter the cell itself is difficult. While biological materials enter the cells readily, synthetic materials do not. Scientists, however, are exploring a synthetic gold *nanoparticle* that may meet this goal.

- Microdevices for controlled drug delivery. Transfer of molecules-- *anti-angiogenesis* (to stop blood vessel growth) and antioxidant (to deliver nutrients) to the eye.
- Bioadhesive microdevices for controlled drug delivery. Oral drug delivery that targets particular tissues.
- Contact lens delivery of drugs. Drugs imbedded in soft disposable contact lens to achieve medication directly to the eye and also correct refraction issues.
- Drug implants. A sustained release of a drug can be injected into various regions of the eye such as the *vitreous* and under the *conjunctiva.*
- Osmotic pump; in experimental stages with animals, delivers drugs through the *sclera* to the *choroid and retina.*
- A plug the size of a grain of rice inserted into the lower tear duct containing enough pressure-lowering medication for about three months.

ENVIRONMENTAL DAMAGE TO THE EYES

It is well known that ultra violet rays damage the eyes. Many eye medications both over-the-counter and prescription may also possess blinding materials that add to the toxic ultraviolet rays. It is hoped that manufacturers will take into account the photosensitizing effects of their products and make them safer to use. To be sure to be protected, however, wear sunglasses. Shining a laser into the eye generates photosensitivity (a toxic reaction.) Cataract surgery before the onset of *ARMD* using a newly-developed *intraocular* lens that screens out blue light protects the *retina* from the sun's damaging rays.

GET THE MOST OUT OF YOUR DROP

Although new drug delivery systems will be broadly launched, glaucoma patients at this writing still need to instill drops in the old-fashioned way. At one time, doctors assumed that given a prescription for a drop, the patient automatically knew how to instill it. Many of us found mastering instillation to be a no-brainer; others achieved success through trial and error. But some of us experienced serious side-effects. I was one of them. While at work, although my colleagues complimented me on my efficiency in instilling my drop, I experienced cold sweats shortly thereafter. At that time, *Carbacohl* was the only drop I could tolerate. If I had to give it up, I worried that I would not find another effective way to manage my IOP. Fortunately, during this period some members of the medical community began to recommend *nasal lacriminal duct* or *punctal occlusion*. Whew! What a relief that was. The symptoms abated and I again found the drop to be effective in my IOP management. Now I recommend this quick technique to all and demonstrate the process whenever I find the opportunity.

Punctal occlusion retains more medication in the eye where it belongs and prevents it from heading for the tear ducts and exiting into the nose. The ducts are located on the upper and lower inside corners of your eyes next to your nose. It's easier to feel the lower duct. It's sort of like a small bump. Medication flowing down into your nose floods nasal tissues and is absorbed by the mucous membrane lining. This lining possesses a number of specific purposes, one of which filters and absorbs substances. Unlike pills which must pass first through the liver before being absorbed, medication entering the nose acts like an intravenous injection. Along with protecting against a systemic reaction *punctal occlusion* retains more medication in the eye enhancing maximum absorption. Furthermore, studies have indicated that patients who regularly occlude can possibly reduce the amount of medication needed and also delay filtration surgery for a number of years. The recommended time for occluding is from one-to-three minutes.

You can avoid the whole occlusion process if you can manage to keep your eye closed for the same time without blinking. This is harder to do, for we are often unaware of our blinking response. I remember being astonished by the number of times I blinked when I viewed a videotape of myself. Blinking acts as a pump sending the stream of fluid from the eye coursing down into the nasal passages.

Everything in the eye is microscopic, including the capacity of the eye to hold liquid. You may believe that more medication insures that you receive a full dose, but the eye will simply discharge excess medication like an overflow of water. This excess fluid runs down your cheek or into your nasal passages. The human eye holds approximately ten microliters (about 5/100 of a teaspoon of fluid). The commercial eyedroppers release from two to five times the amount of fluid the eye can hold. Since the amount in an eyedrop is variable and even at the smallest dose, an overflow of fluid still occurs, do for your own health faithfully occlude your tear ducts whenever you instill an eyedrop. ***Punctal occlusion* is a simple process**

Method 1

1. Tilt your head back.
2. Gently pull your lower eyelid down and away from your eye to form a pocket.
3. Squeeze bottle to release drop into the pocket close your eye, and gently press with your middle or index finger on the inside corner of the eye for one-to-three minutes. Two minutes may be enough according to recent research. Make sure your finger presses both the upper and lower ducts. This action keeps the medication in the eye and prevents it from entering the nasal passages.
4. You're finished. Wipe or wash off any excess medication around your eye.
5. Repeat with your other eye if required.
6. If you need to instill a second drop, wait ten minutes between drops.

Method 2

Provided you are not an automatic blinker. Instill your drop as described above, close your eye and DO NOT BLINK for one-to-three minutes.

Method 3

Start by holding the bottle with the thumb and index finger. If right-handed, hold bottle in right hand, if left–handed, with the left hand. Your non-dominant hand acts as a guide for the thumb holding the bottle. Press your index finger in the center of your lower eyelid to hold it open. Point this finger toward your eye creating a right angle above the knuckle. Slide the bottle aiming it downward on the flat part, and stop at the knuckle. The bottle tip will now be directly above your eye and you can see that a drop falls into your eye. You can view a demonstration of this method by clicking onto *http://www.youtube. watch?v=FhkRAaIbuI.com;*

If you are a first-time user of drops or are unsure if you're doing it right, do ask for a practice session with your doctor or the technician in your doctor's office. If you are concerned that in clear eyedrop bottles the pharmaceutical company is short-changing you because the bottle is half filled, be assured; the amount of medication in the bottle is standardized. The airspace is necessary to allow the drop to issue from the bottle.

Unfortunately, unless a genetic miracle occurs, medication will be with glaucoma patients for a long time. Soon, as described above, patients may be relieved of instilling drops, but some patients may resist implantation of capsules or other devices and still opt to use drops the old way. But with new advances and combination medical therapy, it is easier to take these medications in stride. Doctors are also most eager to find medications that do not impact on life style, for a less burdensome application produces greater compliance. Non-compliance may lead to significant glaucoma progression. Rather than rail about the inconvenience of medication, it's best to regard it as a necessity to maintain vision.

When medication no longer controls IOP, your eye doctor will most likely suggest surgery, usually a *trabeculoplasty* first, although this protocol may differ in countries other than the United States.

CHAPTER 6
The Remarkable Ability of Light

∘ ∘

*The true scientist never loses the faculty of amazement. It is the
essence of his being.*

Hans Selye, Newsweek, March 31, 1958

The vision of using lasers to treat diseases of the eye dates from 1972-to-1979
during which time, researchers attempted various methodologies to reduce
intraocular pressure. One of these, a relatively new tool, the laser, was invented
by Arthur Schawler and Charles Townes working at Bell Labs in 1958. Their
seminal paper "*Infrared and Optical Lasers*" in the journal *Physical Review* and
consequent explorations netted both men a Nobel Prize. The significance of
this technology caught the attention of the scientific community and two
ophthalmologists, J. B. Wise and S. L. Witter who performed a pilot study
with the argon laser successfully lowering pressure in patients with *open-angle*
glaucoma; the use of the argon laser in ophthalmology was sealed. Within a
few years, this operation called *trabeculoplasty* ascended to a viable treatment
for the lowering of *intraocular pressure*. Based on studies consistently
documenting a drop of six-to-ten mmHg or 20% pressure reduction,
trabeculoplasty is generally regarded as an intermediate step between medical
management and filtration surgery (using the scalpel), in the sequence of
therapeutically pressure-lowering interventions.

Laser, an acronym for *light amplification by stimulated emission of radiation*,
harnesses the power of light by creating a narrow intense beam called coherent
light. Atoms are stimulated by a crystal or gas of a specific color. The spectrum
of light composing all the colors of the rainbow is divided by unchanging
wavelengths for each color. For example, the wavelength of blue is different
from the wave length of red. A wavelength is a factor of the distance between

the two peaks of the same waves of light. Light, as you may know from high school physics, combines both a wave and a particle.

In laser technology, a particular wavelength of light excites atoms that then emit energy in the same direction. An atom striking a proton (the smallest unit of light) produces a single wavelength of light, a pure color. By exciting the atoms of a color such as those of crystals or gases on a photon of light, two photons containing the same wavelength are produced. Harnessed in a mirrored chamber, these multiplying photons reflect back and forth but some escape forming a coherent, concentrated stream of light consisting of identical wavelength photons. This channeled stream of light is capable of performing delicate operations on the eye and other parts of the body. In a different venue and with other stimulators, channeled light can penetrate steel. In the ophthalmological community most of the lasers operate within the green zone, the argon being the most commonly used.

The use of channeled light is hardly a new phenomenon. Recall how in grade school, you played with a mirror to capture a stream of light focusing it on a piece of paper, that under the right conditions, burst into flame or at the very least became singed. And, of course, if you've been a scout, perhaps one of your challenges was to start a fire in the wilderness, using a mirror or a pair of eyeglasses to capture the fiery power of sunlight.

The argon laser and the *neodymium: yttrium-aluminum garnet* (*Nd:YAG*), a later development and more powerful laser are the mainstays of glaucoma therapy. Other lasers, the diode, the holmium, the select are also used extensively. An examination of the literature reveals that laser development promising greater precision and a myriad of applications is still energetically pursued by the scientific community.

Lasers are divided into two classes: those using gas to energize the process and those based on solid state technology. They are further identified as low-power, photothermal (heating the tissues), photochemical (chemically affecting the tissues) and photodisruption (disrupting cellular processes). The gases used include helium, neon, argon, krypton, carbon dioxide, argon fluoride. The solid state lasers use the ions of minerals such as yttrium, aluminum, garnet, lithium, fluoride, gallium, and arsenide.

The argon laser is most commonly used for trabeculoplasty, iridotomy, iridoplasty, sclerostomy, photocoagulation, diabetic retinopathy, suturing stitches in ophthalmic surgery, and photodynamic therapy. It also powers the scanning laser and ophthalmoscope systems. It can be either photo-thermal or photo-chemical.

The krypton laser using krypton gas is also used for *iridotomy, trabeculoplasty* and *photocoagulation.*

Carbon dioxide gas is used for *sclerostomy*.

The photochemical excimer laser using argon fluoride gas is the engine of choice for *LASIK* surgery (corrects nearsightedness or reading problems), and *sclerostomy*.

The solid state lasers use the ions in certain minerals. The *Nd:YAG* which can be in either the photodisruption form or the photothermal form uses ions in yttrium, aluminum and garnet to perform *posterior capsulotomy iridotomy trabeculoplasy, sclerostomy, cyclophotocoagulation,* and *retinal photocoagulation,* while the *Nd:YFL* using the neodymium ions in yttrium, lithium and fluoride take care of *iridotomy, capsulotomy* and *sclerostomy.* Two other *YAG* lasers, the *Er:YAG* and *THC:YAG,* only photothermal, essentially do the same job as described above for the other two *YAG* lasers.

The Diode photothermal laser is capable of performing a slew of operations. It is powered by gallium, aluminum and arsenide. *Retinal coagulation* (to correct tears or *retinal detachment* in the *retina*), *iridotomy, iridoplasty, sclerostomy,* cutting sutures, *cyclophotocoagulation, scanning laser, OCT (optical coherence tomography), ophthalmoscopy,* laser pointers and aiming beams are all powered by the Diode that has a major advantage of being portable. This laser is especially valuable to doctors and technicians who are practicing in countries and areas where equipment is not readily available. Studies indicate that *trabeculoplasty* results using diode are comparable to the other two lasers.

A third group uses fluorescent dyes that are injected into the arm and then activated when a laser beam is shone on the diseased area. These are either *photothermal* or *photochemical* and they are generally used for treating *macular degeneration.* They can also be used for *retinal photocoagulation, iridotomy, sclerostomy* and cutting sutures.

As with all technologies, laser instruments continue to evolve. There is a *diode* laser that plugs into a wall outlet and delivers red, yellow and green light allowing surgeons to treat a variety of *retinal* diseases without switching to alternative lasers. Altering wavelengths at the touch of a button increases the versatility of the machine especially when the need arises for specific wavelengths to perform delicate surgery.

Laser ophthalmology is considered to be non-incisional surgery. Traditionally, it has been practiced by ophthalmologists, but optometrists are making a bid to perform this surgery and have gained a foothold in the Veterans Administration.

Basically, the lasers work in ophthalmology by ablating (destroying) a minute amount of tissue in the eye. The energy, beamed into the eye interacting with the tissues of the eye, burns, coagulates or cuts that specific area. For example, laser therapy in *trabeculoplasty* creates a series of burns or fragmentation of tissue on the *trabecular meshwork*, improving drainage. In a healthy *retina*, the *meshwork* cells behave like spiders in a web cleaning up whatever moves. Eventually, however, the number of these clean-up cells is diminished and as the trabecular beams shed cells, they stick together, having lost the electrical charge that kept them apart. Studies on experimental glaucoma produced in monkeys revealed the liberation of bioactive chemicals at the site of the laser treatment; these chemicals stimulate the *phagocytes* to clean up the debris.

Once believed that the thermal effect of laser therapy induced alterations in the *trabecular meshwork* by causing the beams in the *meshwork* to stick together, thus enlarging spaces between beams, current thinking suggests that thermal treatment initiates a cascade of biological events, enhancing outflow that takes place between four and six weeks postoperatively—that is, wound healing producing the effect. The treatment is believed to induce cell division and migration of cells. This action stimulates the *trabecular meshwork* to regenerate and repopulate itself with active and healthier cells.

A more recent addition for *trabeculoplasty*, the *select laser*, is cooler, gentler, and less destructive of tissues. It targets the pigment-containing cells but does not damage the trabecular beams. Studies have found it as effective as the argon and apparently, it can be used more often than the argon.

While the exact sequence of events in laser therapy is still being explored, the use of lasers as technical tools both for research and therapy is expanding. As with all medical instruments, new developments or perhaps improvements in laser technology energize this form of therapy. Although laser therapy is routinely used for *trabeculoplasty*, it is possible that certain laser tools can leap the barrier and be used for filtration surgery. A Japanese company developed an excimer laser with which they performed infiltration surgery on a small number of patients with uncontrolled glaucoma. Results were comparable to filtration surgery with the scalpel. And a more recent development, the *Trabectome* uses laser energy to perform a type of filtering operation (See Chapter 7).

Not everybody profits from laser therapy. Pigment found in the *trabecular meshwork* determines the light energy rate of absorption. Brown pigment is ideal, for it absorbs heat well. Some studies indicate that African-Americans appear to do less well than Caucasians. While the initial success rate was comparable, success rate over time for African-Americans dropped to 55.9% as compared to 82% of Caucasians. Yet the *AGIS* study recommended laser treatment especially for African-Americans. (Go figure).

Another finding of the *AGIS* study broached the sequence of treatment--whether laser therapy should be reserved as an intermediate step between medication and a *trabeculectomy* or if needed, following surgery. This six-year study determined that sequence was not as important as maintaining a safe *intraocular pressure*. All the patients in the study possessed *open-angle* glaucoma and were in need of some form of surgery to lower their *intraocular pressures*. Those patients whose IOP was below 14 mmHg did better but all patients experienced some glaucoma progression albeit those with the lowest pressures had the least progression. In many cases, doctors now routinely advise patients that pressures need to be in the low teens and treat accordingly.

Moorfields Primary Treatment Trial enrolled 168 patients. Their findings indicated that initial *trabeculectomy* treatment achieved the lowest IOP with the least vision loss. These findings have apparently not affected treatment in the United States, for the majority of eye doctors treat medically first before the more invasive therapies. This approach underlies the age-old philosophy of "do as little harm as possible". Intervention therapies requiring ablating and cutting have a greater potential to damage tissues.

Nevertheless, the *Collaborative Glaucoma Initial Treatment Study* that enrolled patients with newly diagnosed glaucoma confirms the *Moorfields* approach. In this study, initially, half of the patients received medical therapy, the other half laser. After nine years, the laser group did better. The *Early Manifest Glaucoma Trial* of 255 patients added an additional fillip. Those patients treated with laser plus *betaxolol (Betoptic)* did better than those without the additional medication. Laser first did appear to be more protective of the *trabecular meshwork*.

Whether laser therapy becomes a routine first line therapy is still a moot question among doctors and it may be a hard sell to patients familiar with the sequence already established. Of the patients in our group, none thus far, have had laser therapy as a first-line treatment. Doctors report in the literature that patients given the choice of adding another drop or taking laser therapy usually opt for the drop. Laser therapy is contraindicated for patients with inflammatory conditions such as *uveitis, juvenile, traumatic* and *congenital* glaucoma also do not respond well to the laser.

That laser treatment has become a remarkable tool for the management of glaucoma and other eye diseases is indisputable. Yet its long-term results are disappointing. IOP on average is controlled from 3-to-5 years with a probability success rate after one year of seventy percent, at five years, forty-nine percent and at ten years three percent. Some patients complain that the effect wears off in a matter of months. The results on the above trials indicate that although laser therapy as a first-line therapy has met resistance in the United States, cases of individuals who, for example, are allergic to all medications, cannot remember to take medications in a timely fashion, or who have certain forms of glaucoma, may benefit from laser first.

Smaller subsequent studies still beg the question as to which therapy works best, but it does appear that if patients have been on medical therapy for a length of time, laser is less effective than when applied as a first-line therapy. The most common laser procedure for glaucoma patients is still the *trabeculoplasty*.

TRABECULOPLASTY

Presently, a *trabeculoplasty* can be performed using three lasers—argon (*ALT*), diode (*DLT*) and select (*SLT*). These lasers have been extensively studied over the past years since Wise and Witter reported on their findings.

ALT, the first and most often selected, shaped some of the methods that ophthalmologists commonly use today. This procedure involves the use of a mirrored lens that enables the doctor to focus on the *trabecular meshwork*. Traditionally, 50-to-100 burns or tiny ruptures are applied to half of the trabecular meshwork, reserving the remainder tissue for future therapy. While the burns are not visible to the naked eye, they can be viewed microscopically. The burn creates a tiny bubble indicating release of thermal energy. Some surgeons advocate as few as thirty-five burns. Typically, the procedure lowers the IOP by four points. If the IOP is in the high 20's this operation may not be viable, for ideal pressures are now targeted at the low teens, and in some cases, single digits. Success rate, initially strong, tapers off to less then 25% within five years in the majority of cases. Patients older than sixty with a lower baseline IOP and who have exfoliation glaucoma most often have favorable long-term results. Ophthalmologists now regard laser therapy as a bridge between medical and surgical therapy.

The operation stimulates a transient increase of IOP (the reason you cannot leave the premises immediately until your IOP is stabilized.) If the pressure remains stubbornly high, your doctor will probably use one percent *apraclonidine* and also possibly a variety of other medications such as *dipivefrin, pilocarpine, Acetazolamide*, and *timolol*. Most often following laser therapy, medical therapy is still necessary although the number of medications may be reduced. More than two *ALT* surgeries are considered risky. More laser therapy may, in fact, worsen the glaucoma as evident in the scientific experiments where animals are given laser treatment to produce glaucomatous conditions suitable for experimental purposes. Several investigators, however, in an attempt to avoid further surgery on patients, have used more than two

ALTs, but the results have been unremarkable—lowered pressures of 33% after one year and only 14% after a little less than two years.

The Diode laser (*DLT*), less expensive than the *ALT*, lightweight, air or electronically-powered using standard current, provides a good alternative to the *ALT*, especially in rural settings or in countries where only minimum medical treatment exists. The Diode differs from the *ALT* in that heat energy absorption is reduced.

Undoubtedly therapeutic, *ALT* or *DLT* treatment does some damage, however minimal, to the targeted cells and the adjacent cells of the *trabecular meshwork*.

The tiny coagulated or scarred areas in the meshwork, nevertheless, can in the future impair fluid outflow through the *trabecular meshwork*.

The *SLT*, which produces short laser pulses (less energy than the *ALT*), selectively targets pigmented (melanin) cells causing a photochemical rather than a coagulative reaction. The laser energy is absorbed by these cells leaving the meshwork undamaged. Less scarring of the *trabecular meshwork* and possibly protection of the adjacent non-pigmented cells may result. In contrast, the *ALT* emits continuous wave radiation. Both lasers apparently work by increasing extracellular matrix turnover in the *trabecular meshwork* through the stimulation of certain enzymes (*matrix metalloproteinase*). The lasers chew up the matrix increasing greater drainage. Studies confirm the *SLT* as effective as *ALT* and in some cases, better tolerated by patients. As with *ALT*, post-operative spikes can be controlled with pre-or post-operative medical treatment. *SLT*, in certain cases, can probably be applied more than twice even for those patients who have had previous *ALT* treatment. Its use may depend upon the preference of the physician and the type of pigmentation in the angle.

A study from the Vision Institute of Milwaukee found that patients who responded well to *SLT* treatment had favorable outcomes. After one year 66% required no medication, 11.3%, reduced medication and a mere 5.6% had no improvement in pressure even with medication. Patients involved in the study did not have previous cataract or glaucoma operations. Improvement in patients who had undergone glaucoma, cataract or a combination followed a similar pattern with 70.9% improved, of which 56% did without medication, 4.2% decreased medication, 10.4% remained on meds, and 29% remained the same. Except for one patient with an inflammatory response that was resolved within a month, treatment was found to be safe. The doctor involved in this research plans to use *SLT* as a first line treatment.

Both forms of laser stimulate an immune system response and macrophages buzz in to clear out the inflammatory debris stimulating greater outflow. Statistically, IOP outcomes are similar. Some researchers have found that the *SLT* may be as effective and safe as a primary treatment for patients with *POAG* and *OHT.*

The fact that laser therapy is therapeutically limited fuels the debate of whether to laser first or medicate first. Some doctors, but not a lot of them, opt for laser first despite the limitations, but the majority of physicians in the United States still use drops for initial treatment.

Usually the choice of instruments depends on availability in a particular setting. Most likely a teaching hospital will have all three instruments. Discuss with your doctor which instrument is most suitable for your condition.

Preparation for laser is minimal. Get a good night's sleep. If you meditate continue your regular practice. Think positively--this treatment will work well for me. The treatment, itself, is quick and painless for most people. You may feel a tiny sting from time to time. One hour before the operation, your doctor will administer a drop of *brimonidine* or *apraclonidine* to reduce the risk of an IOP spike. A local anesthetic will be used and when your eye is numb, your doctor will place a three-way mirror on the eye using a gel interface. With all three lasers approximately 35-to-50 spots are placed evenly along half the angle (180 degrees). If a second treatment becomes necessary, your doctor will place an additional set of spots on the remaining 180 degrees. If you change doctors and should the treatment be separated by a number of years, be sure to bring along your laser history since it may be difficult to identify the placement of the first set of burns.

Unless your pressure is reduced significantly, some or all of your previous medications will still be necessary. For a short time, you will also use a topical steroid or equivalent anti-inflammation drop until the inflammation subsides. The most common steroid recommended is *Pred Forte.* Your doctor will probably want to check your eye the following day, the next week and a month later.

Usually laser *trabeculoplasty* is considered one of the safest forms of therapy, but there is always an exception. Babs has both glaucoma and *nystagmus,* a condition where the eye oscillates involuntarily. This condition impacts on managing her glaucoma and also places her at risk for surgery. Contrary to expectations, her pressure rose dramatically following laser surgery requiring an immediate *trabeculectomy.* Unfortunately, she did lose vision in that eye. Congenital *nystagmus,* the most common form, occurs in from one in four thousand to one in six thousand births. A National Institutes of Health Study documented that a simple strategy involving surgery on four muscle tendons produced positive results in a small group of participants with minimal risk and no adverse side effects.

This case is singular in our Group for an out-and-out failure of a *trabeculoplasty*, but other eye conditions may be contraindicated for laser therapy. These include *Fuch's Endothelial Dystrophy* or other dystrophies (see Chapter 2) that cloud the cornea, fogging up the window of the eye and thus preventing access to view the *retina*. A *corneal* abrasion, something I experienced from the administration of a drop to which I was allergic, can also stop laser therapy cold, but this is a temporary condition, for when the cornea heals, laser treatment can be resumed.

Collateral damage from laser therapy does exist, and this damage is weighed against the benefits. Lasers are powerful tools and regulations do exist that deploy parameters for safe use. The Occupational and Health Administration (OSHA) focuses on health care workers, the FDA and individual states provide recommendations for medical practice. Standards and practice still need to be established nation if not world-wide to insue safety for patients, doctors, nurses and health care workers. An ultra-short laser pulse that produces the necessary effect but with less damage developed by University of Illinois at Chicago: researchers is a positive step in this direction.

IRIDECTOMY/IRIDOTOMY

Doctors, in the early 1900's, envisioned creating a hole in the eye to allow fluid drainage in cases of serious glaucoma. By the 1960's the *iridotomy*, now routine for both relief of *acute-angle-closure* glaucoma and for prophylactic use was introduced. *Acute-angle-closure* glaucoma is potentially blinding, for untreated, extensive loss of sight can occur within hours. The condition seems to come out of nowhere, as it did with Sophia who was watching a movie on HBO in a darkened room. Suddenly, her head ached. She saw flashing lights, and when she turned on her lamp, noticed halos around it. She turned off the television and tried to relax, hoping the sensations would resolve, but after an hour of no remission, she checked in at the emergency room of a nearby hospital where, fortunately, an alert resident sent her immediately to ophthalmology. Most of her sight was saved.

Sophia, with 20/20 vision, had not visited an ophthalmologist ever. Several years ago, a local optometrist prescribed reading glasses, but he neglected to take a pressure reading, and did not remark on her narrow angles. The angle is formed by the meeting of the *cornea* and *iris*. The junction forms the angle and drainage system. Measurement of the angle specifies *open-angle* or *narrow-angle* glaucoma. A 30-to-40 (grades lll, lV) degree opening denotes *open-angle* glaucoma; a 20 degree opening (grade ll) possibly *narrow-angle* glaucoma, and a 10 degree (grade 1) or less is indicative of closed angle and may precipitate an *acute-angle-closure attack*. Sophia's angle measured at 8 degrees. The dilation of her eye, a natural occurrence in a darkened room, brought on the attack. Darkness dilates the pupil, not a problem for open-angles, but for closed or narrow angles, the dilated pupil may push the *iris* into the tiny drainage channel occluding it. An *iridotomy* is not always the solution. In some cases, a filtering operation may be necessary.

An angle closure is highly-correctible. At times, a selfless act produces an unexpected gift. I was asked by a researcher to refer healthy patients for a study comparing healthy eyes with glaucomatous eyes. One of my referrals discovered that he had narrow angles placing him in danger of an *angle-closure* attack. He followed the recommendations for prophylactic surgery in both eyes.

Laser treatment in the form of an *iridectomy* or an *iridotomy* will most often correct the problem. The argon laser heats up the tissue of the *iris* which absorbs the laser energy to form a small hole, and the *Nd:YAG* laser dispatches a bit of *iris* tissue with one blast. Both can be used for this operation. The argon laser may be more stressful for it requires multiple applications, but the *Nd:YAG* may be more risky. Since the *YAG* is powerful, it may not always be the instrument of choice, although for blue-eyed people who have less pigment, it may be more serviceable. Some bleeding may occur following the *YAG* procedure. The argon laser coagulates blood vessels along with the tissues and eliminates bleeding. The *iredectomy* is a surgical procedure where a small piece of *iris* is removed. Now this is a term used interchangeably with the *iridotomy*.

Not everything goes perfectly well and there are cases of failed *iridotomies.* Perhaps the cause was an overly-cautious doctor who did not create a large enough hole that just simply healed itself in time, or perhaps excess scarring closed the hole. The hole, however, can be reopened quite easily. A third reason for failure may be the presence of *plateau iris*, a condition not always diagnosed until an *iridotomy* has been performed. Although occurring in only about five percent of the cases, it is troublesome, but fortunately with the argon laser, a series of low-energy burns around the periphery (*peripheral iridoplasty*) of the *iris* can shrink it. This procedure moves the *iris* away from the angle solving the problem. A fourth problem may be *pupillary block*. If this is the case, a *trabeculectomy* may be necessary. *Pupillary Block* is a structural problem in which the aqueous humor, in its journey from the back of the eye to the front, is blocked in the channel formed by the *lens* and the *iris*. The fluid backs up behind the *iris* and shoves the *iris* into the drainage angle. On the other hand, should you need a cataract extraction, this operation may solve your *closed-angle* problem, for the procedure may lower your IOP and increase the angle width—a neat solution.

Pigmentary Dispersion Syndrome (See Chapter 3) This syndrome also yields to the therapeutic laser. Again, the *iris* presents the problem, but unlike *pupillary block* where the *iris* is pushed forward, in this case, the *iris* is pushed backwards. This condition is called *reverse pupillary block*. Equilibrium is restored with an *iridotomy* that equalizes the pressure between the front and back chambers of the eye by flattening out the eye to a more normal position. In many cases the drug *pilocarpine* will correct the problem. In some cases, however, despite the use of medical therapy, an *iridotomy* becomes necessary.

Contraindications to the laser therapy exist in certain cases. When the anterior chamber is totally flat (no space left between the *iris*, the *lens*, and the *cornea*), or when because of long-term scarring, the *cornea* is completely sealed, *iridotomies* are ineffective.

For the most part, given the statistics (98%-to-99% success rate.) an *iridotomy* usually works. Although it may be successful, you will still need to be followed and perhaps use medication. If you have had first-line therapy with laser, there may be undetected damage that occurred such as scarring. To avoid complications or the risk of failure, your doctor may opt for additional medication or a *trabeculectomy* to lower your *intraocular pressure*.

CYCLODESTRUCTIVE PROCEDURES

We have discussed above various forms of laser therapy to improve drainage. Another method for reducing IOP is partial destruction of the *ciliary body* to reduce the amount of fluid generated. Some doctors consider it as a last resort when all other methods for controlling IOP have failed. Although improved lasers and techniques are available, the problem of precision is not entirely solved. If too much tissue is ablated or destroyed, the result will be too low a pressure (*hypotony*) that will eventually cause adhesions in the eye and lead to loss of vision. If not enough tissue is removed, the problem of high pressure remains. Success rate just barely reaches seventy percent. Prior to the use of lasers, radio signals (*electrodiathermy*) and freezing (*cryotherapy*) applied to the ciliary body were attempted, but little success was achieved. The tissue, not clearly visible, along with inadequate tools, hampered fine-tuning the operation. Either too much tissue was destroyed, reducing the fluid to a trickle debilitating the eye, or too little, while sparing the eye, did not alter the IOP. Nevertheless, the following two procedures may save a failing eye as it did with Janet, who had no other options.

Transscleral cyclophotocoagulation of ciliary body (TSCP)

For *TSCP*, the eye is anesthetized and then the doctor uses a probe, moving it across the *sclera* and positioning it just above the *ciliary body*, Laser energy is then applied to ablate a portion of the *ciliary body*.

Endoscopiccyclophotocoagulation (ECP)

The laser procedure differs from the above only in application. The eye is anesthetized. A tiny probe is then placed directly inside the eye through a surgical incision $1/20^{th}$ of an inch in diameter. The probe contains a minute laser and camera introduced under the *iris* and advanced to a position where the *ciliary body* is visible to the doctor. Laser energy is then applied to destroy part of the *ciliary body*; three-quarters of the *ciliary body* can be ablated with this system. Because the *ciliary body* is a complicated structure containing hills and valleys, enough cells still remain to produce sufficient fluid to nourish the eye. Greater success is achieved if the procedure is performed along with a cataract extraction. Either the *Ned:YAG*, the diode or some of the newer, more sophisticated lasers can be used for these procedures.

Sclerostomy

The *sclerostomy* is a procedure for making a hole the size of a pencil tip into the *sclera* to form an outflow channel for the aqueous humor. While a brilliant idea, it has not as yet proven to be superior to the filtration operation. It is a10-to-20 minute laser procedure performed by directing laser energy through a pencil-point probe that pierces the edge of the cornea at its junction with the *sclera*

Ab interno is a modification on the *sclerostomy*, using the *Er: YAG* laser. An endoscope (probe of silica fiber) directs the laser light from inside the eye by bouncing this light off a mirror in a contact lens placed on the eye. Advantages include viewing the angle where the *iris* and *cornea* meet and positioning the laser light to create a full-thickness hole in the proper location. This method is quicker, but it still has not gained a following.

Photocoagulation

Photocoagulation is the process of heating tissue with laser energy. This system can be used to repair *retinal* tears or detachment and to control proliferating blood vessels found in such diseases as *diabetic retinopathy* and *macular degeneration*.

My first brush with ophthalmic surgery occurred in my early 50's when I was engaged in a very demanding job. I saw flashes of light and after about two weeks when this phenomenon refused to vanish, I visited an optometrist, who after examining my eye advised that I should consider using contact lens. From his viewpoint nothing was wrong. But as the flashes did not abate, I decided to seek a second opinion, this time with a retinologist, who discovered that I had tears in both *retinas*, small holes actually. He advised sealing the holes either by laser or cryo (freezing) therapy. The retinologist used laser therapy in one eye that had a single hole and both laser and cryo therapy in the other that had two holes. Since that treatment, although glaucoma followed shortly thereafter, my *retinas* have remained firm. Discussing my *retinal* surgery with colleagues in my profession, I discovered that two others had also had laser therapy for *retinal* problems, both of whom, as I, were highly near-sighted (*myopic*). I learned subsequently that near-sightedness changes the shape of the eye from spherical to oval causing the *retina* to be more vulnerable to tearing and detachment.

Laser treatment seals back the *retina* by coagulating (creating laser burns) around the periphery of the hole. Any invasion of the eye promotes scar tissue. In this case, the scar tissue acts like a dam or fence preventing the hole from enlarging, for should that occur, *retinal* detachment caused by seepage of *vitreous* gel may follow. This seepage may cause the *retina* to peel away from the wall of the eye, detaching it. If *retinal* detachment is at a stage where laser treatment is ineffective, the retinologist will then attempt to reattach the *retina* with an operation that involves a *sceral buckle*. When a *retina* detaches and cannot be properly reattached, blindness or reduced vision may result.

Photocoagulation Of Blood Vessels

Proliferative Diabetic Retinopathy

Lily has *diabetes* and she also has glaucoma, but, fortunately, Lily's *diabetes* has not affected her vision. She uses her glaucoma medication faithfully, eats well, takes some supplements and rides her bicycle daily. Mathew, on the other hand, is a couch potato who also has *diabetes*. He lives alone, seldom cooks for himself preferring fast food. Although he also faithfully injects a daily dose of insulin, he has developed *diabetic retinopathy*. He has had laser treatment on both of his eyes. His central vision is still intact, but he is troubled by his reduced peripheral vision.

In *proliferative diabetic retinopathy*, the more advanced stage of *diabetic retinopathy*, blood vessels receive incorrect messages. Because *diabetes* affects the perfusion of blood entering the *capillary* systems of the eye, depletion of oxygen (because it is carried by the blood) occurs. The blood vessels emit distress signals that promote development of new blood vessels, which are weak and misdirected. Furthermore, they leak, hemorrhage, and grow where they are not needed. When these vessels pervade the *retina*, the result is called *proliferative diabetic retinopathy;* should the blood vessels occlude the drainage passages, glaucoma results. *Photocoagulation* using a laser beam ablates (destroys) the peripheral cells in the *retina*. This procedure requires about 2,000 pulses. Unfortunately, the outer limits of *peripheral vision* are lost in the process but mid and central vision are spared. Doctors are now attempting to use some newer therapies for *proliferative diabetic retinopathy* similar to those described below for *ARMD* that will, hopefully, spare the outlying *peripheral* cells.

ADULT RELATED MACULAR DEGENERATION (ARMD)

The wet form (*exudative*) of *ARMD* causes ninety percent of the cases of central vision loss attributed to this disease. The problem occurs when blood vessels invade the *Bruch's Membrane*, the tissue underlying the *retina*. These new blood vessels proliferate and cause problems. The pathways to these destructive effects are triggered by inflammation that then leads to oxidative stress, damage to the *Bruch's Membrane* and other parts of the eye.

Photocoagulation is used in some cases of the wet form of *macular degeneration* with varying degrees of success. *Transpupilary Thermal Therapy (TTT)* reduces vision loss in only some thirteen percent of the cases because of the difficulty in treating large or poorly demarcated blood vessels. Unfortunately, these blood vessels are persistent, for fifty percent of those zapped reconstitute. Success rate is less than ten percent of those considered eligible.

PHOTODYNAMIIC THERAPY (PDT)

This therapy may be more effective. It is a two-step procedure. A dye, *Visudyne (verteporfin),* is injected into the arm and in ten minutes it accumulates in the *neovascularization* areas—the site of those errant blood vessels. The doctor then shines a light (cold laser) on the blood vessels destroying them. The treatment is not directed at the healthy parts of the *retina*. It is most successful with the classic form where the problem is visible, as opposed to the occult form where the problem is hidden. Although it is a valuable tool for destroying the errant blood vessels in *ARMD*, it is not altogether accurate, for the doctor must calculate the amount of injected drug and of light necessary for drug activation.

Newer technology may address this problem. A sort of Geiger counter called a *dosimetry system* quantifies the photosensitizing drug concentrations, coordinating the injected drug with the wavelength of light. Trials with animals indicate that this system may overcome the above hurdle. The system also claims to adjust for individual differences in drug absorption.

The drug *Visudyne*, while effective, does have side effects such as clot formation and damage to the thin cell layer just below the *retina*. Addressing this, a scientist has developed a water soluble drug not absorbed by the blood or the other vascular tissues in the eye. This treatment is still being studied.

PDT treatment combined with other treatments promises greater success. Some treatments under study combine *PDT* with drugs that inhibit the growth factor (*VEGF*) (See Chapter 5).

ARGON-LASER SPHINCTEROTOMY

The permanent narrowing of the pupil, a side effect of the miotic medications such as *pilocarpine* and *carbacohl* may not be a problem today, for the newer medications do not affect the sphincter muscle in the eye. But should you be using one of these *miotic* medications, know that your sphincter muscle, if permanently constricted, can be released through *argon laser* therapy. Laser burns are applied around the *pupil's* border widening the pupil. Except in rare cases, the pupil will not, however, revert to naturally accommodate light changes. With a permanently-widened pupil, it is important to wear sunglasses when outdoors for the wider pupil allows more *UV-B* rays to reach the *retina*. On rare occasions, laser light reaches the *retina* and can cause some damage. Glare may be a problem following this procedure but sunglasses do help to alleviate it.

Should you need cataract surgery, widening your narrowed pupil will become part of the procedure. The cataract surgeon mechanically stretches the pupil to accommodate the *lens*. Again, the pupil will probably remain in that stretched position.

TREATMENT FOR NANOPHTHALMOS

Good things like diamond rings come in small packages, but with the eye, it's another story. Some people are born with smaller than usual eyes and this attribute may be problematic, reducing the space necessary to accommodate all the bodies within the eye. Very farsighted people may have smaller than usual eyes and may do well throughout life, but this condition does, however, predispose the eye to *narrow-angle* glaucoma placing the patient at risk of *narrow angle-closure* glaucoma. When the risk exists, the doctor will probably advise a prophylactic *iridectomy*.

BENIGN OR?

Whenever we consider an invasive treatment, we ask our doctors, our friends, and other specialists about its safety, risks, and the possibilities of worsening the condition. We are right to be concerned. There is no procedure that does not leave its mark. Do complications occur with laser surgery? Well, yes and no. For the very susceptible, yes, but for the majority, complications or effects following laser surgery disappear within a day or two, if not in hours. Higher IOP is the most common, but this condition is usually resolved within a few hours especially when treated with *apraclonidine (Iopidine)* drops that reduce the production of aqueous humor. When *Iopidine* fails, the problem may lie with the release of pigment from the *iris* settling in the *trabecular meshwork*. Patients with *uveitis* may encounter adhesions of tissues in the eye because of the inflammation that follows any invasive procedure. Many doctors will advise bypassing laser for a filtration operation for these patients. Distortion of the pupil and in some cases visual field loss can occur. Corneal burns and abrasions are a technical problem and may result from inadequate skill on the part of the surgeon or, in my case, where allergic response to the anesthetic drop caused them. Most complications, however, do clear up within a week.

Laser therapy, as studies have indicated, is comparatively safe as surgical interventions go, but it may be disastrous for some whose condition has not been correctly diagnosed, or who find themselves in the hands of an incompetent doctor as did a friend of mine. She was referred to an eye doctor who performed, I believe, a *trabeculoplasty* (she was never given the name of the procedure). She completely lost the sight of that eye. Her other eye, diagnosed with glaucoma, was sustained on medication throughout the rest of her life. We have spoken of another case of an individual with *nystagmus* (involuntary movement of the eyeball), who lost a great deal of sight after a *trabeculoplasty*. On the other hand, my laser therapy and that of the majority of the members of our Group did just fine. We blew off the procedure as just another step in the process of retaining vision. The main drawback in laser therapy to reduce high IOP is that it is an interim event and within years, a filtering operation is usually necessary when eye pressure again needs lowering.

More worrisome is that any intervention in the eye may cause *free radical* damage. The eye does have a method for zapping the *free radicals* by manufacturing a peptide called *glutathione* that is formed by the precursors of glutamic acid and the non-essential amino acids, cysteine and glycine. In older people *glutathione* is diminished. Protecting the eye from *free radical* damage when surgical intervention is required should be considered.

As a leader of the Group, I encounter many people who quiver at the thought of the powerful laser beam applied to their eyes. While these individuals may accept medical treatment, the thought of intervention of any kind practically sends them into psychic shock. One member has been debating for a year about whether to have prophylactic surgery for *narrow-angle* glaucoma. He has been to three ophthalmologists, all of whom concur that an attack may be imminent. Since many patients have multiple health problems, they are often inclined to put off glaucoma treatment other than drops, although advised by their doctors of the danger of losing vision. Yet there are others who simply will not consider laser treatment under any circumstance, despite their doctor's assurance that while not altogether harmless, laser treatment offers an excellent interim treatment. These and other idiosyncratic observations are legitimate and need to be considered when the physician suggests laser therapy. But the alternative of doing nothing is grim, especially when the danger of rapid progression of vision loss looms.

My experience with laser therapy goes back to the period when ophthalmologists enthusiastically embraced this new treatment for glaucoma. I was frightened at the thought of submitting to this new-fangled technology. Yet when my doctor performed laser therapy to my left eye, I was amazed and relieved that the procedure required only local anesthesia and that I was able, on my follow-up visit the next day, to appreciate my doctor's gleeful appraisal of the results—lowered IOP. I was up and about and ready to return to work following my examination. Needless to say, the use of the laser instruments has seeded many new technologies and has been one of the many arms of the revolution in treatment of many diseases including the eye.

Lasik Surgery

This surgery came of age in the last half of the twentieth century and it has become an option for correction of refraction problems (near-sighted, far-sighted and astigmatic). Some patients with glaucoma, especially those who are younger and who have a milder form may opt to have *LASIK* surgery, but they need to realize that the procedure requires the thinning of the *cornea*. When checking for signs of glaucoma, patients should tell their doctors that they've had *LASIK* surgery for refraction errors, for the *cornea* may register a lower than actual pressure reading that may mask the actual or early glaucoma condition.

Excimer laser, developed by IBM in 1976 for industrial use in etching intricate patterns such as those found on computer chips, is the laser adapted for this surgical procedure. It is a cold laser that breaks down molecular tissue bonds in a tiny, tiny area without producing harmful heat. Each pulse of the computer targets an area the thickness of the human hair, the diameter of approximately 125 microns. Like all lasers, there are a number of versions of the *Excimer*. These are, among others, the broad beam technology that produces a single beam adjustable for various refractive conditions and the fine beam of the scanning laser that moves around the *cornea* removing tiny bits of tissue. Since this is a preset pattern, many surgeons prefer the broad beam system.

The *Excimer* laser sculpts the *cornea* by removing thin layers of the *corneal* tissue to achieve the desired shape. This process requires collaboration between the surgeon and the data fed by the computer to achieve the necessary sculpting pattern. The actual operation requires the creation of a flap from the center of the *cornea* that allows access to the underlying *corneal* tissue. The flap is folded back and laser pulses are applied to correct the refraction problems. Then the flap is unfolded back in place. While the procedure takes only minutes, patients are required to spend several hours in the doctor's office in preparation for the operation, and a few minutes for post-operative instruction.

Retinal detachment has been associated with *LASIK* surgery, and while this result is still speculative, it is wise to have a retinologist examine your eyes before undergoing treatment, especially if you are severely near-sighted. *Myopia*, because it lengthens the eye, predisposes you to *retinal detachment*.

LASER THERMAL KERAPLASTY (LTK)

This procedure uses the *Holmium* laser that unlike the *Excimer* which removes or ablates tissue, creates heat resulting in constriction of *corneal* tissue. It is prescribed for mild to moderate forms of *myopia*. It's called a no-touch procedure and is faster than the *LASIK*. A problem may occur when the cornea heals itself and returns to its former position.

Guidelines issued by Eye Surgery Education Council, a project of the American Society of Cataract and Refractive Surgery, defined in 2002, the criteria for *LASIK* surgery and provides patients with summaries of associated screening examinations and realistic expectations of the surgery. The proper room humidity may impact on the procedure requiring a repeat *LASIK*. Room humidity during the surgery and outdoor humidity may cause the *corneas* of some patients to become more hydrated before the procedure causing difficulty in removing tissue. This situation can be remediated by reprogramming the equipment.

Obviously, laser technology is an enormous field and a great deal of attention is focused on refinement of this technology. There are lasers now capable of observing molecules in action and of three-dimensional viewing of a molecule. Proteins, those molecules that build structures in the body, can now be viewed in their three-dimensionality, opening the doors for building medications that can correct protein errors. The marriage of technology and treatment is ongoing and will certainly have its impact on the glaucoma patient. Two companies have developed *LASIK* treatment, *Z-Lasic* and *ILasic* that reduce glare and the halo effects. All in all, laser treatment, while certainly not a cure, is a way of fighting back the dragon of losing vision and, if it can help with minimum damage to your eye, why not go for it.

Other corrections for near-sightedness include the placement of *interstromal corneal ring segments*. Thickness of the rings determines the flatness of the *cornea*. If they don't work they can be removed. The advantage of this system is that the *cornea* remains intact. Mild to moderate *myopia* is corrected. Implantation of a contact lens presents another possibility. This lens is placed between the *iris* and the natural *lens*. This system may work best for high myopes or high far-sightedness. Another site for implantation of a contact lens is inside the *cornea*. Near-sightedness and reading ability are corrected with this procedure.

THE FUTURE

There is a device called the *Glaucoma Golden Shunt*. It looks like a kind of flatworm, which some of you may remember from high school biology. The *Glaucoma Golden Shunt (GGS)* microscopic 24-carat ultra-thin 30-micron gold shunt containing laser-activated microtubules (channels) is designed to increase aqueous outflow into the supraciliary space. When placed in the eye, half the channels are open and half are closed. The theory behind the procedure is activation of the channels by an instrument called the *SOLX Titanium Sapphire Laser* that was developed by an Israeli-Spanish team. More channels can be opened to attain the desired pressure. No *bleb* results because the fluid is draining into the supraciliary space which is the same anatomical position into which your eye drains. This laser supposedly has deeper penetration with less *trabecular meshwork* damage than with the *ALT*.

This technology, produced by Boston University Photonics Center which owns both the patent on the *SOLX* and the *Glaucoma Golden Shield,* is only obtainable through their auspices. Whether this procedure will take the place of incisional surgery remains to be seen. In the meantime, the next rung on the ladder for management of glaucoma is incisional or infiltration surgery.

CHAPTER 7
The Therapeutic Blade

o o o o o o o o o o o o o o o o o o o o o o o o o o o o o o o o o o o o o o o o o o o

*...hope..."as important as any medication I might prescribe or any
procedure I might perform."*

*Jerome Goodman,
MD the Anatomy of Hope:
How People Prevail in Face of Illness,
Random House, NY 2005.*

In the twentieth century, beguiled by science fiction fantasies, we envisioned
a technological world capable of solving insoluble problems, of finally
establishing a unified theory of everything, and of mastering the medical,
environmental, and sociological problems threatening our existence. Alas, in
the 21st century, our problems have multiplied. While technology continues
to forge exciting possibilities in all walks of life, treatment of a number of
diseases falls short of cure. Change is an incremental process evident most
often when past practices are reviewed. For glaucoma patients, the longed
for hope that "the something on the horizon" will replace surgery, has not yet
arrived. Although researchers and physicians have improved management of
glaucoma immensely, bouncing it from a blinding to a non-blinding disease
in western societies, the fact remains that treatment of glaucoma follows
the same procedures (with refinements, of course) established in the 20th
century.

Because glaucoma utopia is not yet with us, when the visual field continues
to worsen, surgery looms. Methods for surgical intervention, however, have
become more precise and reliable, and while perfection is not yet with us. (Can
perfection ever be attained?), outcomes are considerably improved. There are
a number of procedures that refer to surgery. Laser therapy as described in
the preceding chapter may or may not be considered surgery because it does

not involve the scalpel. Incisional or filtration surgery (*trabeculectomy)* does require cutting into the eye.

In the United States, filtration surgery is generally recommended as the third option for treating refractory (uncontrolled) glaucoma. In other countries, it may be the primary intervention, a decision possibly driven by the lower cost of providing surgery first, thus avoiding the chronic high cost of medication. Surgery first, practiced in Britain however, is claimed by British surgeons to produce better results. And the findings of a British five-year multi-center study did indicate better outcomes with surgery than with either medication or laser as early treatment. At the end of five years, 98% of the surgical patients had IOPs of less than 22 mmHg compared to 83% of medically treated patients and only 68% of those patients who received *trabeculoplasty*. The surgical patients achieved an average IOP reading of 14.6 mmHg, and only one of the 57 subjects in the study had to resume medical therapy. American physicians for the most part still prefer medical treatment first, citing that the effects of drops are reversible. As well, the eye is still intact should a filtration operation be necessary.

The evolution of the operation has taken a number of turns since the early 1800's, when William Mackenzie, a Scottish physician and author of an eye disease textbook, performed a procedure to reduce IOP. He cut a small piece from the *sclera* (a *sclerostomy*) that initially resulted in fluid discharge from the eye but provided only temporary relief. George Critchett, an ophthalmologist practicing at the Moorfields Eye Hospital in London in 1857, slightly improved the operation by cutting a small piece of the *iris* as well dubbing the procedure an "*iridodesis*," but not until Louis De Wecker further refined the operation by producing a filtering scar did the operation become a viable choice for managing the IOP. When Felix La Grange in 1889 combined the *sclerostomy* with an *iridectomy*, the operation took its penultimate form. From the early to the mid-1900s, doctors, in an effort to form a *bleb*, tinkered with methods for invading the *sclera* that included removal of part of the *cornea* and heating up the *sclera*. And by 1968, the operation known as either a filtering, incisional or a *trabeculectomy* operation took its final form.

TRABECULECTOMY

The *trabeculectomy (trab)* is usually the first of the available surgical procedures suggested to the average patient. It is not to be taken lightly. Your doctor has probably weighed a number of options, considering such factors as economic difficulties in paying for medications, your reliability (erratic or responsible for taking medication or returning follow-up appointments), condition of both eyes, timing, age, glaucoma progression, visual potential, cataract or other previous surgeries that have left behind scarred tissue.

With certain glaucoma conditions, surgery appears to be an earlier option than is normally prescribed for various forms of glaucoma. I found this to be the case when my   condition of *exfoliation* syndrome required intervention within the first three years. *Angle- closure* caused by the *iris* adhering to the cornea, corneal disease, and a form of juvenile or secondary glaucoma caused by displacement of the ciliary body pushing into the front chamber of the eye, *uveitis*, or *Aniridia*—all may require early surgery.

Essentially, the decision to have surgery rests both with your doctor's advice and with your own perception of the worsening of your condition. Your visual field may develop more *scotomas* (diseased areas), medications may no longer be equal to adequately lower of your pressure, and the effects of laser therapy may have worn off. Each member of our Group spoke of his or her idiosyncratic reasons for going for the operation. Marie kept losing vision although her pressures were mid-range (*normal-tension* glaucoma); my pressures wavered around 22 mmHg and my visual field continued worsening. Fred, having lost one eye to glaucoma, determined that his remaining eye needed to be protected. If you have doubts about undergoing the knife, by all means get a second opinion.

What You Need To Do Before Surgery

Now that you've decided to have the surgery, your doctor will advise you of the steps to take prior to the operation. You will be told to stop some drops you are using such as *miotic* drops. These tend to promote inflammation and a breakdown of the blood-aqueous barrier (a system governing the materials in blood allowed to enter into the aqueous humor) and constricting the pupil, which *may* cause *pupillary block*. Another medication rarely prescribed today, *Phospholine iodide (Echothiophate)* should be discontinued two weeks prior to sugery for it inhibits an enzyme that ordinarily breaks down commonly-used anesthetics, which need to exit the body as quickly as possible. Drugs that decrease the aqueous flow, such as the *carbonic anhydrase inhibitors* and *beta-blockers* (see Chapter 5) before and after surgery, may also make the list. Decreasing too much fluid production may hamper the formation of the bleb. In my case, because of the fear that my IOP would rise should I discontinue my drops, I continued my medical routine. The hope is, of course, that medication will not be necessary following surgery. Other drugs not associated with glaucoma, such as aspirin or anticoagulants (thinning of the blood) that may cause excessive bleeding during surgery, are most often discontinued as well. Supplements such as gingko biloba, vitamin C, bilberry that also thin the blood should be discontinued a week prior to surgery. Many doctors will recommend that all supplements be discontinued.

If you take a number of prescription medications other than glaucoma drops, it is wise to have your surgeon consult with your family physician as to which medications will impact on the surgical procedures.

Prior to surgery to prevent infection, doctors prescribe a regimen of antibiotic drops.

On The Operating Table

Most filtering operations are now performed under local anesthesia. When I had my first operation, I was admitted into the hospital, supposedly, only for overnight, and received general anesthesia. However, in my case, my pressure dropped dangerously low, and my doctor extended my hospital stay to five days in order to monitor my progress. Except in rare instances, a long hospitalization is not required, especially since a *trabeculectomy* has joined the ranks of out-patient procedures in the United States. In other countries, patients may still be pampered with a hospital stay that in the parlance of medical terminology is not cost-effective.

By the time of my second *trabeculectomy,* the outpatient procedure was firmly established. The decision of whether to remain overnight is yours (some medical plans will pay for this). Preparation for the procedure requires current blood work and a physical that can be performed by your general practitioner or at the hospital. A *retrobulbar* injection of anesthesia (injection into the eyeball—only a little sting) begins the process. Almost instantly, the eye is numbed. You sink into a sort of twilight sleep but you can still hear the medical team conversing, and if you're curious about the procedure as it unfolds, you can also ask your surgeon questions. Should you opt to stay in the hospital or return home, whatever your decision, your doctor will still want to examine you the following morning in order to check your pressure and for any possible complications.

There is always concern that any product injected into the eye may be toxic and anesthesia is no exception. *Lidocaine* and *bupivacaine* are the anesthetics commonly used. A study on rabbit eyes determined that these drugs were not toxic to the rabbit *retina* at concentrations effective for retrobulbar anesthesia.

Creating The Bleb

The eye is small and your doctor must perform microsurgery. The view is, of course, magnified. Creation of the *bleb*, the cornerstone of the operation, usually takes about a half hour. In the first step, in most cases, a partial thickness incision is made through the *conjunctiva* (outer skin of the eye) which has the consistency of plastic wrap. Usually a full thickness incision that goes right through the *sclera* is reserved for younger patients. A flap (think trap door), is then created by making a three-quarter cut through the wall of the eye. The flap is positioned just above the location of the *trabecular meshwork* and the *Schlemm's Canal*. The surgeon then cuts an opening through the bed beneath the flap (basically a hole in the eye), calibrating the operation to control the amount of fluid to be released, an important step: excess fluid results in a condition called *hypotony* (a flattening of the eye because too much fluid drains out) or not enough flow to adequately lower the IOP.

At this point the surgeon may or may not elect to apply an *antimetabolite* to prevent scarring. Two kinds of *antimetabolites* are used--*mitomycin C (MMC)* that is sponged into the eye at the time of the operation and *5-fluorouracil (5FU)*--either injected at the time of surgery or injected directly into the bleb following the operation. These substances prevent the wound from scarring over. Although the *antimetabolites* are used primarily for cancer therapy, application to the eye has helped maintain the *bleb* formation. The *antimetabolites* prevent the *fibrinogen* cells from dividing and clotting together to form a scar. Studies indicate that both drugs yield comparable results and despite the destruction of the fibroblasts cells, *antimetabolites*, for the most part, keep the *bleb* patent.

My own eyes provide a sort of test case. One eye had a *trab* with *MMC*; the other eye with a *trab* did not have *MMC*. The eye with the *antimetabolite* has maintained a low IOP to this date, while the eye without it required subsequent interventions. *Antimetabolite* treatment, however, is not without risk. These are powerful medications which leave behind weakened tissue. They may also cause some blurring but that effect usually resolves after a period of time. Nevertheless, studies describe attempts to balance their long-lasting toxic effects with the maintenance of the *bleb*. Researchers have tinkered with reducing the length of time the sponge remains in the eye and also the use of lower concentrations. Findings indicate that these adjustments provide the same effectiveness in controlling scar formation. This is good news for while the use of *antimetabolites* has improved *bleb* longevity, the less used, the better for the eye. Toxicity to the eye may also be reduced through a system called *trephination*. This consists of excising a tiny, thin disc of the *scleral* tissue and dipping it into *MMC*, irrigating it and then reimplanting it into the eye during the *trabeculectomy*. A study of this technique produced the same lowering of pressure as the standard method.

As with any medication, there are pros and cons. A study of 213 high-risk-for-failure patients was divided into those receiving *5-FU* and those without.

The have-nots achieved a twenty-five percent success rate, but the haves doubled that to fifty percent. Management with *antimetabolites*, especially *5 FU* may be needed months or years following the initial operation. Eye surgeons have found that a shot of *5 FU* can revive a failing bleb and *5-FU* may be viewed as a maintenance drug to prolong the life of a *bleb*.

Doctors often make a distinction between high-risk and low-risk patients. For example, I'm a high-risk patient and to keep the *trabeculectomy* viable, *MMC* was used. But Gerri is a low-risk patient. She is in her 90's, and has been on medical therapy for only several years. For her, a *trabeculectomy* without the antimetabolites was deemed advisable. In some cases, given the slow progression of loss, no intervention is advised.

With or without the application of an *antimetabolite*, the next step consists of removing a wedge of the *iris* (*iridotomy*) to prevent the *iris* from prolapsing (slipping) into the opening. This step is important for the *iris* is a sticky, floppy body that would tend to prolapse into the newly-created opening and muck up the works. To prevent the fluid from gushing out as fluids are wont to do when a new channel is created, the trap door is anchored back in place using 2-to-5 stitches, a procedure that also serves to create the filtering bleb. Alternatively, glue may be used, which some researchers find superior for anchoring down the trap door. Glue is quicker and causes the patient less pain. Glue, however, limits the option of releasing stitches if the pressure rises.

The flow of aqueous humor fills the new space causing the tissue to rise into the likeness of a bubble or blister forming the all-important *bleb*. Shortly thereafter, the *bleb* becomes diffused. The size of the *bleb* varies. Following the operation, it may cover as much as a quarter of the eye, but it usually contracts to about three-eights of an inch in about a week. Believed to aid in drainage, small cysts form as the *bleb* matures. The anterior chamber stabilizes along with the *bleb*.

ALTERNATIVES TO ANTIMETABOLITES

In some cases, the patient may possess certain proteins that resist the action of the *antimetabolites*. Given these circumstances, it would be to the patient's advantage if another group of drugs could be identified as *bleb* preservers. Under investigation is a recombinant *anti-TCF-B2 human monoclonal* antibody (specific antibodies of exceptional purity that are used in a variety of medical procedures). Genistein (a derivative of soy) has been under investigation for some time but it still has not made the cut. Yet genistein does inhibit the action of an enzyme involved in scar tissue formation, and it may one day give additional support to *TCF-B2* that is less toxic than *mitomycin-C* and may be just as effective. An antibody called *CAT-152* appears to be well-tolerated and some surgeons have chosen it over the *antimetabolites*. With this treatment, the *blebs* were diffuse, non-cystic and non-avascular unlike those associated with the *antimetabolites*. Four injections prior to and following surgery are required and *5-FU* is added where needed.

The use of *cellular photoablation* is in the exploratory stages. Only the cells responsible would be targeted sparing other tissues. A group of German researchers have developed a novel approach using *PhotoDynamic* therapy. Prior to the *trabeculectomy* a *PhotoDynamic* medication is injected under the *conjunctiva*. The area is then treated for eight minutes with a diffuse blue light. After six months the IOP of the patients receiving this treatment was significantly lowered and no toxic effects were observed.

Managing the Bleb

The battle to save the *bleb* is ongoing. Should the *bleb* show signs of releasing insufficient fluid to adequately manage the IOP, your doctor will take steps to rejuvenate the *bleb* by lysing (cut with a laser) one or more stitches widening the opening. This procedure usually takes place during the first few weeks following surgery.

Contrarily, the wound may be too wide, causing an excess flow of aqueous fluid resulting in *hypotony*. Should this occur, a *Simmons shell* (a dome-shaped shell of transparent plastic about three-quarters inches in diameter) can be placed on the *bleb*. This device creates pressure on the *bleb* stemming the flow of fluid. Controlling the excess flow of fluid protects the anterior chamber from flattening out and preventing parts of the eye from adhering to each other due to loss of aqueous.

Restitching the flap may be another solution, but this procedure requires reopening the eye. Massaging the area to manually force more fluid through a recalcitrant *bleb* offers another possibility. If this is a recommendation, be sure to have your doctor or the technician demonstrate the technique. Under development is a device that will both measure your *intraocular pressure* and massage the *bleb*.

In the following months or years, should the *bleb* show signs of flattening out and in danger of scarring over, doctors may use several strategies to redress this unfortunate situation. Depending upon the position of the scar formation, doctors may vaporize the scar tissue using a laser or break it up either by needling or cutting it open. Special instruments have been designed for this procedure. When I had my first *trab*, reopening the bleb had not become routine and it clamped down in less than a year. With my second *trab* on the other eye, *mitomycin-C* has kept the bleb patent. Like a game of chess, moves and counter moves—the doctor pits strategies against the body's intelligence to repair damaged tissues.

Bleb failure may occur in patients with *neovascular* glaucoma because their proliferating blood vessels tend to promote scarring. Surgeons recommend laser treatment (See Chapter 6) before undergoing *trabeculectomy* to prevent such scarring. Patients with *uveitis* (inflammation of the uvea), may experience increased inflammation that may result in scarring at the site of the *bleb* sealing it.

Medical treatment following a *trab* is a given. Inflammation, the body's response to injury, is inevitably a byproduct of any invasive procedure. The eye is angry that it has been tampered with but it calms down with the application of topical steroid drops such as *Pred Forte*. There are also non-steroidal drops available. To protect the eye from bacterial invasion (for the eye is now open to pathogens), the antibiotics prescribed prior to the procedure continue to be used for a period of time. From here on, you should avoid touching your eyes with unclean hands, for an operated eye, although healed, remains more vulnerable to infection since it is no longer completely closed.

Gene therapy is also percolating but its time is yet to come. *Atropine*, an antispasmodic drug that normalizes the permeability of the blood-aqueous barrier, also offers a possibility. It would dampen the body's trauma response that in the face of injury increases permeability, in turn, increasing clotting factors. The results of a study using *p21WAF-1cip-1* in ocular hypertensive monkey eyes demonstrated that the wound had not closed and the side effects seen with *MMC* did not occur with this treatment.

Because the *antimetabolite* liquid is colorless, some researchers suggest that more precise application may be improved with staining. Studies are underway to determine if the dye or dyes in question are safe to use in the eye.

Post-operative care requiring careful monitoring of each patient is very important, for no two patients heal alike. One patient may do fine after one or two postoperative visits while another may need about six visits.

SSS Safety Surgery System

This system was developed by **a** group in England. Rather than focusing on developing new procedures and new instruments, the researchers sought to improve surgical techniques and safety issues. The strategy involves preventing the pressure from plummeting to zero during the *trabeculectomy*, thus preserving the eye pressure and retaining the anatomy of the interior chamber during an operation that may require some fifty minutes or so. A pressure of zero for an extended period of time is not good for the eye. To achieve a constant pressure in the neighborhood of 10-to-12 mmHg, the interior chamber of the eye is filled with fluid that remains in the eye during the entire procedure reducing the specter of hypotony. This group has also invented adjustable sutures. Three weeks following surgery the sutures can be adjusted. Rather than simply cutting them, the sutures can be relaxed gradually until the mean pressure is achieved. This improved technique has reduced complications and maintained pressures in the target range of 12 mmHg.

Non-Penetrating Surgery (Deep Sclerectomy And Viscocanalostomy)

Unlike the *trabeculectomy, non-penetrating surgery* designates that the anterior chamber is not entered. In theory, this should make the operation safer than the *trab* and some ophthalmologists feel it does. It is regarded safer because the eyeball is not penetrated as it is with a *trab,* thus protecting the eye from contamination of opportunistic microbes or bacteria. It has not, however replaced the *trab.*

This surgery results in an IOP range of between 14-and-18 mmHg. Final pressures are not as low as those acquired with a *trabeculectomy,* but complications are minor. In essence, this operation bypasses the sluggish *trabecular meshwork* by filtering aqueous through the *Descemet's Membrane* (a thin, transparent tissue that forms the innermost layer of the *cornea*). The fluid then spills into the *Schlemm's Canal,* exiting through the normal pathways.

Two methods have been developed--*deep sclerostomy* and *viscocanolostomy.* Both require the same initial procedure. The surgeon enters the eye through the *sclera (a sclerostomy),* creating an inner *scleral* flap and dissects right down to the *Descemet's membrane.* This is the part of the procedure that requires exquisite skill. For the operation to be effective, the surgeon must not penetrate the delicate *Descemet's membrane.* Because the *Descemet's membrane* is so thin, aqueous fluid seeps through it bypassing the clogged *trabecular meshwork,* thus enabling the fluid to flow directly into the *Schlemm's Canal.* Should the anterior chamber be breached, however, the operation is then converted into a *trabeculectomy.* Hard to visualize this procedure? Think about home repair and a sheet rock ceiling. A sheet rock is manufactured by encasing rock particles between two pieces of thick paper. Imagine going up to your roof and cutting through that first piece of paper and through the rock layer right down to the last piece of paper. That last piece of paper can be compared to the *Descemet's membrane.*

DEEP SCLEROTOMY

This form requires dissecting the *sclera* as described above. To prevent collapse of the *scleral flap*, an absorbable collagen implant is sutured into the space vacated by the removal of tissue. Fashioned from porcine (pig) collagen, this implant dissolves within six-to-nine months. Aqueous humor percolates through the *Descemet's membrane*. The space remaining when the implant dissolves becomes a collecting aqueous reservoir prior to the final exit of aqueous. The last step consists of tightly suturing the *conjunctiva* opening. Minimal post-operative care is needed, and at 12 months, fewer glaucoma medications were needed in eighty-three percent of the eyes.

VISCOCANOLSCOPY

This is the procedure developed by Professor Robert Stegman of South Africa. He found it highly successful, especially with black patients. A success rate of lowering *intraocular pressure* to 22 mmHg without glaucoma medication has been reported. The procedure involves redirecting the fluid immediately into the *Schlemm's Canal* and the *episcleral veins*. The surgical technique follows the dissection of the *sclera* described above, but additionally, a portion of the *Schlemm's canal* is unroofed allowing the aqueous to slowly seep through the anterior *trabecular meshwork* and beneath the remaining membrane. Following the unroofing of the *Schlemm's canal*, the surgeon places a cannula (a small tube) into that space followed by an injection of *viscoelastic* (an elastic substance) on both sides of the opening of the *Schlemm's canal*. The *viscoelastic* expands the diameter of the canal considerably—from 30-to-230 microns, promoting increased outflow of aqueous.

Compared to the *trab*, *viscanolostomy* is more complex and requires a longer training period. Theoretically, this procedure should be a step forward because the anterior chamber is not entered preventing scarring. Also, because no filtering *bleb* is created, a sudden drop in IOP resulting in *hypotony* and *flat anterior chamber* is avoided. This procedure also limits risk of cataract and infection.

Drawbacks, however, include IOP lowering to only the mid-to-high teens rather than to the low teens or single digits that are routinely expected from a *trabeculectomy.* Experimental studies on the mechanism of action revealed evidence of micro-openings throughout the wall of *Schlemm's canal* which may be responsible for the outflow. A study of the effect *of viscocanolostomy* suggested viscose material may enhance the outflow of aqueous fluid. Short-term studies have found comparable results to the *trab* and success in combining this operation with that of cataract. Whether this option becomes routine remains in the hands of the clinicians. Some doctors are very enthusiastic about the operation and cite good control of glaucoma in their patients. Other doctors are wary, especially for advanced glaucoma cases where patients need pressures in the low teens or single digits, a condition not readily attainable with non-penetrating operations.

This approach does appear to eliminate some of the problems associated with a *viscocanolostomy,* although it is not suitable for all cases as is the *trabeculectomy.* Patients with *closed-angle* or whose *Schlemm's canal* is damaged from previous operations are not considered good candidates. Refinement in technique and equipment continues to evolve, such as a milling drill developed in Spain that surgeons can use to quicken the pace of the operation.

Several members of our Group opting for this operation reported different outcomes. Dave, intrigued with the operation and the published results and wishing to avoid a *trabeculectomy,* opted for it. Since his *viscanolostomy,* he has been extremely pleased with the result. Ordinarily, pressure from this operation stabilizes at about 14-to-18 mmHg. Dave's IOP registered in the middle of that range. A year later, concerned after reading about the more recent guidelines linking a lower IOP to optic nerve protection, he discussed with his surgeon the possibility of lowering his IOP further. His surgeon performed a laser procedure reducing the pressure to the range of 11-to-12 mmHg along with the addition of two drops—Timoptic and Travatan. Six months later needing a cataract operation, his surgeon revisited the *viscanolostomy* site, touched it up, according to Dave, and Dave's eye responded with a lowering to 9-to-10 mmHg using just Timoptic every three days. Dave is one happy glaucoma patient. Bill, on the other hand, had his operation performed by another surgeon. Within three months, his pressure rose to high levels threatening the health of the *optic nerve,* even with the addition of maximum drops. He checked in for a *trabeculectomy* that resolved the problem at a comfortable IOP of 9-to-l0 mmHg.

The fault may not have been the procedure, but the inexperience of the practitioner. Training apparently is the key, for the operation, which when successful, eliminates a host of secondary problems that, unfortunately, plague *trabeculectomies.*

While non-penetrating surgeries haven't taken the ophthalmologists in the United States by storm, surgeons reporting from Italy, France, and other countries generally regard this procedure favorably. Theoretically, since these procedures eliminate the dread of flat anterior chamber, those surgeons practicing them have become converts. Can it work for everyone? In the hands of a competent surgeon, yes indeed. But the surgery does require additional training and the procedure itself is so painstaking that it may take too much time for a doctor to become skilled enough to achieve a confidence level that equals the *trabeculectomy*. Studies comparing both the *trab* and the non-penetrating procedures found that after two years *viscocanolostomy* produces IOPs at 16 mmHg. trabs at 14 mmHg. If your condition requires an IOP below 16 mmHg, a non-penetrating operation is not your game.

THE TRABECTONE

A new procedure using a specially designed surgical instrument called the *Trabectome* may improve the standard *trabeculectomy*. This instrument ablates (removes) the *trabecular meshwork* allowing the fluid to drain directly into the *Schlemm's canal*. A small incision is made in the *cornea* through which the instrument is inserted and gonioscopy is used to visualize the *trabecular meshwork*. This operation, while it does not replace the *trabeculectomy*, with certain patients, it may be more advantageous, for because drainage flows directly into the *Schlemm's Canal*, the creation of a *bleb* is unnecessary. It may be the most appealing of operations for early glaucoma patients who need a procedure to adequately lower their pressures.

THE SHUNTS: MICROPROSTHESES

There may come a time in the progression of glaucoma damage that medication, laser or filtering operations no longer work. This is when your doctor may suggest the instillation of a Seton or shunt. Or, your condition may be such that your doctor advises the shunt rather than more surgery to save your vision. The shunt, in existence for over thirty years, is used primarily with advanced glaucoma patients who have already had one or more *trabeculectomies*. Patients with surgeries, *diabetic retinopathy*, the very young (*congenital glaucoma*), traumatic eye injury, and non-compliers—all may benefit from the shunt. It is estimated that several thousand implants are used in the USA each year. The shunt may also be an option for patients in third-world countries where access to a clinician is limited.

The theory of shunt technology is simple--place an artificial drain into the eye to siphon off excess fluid. The devices commonly used require a two part procedure. One or two plates (the drainage system) are sutured on the outside of the eyeball toward the back of the eye under the *conjunctiva*. A silicone tube or filament is carefully inserted between the *cornea* and the *iris*. The fluid drains through the tube or along the filament (like liquid draining off a fringe), into the area around the back end of the eye to a drainage plate (s), where it is absorbed by the tissues in that area. Scar tissue forms around the drainage plate anchoring it firmly in place and transforming the plate into a sort of thick *bleb*. Unlike a *trabeculectomy*, this scar tissue does not close off egress of fluid.

The most commonly used shunts come in four flavors: *Moltino, Baerveldt, Ahmed and Krupin*. But, as with other aspects of medicine, scientists are constantly engaged in developing better, more effective and less-disruptive Setons. A number of different devices exist and they all perform the same function. Different materials address the problem of biocompatibility. A Seton, under study, is made from Gore-Tex coated with laminar (an extracellular matrix) that appears to be more biocompatible than other materials.

While the above mentioned shunts are considered effective in controlling IOP, doctors do have their preferences, and if you are scheduled for a shunt procedure, your doctor will probably use his or her favorite. Both the plates and the tubes differ in each of these systems. The *Ahmed* and the *Krupin* implants possess a valve that maintains the pressure during the period of scar tissue formation. Once scar tissue anchors the plate, the valve becomes unnecessary. The *Molteno* and *Baerveldt* implants do not have valves and to prevent excess outflow of fluid, the tube is temporarily closed off (temporary stitches) and then reopened several weeks later. The *Molteno* uses two plates and a silicone tube. Since the tube has no valve, the two-plate method better controls the free flow of fluid, possibly avoiding *hypotony*. The *Baerveldt* uses a thin plate, less than one millimeter thick but with a large drainage surface. In this procedure, the tube is sutured shut until the plate is encapsulated. The *Ahmed* is positioned in only one quadrant of the eye and can have either a single or double plate. *Ahmed's* valved system significantly reduces overfiltration, but some studies have suggested that more complications occur with the *Ahmed*. The *Krupin* has a pressure-sensitive one-way valve.

New shunts promising better and safer results are being evaluated. Two of these, the *Express* implant and the *Eyepass Glaucoma Implant* are worth examining.

Postoperative care follows the general rules of surgery—topical steroid drops, antibiotics, and dilating drops to relax the muscles of the eye. This routine produces better focus. After the tube is opened, pressure tends to rise and pressure lowering medications may be necessary for several weeks until the eye stabilizes. Some patients need no further medications, and others may need only one.

Those doctors who specialize in Seton implants are enthusiastic about the use of this tool, and statistics show a respectful success rate between sixty-five-to-eighty-two percent.

I have now had a shunt implanted in my left eye, the one that has been plagued with difficult-to-control IOP, and which as a result, has had a number of different procedures. As a high-risk patient, the implant did not work for me. Or it worked too well, for I developed uncontrolled *hypotony*. I also experienced significant loss of sight, my vision going from 20/25 to legal blindness. Other members of the Group have had successful implants, even Sophia who has *uveitis* which should have created greater problems than mine, but perhaps because she is fifteen years my junior, her eye may be more resilient or who knows why?

EXPRESS IMPLANTATION

This is a relatively new procedure that has been used with a small number of patients. The implant is positioned under a *scleral flap* with an application of *mitomycin C*. It has been compared to a *trabeculectomy*, a *sclerostomy* or a peripheral *iridectomy*. Twenty-four open-angle patients, 16 of whom had failed *trabeculectomy* surgery, were recruited to receive this procedure. *Hypotony* was the major complication occurring in three patients but it resolved spontaneously. Management of IOP with no adjunctive medication still functioned a year later with twenty eyes.

The *Eyepass Glaucoma Implant* at this writing is in its final Phase III clinical trial and has yet to attain FDA approval. This is a Y-shaped tube. The main stem is inserted into the anterior chamber and the two arms inserted in opposite directions into the *Schlemm's canal*. It differs from other devices by draining internally using the natural outflow system. Researchers involved in this device claim that complications related to external drainage such as *hypotony*, late infection and scarring are avoided.

RISK FACTORS

The same complications can occur as with any surgery to the eye (see below). In addition, the implant may cause traction of the *conjunctiva* over the implanted area and/or implant intrusion into the *iris* or the *cornea*. Success may depend upon the drainage plate size. A large drainage plate, although preferable, may drain too much fluid resulting in *hypotony*. These problems although uncommon may be traced to improper positioning of the tube. Because of its proximity to the *extraocular* muscles of the eyes, left and right movements of the eyes may be restricted. Loss of one or two lines of acuity may occur, and there may be scarring, other than that of encapsulating the plate. Less frequent are infections, for the eye is closed up foiling bacteria from entering. Other problems include insecure anchoring of the shunt that then erodes the *conjunctiva* and also improper tube placement possibly injuring the *cornea*. Common to all surgeries is the loss of *corneal* cells. Unfortunately, patients who have had a number of surgeries experience some loss of cells with each operation. Another complication involves injury to the *cornea* due to mechanical contact between the tube and the tissues of the eye. How this situation affects the eye in the long run is unknown since there is little research into this side effect.

TO TAME INFLAMMATION

Inflammation, a natural consequence of surgery, if not tamed, can cause serious side-effects. Inflammation is the eye's response to invasive treatment and trauma to the body. To manage inflammation, ophthalmologists traditionally prescribe steroids despite the known risk that steroids can promote a rise in the IOP. Patients with *angle-recession* are most likely to be at risk for *steroid-induced* glaucoma. As with any drug, steroids have a multiplier effect and should you be using steroids for treatment of allergy and asthma, advise your surgeon. Most commonly, a steroid such as *Prednisolone Acetate (Pred Forte)* is prescribed. If your pressure does rise as a result of steroid therapy, your doctor may switch to a non-steroidal drop. Generally, however, steroids are safe and effective and are required only for a limited time. Within this short period, potential side effects such as *corneal* and *scleral* thinning and fungal infections generally do not occur. Women who are either pregnant or nursing should consult with their obstetricians or pediatricians for the best course of action since steroids may affect the fetus or the neonate.

An interesting study conducted in England that documented the side-effects of inflammation following either a *trab* or a combined *trab* and cataract extraction found a quieting down of inflammation of the anterior chamber after four weeks in the *trab* group. In the combined operation group, inflammation and breakdown of the blood-aqueous barrier continued for four months. Be aware that this is single study. It is well known that steroids are helpful in either procedure, for in addition to quieting the inflammation, steroids bolster the formation of the *bleb*. I, for one, did not experience long-term inflammation after a combined *trab-cataract* operation but did suffer it from a shunt implant.

As with any medication, *Pred Forte* does have side-effects. The side effect of the onset of glaucoma is irrelevant for those already diagnosed with glaucoma. Long term use, however, poses risks such as damage to the *optic nerve*, visual field defects, fungal infection, and formation of cataracts. Steroids also lower the immune system response. It is important when using a steroid medication to continue follow-up visits with your doctor who will be able to evaluate steroid's effects on your eye(s) and advise you accordingly.

Physical Restrictions Following An Operation

- Wear the rigid eye-protecting shield that your doctor provides for the length of recommended time especially at bedtime. Your doctor or technician will show you how to tape it on your face.
- Do not stoop or bend your head below the waistline or engage in physical exercise.
- Leave the lifting of heavy objects to your mate, children or anybody else. Above all, don't lift.
- Drink lots of nonalcoholic fluids.
- Discontinue the use of regular eye drops unless advised otherwise by your doctor.
- Reduce movement in both eyes.
- Continue with all the medications that your doctor prescribed until advised to discontinue.
- Should your eye feel "sandy" or if it feels like a foreign body is in it, close your eyes and rest in a darkened room.
- Usually painkillers are not required, for although the eye may feel bruised for several days, almost no one experiences severe pain. But if you do need relief, try Tylenol (*acetaminophen*) or the equivalent rather than aspirin, since aspirin is a blood thinner, and you want to avoid any chance of bleeding. If you are still in discomfort with the recommended dose of *acetaminophen*, do not increase the dosage, but consult with your doctor.
- Should your eye become sensitive to bright light or sunshine, do wear sunglasses. Many doctors now provide you with an aftercare kit that contains sunglasses.
- If you are constipated use a stool softener such as *Colace* or other product to avoid straining. Continue for about two weeks or until your doctor tells you that your eye has stabilized.
- Follow the instructions faithfully. Usually, you will receive a printed sheet to reinforce verbal instructions.
- On the days following an operation, the eye is sometimes sensitive to the heat and other substances such as plant phenols, generated by food preparation (cutting up an onion), escaping steam and cooking odors in general, Doctors sometimes advise staying out of the kitchen for a few days giving the eye time to heal and to desensitize.
- Finally, check in with your attitude. It is natural to be fearful, anxious, and concerned about having a major operation on your eye,

but do bear in mind that a positive frame of mind is a great asset in the healing process. One member of the Group self-hypnotized himself before going in for an operation on his leg and prevented heavy bleeding during the procedure. Not many people are capable of this level of self-hypnosis, but one or several visits to a therapist prior to the operation may root out a deep-seated fear. Yoga, too, can help to soothe jittery nerves. Or a simple measure might be to listen to a calming tape on mind and spirit. Before submitting to any operation I quell my anxiety by listening to such a tape and I increase my meditation time. Tapes can now be found in large bookstores, on the internet, mail-order and in some health food stores. (See resources). Remember, that your entire being is involved in the successful outcome of this operation. Psychologically and spiritually, your attitude toward the operation and your postoperative frame of mind are critical for the healing process. Negative and fearful thoughts often melt away when you believe you've chosen or been referred to a doctor you can trust, for trust in your doctor's ability to solve your problem may be one of the paramount determinants in the success of the operation. I've had several operations and my unwavering trust in my doctor helped, I believe, in the success of some of my operations.

DID IT WORK?

If IOP drops to the desired level suitable for your condition, even if you still may need a drop or two, your operation can be rated successful. You may well fall in the successful cohort of eighty-to-ninety percent of the cases. The few people who do not profit may be long-term glaucoma patients who have considerable visual loss. But even in these cases, with the exception of patients who may be in their nineties, doctors will often recommend surgery in an attempt to save remaining vision. Success rates with combined operations have also improved. With advanced techniques for eye operations and state of the art technological equipment available for cataract operations, success rate should equal virgin operations on the eye. Of course, your doctor will help you decide the best procedure for you.

In many cases, according to published sources, surgical procedures cause an unavoidable loss of one of two lines of vision. If you possess 20/20 vision, you may find your acuity has dropped to 20/25, 20/30 or even 20/40. While a reliable explanation for vision loss is up for grabs, many patients will trade loss of several lines for a stabilized IOP. Furthermore, your lens prescription can be adjusted. In my long experience with managing my glaucoma, I've lost vision in one eye and gained it the other eye. Other post-operative problems may include an increased sensitivity to bright light, especially sunlight.

RISKS AND COMPLICATIONS OF MOST SURGICAL PROCEDURES

What would life be without complications? They occur frequently if not everyday. We should be prepared to take them in stride, for in our daily activities we are constantly shifting priorities to meet daily disruptions and emergencies. When complications occur following an operation, however, we may be shattered by the experience. Complications resulting from eye operations can be harrowing, especially when vision is weakened or lost. Of course, we know we've chosen a surgeon in whom we have confidence, and we have been persuaded that the procedure will improve our situation, but, nevertheless, many of us worry about the outcome.

When complications do occur, the surgeon will fix them, but perhaps not as rapidly as your computer fixes errors. Some complications resolve without intervention in a few weeks; others need additional treatment, and unfortunately, there are some that cannot be fixed. Below are some of the more common complications and methods for restoring the integrity of the eye.

- **Scarring**: Make a cut. A scar forms. A fact of life. In eye surgeries, the amount of scarring can be beneficial for placement of a shunt or detrimental when the *bled* scars down. An acute problem may occur when the *Schlemm's Canal,* because of an accumulation of small fibers, shortens. This situation may occur in as many as forty-one percent of patients. Scarring may also occur in patients who have had prior scarring from a failed *trab*, or who have had cataract surgery. Certain types of glaucoma such as *neovascular, uveitis*, and glaucoma in young patients, children, and African-Americans are all at greater risk of scarring. Some patients develop a thick layer of scar tissue called an *encapsulated bleb* preventing a free flow of fluid. Pressure rises accordingly and further treatment such as needling to reopen the bleb and possibly additional medication are recommended.
- **Bleb Leak** may occur early in the post-operative period. It may also occur six or more months down the road. Don't be alarmed. *Bleb* leaks are manageable, for although they are potentially serious exposing the eye to grave risks such as infection, when diagnosed, your doctor will take immediate steps to remediate the problem. You may be the first, however, to notice that something is not quite right--your eye tears

and your vision is not as good as it was. If you suspect that all is not well, schedule an appointment with your doctor. Upon examining your eye, your doctor will evaluate your condition. A number of factors may be causing the leak. These include corneal problems, cataract, or *optic disc* swelling. A *bleb* leak may also be associated with *antimetabolite* use. A full thickness procedure can cause a leak as well, although doctors rarely use this procedure now. Your surgeon will also evaluate whether the anterior chamber is too shallow, *hypotony*, or a low *bleb* problem. Sixty percent of bleb leaks resolve using a topical antibiotic. Other medical treatments for *bleb* leaks include reducing the steroids, application of aqueous suppressants such as *trichloroacetic acid*, or *cryotherapy* (freezing). Early in the post-operative period, your doctor may turn to treatment that may include pressure patching, a collagen shield, compression sutures, or a *Simmons shell* but that may be uncomfortable. Various adhesives may do a nice seal. These include fibrin tissue glue, or *cyanoacrylate* (a toxic glue and should only be a last resort). More compatible is using your own blood (*autologous* application). I had a *bleb* leak that resolved in a week using my own blood. My eye looked terrible for it turned all red, but when the blood reabsorbed into the system, my *bleb* was fine and it's still functioning well. The laser, also, may repair the problem. And lastly, there may no alternative except to revise the *bleb* through additional surgery.

- **Failing Bleb** is different from a *bleb* leak. Ideally, the *bleb* should be diffuse with few vessels and correspond with a low IOP. Early signs of failure include a thickened *bleb,* normal or high IOP, or a cyst in the back of the eyeball. Failure may be attributed to a *scleral flap* that is too tight, scarring of the *conjunctiva* beneath the *bleb*, an internal obstruction, tissue covering the *bleb*, blocking underneath the *bleb*, and scarring down of the trap door. Treatment for this condition includes massaging the eye, useful primarily in the early post-op period, suturing (cutting) the stitches, needling of the *bleb*, a procedure that carries its complications such as infection and a risk of a *conjunctival* leak, intensive steroid treatment, injection of *5 FU* or application of *mitomycin-C* and reopening the trap door using a spatula-type knife. If none of these strategies work, then a surgical revision of the *bleb* is in order.

- **Bleb Infection** (*Endophthalmitis*). Medical history is rife with errors, some of them caused by adhering to protocol while ignoring the evidence. At one time women routinely died giving birth because doctors neglected to wash their hands before examination. Perhaps doctors should also wash their ties. A recent study found that doctors' ties become contaminated through contact with the bed sheets of patients. The authors advise tacking the tie or wearing bow ties. Ocular infection is the most feared for *bleb* survival. The use of *antimetabolites* may render the *bleb* more prone to infection, but infection can occur at any time even some years down the line from the original operation. Whatever the cause, infection is <u>bad news</u> if it occurs in the eyes. One reason is that an operation exposes the eye more readily to infection, for bacteria can more easily penetrate the *conjunctiva* that now communicates directly with the interior of the eye. A *bleb* leak must be monitored immediately upon detection for infection is twenty-six times higher when the *bleb* leaks. Cleanliness is a factor. If you wear contact lenses and do not clean them properly, infection can occur. In general, it's wise to be on the alert for any signs of an infection in your eye. If you notice **<u>redness, irritation and change of vision, advise your</u> <u>doctor immediately.</u>** This is a medical emergency. A dangerous infection may result in significant visual loss. Early recognition is the key to management of a *bleb* infection followed by aggressive treatment. The most common organisms causing infection are *streptococcus* and *staphylococcus*. If recognized in time, a broad spectrum of antibiotics, both topical and oral and possibly steroids may resolve the problem. If attended to in a timely fashion, destruction of vision caused by infection is usually avoided. While this particular risk occurs in a small number of patients in the neighborhood of one-to-two-percent, be alert to the possibility. If the infection is not caught and squashed in time, *endophthalmitis* may develop.

- **Conjunctival Buttonhole.** At a recent eye conference, I overheard a doctor tell a colleague how everything in the surgery on a particular patient had gone well, yet a buttonhole erupted. In the best of worlds, errors or inherent weaknesses of the tissue may cause a tear in the *conjunctiva*. This situation needs immediate repair (and it can be done with little consequence). But, if left untreated, it can cause excessive runoff of aqueous that will then hamper *bleb* formation.
- *Scleral* **Flap Disinsertion**. In this case part of the *scleral flap* (the trap door) is torn during the operative procedure. A minor surgical procedure will correct the problem to insure proper filtration.
- **Vitreous Loss**. This situation primarily occurs in eyes that are highly *myopic* (nearsighted), enlarged, having a thin *sclera*, or *aphakic* (minus a natural lens). If not corrected, this condition may cause the

vitreous to plug up the drainage site. The problem may result when the surgeon is not diligent in cleaning up the escaped *vitreous*.

- **Hypotony** This is the medical term describing a condition where aqueous has leaked out of the wound causing a flat anterior chamber, or following a shunt operation that is too effective in draining the aqueous. After most filtering operations, *hypotony* usually resolves in several days as the chamber reforms spontaneously. During the period of the chamber righting itself, doctors grade the reformation: Grade 1--chamber reforms spontaneously: Grade 2--chamber needs close watch and possibly additional help in reforming; grade 3--chamber requires reformation help that consists of injecting the eye with a balanced salt solution of *sodium hylaronate*, an injection of your own blood and/or a compression suture, and as a last resort, a graft that requires opening the eye again. Bill's doctor tried all the above srrategies, but to no avail, and finally he reopened the eye and repaired the *trabeculectomy* by stitching a graft to the damaged site. Complications can also occur years after surgery such as chronic low pressure. Over an extended period, too low pressure may develop into secondary problems such as folding of the *retina* or *choroidal* adhesions—fusing of the outer and middle layer of the eye. Low pressure may not necessarily be negative for some older patients with IOPs below 6 mmHg who, because their *scleras* are more rigid, may tolerate minimum pressures better than younger patients. Generally, however, a very low pressure needs to be corrected.

- **Hypotony Maculopathy** This is a condition that consists of folds in the *retina*. It decreases visual acuity. Those most at risk include patients who are *myopic*, young, male, previously treated with *mitomycin C,* have systemic illness such as hypertension or coronary artery disease, or have high preoperative IOPs. It is not a clearly understood condition and doctors speculate that in younger patients it may result from a more elastic *sclera;* in *myopic* eyes from a thinner *sclera.* When associated with surgery, *bleb* leaks, overfiltering *blebs*, shunts, or inflammation may occur. If *hypotony* continues for some time, irreversible damage may result in the *retinal* folds, as well as scarring of the *retina, choroid* and *sclera.* Conservative treatment consists of medical therapy or a large bandage contact lens. If this doesn't work, the next step involves surgically correcting the problem.

- **Malignant Glaucoma**. *Angle-closure* patients are subject to this post-operative condition, but only two-to-five percent are susceptible. The term malignant in this case refers not to cancer, but rather to the action of the *ciliary body* that rotates and blocks off the normal flow of aqueous fluid. Pressure rises sharply. This situation may occur hours, days, weeks or even months following a procedure. A wide variety of ophthalmic procedures that may be responsible for this condition include *miotic* use (drops that constrict the pupil) after filtration surgery, cataract surgery where the lens is implanted in the back chamber of the eye, the use of *Nd:YAG* laser for *cyclophotocoagulation*, *iridotomy*, and laser release of the *scleral flap* sutures. Other conditions are spasm and swelling of the *ciliary body*, *central vein occlusion*, *retinopathy of prematurity* (a childhood disease, (See Chapter 3) and a shallow anterior chamber. At times, this condition may be confused with *pupillary block*. Management of this condition consists of topical steroids to decrease inflammation, reversing the anterior rotation of the *ciliary body*, decompressing the *vitreous*, and suppressing the flow of aqueous. Should medical treatment fail to resolve the situation, laser treatment such as peripheral *iridoplasty* may be used to break the attack. In this approach, the surgeon uses the *ALT* laser to make a series of burns around the periphery of the *iris* causing it to shrink away from the blockage, or the surgeon may elect to use the *Ned:YAG* laser to rupture the tissue between the anterior and posterior segments, which then equalizes the pressure in both chambers of the eye. A third option is a *vitrectomy* (removing the vitreous fluid). If none of these procedures resolves the situation, surgery may be necessary.

- **Bleeding**. High blood pressure, blood clotting disorders, the use of blood thinners such as aspirin, vitamin C, gingko biloba, bilberry and other vitamins may reduce the body's ability to successfully clot at the site where the incision is made. Ordinarily, a bit of bleeding resolves within a few minutes, but if the bleeding continues, the surgeon intervenes by medically coagulating the site.

- **Hemorrhage**. This situation differs from simple bleeding. As the name implies the bleeding is more excessive. Usually hemorrhage occurs in the *choroid*, that highly vascular tissue that nourishes the eye, or in the eye socket itself (orbital hemorrhage) after a local injection of the anesthesia that tenses up the eyeball and possibly compresses the optic nerve. Both situations are correctable. Pain may signal the hemorrhage's occurrence in the *choroid*, a pain that, unfortunately, may resist palliatives. When this situation occurs, the surgeon must immediately close the incision and intravenously administer *Acetazolamide (Diamox)* and *Mannitol* to lower a skyrocketing IOP. Surgery in both cases will be postponed until the hemorrhage has resolved.

- **Superciliary Effusion**: In this condition that follows filtration surgery, the aqueous fluid collects beneath the *ciliary body* causing a swelling of the *choroid* because of an imbalance of fluids between the front and back of the eye. Steroids are used to reduce the swelling and normalize this imbalance.

- **Cataract Formation**: This is an unfortunate consequence of many filtering operations, although younger patients with their nice clear lenses usually avoid this situation. Here are a number of possibilities as to why so many of us do develop cataracts following a filtering operation: a nick from a surgical tool damages the *lens; hypotony* (see above); forward movement of the *lens* and touching the *cornea*, the contact causing damage, and use of steroids, especially when topically and systemically combined.

- **Corneal Dellen**. This is a condition whereby the adjacent area to the *bleb* dries out. This is not serious and it is easily treated with a topical lubricant until it resolves.

- **Internal Sclerostomy Blockage**. Internally the *iris* or a membrane blocks the opening. Laser treatment effectively reopens the site.

- **Second and Third Surgeries**. If at first you don't succeed, try again. This familiar adage does not apply to glaucoma operations. With each succeeding attempt to create a working filter, chances of success are lowered. One of the problems is location of a site for surgery free of scar tissue. Inevitably, the second or third site will not be as advantageous as the first, and chances for a successful outcome are reduced. In the hands of an experienced surgeon, however, a second and even a third operation may yet beat the odds.

- **Wipe-Out**. We've saved this complication for last, for hopefully it will not occur in your case. Both patient and doctor fear wipe-out for unlike many of the other complications, wipe-out cannot be fixed. When it does occur, it may happen with patients who have a history of difficulty in controlling the IOP. After a surgical procedure loss of central vision affecting fixation and/or blinding in a section of the eye or the entire eye may result.

Naturally, anything to do with the eye or any part of the body may cause complications. It's a fact of life that we all accept when we submit to surgery.

Those complications listed above make up a small percentage of the cases when compared with the number of filtering or other operations performed daily that are considered successful. That they can occur is not debatable, but in most cases, the filtration surgery goes well and the patient is pleased that the IOP is lowered and all or most medications can be eliminated. Also, the prospect that, with the exception of wipe-out those complications can be fixed, is comforting. When glaucoma strikes and IOP no longer can be controlled by means other than surgery, many patients negotiate a bargain with themselves submitting to a destructive process to save their sight. Destroy to save permeates all medical treatment, whether topical, systemic, use of lasers, or surgical. The driving force behind submitting to a procedure is to retain function as long as possible. I've had a lot of surgery in one of my eyes and while that eye has lost most of its function, it's not completely wiped out. And for that, I'm thankful. Amazing how we settle for tiny victories. Denise, on the other hand, refused additional surgery arguing that since the original surgery failed, why should a second succeed? Denise is now legally blind. Rachel, another member of the Group, with very serious glaucoma complicated by deteriorating *corneas* did submit to several surgeries, one of which was a *cornea* implant and while her vision is greatly reduced, she is still able to work on her computer and cook meals for herself and her husband. Successful surgery usually combines your attitude (positive) with your surgeon's skill, at expertly solving whatever problems may occur during surgery.

TELEMEDICINE

Patients living in metropolitan western societies most often have access to competent practitioners who also practice some of the more advanced medical strategies, but in many parts of the world, such services may not exist. All this may change as telemedicine becomes more available. High resolution video images and health data are sent through communication lines providing patients throughout the world access to a skilled physician. Diagnosis, surgery and post-op care can be carefully monitored long-distance. The first step in diagnosis can be as simple as stepping into a kiosk in a shopping center, placing your chin against a frame, and without need for dilation, having a camera take a picture of the back of your eye. This information is then sent off to the University of Maryland's ophthalmology department. If a problem is detected, the next step is to visit an eye doctor. Surgery can also be performed in remote areas such as the Amazon. Portable equipment is trucked in and the doctor performing the operation on site is in communication with a skilled ophthalmologist if an eye operation is necessary. Several obstacles need to be overcome for telemedicine to become routine. World-wide guidelines and standards need to be put into place, equipment needs to become more readily available and free from errors, and in cases for monitoring a particular condition, patient compliance needs to be strengthened.

CHAPTER 8

Cataract—Clear View Ahead

○ ○

"The eye altering alters all"
William Blake, "The Mental Traveler" (1800-10)

Mabel prepared for her cataract operation in high spirits. A world traveler and seldom ill, she saw no reason to worry about this small operation especially since many of her friends had had successful procedures. She lost ninety-five percent of the sight in that eye which previously had read the 20/25 line on the *Snellen* chart.

Joan who worried excessively about her health required constant reassurance from her doctor that her cataract operation would be successful. She lost seventy-five percent of her vision in that eye through a physical mishap on the part of the doctor. The *intraocular* lens slipped and damaged the *optic nerve* during the retrieval efforts.

Felicity was assured by the ophthalmologist who was treating her for glaucoma that she would see well if her cataract was removed. Following the operation, she was informed that her eye had developed complications. She learned later that the complications were a result of her ophthalmologist not recognizing the impact of *exfoliation* on the *zonules* (fibers) holding the lens in place. Uncontrolled pressure, bleeding, and loss of sight followed this sad scenario.

What knits these stories together? All three women have glaucoma. Conditions created by glaucoma raise the bar for complications to occur during a cataract operation. Patients with no disease may experience a rise in pressure following the operation but this condition soon subsides with no evident damage. For those with glaucoma, however, a rise in pressure can be disastrous. Furthermore, if the patient has *exfoliation (XFS)* as does Felicity, the odds for a successful operation decrease. Patients affected with both glaucoma and *(XFS)* who have cataracts are vulnerable to a number of problems that may occur during the operation. *Zonules*, the fibers holding the capsule in which the lens nestles, are often weakened by an accumulation of the exfoliation material causing the fibers to stretch, break or become detached from their moorings. When this occurs the capsule destabilizes and recedes back *(subluxation)* into the eye imposing difficulties in removal of the diseased lens. Mechanical stretching of the pupil, not without risks, is another procedure for glaucoma patients who have been using *miotic* drops. This is necessary when the pupil no longer responds to dilation drops and must be stretched wide enough for insertion of the *intraocular* lens. Pre-operative and post-operative treatment is essential. I've had two successful cataract operations and although I have *(XFS)* and pupils that no longer dilate because of long-term *miotic* drop use, I experienced only the common side affects. With both operations my doctors, knowledgeable in both glaucoma and cataract extraction, were able to avert any unforeseen problems. While the eye is restabilizing, follow-up visits for glaucoma patients are essential.

Cataract formation is not necessarily associated with glaucoma. A longitudinal study found that age-related cataract to be the first cause of visual impairment in the world. In the *Framingham Eye Study*, lens changes affected 42% of those between the ages of 52-and-64. Comparable statistics were reported in the *Beaver Dam Study*. Factors associated with cataract development include a lower socio-economic status suggesting environmental influence, long-term use of steroids that might lead to *posterior subcapsular cataract*. Smoking may lead to *nuclear cataract*. In some studies, a higher use of multivitamins and other nutritional supplements lowered the risk. The study also found that once opacities are present, the *nuclear* and *posterior subcapsular* forms frequently tend to worsen. The risk of *nuclear* opacities increased with each year of age, and was three-folds higher in whites than in other patients. Users of gout medications also had a higher risk. Cataracts are most often diagnosed when a opacity occurs, but a test developed by National Eye Institute in Cleveland involves measurement of a protein related to cataract formation. When available this test may signal a change in life style to stem further development._

THE INCREDIBLE LENS

Sight requires a transparent medium for light to reach the photo-optic cells in order to boot up the process of vision and herein lies a potential problem, for the cells, the building blocks of the tissues, contain a number of components--the nucleus, the mitochondria, etc., all of which scatter light. If the lens, the largest and the major focusing body in the eye, were composed of cells, light would scatter compromising the ability to see. But, the lens, unlike every other tissue in the body that contains its full complement of cells, harbors only a single layer. Yet despite nature's provision for clear sight, the aging process still exacts a toll on clarity of sight, and although vision is still adequate, it may be necessary to use stronger prescription glassses to enhance vision even in the absence of cataract formation.

THE BESIEGED LENS

Essentially, there is no fallback system when the cells in the *lens* are injured. Almost one in five persons between the ages of 65-to-74 will need a cataract operation; one of two people over the age of 74 will be affected. Worldwide, cataract is the leading cause of blindness, believed to be a result of both environmental and genetic factors. Environmentally, ultra violet (UV) radiation is the leading cause. Together with the major hole in the ozone layer, air-borne pollutants, and global warming, the atmospheric problems exact a toll and will continue to do so. Evidence of this major environmental problem already affects Antarctica. In Patagonia, a South American region, evidence now exists of abnormalities such as blindness in animals. While sunlight in certain areas of the world is responsible for major radiation peril, increased use of medical equipment, personal computers, photocopying machines, electronic equipment, kitchen appliances, and even electrical light bulbs, multiply the radiation exposure for all living things. In addition, the increasing use of drugs, especially long-term steroids taken by many seniors, foods contaminated by pesticides, fungicides, herbicides, heavy metals such as cadmium, arsenic, lead, PCB's, dioxins and other chemicals present in the soil, water, and air, *x-rays* such as radiation therapy to the eye, inflammatory and infectious diseases, and complication of diseases such as *diabetes*, cerebral calcification, an associated problem that reduces the brain volume--all contribute to a myriad of medical problems, including cataract plaguing the human condition.

Yet our vulnerability to cataracts may reach back into prehistory and yield to unique treatment methodologies. Far back in the history of our developing planet, as anaerobic life forms emerged, oxygen did not exist. Micro-organisms lived and grew in the absence of oxygen. But with emergence of oxygen, new life forms developed. In deep time, therefore, these new life forms, dependent on oxygen for existence, may lay the root of cataract development created by an interplay of oxygen and light that produced *reactive oxygen species–ROS.*

THE CONUNDRUM OF SUNLIGHT

Sunlight or full spectrum light contains all the wavelengths of light radiation. Sunlight interacts with oxygen to form *reactive oxygen species (ROS)* a toxic substance to the lens. *ROS* is an oxidizer. It acts on protein, DNA, lipids (fats) to form *free radicals*--those particles that snatch molecules from healthy cells destabilizing them and eventually causing cell death. Some of these harmful effects are generated by the non-essential amino acid arginine, nitrous oxide synthase, superoxide, and hydrogen peroxide a relatively nonreactive substance when compared to superoxide, except when it is exposed to a substance found in many proteins that have escaped the binding action of nucleic acid transforming the substance to dangerous hydroxy-radicals.

Studies on animals have shown that continuous exposure to light even at low levels can cause light-induced blindness--researchers at Johns Hopkins determined in animal studies that it was caused by a gradual loss of *rhodopsin*—a key light detecting protein found in the photo-optic cells in the eye. These results were unexpected, for they overturned the assumption that blindness from chronic light exposure is a direct result of *retinal degeneration.*

Nature, however, in its wisdom, counterbalanced the above dire situation by having created a new set of compounds that attacks the ravages of oxygen. Most important is the compound glutathione (GSH), a reducing agent. High concentrations of glutathione present in the lens cells of the eye balances the oxidative effects of *ROS*. Unlike other cells in the body, the cells in the *cornea* and the *lens* (having no blood supply) synthesize high concentrations of glutathione. With age, however, the level of glutathione decreases. In healthy eyes, the ratio of reduced glutathione in the cells of the *lens*, the *cornea*, the *trabecular meshwork* and other regions of the eye is 100-1. In eyes subjected to oxidative stress, this ratio is reversed. Caught in time, if the oxidative stress is removed and the cell is still viable, it will revert to its healthy ratio. This research has opened a window on the level of glutathione affecting other regions of the eye especially the *trabecular meshwork*. This finding raises the yet unexplored question of whether the *ROS* effect provides yet another link to those factors damaging the *ganglion* cells. There is already ample evidence that *ROS* is implicated in one of the factors causing *macular degeneration.* Several substances may help remedy the problem. These include: riboflavin, a B vitamin that acts as a photosynthesizer--trapping the energy of the light that chemically produces reactive ions, and n-acetyl cysteine, an amino acid made inside the cell along with glycine and glutamic acid. Because glutathione is difficult to get into the eye, protection from *ROS* may be increased by taking the above vitamins.

Increasing glutathione levels may be one solution and genetic therapy may be another remedy for the cataract problem. Two major genes, *catalase* and *glutathione transferase*, enzymes that are active in healthy eyes, are detoxifying agents. The trick is to turn these genes on in sick eyes. (See Chyapter 9 for information on gene therapy.)

Other environmental conditions may also lead to cataract development. Low-level lead exposure, according to a study of men in the United States reported in the *Journal of the American Medical Association (JAMA,)* increases the risk of cataract. Exposure may also derive from cigarette smoking and even drinking water contaminated by lead. This eight-year study involved 642 men sixty years and older who participated in the Boston-based *Normative Aging Study (NAS)*. Men with the greatest concentration of lead in their bones were 2-to-7 times more likely to develop cataracts than those with less concentration. Bone lead levels, a more stable source, were used rather than blood levels.

And would you believe? Ducks get cataracts when fresh lakes and ponds become too salty. This condition leads to premature death of the birds.

Many patients turn to vitamin supplementation hoping to reverse or at least stem rapid cataract development, and there is some evidence in the medical literature that specific vitamins do help. At Tufts University, Boston, a study found that women who used vitamin C (140-to-300 mg) and lutein and zeaxanthin (2.4 mg daily) for ten years or more had a lower risk of cataract development than women who took no supplements at all.

How Cataracts Affect the Eye

With an unaffected lens sight is a straightforward process. Light passes through the *cornea*, which helps to focus it, through the expanding and contracting pupil that accommodates to available light, through the fine-focusing *lens*, onto the *retina*, a tissue no thicker than wet Kleenex, and thence onto several layers of specialized cells, journeying to the *ganglion* cells, that as previously stated, form the *optic nerve* responsible for carrying the precious signals to the brain. But light has its detrimental side. It causes light scatter, glare and a clouding of the *lens*. As well, glaucoma conditions intensify glare, a common complaint among members of our Group. The excesses of light scatter is controlled somewhat when riding in a roofed vehicle, wearing a brimmed hat, sunglasses or sitting in a darkened room with only one central light source. I find watching theatrical productions quite comfortable for only the stage is lit.

Cataracts affect different parts of the eye. A central cataract is called *nuclear*. Glare is often a problem with a *nuclear* cataract especially when driving at night, for with the expansion of the pupil to accommodate to dim light, the headlights of cars scatter light at the edges of the cataract causing glare and halos. Also, *miotic* drops narrowing the pupil worsen the effect. In normal light, the *nuclear* cataract acts as a stronger lens enabling far-sighted and older people especially to read print again without corrective lenses. But as the cataract thickens, this so-called second vision vanishes.

Another form, *posterior subcapsular cataract,* is formed in the back of the eye. In this form, vision is affected almost immediately, for the clouding occurs where the light rays converge to form a narrow beam, impairing vision in bright light and also possibly causing more glare and halos. Big bellies appear to be associated with this form of cataract. Women with waistlines larger than thirty-five inches and men with "beer belly" are the most prone. The link, common in cases of obesity and *diabetes*, involves high blood sugar levels that are apt to damage proteins in that part of the l*ens.*

A third type, *cortical cataract* affects the *cortex* or covering of the eye.

Epidemiologic studies have demonstrated that estrogen-deprived women (post-menopausal) have a higher incidence of cataract formation. This has given rise to research in this area. A study to determine the protective effect of estrogen in cultured *epithelial* cells revealed that estrogen preserves the mitochondrial function during oxidative (free radical release) insult. This implies that estrogen may be a useful protectant against cataract formation in women and that a non-feminizing estrogen may do the same for men. This study, while interesting and advocating a hormonal approach was, nevertheless, conducted in a Petri dish. We do not suggest estrogen replacement except under the care of a physician, preferably an endocrinologist.

GENETIC FACTORS

Not all cataracts are a product of environmental toxins, age and/or invasive procedures. Genetic mutations may also be responsible. When an infant is born with cataracts, the cause may be genetic. *Fanconi syndrome*, a rare disorder, causes excessive amounts of glucose, bicarbonate, phosphates, uric acid, potassium, sodium, and certain amino acids that are excreted in the urine. Damage to bones (bones need phosphates) and kidneys may occur before the disease is diagnosed. Not curable, but with treatment damage can be contained, but the infant may already have cataracts and rickets. Usually infants so affected rarely make it into adulthood.

Another rarer condition, *galactosemia,* an inborn error of metabolism manifesting in an inability to break down the enzyme galactose necessary to digest lactose (milk sugar), before it is converted into glucose, may cause cataract and other problems. This is a correctible disease but if not diagnosed, either in utero (found through amniocentesis), or in the neonate, problems will result. If not diagnosed within a week after birth, the infant will fail to thrive due to anorexia, vomiting, and diarrhea unless galactose and lactose are removed from the diet. The mother is advised to exclude milk products from the diet.

Glaucoma patients also are more prone to complications arising from cataract extraction as described in the opening of this chapter. Just about all the interventions to stem the progression of nerve damage—from drops to surgeries—may affect the health of the *lens*. Filtration surgery may cause a cataract to pop up immediately following surgery, but most often cataracts associated with surgery usually develop within one or two years. A number of theories possibly explain this unfortunate situation. The problem may stem from the loss of fluid from the eye during the surgery. Rapid drainage causes a precipitous drop in the IOP resulting in a flattening of the eye, which impacts on the *lens*. Another possibility involves an accidental nick to the lens during surgery and this damage sets the cataract process in motion. And the age factor cannot be ruled out.

Following surgery, cataracts are more readily formed in older patients than in those younger. Every person in the Group speaks of events leading up to the need for cataract surgery especially following a filtering operation. Yet, as with all scenarios, there are exceptions. Dorothy, who because of progressive glaucoma in both eyes had to have filtering operations, surprisingly did not develop blinding cataracts, while William, in his early fifties, developed cataracts before his fields showed glaucoma progression. At times there may be confusion about which of two eye conditions is causing fogginess as happened with Rose who, after a *corneal* implant that did not resolve the foggy problem, found she also needed to have her cataract removed.

Cataracts lower visual acuity and you may wonder what you'll be able to see when the cataract is removed. Two screening tests may possibly provide clues. One is called a *PAM* test that probes behind the cataract and gives some indication of potential vision, but some doctors claim that this reading is tenuous at best. This certainly proved to be my case. My ophthalmologist, after giving me the *PAM* test, said that I would probably have 20/50 in my eye, but when my cataract was removed; my vision registered a respectable 20/25. The diagnostic instrument *Scanning Laser Acuity Potential (SLAP)* according to a small clinical report may provide a more accurate reading of acuity following cataract surgery. A third system has been developed by scientists at the University of Auckland, New Zealand, called the *wavefront sensor system*, produced by Bausch & Lomb. According to this group, the system objectively determines the degree of visual impairment caused by the cataract. They found different aberrations between the *nuclear* and *cortical* cataracts. This system has yet to undergo large trials to prove its effectiveness, but if it meets its goals, it will provide a rapid assessment of the visual potential hidden by the cataract.

Cataract removal, especially before a filtering operation, may reveal a more stable visual field, for the cataract impedes your ability to see all the targets. As well, the opacity of the *lens* hampers your doctor to precisely establish the health of your *optic nerve*. Following cataract removal, you may discover that for the time, a filtering operation may be postponed.

READY FOR CATARACT SURGERY?

When should a cataractous lens be removed? Usually you're the first to know. When colors mystify you, especially differentiating between the blacks and browns, when you turn on strong lighting, can't thread a needle, see double, experience distracting glare, see halos around lights, can't read street signs (as happened with Yvette), can't read light print, when stronger glasses don't correct the problem, and you surrender your driver's license (as I did) convinced that you'll never see well enough to drive again—you may be ready for cataract extraction. You may also become aware that your doctor is suggesting more often that you should consider a cataract operation, especially if the cataract is swelling, a condition that may increase pressure in your glaucomatous eye.

Cataracts also occur in babies' eyes. Should your infant be affected and you want to know whether your infant possesses any vision, you can obtain such information from a series of simple tests. Specialists in this field check the infant's level of preferential viewing—testing the baby's response to a set of objects, and/or by a test called the *Visual Evoked Potential (VEP)* a measurement of electrical impulses of the *visual cortex* generated during the baby's viewing of patterns on a screen.

CATARACT REMOVAL

Those who have had successful operations call it a cinch. Modern equipment has reduced the cataract operation from hours to minutes, from hospital overnights to outpatient treatment, from heavy lens eyeglasses to lens implant with an adaptable focus. World-wide, however, in countries where medical services are limited, cataracts are one of the major blinding diseases.

Simply, a cataract operation involves the removal of the diseased lens and in most cases (with the exception of some but not all highly *myopic* individuals) replacing it with an *intraocular* lens that is implanted in the eye. Implants are usually manufactured from silicone or plastic materials, but as with every feature in medicine, scientists are searching for new and possibly better materials.

Preparation for a cataract extraction involves a series of tests to calculate your refraction, the shape of your eye, its axial length and the condition of your cornea. You are entitled to add your "two cents" to this assessment for the strength of the *intraocular* lens will depend upon whether you prefer close or distant vision with corrective glasses since accommodative lenses may not be recommended for you. For example, people who have been near-sighted most of their lives are accustomed to seeing at close range and using corrected lenses for distance. If you are having implants in both eyes, some surgeons suggest correcting one eye for distance and the other for near vision. This procedure may or may not be an option for you, especially if one of your eyes is more compromised from glaucoma than the other.

The first step of course, with any invasive procedure, involves anesthetizing the eye. Most often the anesthesia is injected into the eyeball, but a Spanish study found that immobilization of the eye could be similarly obtained with the same local anesthesia applied before taking a pressure test, thus reducing possible side effects. With the speed of modern equipment the more potent anesthetic agents may no longer be necessary.

The *lens* nestles in a capsule—like a baseball mitt holding a ball. To perform cataract surgery, the faulty *lens* must first be extracted. Two methods evolved over the years—*intracapsular* extraction and *extracapsular* extraction. *Intracapsular* extraction, hardly in use today, consists of an *iridectomy*--the entire structure, *lens*, *capsule* and *zonules*, are removed. This procedure, although it did prevent *pupillary block*, is more drastic than *extracapsular* surgery, which together with *phacoemulsification* has revolutionized the cataract operation. With *extracapsular* surgery only the diseased *lens* is extracted. The back of the *lens capsule* and the *zonules* remain firmly in place. Furthermore, only a tiny incision is necessary. This procedure is called "no stitch", for as implied, stitches are not required.

A more recent development that may supersede ultra sound *phacoemulsification* and be safer is using a laser. Heat is not generated and furthermore, the incision required for the instrument is smaller promoting faster healing. Corneal burns are avoided with laser. Depending upon the patient's condition and the doctor's bias, this new technique may not always be applied even when it becomes generally available.

A surgeon using *phacoemulsification* divides the *lens* up like a pie, and then fragments it with ultrasonic vibrations. The bits of lens are then vacuumed up. Because the eye loses fluid when entered, a solution (usually *viscoelastic*) is injected before the *phacoemulsification* procedure.

Some glaucomatous eyes pose problems that require special attention and careful positioning of the *intraocular* lens is necessary. Medical therapy may have permanently narrowed the pupil (*sphincter sclerosis*). In this case, the surgeon uses special clips to perform a *sphincterectomy* on the muscle sphincter that controls the action of the pupil. An incision is made in the sphincter to release its hold. This procedure is not altogether without its risks, for the hooks may pull the *iris* plane forward. Enlargement of the pupil may become permanent as it did with me and several other long-time users of the *miotic* drops. I have not found this to be a problem, and indeed, I consider it an advantage, for my doctor can now view my *optic nerve* without using dilating drops.

Exfoliation syndrome (See Chapter 2) may require positioning the *intraocular* lens in a place in the eye other than in the capsule that may have been rendered unstable because of *zonules* deterioration. This situation may be resolved, however, with a capsular tension ring called the *Morcher capsular tension ring*, a flexible horseshoe-shaped filament that is inserted into the capsular bag stabilizing it, like, if I may be so bold, an underwire bra. This ring increases the safety measure for *exfoliation* patients. If the patient has a leathery *iris* or a flaccid or misplaced *iris*, an *iridotomy* may be necessary to stop the *iris* from prolapsing into the drainage channel.

Certain forms of glaucoma, especially *uveitis* need special attention when cataract removal is contemplated. *Uveitis* may be caused by a number of abnormal eye conditions. One form of *uveitis* is called *Sarcoid Uveitis*. The symptoms of *sarcoidosis* are associated with the presence of granular-like lesions in the eye. *Sarcoidosis* may also affect other tissues of the body. With removal of the cataract and replacement of an *intraocular* lens, doctors prescribe an aggressive regimen of steroids to prevent a *uveitic* attack.

Persons with *diabetes* get cataracts more frequently and they may experience special problems such as *retinal detachment* or other *retinal* abnormalities. In some cases a *vitrectomy* needs to be performed with subsequent injection of silicone oil to fill the vitreous cavity. London researchers monitoring 1,500 *diabetic* patients found that cataract operations could still be successful despite problem cases requiring the injection of silicone oil.

Implantation of the folded plastic lens into the now-empty capsule is the final step in the cataract operation. Inserted into the capsule the lens opens like a flower. Half the size of the normal lens, it is secured in the eye by haptics (tiny arms) that extend from both sides of the lens to the wall of the eye. The *viscoelastic* solution is then drained from the eye and replaced with a fluid virtually identical to the aqueous humor.

Possibly, *phacoemulsification* can lower your IOP. A small study of 52 patients indicated a decrease in pressure. There appears to be a scientific foundation for this finding. The *trabecular meshwork* cells synthesize a substance called *interleukin-1-alpha* that has the property to increase the outflow of fluid. *Phacoemulsification* stimulates the production of *interleukin-1-alpha*.

THE INTRAOCULAR LENS

A lens implant should vastly improve your vision. As with every technological feature (note the obsolescence of your computer after several years), lenses also undergo advances in technology. In the good old days, an *intraocular* lens might have caused acute inflammation rendering the eye susceptible to *uveitis*, scarring and compromising the blood-brain barrier. In common use now is a heparin-coated lens that resolves some of these issues. This particular lens is in a state of constant molecular motion, the negative charge repelling bacteria and white blood cells, because they share the same surface charge.

Even so, an implanted lens may not be suitable for people who are allergic to the implant material, including *uveitis* patients. An allergic reaction can provoke inflammation. Should this be a problem, the diseased cataract may still be removed and the site restored by using a contact lens.

The manufacture of lenses continues to evolve. Multifocal lenses are now available. These lenses include the *REZOOM* lens and the *RESTOR* lens. Basically, although somewhat different, these lenses provide the same acuity by splitting the oncoming light for near, intermediate and distant vision. As well, an accommodating lens, known as the *Crystallin* lens, works by a slight movement of the lens optics when something up close is viewed. In addition, *aspheric* lenses improve the quality of post-operative vision by enhancing contrast sensitivity. At the time of cataract surgery, treatment for *astigmatism* may include either a *Toric* lens or a *Limbal Relaxing Incision*. Generally one or the other suffices, but if there is a great deal of *astigmatism*, the procedures can be combined. There is also a lens that blocks the blue light rays that are believed to cause *macular degeneration*. This particular lens blocks the blue light spectrum found in both natural and artificial light and as an added bonus, reduces troublesome glare that some glaucoma patients experience after cataract surgery. Another positive feature of an implant serves the mechanism of the eye well by creating a natural barrier between the front and back of the eye. Poised for marketing is a lens set in glasses called "heads-up." The technology allows for an overlay of such information as maps, specific directions, and sidewalk dynamics. In development, these glasses may aid those with visual handicaps.

Under study is a bionic eye designed to provide varying shades of light to the blind. Depending upon the success of this trial at Moorfields Eye

Hospital, Great Britain, this technology may become available widely for the blind and severely visually handicapped.

Equipment Improvement

In general, the new advances in medicine aim to improve success rates by increasing the safety parameters of an operation and sharpening the surgeon's skills. A nifty instrument called *The Infiniti*, an Alcon product, fits this bill. It is one smart hunk of technology. The system helps the surgeon perform all the steps of the operation in record time. It automatically checks the pressure in the small tube (through which the cataract is removed) 500 times a second, assuring that the IOP does not drop precipitously during the surgery—a condition that would injure eye tissues. *Phacoemulsification* is replaced with Aqualase, a technology using a heated saline solution to break up the cataract. High-velocity pulses of water speed up the process. The Aqualase is equipped with a gentler plastic needle rather than a metal tip that in the past could get stuck in very hard cataracts, something like a drill clinched in tough wood. The *Infiniti* possesses an oscillating feature (back and forth movement) that rectifies this problem. The debris is aspirated through a tiny incision. Smaller softer bits left behind are then removed with a gentler instrument.

What makes the *Infiniti* special is the *servomechanism*--a feedback system that detects when the pressure in the eye is about to drop dangerously low and instantaneously halts the removal process. Throughout the operation fluid identical to the eye's natural fluid bathes the eye. This automatic system informs the computer when to safely increase vacuum force to suck out the bits of debris from the diseased lens. This stronger force benefits the eye by shortening the operation, thus vastly decreasing to a fraction the volume of fluid passing through the eye. Fluid is reduced from a cup to approximately 20 tablespoons; a mere one-tablespoon of fluid often does the job. One of the major benefits of reduced fluid is protection of the *cornea*. Complications may arise should excess fluid flow through a vulnerable *cornea*. A long operation requires a constant flow of fluid moving through the eye subjecting the eye to possible damage.

The procedure from start to finish in an uncomplicated eye takes no more than five-to-six minutes. Every detail of the operation has been calibrated to de-stress the surgical effects on the eye for the less time spent in the eye increases the margin of safety. An added advantage of this speedy operation is the possibility of using the same anesthetic drop as for a pressure check, dispensing with the injection of anesthesia into the eye. This development is a far cry from merely 10-to-15 years ago when hospitalization was the norm, and the patient received systemic anesthesia or more recently injection of anesthesia directly into the eye, a procedure that, in some cases, produced an unsightly black eye. Inflammation, while not entirely reduced, does take a back seat with this system.

Is this machine taking over cataract removal? Never fear. Unlike Hal in the film *2001: A Space Odyssey* by Arthur C. Clarke, the *Infiniti* does not supplant the doctor. Fully in command, the surgeon practices his/her skills with utmost precision while directing the technician to activate critical features on the console. The *Infiniti*, success rate registers greater than 99.9%. In the words of an 85-year-old friend who just had a cataract operation, "I thought the doctor was doing the preparation, and then she said, "all finished."

Combining Cataract and Glaucoma Surgery

Whether to perform a combined *trabeculectomy* and cataract operation or opt for separate operations depends primarily on your glaucomatous condition. During a combined operation most doctors preferentially use the same site and they may also apply *antimetabolites* to insure a functioning *bleb*. These decisions and that of justifying either single or combined operations depend upon your doctor's evaluation of your condition. Especially in the case of glaucoma damage, no size fits all. Some doctors base their decisions on the following assessments:

Moderate--Glaucoma controlled with two medications--only cataract operation.

Mid-Moderate--Glaucoma controlled with more than two medications—*trabeculectomy* & cataract operation.

Advanced Glaucoma--trabeculectomy & cataract operation

In western nations, everybody can benefit from cataract removal and implantation of an *intraocular* lens. Blindness from this disease no longer haunts those with cataracts. Once excluded, children born with cataracts and people who have crossed the century divide can receive this surgery.

Your Role in the operation

You are an active participant in the surgical process. From the time that an operation is scheduled, you will be engaged in the process. Beginning with the pre-op, you will most likely be required to have a medical workup. Usually, this assessment can be performed by your general practitioner or in the hospital where the operation is scheduled. Most eye operations are now out-patient procedures in USA, although Medicare does allow for an overnight stay. Each country however, and in some cases, each hospital, has its own rules, and patients in those hospitals that allow for a day or so of recuperation consider the American method of immediate release barbaric. Nevertheless, if you are anything like me, you will probably appreciate going home the same day, especially if you live near the hospital and can easily return should complications arise.

When your operation is scheduled, your surgeon will prescribe both steroids and antibiotics to be taken several days before the operation. Continue using your glaucoma drops along with these new medications unless otherwise advised by your doctor.

In the operating theater only your eye will be anesthetized with either a *retrobulbar* injection directly into the eye (it may hurt but the discomfort lasts less than a minute), or an anesthetic drop commonly used when your doctor measures your IOP. A combined operation expands the time required and *retrobulbar* anesthesia may be required.

Upon discharge, continue all your medications as instructed until advised to discontinue. Note that steroids are included in the mix. Remember that following an invasive procedure, the body protects itself by sending its healing messengers to the site causing an inflammatory response that if not dampened by steroids will cause an additional set of problems. Usually, your eye will be patched overnight and you will be advised to wear a protective shield on your eye while you sleep.

Some surgeons feel restrictions are unnecessary; others advise against bending the head lower than the heart, resisting lifting heavy packages, using a stool softener if necessary, waiting several days before showering. If you're good at squatting to pick up things from the floor, you can regard this activity as an exercise that will strengthen your thigh muscles.

Stabilization of your eye requires from four-to-five weeks before you can be fitted with corrective glasses or contacts. Your sight will be imperfect during that period. Should you be in the forefront of bifocal implantable lens, this period may be shortened.

COMPLICATING FACTORS

While most problems become immediately evident, there are some that may arise a week or more following surgery. In a study of 1,000 patients who were examined a week after surgery, problems surfaced that had not been apparent at the time of surgery. Although this was a small study, the fact remains that problems can occur even in the best of circumstances, and the need for close medical monitoring is essential.

- **Inflammation.** Foreign objects in the body may precipitate inflammation that may affect different parts of the uvea as in *uveitis* or *iritis* (inflammation of the *uvea* or *iris*) especially if the lens is improperly positioned. Whenever inflammation occurs, you will most likely be treated with steroid drops until the eye quiets down.
- **Adhesions.** Should your IOP drop to the *hypotony* level (below 5-to-6 mmHg) and remain so for an extended period of time, you run the risk of various parts of the eye adhering. Normally, parts of the eye like the *iris* and *cornea* are kept separate by the circulating fluid.
- **Macula Edema.** Swelling of the *macula*, a condition caused by excess fluid in the *macula* can be resolved with steroid therapy.
- **Bleb Function Threatened.** Many glaucoma patients who opt for a cataract operation have already had a *trabeculectomy*. In this case the doctor may choose to protect the *bleb* by applying an injection of *5-FU*, an *antimetabolite* that discourages scarring at the *trabeculectomy* site. Nevertheless, there are risks that include *bleb* rupture. As well, microscopic lens particles may enter the filtration site affecting the quality of *bleb* function. Should a *bleb* be compromised during cataract surgery the surgeon can at the same time perform a revision of the *bleb*.
- **IOP Elevation.** In some cases IOP can rise dangerously if preexisting conditions such as *exfoliation* are not taken into account. Also, although a cataract operation often reduces IOP, it may, on the other hand, raise it.
- **Pupillary Block.** This condition, although rarely occurring, prevents the aqueous fluid from squeezing through the space between the *lens* and the *iris*. Pressure builds pushing the *iris* forward so that it blocks the drainage channel resulting in increased IOP. This condition will need correction with an *iridectomy* or *iridotomy*.
- **Bleeding.** Disruption of blood vessels can cause bleeding. Generally, bleeding vessels can be cauterized or will self-seal, but if the situation does not resolve within several days, your doctor might need to intervene. Released blood into the eye may cause blurry vision. This in itself is not dangerous but if there is recurrent bleeding, *neovascularization* may develop, promoting a condition similar to neovascular glaucomas.(See Chapter 2).
- **Corneal Decompensation.** Many glaucoma patients' *corneas* have become fragile, both from medication usage and surgical treatment. If your *cornea* has lost cells, your sight may be blurry for a while. Before the operation, your doctor has most likely performed a *corneal* cell count, a noninvasive procedure that determines your

vulnerability for a *corneal* problem and advises you accordingly. Most often even with a reduced number of *corneal* cells, an operation can go forward. In my case, my weak eye has half the *corneal* cells of my good eye. Yet my *cornea* has been able to bounce back after a number of procedures. On the other hand, Felicity's *cornea* took six months to heal.

- **Narrow Angle Glaucoma.** Should there be a slight shifting of the eye's bodies—the pupil or the *ciliary body, narrow angle* glaucoma may result. Trapped air acts like a firm body (think air mattress) and it, too, can cause problems.

- Retinal **Detachment**. Highly-*myopic* patients, because of the length of the eyeball (long eyeballs stretch the *retina*), are at risk for *retinal detachment* during or following a cataract extraction. Should detachment occur (you notice a section of your sight is occluded), your doctor will take immediate steps to remediate the situation.

- **Ghost Cells** (See Chapter 2)

- **Drug Interaction:** The drug Flomax may cause *floppy iris syndrome*, a post-surgical complications.

- **Secondary Cataract** While you may escape many of the above problems, you may still be subject to what is called in common parlance, a secondary cataract. In the year 2000, 863,567 cataract operations were performed in United States and 601,850 neodynamic *(Nd:YAG)* laser posterior *capsulotomies* were also performed because of *posterior* capsule clouding, the site for the *intraocular* lens implant. Statistics have improved, but by current estimates, some ten percent of the cataract removal cases will still develop opacification of the *capsule*. This situation develops because cells from your own *lens* are still present after the lens extraction. Elimination of these *cells* is tricky because application of a disabling pharmacological substance will be toxic to the surrounding cells. The severity of the haziness varies with each individual. In my case, one eye remained perfectly clear and in the other eye minor dimming developed, but I found it did not interfere with my acuity. David, on the other hand, experienced considerable haze and was deeply disappointed that his former dim vision returned. If the cloudiness becomes very uncomfortable, this situation can be remedied with a *capsulotomy*, a laser procedure {neodynamic *(Nd:YAG)* laser} that penetrates the *capsule* allowing unfettered light to again reach the *retina*. Like all methods of intervention, this procedure can cause problems in susceptible patients.

WHAT GLAUCOMA PATIENTS WORRY ABOUT

Much as you would like better vision after surgery, you may be disappointed when you experience a time lag compared to people not affected with glaucoma. Depending upon your condition and the number of procedures you have experienced, the healing process can take weeks and even several months. With the most up-to-date equipment, this time period is considerably shortened. Since I have experienced two cataract operations years apart, I waited out my first for six weeks, but for my second, only one week. People without glaucoma report good sight within days.

Worrisome, of course, is whether your IOP will be affected. In most cases, it will remain the same, and in some fortunate people, drop down a notch; in others, rise slightly, and with the current low values of IOP generally recommended, you may need to add another drop to your routine. One study, however, found that 70% of glaucoma patients undergoing cataract surgery retained their former IOPs. Vision improvement with or without glaucoma is usually considered remarkable. Recently, three of my close friends who do not have glaucoma reported instant success and I shared their joy at renewed sight. Studies have indicated that glaucoma patients, for the most part, equally share in the thrill of renewed sight. Cataract operations have become routine for glaucoma patients. There is no reason to suffer in a dim world. For glaucoma patients especially, when contemplating a cataract operation, do seek out a doctor who is aware of your particular condition, especially if you have secondary glaucoma such as *exfoliation*. With the experienced physician and a positive attitude on your part, your cataract operation should be a cinch. Go for it!

CHAPTER 9

The Next Big Thing: Retooling and Protecting The Eye: Neuroprotection, Genetics & Stem Cells

○ ○

"Remember that the future is neither ours nor wholly not ours, so that we may neither count on it as sure to come nor abandon hope of it certain not to be."

Epicurus, Letter to Menoeceous (3rd c. B.C.) in Letters, Principal Doctriness and Vaican Sayings, tr. Russell M. Geer

At annual ophthalmology conferences, sections are devoted to *neuroprotectants*, genetics and regeneration of neurons. The quest for a cure for glaucoma and other *neurodegenerative* diseases may finally reach its goal should the reported studies evolve into effective methods for saving vision in glaucomatous eyes. It is now a given that successful lowering of IOP at the very outset of the disease will protect vision and/or slow down the progression of the disease despite the tolls of the aging process. Much is at stake for preserving vision. Teams of researchers gathered throughout the world are engaged in solving fundamental questions as complex as, for example, the need for the some twenty-five different types of *optic nerve* cells—why this variety? At birth the eye possesses approximately 1 million neurons grouped into several hundred bundles that comprise the *ganglion* layer of cells located in the *retina*. The *optic nerve* is composed of another million or so. Older people lose about half of these cells. Death or injury to these cells in glaucomatous conditions is characterized by an enlarged or excavated cup and a thinned nerve fiber layer in the optic disc. Injury may occur from high *intraocular pressure*, blood flow problems, stroke, mechanical trauma, degenerative disease, and/or toxic elements. A process called "dying back" also occurs. The axon at the end of the nerve, responsible for the synoptic leap from one neuron to another, dies back, disrupting connections between cells. While loss of neurons may be divided into three stages, like a house of cards, they are linked together. When the first stage is affected, the second stage becomes vulnerable, and so on. Generally, the first stage occurs when there is a defect in the aqueous flow dynamics resulting from a blockage of the *trabecular meshwork* and/or with certain susceptible individuals, elevated IOP affects the flow of nourishing blood to the *retina*.

Researchers delving into all aspects of the neuron are investigating the regulation of the precursor cells in the developing nervous system that facilitates the maturation of neurons. When formulated, this information should lead to a deeper understanding of how genes contained in these cells are activated to produce mature neurons.

A variety of *neuroproctective* agents under investigation may interfere with different molecular pathways leading to cell death. One of the goals sought by researchers focuses on *neuroprotective* agents to marshal the body's own ability for tissue regeneration by stem cells, a process comparable to the ability of the zebra fish or newts to regenerate specific organs and body parts. Cell death or *apoptosis* is not a bad thing, for *apoptosis* involves normal cell turnover. When it occurs prematurely, however, cell loss seriously impacts on the health of the organ. During the normal remodeling of the *ganglion* cell layer, the signal for cell suicide is triggered by *neurothropin deprivation* (nutritive elements). It appears that with glaucoma, the *ganglion* cell unfortunately receives the "destroy" button before its time. On the other hand, in some diseases, such as cancer, the destroy signal goes awry and cells proliferate. Toxic factors in glaucoma such as excessive glutamate also impact on the cell dynamics, although definitive pathways appear to need further elucidation.

The problem of cell death may begin in the *mitochondria*. Insufficient mitochondria, tiny, thread-like bodies within each cell that serve as the body's energy source, may be partly responsible for cell death. Problematic mitochondria has been linked to several *neurodegenerative* diseases such as *Alzheimer's, Lou Gehrig's* and *Huntington's*. Glaucoma is considered a *neurodegenerative* disease. Insufficient mitochondria can lead to increased permeability of a specific calcium channel located on *n-methy-d-aspartate (NMDA)* receptor, the main *neurotransmitter* in the *retina*. Evidence suggests that the inability of mitochondria to churn out sufficient energy results in permeability of the mitochondria membrane that then releases several chemicals that may cause excitotoxity and programmed cell death.

Escape of these chemicals is thought to transpire either through open pores, or from chemicals outside the membrane, both of which increase the cell's permeability. When this receptor is stimulated by glutamate, it produces an inappropriate influx of calcium further compromising the mitochondrial cycle and eventually leading to *apoptosis*. The loss of mitochondria along with the diminishing function of mitochondria is a consequence of aging. These studies may reveal an important factor in degeneration of the nerve cells. There is a possibility that potassium channels in the mitochondria may also be involved as one aspect of dysfunction.

Autoimmune disease has been linked to certain forms of glaucoma. The process may begin with the action of the T cells. People with normal pressure glaucoma may be more susceptible to autoimmune diseases such as *rheumatoid arthritis* and *insulin-dependent diabetes*. Also, inflammatory diseases such as *uveitis* may be a sign of autoimmune disease. Subtle effects of inflammation may be also present in other forms of glaucoma. One researcher that I talked to working on *exfoliation* glaucoma asked me about arthritis, and I showed her deformed knuckles on my hands. Relationship? Some glaucoma specialists believe that in glaucoma, the *optic* nerve suffers from inflammation.

Inflammation has been identified as a major cause of all illnesses. In some cases inflammation is not necessarily harmful, for it is the immune system's method for striking down foreign invaders by producing cytokines and proteins that attack germs and repair damaged tissue. When inflammation is excessive however, the protective agents become overwhelmed and therefore, are possibly partly responsible for the buildup of plaque found in the brains of people with *Alzheimers* and other degenerative diseases. It has taken center stage in heart disease and osteoarthritis. The immune system of older people appears to lose its self-regulatory ability resulting in mobility loss, weight gain, muscle strength loss, and disease-fighting capability.

NEUROPROTECTION

Neuroprotection is hot. If drugs can be developed to protect the neurons from committing premature suicide, then possibly, the *optic* nerve will be spared its slow glaucomatous decline. The following three examples are some of the goals that scientists are working on.

- Block destructive events affecting *retinal ganglion cells*.
- Enhance *optic nerve fiber* survival mechanisms.
- Repair damage

Patients blinded by glaucoma have lost ninety-five percent of their neurons. One *neuroprotection* goal aims to block the mechanisms leading to blindness. Unlike other repair systems in the body, when a neuron dies, it's gone forever. Neuroproctective agents will be set to interfere with various cell death stages--halting progression from Stage 1 to Stage 2, the sequence where a molecular change in the *retinal ganglion* nerves and surrounding tissues occur, thus avoiding cell death at Stage 3. This plan would primarily emphasize pressure control to remove the effects of Stage 1, thus disrupting the chain of events. In cases of uncontrolled IOP, however, it is uncertain if the chain of events has not already occurred. For that reason, scientists are also concentrating on Stage 2 where two damaging stimuli have been identified that possibly activate *ganglion cell death*. The first of these is *neurotropic deprivation. Neurotrophins* are small peptides (a class of nutritional substances synthesized from amino acids) grouped together in a class of molecules that also include *growth factors* and *neurotrophins*. Survival of all cells requires a steady supply of *neurotrophins*. The peptides interact with cell surface receptors that when activated control cell growth and abnormal activity. The *neurotrophins* come from other cells that, when contacted, are thought to update the status of neuronal connections. *Retinal* ganglion cells get their supply of *neurotrophins* from other neurons in the brain, which appear to be primary to their health. These are called *brain-derived neurotropic factor (BDNF)*. The *ganglion* cell absorbs secreted *BDFN* and transports (retrogrades) it along its axon to the *retinal ganglion body*. In the presence of glaucoma, the retrograde flow of *BDFN* is thought to be blocked--that is, the nutritional factors generated in the brain do not reach the *retinal* cells. Another growth factor, *ciliary neurotropic factor (CNTF)*, has been experimentally shown to reduce *retinal* ganglion cell death when the axons have been severed in an animal model. Yet, another growth factor, *pigment epithelial-derived factor (PEDF,)* has been shown to protect cultured *retinal* neurons against the effect of induced cell death due to hydrogen peroxide. A naturally-occurring growth factor called *oncomodulin* stimulates regeneration of *injured* (axons). Inflammation occurs with injury stimulating macrophages (the immune system) to enter the site. Macrophages produce *oncomodlin*, which stimulates axon regeneration.

How long a *ganglion* cell can survive without nourishment is unclear, but it may be a matter of days. Scientists seeking *neuroproctective* strategies are investigating a different source for delivering *BDFN* to the *ganglion* cells. They have demonstrated in animal models the possibility of *intravitreal* (directly into the eye) injections of *BDFN*, but side effects may occur. In other experiments, the *neuro growth factor (NFG)* was directly administered into an animal's degenerated optic nerve. The possibility exists also that *neurotrophins* may function as *neuroregenerative stimulants*—that is, MAKE NEW CELLS. How wonderful this will be if this branch of cell technology takes off!

Dependence on human cloning hampers advancement towards finding a cure. Stem cell research is fraught with ethical questions concerning the beginnings of life, although in some countries, Britain, for one, the granting of a license to the scientists who cloned "Dolly the sheep" to clone human embryos for research has occurred. This is the second license approved by the British to legalize cloning. Nevertheless, human cloning legislation varies widely among other countries. Belgium, Singapore, and Japan allow its use for human research. Switzerland and Italy prohibit it. Australia has a moratorium on it. And the United States has loosened its restrictions of the use of federal funds for this purpose, although no restrictions apply to privately-funded laboratories. The United Nations, deadlocked at this writing, will be reconsidering it.

Harnessing the body's own resources to provide protection from dysfunctional problems would, of course, be ideal. A promising line of research involves Ribonucleic acid *(RNA)*, the molecule responsible for carrying out the genetic code. It has been recruited to interfere with the activity of a mutant gene. A study of the effects of an *RNA* injection in patients with *macular degeneration* is underway. Also, under study is coaxing the body to make its own *RNA* interference. Should this strategy be successful, injections will be eliminated.

Like the *neurotrophins*, excitotoxins interact with receptors on the cell surface. Three sub-types of glutamate receptors are located on neurons, but the problematic one is the *N-methyl-D-aspartate (NMDA)* receptor. Glutamate binds to this receptor opening up the channel that allows sodium and calcium to enter the cell. At high concentrations of glutamate, an excess of calcium crosses the cell membrane, the action of which is then believed to trigger a whole series of events, one of which activates the enzyme *nitric oxide synthase*. Other studies have linked high levels of glutamate and calcium to a decrease in the uptake of cysteine, an amino acid that is an important component of *glutathione* synthesis, an agent vital for *free radical* elimination.

The National Eye Institute, along with pharmaceutical companies and organizations devoted to curing eye diseases, is constantly on the trail of new and better medications for both controlling *intraocular pressure* and protecting the *optic* nerve. *Memantine,* an open channel blocker and antagonist to *NMDA*, a short-life drug, was launched in an extensive trial, but it did not demonstrate immediate protective effects, although the data is still being analyzed. In Europe *Memantine* has been used to treat degenerative diseases such as *Alzheimer's.* In a laboratory study *Memantine* has been shown to decrease glutamate concentration. The Public Citizen Health Research Group reviewing the literature, however, found that, at best, there was but a small reduction in the rate of deterioration in the *Alzheimer's* trial. *Memantine's* potential side effects can be severe. These include dizziness, headache, constipation, pain, and difficulty in breathing. Three cases of inflammation of the pancreas and four cases of renal failure have been reported. In Germany where the drug is marketed, the company has received seventy-three adverse events including seizures, high blood pressure, circulatory failure, jerky movements, rash, skin lesions, tremors and nausea. Side effects of the *Memantine Glaucoma Study* have not yet been reported.

Heat Shock Proteins, intrinsic for neuroprotection, are synthesized by cells subjected to stress resulting from reduced blood flow, depletion of oxygen, or exposure to harmful light rays. These proteins increase cellular resistance to glutamate but antibodies that block *heat shock proteins* may weaken the protective effects of this molecule. Apparently, quercetin is one of the culprits diminishing the effect of *heat shock proteins*. Scientists found that by adding quercetin to the *heat shock protein* molecules in a Petri dish that quercetin reduced the synthesis of *heat shock proteins*, lessening its protective effect. *Heat shock proteins* may have a protective impact on the *retinal ganglion* cells. To increase the levels of *heat shock proteins*, researchers have intravitreally injected *N-mythl-D-aspartate (NMDA)*, an agent that may also be responsible for cell death in other situations. This research is still in its infancy, but it looks promising for, by surrounding the protein with *NMDA* as the protein assembles its amino acids from food intake and also replays its genetic expression, *heat shock proteins* act to protect the still vulnerable protein from outside insults.

Excess glutamate, and its role on glaucoma, is regarded as a serious problem. It is linked to hypoxia (decreased oxygen) leading to toxicity that damages or kills neurons. Glutamate toxicity is implicated in *neurodegenerative* diseases that include glaucoma along with *Lou Gehrig's, Alzheimer's, Parkinson's, Huntington's*, and even AIDS. It is the most abundant *neurotransmitter* in the brain. Studies of the glaucoma effects on the brain indicate that visual pathways are lost in the *lateral geniculate nucleus*, a part of the *visual cortex*. The brain shrinks in size reflecting this loss. A class of drugs, "open channel blockers" limits the release of glutamate by binding to *NMDA* receptor channels, thereby blocking calcium entry. Open-channel blockers enter and bind to the inside of the channel, blocking excess calcium from entering the cell, but like all drugs, side-effects may cause more damage than cure. *Naftidrofuryl,* a drug used to treat stroke victims is reported to improve neurological recovery, as well as increase blood flow by dilating the arteries, inhibiting platelet clumping and increasing oxygen supply. The calcium channel blockers—*SNX-III, Flunarizine, Nimodipine, Nicardipine* and others;

Calcium Chelaters--*BAPTA-AM, phencyclidine hydrochloride*, (angel dust) are all being explored, but their effect on protecting glaucomatous eyes remains to be documented.

Sodium channel blockers may also become candidates in glaucoma therapy. These substances may slow down the *retinal ganglion* cell death by inhibiting sodium channel action during *retinal gangling* cell injury. These blockers act by decreasing intake of *adenosine triphosphatase (ATP)*, an enzyme providing energy, particularly to muscle cells. Drugs in this class include *Lamictal, Topamax and Riluteke*. A group of Columbia University researchers have targeted the red blood cells as a possible site for *neuroprotection* activity. On the cell's surface, a molecule linked to the development of red blood cells accepts a signal of the gene, *erythropoietin receptor (EpoR)* to produce more red blood cells under low oxygen conditions. Production of red blood cells increased in the bone marrow and it was found that the neurons were also protected.

Other sodium channel blockers being studied include: 619C89. Lamotrigine, Riluzole, Lubeluzole, CNS 1237, kappa opiod agonist, C197, NMDA (N-methyl-D-aspartate) blockers-Aptiganel HCI, Phencyclidine hydrochloride, Ketamine, Dextromethorphan derivatives, Remacemide hydrochloride, magnesium, Dizocilpine, as are the Nitric Oxide inhibitors—Nitroarginine, Benzamine derivatives, FK 506, Cyclosporine. Eliprodil, a drug that is a NMDA antagonist, according to a study by researchers in Texas, may prevent the retinal pigmentary cells from oxidative stress. Obviously, a good many drugs are candidates for neuroprotection, but require painstaking research before their promise transforms into therapy.

Protease inhibitors offer another class of drugs that may also prove useful for blocking toxic actions. *Proteases* are enzymes critical to the synthesis of protein, and a subset of this chemical family is involved in cell death. Drugs in this category include *saquinavir mesylate, ritonavir, indinavir* and *nelfinavir mesylate,* the latter drug used for treating AIDS. Other drugs in this family that may be promising include *monoamine oxidase* and *selegiline*. Scientists reported in one study that rats with experimental glaucoma lost less than ten percent of their *retinal ganglion* cells as against thirty-six percent of the rats not treated when the drug *aminoguanidine* was put into their drinking water. Glaucoma medications, especially *betaxolol (Betagan)* and *brimonidine tartrate,* (Alphagan, Alphagan P) according to research, do have protective effects.

Two drugs, *Tarceva* and *Iressa* currently used for cancer treatment have been found to block reactive *astrocytes*, usually benign, but when they become destructive, can affect the *optic nerve* and the brain. Demonstrated in a rat model both drugs protected the optic *nerve*. The two companies manufacturing the drugs, however, are not interested in conducting a glaucoma trial and the researchers would like to see a doctor take on this challenge with a small group of glaucoma patients. Another drug, *rasaline,* approved for treatment of *Parkinson's,* may protect the *retina.*

Chondroitin sulfate-derived disaccharide has been shown in the rat model to protect *retinal* cells from elevated IOP in suppressed immunity aged rats. Looks like this supplement we take for arthritis may also benefit the eye.

Injection of a harmless virus that contains *rhodopsin-2* (used by the photosensitive cells) into a rat model indicated that this protein made the *retinal neurons* sensitive to light. The authors speculate that this model may restore vision in patients experiencing photosensitive cell degeneration.

Free radical scavengers well known to those of us who faithfully take our antioxidants are gaining respectful attention in conventional medical practice. *Free radicals* have been implicated in the slow, chronic *neurodegenerative* diseases described above. Several drugs, among them antioxidants, have been found useful. One class, blocking lipid peroxidation (the *Lazaroids*), has been shown to delay *retinal ganglion* cell death in test tubes--oxygen radical scavengers--*DL-6-8-dithiol octanoic acid (DHLA) lop urinal* and *dexanabinol* are being studied. The antioxidants vitamins C, E, beta-carotene, and the enzymes *catalase* and *superoxide dismutase (SOD),* as well as the herbs *ginkgo biloba, Reservatrol, bilberry, alpha lipoic acid* and *lipid peroxidation* inhibitors may help to protect the *optic nerve.* Free radical production is related to increased intracellular calcium that leads to oxidation of *arachidonic acid.* High levels of intracellular calcium also activate the enzyme *xanthineoxidase* that then produces uric acid and the superoxide radical.

A third cause of *free radical* production is in response to oxidation of proteins resulting from insufficient blood flow. A drug, *Carvedilol,* an antihypertensive drug may cause *free radical* activity. *Nitric Oxide,* a *free-radical* gas first identified in 1987, is manufactured from *L-arginine,* an amino acid. Contrary to a widely held belief, researchers have discovered that *nitrates,* long considered insignificant if not downright dangerous when associated with foods, convert to *nitrous oxide* that serves many functions. Some of these include inducing *vasodilatation* (widening of the blood vessels), dilation of the uterus during pregnancy, inhibiting bone resorption, affecting penile erections, and much more. It also kills bacteria, fungi and even tumor cells. But at high levels it becomes a potent nitrogen *free radical* capable of killing neurons and in this form is implicated in some of the degeneration of the nervous system that occurs with some diseases. Its dual action lies in the amount it produces. While it may act as a *neurotransmitter* to the brain, an oversupply becomes toxic to the cells. If a lot of glutamate is released, *nitric oxide synthase* molecules act like macrophages, releasing large amounts of *nitric oxide* that also kill neighboring neurons which may be perfectly healthy but too close to the action. *Nitric Oxide* can also interfere with the repair of Deoxyribonucleic acid (*DNA*). *Nitroglycerine* provides a source of oxidized *nitric oxide* and this has been found to reduce neuronal damages in animal models affected with stroke. The role for *nitroglycerine* retarding glaucomatous damage was demonstrated in a study that followed sixty patients with open angle glaucoma for a period of eight years. Results of the study revealed that patients receiving systemic nitrate medications had better preservation of the *optic nerve* and visual field.

Inhibitors of *nitric oxide synthase* can protect neurons from *nitric oxide* toxicity. Three forms of nitrous oxide are found in the eye. NOS 1, NOS 2 and NOS 3. One and two, when excessive, interact with *superoxide* and may be toxic to the neurons. Number 3, however, is beneficial for this is the form that dilates the blood vessels increasing the flow of blood to the tissues. Theoretically, if One and Two can be suppressed with medication, the axons will be spared. In the physiology of the eye it is one of the good/bad guys— good if *L-arginine*, nitric oxide's precursor, lowers eye pressure (animal studies indicate the activity of *L-arginine* lowered *intraocular pressure*.) Good, also as a vascular dilator to increase blood flow to the *optic nerve*, but this exploration has not been actively pursued.

If *nitric oxide synthase* can be tamed, researchers argue that glaucoma effects can be lessened. Still in the animal stage but promising, researchers are examining the effects of a promising drug called *SC-51*. Over a seven month period, rat eyes treated with this substance remained stable, while those untreated lost approximately 20,000 *retinal ganglion* cells.

Meanwhile, to avert the negative effects of *nitric oxide*, consider some of these precautions: *Nitric oxide* levels may rise when allergies are present and in cases of iron deficiency (oxygen is conveyed on iron molecules). When a deficiency of iron occurs, reduced oxygen circulates in the body, increasing carbon monoxide exposure and estrogen levels, (a consideration for women on hormone treatment), and possible fluoride poisoning. *Beta-blocker* drugs are suspected of causing an increase in *nitric oxide*. Obviously, *nitric oxide* is such a multifaceted substance that remedies for preventing its harmful effects may impact upon other treatments that have proven successful.

The *carbonic anhydrate inhibitors* (*Trusopt* and *Asopt*) and the herb *ginkgo biloba* may also improve blood flow. Studies, however, do not indicate significant differences in the visual field, although patients have reported enhanced visual acuity. *Nimotop (Nimodipine)* is a *neuroprotective* agent used to treat hemorrhaging in the brain. The *beta-blocker, Betoptic* may be one of the better glaucoma medications in that class for it has exhibited calcium blocking activity through a secondary receptor other than that involving the glutamate receptors.

Promising is the work conducted by Michal Schwartz of the Weizmann Institute, Israel,who has developed a vaccination that contains antigens that boost the immune system to induce autoimmunity and promote ocular blood flow. Dr. Schwartz has demonstrated that a sub-toxic level of glutamate injected into rat eyes induced cells to self-protect against glutamate toxicity. Another of her studies focuses on the drug *Copaxone (Cop-l)*, a drug developed to treat *multiple sclerosis*. Based on research conducted at the Weizmann Institute with rat models, *Cop-1* provides protection of the *ganglion nerves* from injury caused by excessive glutamate. Human trials are now underway. A neuroprotective drug based on a Chinese herb has been developed in that country. It is approved by the SDA in China that is equivalent to the FDA in the United States. The drug *Erigeron Bremscopus Hand-Mazz (EBHM)* needs to be taken for six months to determine whether it has a protective effect. As well, the IOP needs to be controlled before the drug can be administered. Chinese studies indicate a lessening of vision loss, and in some cases better vision. This medication can be ordered directly from a Chinese pharmacy in Changsha, Hunan. China. (See Resource Section)

A drug *erythropoietin (EPO)* developed for anemia is under study at Columbia University. In animal studies an intravitreal injection indicated promise of nerve protection

Pioneering work led by researchers from the National Institutes of Mental Health (USA) on the effects of lithium on brain cells provides intriguing possibilities of this compound's role as a *neuroprotective* agent. The researchers have found that lithium protects brain cells against damage caused by toxic molecules that are naturally formed in the course of metabolism of excessive glutamate in the brain. The over stimulated *N-methyl-D-aspartate (NMDA)* is the pathway to brain cell injury. Lithium, apparently, inhibits *NMDA* receptor activity. Scientists call lithium's effect for protecting nerve cells robust. Lithium also increases production of a major brain protective protein called *bel*-2 in both human and animal brain cells. In animals regeneration of axons has been noted. And it is possible that lithium can enhance nerve cell *DNA* replication. Lithium is an effective chelater of aluminum (removing it from the body). The authors of the paper do not recommend taking lithium without medical supervision since an overdose can be toxic although there are some low-dose lithium supplements on the market, but even these, should only be taken with your physician's approval.

Alphagan and Xalatan, the *beta-blockers* and possibly other glaucoma medications may provide some level of nerve protection through improving the neurotropins (beneficial substances) that flow to the *retinal ganglion* cell bodies, which, in turn, aids these cells to dampen the effects of overactive glutamate.

GENETIC THERAPY--AT THE BASIC LEVEL

A gene is a biological unit of heredity that stakes out a particular location on one of the 23 sets of chromosomes, 22 of which are called autosomes. The 23rd defines the sex--X for females and Y for males. There are approximately 30,000 genes in the human body. They are microscopic structures, self-producing, and under certain circumstances, give rise to a new character—called a mutation. Genes are inherited, mutations and all. Heredity traits are controlled by pairs of genes in the same position on pairs of chromosomes. The gene pairs are called *alleles* and they comprise our *DNA*. A *phenotype*, on the other hand, is what we express, our physical makeup. Each person has a specific *phenotype* that determines how physical characteristics develop. We may carry a gene for glaucoma, for example, but if it is not expressed, we will not develop glaucoma. *Pedigree* denotes your family history. To study the genetic mutation highway, for example, scientists prefer examining four living generations. Those particularly susceptible are identified as *Autosomal Dominant* carriers whose mutations will be transferred in every generation. The next type of inheritance is called *Autosomal Recessive*. It skips a generation. Children born with this defect present a severe medical management problem, but congenital glaucoma is rare. To complicate matters, a separate set of genes is found in the mitochondria, but this avenue is still being explored. *Polygenic Inheritance* refers to more than one gene responsible for a condition. With the exception of *exfoliative* glaucoma, all the other glaucomas are thought to be caused by multiple genes. Three or four mutations may blend together and act upon one another. Although two people may have the same set of mutated genes, expression of the genes may be different resulting in different treatment. Furthermore gene expression in different countries (*Complex Mutlifactorial*) further muddies the waters for the same gene in an individual in France and one in the United States may be expressed differently.

Functional genomics is the study of gene function and the molecular and cellular consequences of disease-causing genetic mutations. Genes are the teachers for every cell in the body. They instruct cells to manufacture specific proteins, the building blocks of the body. Because the cells faithfully follow the gene's instructions, the cells manufacture mutated proteins that screw up a particular organ's function.

When a mutated gene is located, it is subjected to a micro array analysis to provide a better understanding of the consequences of its mutations. Computers then analyze the simultaneous expression of thousands of genes.

The next step traces the effect of a particular gene on the function of a set of cells. Most of the studies still occur at the animal level using *transgenic* mice as subjects for experimentation (human genes transferred to the mice). Scientists study how these genes affect the function of a particular organ. As features in the structure of cells become clearer, scientists are able to trace the damaged gene's impact on cells. For example, should a gene responsible for oxygen inflow to a cell be malfunctioning, deprivation of oxygen suffocates the cell to death.

Genetic research into glaucoma is quickening. With the initial draft of the identification of the genes in the human genome in 2001, scientists have found over ninety genes responsible for inherited eye disorders--nine for the *cornea* and the front of the eye, twenty-one for *glaucoma*, sixty-two for the *retina*, and one for *exfoliative glaucoma*. At least eight genes are related to different forms of glaucoma. Excitement was high in the medical community and in patients when the gene for *Juvenile Open- Angle Glaucoma (JOAG)* was identified. It was labeled *GLCIA*. The *GLC1* stands for open-angle glaucomas, the *A*, for chromosome 1q25, the location of the gene. The gene (*MYOC*) *myocillan* on *chromosome 1* obstructs the aqueous flow through the *trabecular meshwork*. Only ten percent of the families with *JOAG* were found to carry this gene, which also turned up in five percent *adult-onset open-angle* glaucoma patients.

In one study researchers found 16 different *GLC1A* mutations located on chromosome 1 in 4.6% of a group of glaucoma patients. It is not clear how *myocilin* works in the eye, but researchers speculate that because it is found in the *trabecular meshwork* cells, fluid outflow may be involved. *GLC1B* located on chromosome 2 is associated with normal to moderate elevated eye pressure and damage to the *optic nerve*. Two genetic defects on chromosomes *GLC3A* and *GLC3B* have been identified as responsible for congenital glaucoma. Both parents must be carriers of this gene for this anomaly to occur, but as with a number of other gene-related diseases, each parent carrying only one copy may be perfectly fine.

The *GLC1C* gene on chromosome 3 is associated with increased eye pressure plus cup-to-disc abnormal ratios, the *GLC1D* located on chromosome 8 and the *GLC1G* gene on chromosome 10 are associated with mild-to-moderate elevated pressures in people with nerve damage. Also the *GLC1F* gene located on chromosome 7 is associated with elevated pressures or visual field loss and an enlarged cup. Two genes have been associated with some forms of *angle-closure* glaucoma. The first discovered gene *12Q21* and several years later another located on chromosome 11 have been identified.

Another gene affecting *open-angle* glaucoma is called *optineuron* (*OPA1--optic neuropathy-inducing protein*). Active throughout the body, in the eye, this gene affects the *trabecular meshwork, ciliary body*, and *retina*. Abnormal *optineuron* appears to be at least partly responsible for *retinall* cellular death, perhaps by inhibiting the flow of oxygen to the *retinall* cells. It may be involved in *normal-tension* glaucoma. Early onset primary open-angle glaucoma occurs after the age of sixteen and before forty and is caused by two genes, the *CYPIBI*, known to cause congenital glaucoma before three years of age, and the *MYOC* gene in adults.

The *fibulin 5 and 6* genes have been associated with *macular degeneration*. *Fibulin 5* has been identified in persons who have *macular degeneration*. This gene is involved in a protein that manufactures elastin, the fibers that help maintain the integrity of tissues like skin and blood vessels. The fibers are also found in *Bruch's membrane*, the tissue that underlies the *retinall pigment epithelium*–cells vital for support and nutrition. And genes have been located for *Axenfeld-Rieger Syndrome, Aniridia, Nail patella syndrome*.

Three genes, *bcl-2, bax* and *p53*, are involved in the life-death cycle of cells. The *bcl-2* gene promotes cell survival but the *bax* gene promotes the death (*apoptosis*) of the cell. In lively, healthy cells, *bcl-2* binds with *bax* to form a state of equilibrium. In a sick cell, elevated *bax* levels outnumber *bcl-2* initiating *apoptosis*. The tumor suppressor gene *p53* plays a role in this scenario. It has two major functions--to check abnormal cells from dividing and to promote *apoptosis*. It does this by de-activating *bcl-2* and promoting *bax*, thus destroying the equilibrium between *bcl-2* and *bax*. Scientists at the Schepens Eye Research Center, Boston, using neonatal animals, have found that when inhibitory factors in *bcl-2* are removed, the *optic nerve* regenerates. Lithium (see above) is a drug that can stimulate *bcl-2* to regenerate. Studies have indicated that *ganglion* cells in animals with glaucoma had a predominance of *bcl-x*, rather than *bcl-2*; furthermore, analysis revealed that *bcl-x* could possibly override the *apoptosis* syndrome of *P53* and be harnessed for glaucoma therapy. Should any of these therapies prove fruitful for glaucoma maintenance, it will be necessary for the patient to contend with a host of side effects if the gene is of foreign origin.

The possibility of eventual gene therapy to correct protein expression in the eye is enhanced by immune privilege. This means that the tissues in the eye do not react to foreign tissues, such as the immune system ousting the offending intruder. It might, therefore, be possible that use of foreign products may bypass the Cerberean immune system and provide access to genetic therapy. Animal studies are encouraging. By transplanting the *GDNF* gene in the *optic nerve* fibers of rat eyes, some regeneration did occur.

Research suggests that the signal that occurs in glaucoma also increases *free oxygen radicals* that chemically react with almost everything in the cell, eventually leading to the activation of enzymes that degrades *DNA* (nucleases and proteases-- protein components). Triggers to that cascade of events are now under the microscope. Still at the laboratory stage but most promising, is programming cells to repair tissues within the body through guiding stem cells to locations where repair is needed. The hope is that these cells will knuckle down and build new nerve or bone cells. While this research is at the Petri dish exploratory stage, its basic concept of manipulating cells to communicate with each other in a repair mode is promising.

Eventually, gene delivery for glaucoma will involve a number of potential target cells in the *trabecular meshwork, ciliary epithelium* (surface layer of cells), *ciliary muscle, retinal ganglion cells,* the *cornea, Muller cells, extracellular matrix* architecture (tissue that maintains resistance to aqueous flow and keeps eyes inflated) and the *iris.* In the *trabecular meshwork,* so vital for outflow, the possibility of replacing or adding cells necessary for function would eliminate medications now used to suppress the manufacture of vital aqueous fluid. It is now possible to bypass the *trabecular meshwork* entirely by ablating it with a laser (See Chapter 7-Trabectome). This procedure eliminates the need to correct its function. But transplanting genes is a tricky business, for genes apparently are responsible for a variety of functions--some fine-tune the end product, some provide subtle adjustments, others act as nursemaids, and there are those, of course, which are the major players of tissue building. As definitive studies emerge, scientists will be better able to target those tissues in the eye that will respond effectively to genetic manipulation, and as scientists learn more about the body's own mechanisms and the multiple functions of cells, the prospect of gene manipulation moves closer to reality.

One such relatively recent discovery involves *RNA.* It comes in multiple flavors, one of which is called small *RNA.* This strand can turn off a gene's action and it is in the investigative stage for *macular degeneration* therapy. *RNA* transcribes the *DNA* recipe when there is need to manufacture a particular protein—in this particular case, small *RNA.* But *RNA* is responsible for a number of functions, in addition to its transcribing functions, and these are are now being assiduously examined.

Possibly, genes can be delivered that will lower IOP eliminating the need for daily drops. Most important is the protection and possible resurrection of the *retinall ganglion* cells. Injection of *neurotropic* (nutritional) factors discussed earlier in this chapter show promise. There is evidence that the *brain derived neurotropic factor (BDNF)* rescues *retinall ganglion* cells but a method still needs to be developed to eliminate repetitive inoculations.

The use of zinc, involved in the transcription process is another exploratory approach. Proteins known as *zinc-finger transcription factors* found naturally in the human body turn genes on and off. These zinc fingers can attach to any particular *DNA* sequence. Researchers are studying a drug promoting the body to make its own zinc fingers to correct blockages in leg arteries.

Gene therapy may also be recruited to serve in the healing process following eye surgery. Using animal models, genetic therapy prevented scarring in post-operative wound healing following a *trabeculectomy*.

Studies are underway on a number of fronts. At this writing an innovative gene therapy to cure blindness in children is into three Phase I clinical studies. A tiny implantable capsule that may halt or reverse vision loss for people with a variety of *retinal* diseases is in three Phase II/III studies across the United States. A stem cell company, Advanced Cell Technology, is poised to begin a human study of a promising *retinal* treatment derived from human embryonic stem cells.

Optimism that new and revolutionary therapies will one day become available and that perhaps today or tomorrow, doctors will be discarding old treatments and issuing new protocols, is in the air. This does not mean that drugs already on the market will be set aside, but it does suggest that newer remedies with fewer side-effects will be introduced. Along with the expansion of the medical arsenal, technology, providing more precise diagnosis, may redefine the underlying causes of glaucoma. Hope that new procedures developed from genetic and stem cell research will cross the divide from theory into practice remains high.

DISCOVERY INTO PRACTICE

Delivering a gene to the body requires specific tailoring. Scientists adhere to basic principles that include an efficient and nontoxic delivery system, a sound genetic basis for introducing the approach, control of the gene's expression, and access to an animal model for preclinical testing of the gene and its delivery. Genetic transfer proceeds via a vector that delivers the gene to a specific site. There are possibly six different delivery systems that include four viruses stripped of their toxic products—*adenoviruses, adeno-associated viruses, herpes simplex virus,* and *lentiviruses; liposomes* (shells formed when fats are in aqueous solution—may be manufactured and filled with medicine); a man-made virus called *recombinant adeno-associated virus (rAAV)* and naked *DNA.* The use of a virus vector, however, is complicated. Should the immune system react, the patient may experience septic shock and even death. The possibility exists that synthetic gene delivery vectors may be developed that will not activate an immune response. Toxicity has not been a problem, but inflammation, which may be severe, does result and researchers have found it occurring more frequently in primates than in rats. Tinkering with dosage levels may resolve this issue. Perhaps the use of nanoparticles of organic modified silica (*ORMOSH*) capable of carrying *DNA* to cells may solve the problem. Fluorescence imagery tracks the progress of these particular particles. They are comprised of fifteen nanometers (a nanometer is a billionth of a meter) and are capable of penetrating cells. Results from human studies for diseases other than those affecting the *retinal* have proven to be effective. No adverse effects were reported. Researchers are poised to explore the use of this gene delivery system for *retinal* problems.

Another approach involves multilayered, smart nanosystems containing cell targeting, entry facilitation, and localization molecules with molecular biosensors controlling delivery of therapeutic genes into single cells. Other possibilities are being explored for injecting specific genes into the *retinal pigmentary epithelium*. If successful, these healthy genes should form new proteins that would wipe out or absorb damaged cells.

Should a gene correct a deficiency or maladaptation in the research animal, scientists then prepare to test the therapy on human eyes. In 2002, the first breakthrough in sight restoration in an animal occurred. Scientists announced that through genetic transfer a dog born blind from *Leber's Disease* had a 49% sight restoration. This disease also occurs in humans and at this writing, it remains to be seen if gene transfer can have an equal affect in those afflicted.

With the growth of knowledge about genes and the potential for illnesses arising from mutant genes, when faced with a family history of glaucoma, you may want to determine if you are a carrier. Currently available is the Ocugene Test. It tests for *myocilin* mutations. Other tests will no doubt follow as testing for mutations gains purchase in the community.

The picture of how genes influence the development of particular proteins may be changing. *RNA*, once believe to be a rather simple transcriber of the *DNA* code has been found in recent research to to be responsible for many functions. The cell itself also puts in a word or two on how a gene will be expressed and the *DNA* adds its two cents. This new research still needs to establish a theory comparable to the description at the beginning of this section, but it is being built on a solid foundation, and it will, without doubt, be integrated into the existing genetic information. Do not be surprised to hear about new medications, both pharmaceutical and alternative touting positive effects of *RNA* therapy!

STEM CELLS

As important as finding the mutant gene responsible for anomalies in the eye, coaxing the eye to replace neurons that have died is another step on the ladder of eye therapy. Stem cell research travels hand-in-hand with genetic research.

A stem cell as defined by National Institutes of Health is able to divide for an indefinite period of time in culture and give rise to specialized cells. In other words, a stem cell is *pluripotential* (able to differentiate into a wide variety of cell types). Stem cells are found in the embryo, embryonic tissues, umbilical cord blood and some differentiated adult tissues. They can develop into any tissue in the body given an environment conducive to regeneration. But stem cells are complex. They must orchestrate 25,000 genes to develop into a mature cell of the brain, the heart, the eye or any other body part. This intricate dance is carried out by a number of factors intrinsic in the cell that controls which gene should be turned on and which gene suppressed. Scientists need to gain an understanding of how stem cells proliferate, migrate, differentiate, and establish functional cell contacts. As well, when stem cells are derived from donor tissue, problems of immunity need to be resolved.

Stem cells are easy to grow in a laboratory provided they are removed from the inner cell layer of the blastocyst (a ball of 4- to-50 undifferentiated cells formed in the first few days after the sperm fertilizes the egg.) These are the progenitors of your entire body, that when given the proper signals, become your hands, feet, eyes, organs, blood vessels and so on. Best understood are those derived from cells in early fetal development (during the first few days of fertilization). A challenge facing scientists, however, is to unravel the nature of the nerve cell. For example, a single nerve cell in the toe might travel the entire length of the leg. Regenerating nerve cells necessary for sight restoration is complicated, since the wiring of the brain is not fully understood.

Ethical concerns swirl around the use of stem cells. Research and application has been curtailed in some countries but worldwide, stem cell investigations are progressing wherever governments allow. The limited lines of stem cells that scientists are working with further complicates the stem cell picture, for the stem cells used carry their own antigens that may result in rejection by the host. To establish a match between host and an implant, a bank of cells from several million of discarded embryos would need to be established. Another source for stem cells lies with those harvested from cord blood and a company has been established that promises to provide stem cells for drug delivery and research. Meanwhile other avenues continue apace. There is evidence from laboratory studies on mice that stem cells may be obtained without destroying the embryo. This method involves allowing the mouse egg to divide three times, just before it becomes a blastocyst. Scientists then remove a single cell that contains all the information for developing into a cell line. As this technique is expanded to human embryos, controversial noise may quiet down.

Cases of stem cell transplants already exist worldwide to improve or even to save the lives of persons suffering from diseases such as *leukemia, lymphoma* and immune deficiency. These are bone marrow stem cells that when implanted do help but also relegate the patient to life-long immunosuppressant drugs. Laboratory studies have confirmed that bone-marrow stem cells give rise to daughter cells that specialize in muscle, liver, connective tissues, fat, nerve and other cell types. The use of electron microscopy has enabled detection after a day of culturing, the pulsing of newborn heart muscle cells. Adult stem cells, taken from your own body, are not rejected, and some cells have been identified as having potential for promoting therapy in other organs in the body. And restoring eyesight lost to certain diseases is already a reality. The Foundation Fighting Blindness reported that three young adults with *Leber congenital amaurosis (LCA)*, a severe form of *retinitis pigmentosa* benefited with some sight from the delivery of an *RPE65* gene via an *adeno associated virus*.

Under exploration are skin, *iris* and cells from other organs. Stem cells derived from the central nervous system and ocular tissues using the body's own tissues may one day be used to repair eye diseases, thus bypassing both the ethical use of fetal stem cells and the autoimmune problem associated with implanting foreign tissue. Adult stem cells reside in many tissues found in the body. Skin cells, for example, cannot replace themselves by dividing but rely on skin stem cells to replace those skin cells sloughed off in the constant process of cell renewal. Scientists have succeeded in transforming skin cells to embryonic cells by adding four genes, and while there are still some drawbacks in this breakthrough discovery, the scientists involved are confident that they can overcome them. In the case of glaucoma, we now understand that glaucoma is both a polygenic (a number of genes causing the disease) and mutlifactorial (external environmental factors) disease. This daunting analysis suggests that even if the proper gene combination is identified and injected into the eye, cure might still be elusive. But, should an adult stem cell be stimulated to proliferate through chemical and genetic strategies, cure may then be possible. In August, 2005, scientists from the Universities of Milan and Edinburgh reported that they had created pure stem cells from human embryonic tissue. Needless to say, this dispatch raises high hope that degenerative diseases can be addressed as never before.

The possibility that stem cells are present in the eyes has been confirmed by a number of studies. About one hundred stem cells exist in a rat cell *retinal* while the human eye clocks in at 10,000. These cells can be isolated from eye bank eyes. Capable of producing all the different cell types, they require no growth factor and can be easily generated in the laboratory. *Corneal* stem cells have also been identified. These are limbal cells that can be transplanted onto *corneas* and which require no autoimmune suppression. Regenerating the eye's own tissues from the *cornea* may one day replace *corneal* implants. *Trabecular meshwork* cells are also under study as are cells from *conjunctival* tissue. Most important for glaucoma patients, however, is regeneration of *retinal* ganglion cells. These cells may one day be derived from the *pigmented ciliary epithelium* (lining cells). As described above, an outside source of stem cells found in eye bank cells may be used for both experimental purposes and repair of various eye structures once the problem of rejection is mastered.

Repopulating the *optic nerve* with stem cell-derived normal *astrocytes* and fibroblasts cells might be an alternative therapy for glaucoma. Investigation with animal models reported some success in young pups, but not in mature animals. Discovery of how these lower animals maintain *neurogenesis* (regenerating new neurons to replace injured or lost cells) will reveal important data for stimulating human tissues to follow suit. Research with animal models has also revealed that *retinal stem cells*, while not differentiating from brain cells, do have the unique ability to produce all the *retinal* cell types. They grow easily and rapidly in the laboratory. *Retinal stem cells* have been found in the *pigmented ciliary* margin of the adult mouse *retina*, and in the border of the *cornea*, promising that use of these cells may one day heal *corneal* diseases. Other predictions include the possibility that *trabecular meshwork* stem cells will be found and that they will have the ability to restore *trabecular meshwork* function. In animal models, especially with young animals, transference of *retinal stem cells* did develop into the various *retinal* cell types. Animal models provide information of the location of stem cells in the eye.

Excitement is high at Schepens Eye Research Institute in Boston, and Children's Hospital in Orange County, California, for they have been able to witness the process of transplanted stem cells developing into mature neurons. The researchers extracted *retinal* progenitor or stem cells from day-old transgenic mice, (a mouse that has human genes) whose cells had been altered to glow green under an excitation light. Some of the cells became neurons and photoreceptors when transplanted into mature mice.

Normally during early development, stems cells growing within the milieu of cells destined to become the eye detect and respond to chemical and physical cues from surrounding tissue that tell cells where to go and when to increase their numbers, and help determine the necessary specialization. Scientists are working on a kind of scaffold to act in part as the natural cues present during early development. The aim of the scaffolds is to provide the orientation necessary for the photoreceptor cells to develop and integrate the special connections with other cells and the central nervous system.

Knowledge that the brain is capable of growing new cells has appeared in the literature. Birds, rats and monkeys do it. Why not humans? The new cells in mammals appear in a region of the brain known as the hippocampus and they replace dead cells. In mice genetically predisposed to eye disease, a team of researchers targeted the blood vessels in the *retina* for a rescue mission. Selecting adult stem cells capable of becoming *endothelial* cells that line the blood vessels, the researchers injected the stem cells into a mouse eye. *Astrocytes*, the body's support cells, guided the stem cells to blood vessels in the back of the eye. The stem cells appeared to protect both the blood vessels and *retinal* neurons from death. Researchers have yet to harness the human body's capability of brain regeneration and nervous system.

Bone marrow cells have been explored for their ability to deliver cells to the eye and this cell-to-cell interaction may possibly treat *diabetic retinopathy, macular degeneration* and other inherited *retinal degenerative* diseases. Researchers from the US National Institute of Neurological Diseases and Stroke have found evidence that stem cells from bone marrow can develop into brain cells. Four female patients received bone marrow transplants, and researchers found clumps of brain cells that contained the male Y chromosome in each woman's brain. Some progress has been made on umbilical cord blood stem cells. A single cord produces about a thimbleful of blood but contains 100,000-to-300,000 stem cells. The Steenblock Research Institute, a nonprofit organization, is following cases that have been treated with this therapy.

Scientists have also discovered in the light of lens injury, the subsequent inflammatory response summoned macrophages, and these molecules in turn produced a *growth factor*. Growth factors are a good thing in many cases and researchers are studying how to induce various growth factors into useful therapy.

Introducing stem cells into the eye should theoretically repair damage or replace lost cells in the eye. A precise mixture of proteins is necessary for maintenance of the embryonic stem cells' ability to develop into different cell types. Scientists are working on methods for distinguishing these proteins. A possible therapy already exists called therapeutic cloning, a technique where the nucleus of a skin cell, is inserted into an egg from which its own nucleus has been removed, enabling the creation of an embryo that has almost the same genes as the skin cell donor and will act as an embryo and begin the process of dividing itself into multiple cells. Scientists at Harvard and the University of California, San Francisco announced in 2006 that they will attempt to make a human embryo that will be pluripotential and capable of correcting certain forms of disease. Cells necessary for nerve replication would then be isolated for therapeutic use in the eye. In other words, scientists would use your own cells from another part of the body to make embryonic cells to replace those missing cells in the eye. This system would bypass the use of a virus vector to insert genes and reduce the risk of future problems. Yes, in this century we will no doubt witness, through genetic manipulation, the body's own ability for healing.

Will stem cell therapy work for me is of utmost concern for the glaucoma patient.   Hopefully, yes. Scientists have identified a number of different sources and types of stem cells and precursor cells that can target three areas for cell restoration —the *retinal ganglion cells, optic nerve head* and *trabecular meshwork*. The issues to be resolved include survival and differentiation of the stem cell, establishing functional connections, maintaining the site of the surrounding microenvironment, and activating synaptic connections. If this therapy comes to pass, use of these cells would require immune medication. *Retinal ganglion cells* have already made the connection from the *retina* to the optic nerve in an animal model, but scientists do not yet know whether this connection has produced vision.

Safety problems associated with the stem cell therapy need to be resolved, however. Technically, the requirement for cell delivery into the eye or any other organ in the body is complicated, for scientists need to ascertain that a stem cell will do what it's chartered to do—perform the desired functions while remaining at the targeted site, overcome a hostile environment present in the adult eye, will not reproduce the same symptoms as the original disease, will remyelinize (myelin is a fat like sheath found around the axons), and not reject the transplanted cells. It's a tall order. Unquestionably, the eye, as with the entire body, is built from a genetic code found in the *DNA* that is both universal and specific to the individual. The work of building a body relies on the messenger *RNA* that controls protein synthesis in all living cells. But this process does not proceed in an environment free from harmful effects that may and do cause mutations.

IMPLANTS

Prostheses to restore sight have long been a dream of researchers. Theoretically, a chip could be developed to efficiently reclaim vision. Scientists have already developed chips that either sit atop the *retina* or are positioned under the *retina*. To be effective, the chip must possess an incredible amount of information. Think of it. Our visual system receives greater bandwidth by many orders of magnitude than any other sensory system. There is no computer system today capable of performing what our visual system does with such ease. Nevertheless, researchers now have tools drawn from a plethora of miniature electronic parts that up the ante for the possibility that an implanted prosthesis in the eye can stimulate the *retinal* cells or act as an artificial *retina*. Mainly, research has been directed to those diseases where the *ganglion* cells are unaffected. But some of the experimental results look promising. Size of the implant is crucial. A larger implant offers the opportunity for increased energy supply, especially in cases where available ambient light is insufficient to produce the required energy for *retinall* stimulation. Implanting a larger chip, however, does require more surgery.

A chip containing 5,000 microscopic solar cells has been used in a trial involving a small number of *retinitis pigmentosa* patients. This chip was inserted in the *subretinal* space. Light striking the chip is converted into minute electric currents that stimulate the functioning *retina* cells. Powered by ambient light, this chip is ideal for implantation. Within two -to-four weeks following insertion, vision improvement was noted in these patients. The patients in this study had lost most of their vision, and while the chip improved the vision somewhat, it by no means restored full vision. Nevertheless, those patients involved were grateful for even a tiny uptick in their vision.

Researchers at Stanford University in California have developed a chemical chip that releases small amounts of neurotransmitters that actually mimic natural synapse stimulation. Electro-osmosis drives the implanted chip in the eye. By using electro-osmosis to move the fluid, no moving parts and little power is required. When the technical problems are resolved—such as biocompatible materials and a chip large enough for information processing but small enough to fit under the *retinal*, this innovation may see the light of day.

To harness the power of nanotechnology, scientists are exploring therapeutic molecules to transfer antioxidant and antiangiogenesis (anti blood vessel growth) into cells in the eye. The use of tiny structures (micro fabrication) for drug delivery of a medication normally taken by mouth to travel directly to a site in the eye has been developed. Soft disposable contact lenses are ideal, for the lens can both incorporate medical control of glaucoma and correct refraction problems. Under study is the growing of *retinal* cell dendrites and axons directly onto a microchip and then stimulating them with packets of neurotransmitters mimicking the natural vision processes. Other research investigations, most of which are barely off the drawing board, stagger the imagination. Cages, a process that involves using molecules to act as cages for other molecules, offers the possibility of a *neurotransmitter*-based visual prosthesis. Light triggers these caged *neurotransmitters*, and the ultraviolet rays of light striking the molecule cleave away the cage, thus freeing the stimulating transmitters to go to work. Obviously, this possible therapy has a long way to go before it can be applied.

Both Harvard University and the University of California, San Francisco announced plans for developing stem cells from adult cells. These are privately funded programs and so are free to use donor eggs in whatever fashion they choose. One thrust of the research is to clone the cells. This process involves transferring the nucleus of an adult cell into an unfertilized egg where the nucleus has been removed.

WHAT DOES THE FUTURE HOLD?

Progression of glaucoma varies as does the age of the individual who retains or loses functional vision. Because a large portion of the *retinal ganglion* cells is lost before functional vision disappears, scientists hope that restoration of the *retinal ganglion* cells and possibly the *optic nerve head* and the *trabecular meshwork* might be possible by repairing only a small portion of these bodies or simply establishing new connections. Some headway in restoring the *optic nerve* in animsls has been made at the Schepens Eye Research Institute, Boston, but this research is still in its infancy. The scientific community is drawing closer to establishing paradigms that will work for repairing many body parts through the use of the above modalities. With the increase of longevity, we eagerly look forward to the promise of cure.

PART II

CHAPTER 10

Therapies That Complement Medical Treatment

○ ○

Each man must look to himself to teach him the meaning of life. It is not something discovered: it is something moulded.

> Saint Exupery, Wind,
> Sand, and Stars (1939)
> 2.1.tr. Lewis Galantiere.

The divide between complementary therapies and traditional medicine may one day narrow to the trickle of the Rio Grande in times of drought. Certainly, the Office of Alternative Medicine (OAM) of the National Institutes of Health (NIH) with a yearly budget of over a million dollars is a positive development. It sponsors grants up to $30,000 each to fund exploratory pilot practices, specialty studies on complementary and alternative medical treatments with average funding of approximately $850,000 over three years for each project. Vigorous methods are now in place to study what is effective, useless and even may be dangerous. With this added emphasis on transparency, it is hoped despite the high costs of trials for various therapies, the public will be better informed as to those therapies that have undergone rigorous study.

A number of hospitals offer alternative or complementary therapies as well as diet and lifestyle recommendations. This trend is affecting the way doctors are trained. Two-thirds of the nation's medical schools provide courses on alternative medicines and research into alternative therapies. As well, doctor's training may include alternative health treatment and integrative medicine. In such centers, a primary care physician evaluates a patient's health and lifestyle with recommendations for designing and implementing a wellness plan. Many clinics now offer massage therapy, acupuncture, nutrition, meditation, and the like. The Bravewell Collaborative is an organization that knits together the integrative medicine centers throughout the country. See resources for centers in the network.

The spread of multicultural practices is also penetrating the medical systems in the United States. In Albuquerque, New Mexico, *curanderos* from Mexico have conducted a two-week course called "Traditional Medicine Without Borders" that takes place on the campus of the University of New Mexico. The visiting *curanderos* are master teachers and working with faculty members, train medical practitioners to create an integrative approach.

The interplay of the brain and mind on the physical body underlies the heart of complementary therapies. These ephemeral connections have fascinated psychologists, philosophers, and thinkers over the ages and have given rise to both a materialistic and a consciousness or willful view. The materialistic aspect took particular form when Descartes, the influential 17th century philosopher, separated mind from matter. Within his time, other philosophers questioned this division, generating two schools of thought that exist to this day. Matter, the material, is real, something you can touch, probe, reshape like the brain itself. The mind which is immaterial—who can hold a mind in the palm of a hand?—is illusory, but philosophical thinkers on this side of the divide have given much thought to it. A prime example concerns Buddhism, derived from the practices of Siddhartha Buddha who was born in 483 BC, and whose teachings up to this day, bind together a world-wide community seeking oneness of mind and body.

Biophotonics imaging systems such as the *MRI (magnetic resonance imagery) CAT* scans (*computerized axial tomography*), and other sophisticated systems bury the notion that activities generated by the mind are not observable. Inconceivable in the middle of the twentieth century, the plasticity of the brain influenced by thinking and action is readily now apparent with the advances of technology. The surprise finding that human beings possess some 30,000 or so genes, not a great deal more than the common insect, led to the conclusion both that the genes are multi-potential and that the one-hundred trillion synapse system in the brain account for our higher order of thinking. Neurons stimulated by sensory input of thought, feelings and action make us what we are.

We now understand that everything we do, feel, think, believe, etc. is a product of the brain's circuitry. A finger movement, a toe pain, digestive processes are all governed by the nervous system. Neurons (cells) in the brain busily remap and encode new information. In the human body there are fifty trillion cells. Each cell wall contains receptors, chemicals particular to a cell enabling it to capture the material necessary for stability and function. These receptors are not static, for in response to instruction from the cell, they change shape when necessary (part of the remodeling process). Each cell, a world unto itself, contains a swirling mixture of water and other chemicals along with the mitochondria (the base of energy production), and the nucleus containing the spiral twists of *DNA*.

All cells emerge from stem cells but to build a body part, must differentiate. As a result each cell possesses its own specific function, such as the cells on the beams of the *trabecular meshwork* that are designed to allow aqueous fluid to flow out of the eye, or cells in the *retina* that transmit signals to the brain. Every organ in the eye along with every organ in the body is a confluence of cells. Those in the ciliary *body* are responsible for producing aqueous fluid to nourish the eye. With the exception of the neuronal cells, all the other cells periodically replace themselves.

Balance, an important consideration for both glaucoma patients and the aging population, relies upon the interplay of vision, hearing and the governing body of the brain. Tiny inner ear hair follicles working closely with the eyes achieve balance. The inner ears, however, do not always work harmoniously with the eyes. For example, spinning with closed eyes for five or more times causes wooziness for a few seconds until the fluid in the inner ear stops sloshing about, signaling the brain that the movement stopped. Repeating the movement with open eyes stimulates nausea for the visual cues are subverted and the brain can't register the movement. Often, balance problems may be helped with physical therapy that uses vestibular rebalancing exercises.

Another often overlooked ingredient in this healing mix includes the inner strength of self-empowerment. Dating back to the Greeks and Romans, physicians have been viewed as teachers prepared to educate, empower and motivate patients to take responsibility for their own health. Even today, such a relationship can benefit. Positive thinking, long touted as important for healthy living and confirmed by brain scans, has a direct influence on the immune system. Claims that even the very sick can heal have been documented.

Plasticity of the brain is responsible for retaining information. Neurons present in the brain from birth while weaving themselves into circuits possibly remaining for a lifetime, are, nevertheless subject to remodeling, for parking space in the brain is limited. The brain, needing space, replaces unused or dormant material with newer, more relevant stuff. Neuroplasticity, a twenty-first century concept, is more active in the young growing brain, but doesn't end there. Experience with stroke victims demonstrates that plasticity in the brain even in the event of neuronal loss is still present. According to Dr. Jerome Groopman of Harvard, whose latest book *The Anatomy of Hope* (Viking), "true hope is clear-eyed. It sees all the difficulties that exist and all the potential for failure, but through that carves a realistic path to the future." Hope, according to Dr. Groopman, can change brain chemistry through reduction of pain, for hope, as experimentally demonstrated, releases *enkephalins* and *endorphins* (mood enhancing hormones), thus improving muscular, cardiac, and respiratory functions. Another important thinker, Dr. Bernie Siegel, in his book, *101 Exercises for the Soul: A Divine Working Plan for Body, Mind, and Spirit (New* World Library), "posits that our internal environment selects the blueprint that affects our physical health and bodies." Dr. Siegel has witnessed spontaneous reversal of disease in cases of cancer and other debilitating conditions.

Which brings us to the various forms of complementary therapies described in this section of the book, some of which may help to retain vision. Remember, however, action produces the best result. Notwithstanding the role you play in medical treatment whether passive or active, a good percentage of the cure can be attributed to medical treatment. Clearly, conventional treatment of glaucoma has transformed a blinding disease into one of preventable blindness. Fortunately, however, to maximize your eye's capability, the medical profession's acceptance or at least tolerance of complementary therapies (herbs, acupuncture, relaxation, etc.) has gained purchase notwithstanding the dearth of double-blind studies. While this situation is improving, the high costs of testing all products and therapies that find their way into the market limit access to reliable information.

Self-healing partners with the immune system. Research into eye disorders such as *uveitis, macular degeneration* and possibly glaucoma, indicates they may be caused, in part, to malfunctioning of the immune system. Thousands of different chemicals exist in the immune system that is geared to rid the body of toxic materials, heal injury through the action of white blood cells, provide antibiotics, and engender countless other protective activities. Phagocyte cells produced by the thymus gland ingest and digest parasitic invaders and the T. lymphocytes destroy foreign or infected cells. The B. lymphocytes produce antibodies. T. lymphocytes stimulate macrophages. B. lymphocytes produce cytokines (substances that reduce inflammation) and antibodies that mark parasites for destruction. These two types of cells work together.

In a world where pollution and the emission of toxic chemicals are minimal, the immune system might be capable of maintaining health, but today, the immune system is seriously challenged by toxic effluents in the air, water, soil, and food. Strengthening the immune system is a claim made often in complementary therapies, and indeed, people who exercise, eat the right foods, meditate, etc. do seem to fare better than those who neglect self-care practices. Harry took matters into his own hands when diagnosed with cancer. He spent a year juicing tons of vegetables, exercising religiously, detoxifying—in other words, the whole nine yards. At the end of a year, he was cancer free.

Genetics, environment, unsafe and empty caloric foods, life style, attitude, and stress, in part, weaken the immune system. Strengthening this complex system at this time relies mainly on diet, exercise and stress reduction. In the future, the medical community may develop vaccinations to do this job.

Scientists have documented physical changes in the body resulting from stressful conditions. *Diabetes* is one example. This disease can lead to *diabetic retinopathy* (See Chapter 2) and possibly blindness. Stress increases the hormone cortisol secreted from the adrenal gland, necessary for conducting everyday activities. An excess of cortisol, however, depletes the adrenal gland and increases insulin insensitivity and resistance. Stress also increases small vessel contractions that may lead to *intraocular pressure* and systemic blood pressure. Negative emotions such as anxiety, anger, fear, and helplessness all activate overproduction of cortisol. While the regulatory action of cortisol is necessary for its role in metabolizing fats, carbohydrates, sodium potassium and protein, an excess can weaken the immune system and damage the hippocampus, the area of the brain responsible for memory and learning. As with glaucoma and high blood pressure, stress, in its first phase, emits few physical signals. But when a physical breakdown occurs, possibly a stressful condition may trigger the event. I spoke to a friend the other day about his angioplasty and he told me in no uncertain terms that his heart problem had developed from stress associated with the failure of his business. I recognized stress in my life when struggling to balance a demanding job with family needs. I developed *retinal tears*.

In its second phase stress depletes magnesium, potassium, zinc and B6 while at the same time creating an imbalance by retaining water, sodium and calcium. In the third phase, the imbalances may provoke a number of physical problems including those found in the eyes. Water retention and adrenaline increase ocular pressure. A low magnesium level causes tiny vessel spasms that also increase ocular pressure. Poor digestion of vital nutrients deprives organs of the body (including the eye) and produces premature aging. Stressful factors also promote vital mineral disruption and greater release of glucose (sugar), leading to *diabetes*, hypertension, and possibly further damaging the small blood vessels in the eye.

Many of us are unaware or not tuned in to what causes our stress athough we do know that stress causes harm. We may, in fact, choose to soldier on, rather than modify our fast-paced lives. Indeed, a bit of stress may be beneficial, for stress is cited with spurring on unusual achievements. This ancient stone-age survival tactic known as a "flight or fight" life-saving mechanism, however, is detrimental to health today. Stress may develop during infancy, school interactions, or be job-or-family-related. Considering my own childhood, I suspect my adaptation to stress began by channeling resentment of being the youngest in the family, where I was called a pest because of my insatiable curiosity that impinged on my siblings' activities. To overcome this, I developed what is commonly called an A personality. Even in retirement this trait still spurs me on.

How do we generate these negative emotions that cause stress? Any one of you can name a dozen things that drive you up against a wall. Everyday situations may be the stimulus. Some of us shrug off unpleasant events and get on with our lives while others experience emotional trauma. Albert Elkin, Ph.D., director of the Stress Managing Counseling Center in New York City, suggests that a person should try to gain perspective. Most situations are not life-threatening or disastrous but thinking they are causes an overwhelming reaction.

Stress may also result from admiral coping skills such as multitasking. Some high-energy people do, indeed, benefit from multitasking, being blessed with an ability to process a number of things seemingly simultaneously, but others are overwhelmed. Some experts, however, equate multitasking with stress, illness and inefficiency. David Meyer, a psychologist at the University of Michigan suggests that multitasking strains the brain. Meyer compares the brain to a computer with a central operating system governing tasking. The system needs to rev up between tasks for the most efficient output. Even unrelated tasks such as listening to the radio while cooking (I do it all the time) can stress the brain. You may neglect chopping up garlic when you hear a captivating program coming over the airwaves, or when your husband or a child needs attention. According to Meyer, multitasking can damage memory and curtail the ability to absorb new information and retain recently acquired memory. But perhaps most important, multitasking can weaken the immune system, for it creates stress hormones that divert energy from the brain.

Stress from extraordinary demands or severe trauma can age an individual by as much as ten years. A team of researchers studying severe emotional stress resulting from divorce, loss of job, caring for a chronically-ill individual found that blood cells in a group of these individuals were genetically about a decade older than a control group of their peers. This more current understanding goes deeper than simply linking chronic stress to a weakened immune system and an increased risk of catching cold. "It is a new and significant finding," said Bruce McEwen, director of the Neuroindicrinological Laboratory at Rockefeller University, New York. Findings from this research established clear evidence that stress affects wear and tear on human tissues. This group is studying whether cognitive therapies such as those described below will retrain the aging process that has taken hits from stressful conditions. Furthermore, that the nervous system in your gut reacts to stress clearly identifies the role of neurotransmitters such as serotonin in that organ.

Keeping your mind active may be a successful antidote to stress. It may also help to prevent debilitating diseases such as *Alzheimer's*. A study examining the association of the quality of written material in a nun's diaries that when matched with findings of her autopsied brain reported a correlation between the richness and complexity of her diary entries with her mental health. Keep that brain active.

The art of healing is varied. At Columbia College of Physicians and Surgeons, New York City, Rita Charon, MD, founder and director of the Program in Narrative Medicine uses literature to sensitize hospital staff, including doctors and medical students, to deepen their understanding of how a patient's fears, expectations and disappointments impact on health and recovery. Literature helps medical personnel to bridge the gap between the intake information and the patient's emotional responses, an important factor in the healing process.

There are many anecdotal stories of healing but one of the most dramatic involves Meir Schneider who heads an organization for self-healing in San Francisco based on methods he developed for restoring his own sight. Born with glaucoma, astigmatism, nystagmus, and cataracts--in other words, blind, he now sees at a respectable 20/70. He attributes this miracle of vision to combining medical treatment with massage therapy, eye exercises, palming, nutrition, spirituality and physical activity, all of which is now practiced at his center.

WILL ALTERNATIVE OR COMPLEMENTARY THERAPIES WORK FOR ME?

It is human nature to want guarantees. Whenever we purchase a piece of equipment we receive a warranty that at the least provides support and repair for a period of time should there be a problem. So why not require a warranty from practitioners to whom we turn for healing? Alas, the complexity of the human body and its idiosyncratic responses to intervention whether pharmacologic, surgical, herbal, or physiological subverts such a response, although lawsuits abound against practitioners in the healing arts, especially in cases of surgery and obstetrics, despite modern medical technology. For myself, I have sought out complementary therapies in the hope of preserving my vision. And while it is difficult to judge whether any of the therapies listed below actually worked to better my chances for maintaining my vision, I did find that my life style changed for the better. Both my physical and mental health improved. I still have stamina despite advancing years and family problems. But, best of all, I'm still among the sighted.

Uniting medical and complementary therapies for treatment of glaucoma is a work in progress, for unlike cases of stroke where rehabilitation includes relearning what has been lost, the use of complementary therapies for achieving improved *optic nerve* health is difficult to assess. Anecdotally, persons practicing certain forms of complementary therapies, myself included, speak of benefits. Embarking on a course of such therapies, however, is self-generated, but when these therapies include the use of herbs, it is probably wise to consult a nutritionist or herbalist. Certain herbs pose a danger of toxicity, especially those grown in foreign countries. Lead and other dangerous minerals have been detected. Furthermore, herbs are in no way benign. They are the raw forms of medicines and as such, may have a powerful effect on the body.

Whatever complementary therapy you choose to practice, please share this information with your eye doctor. We have found that doctors are generally open to their patients' participation in the healing process, especially if they appear to profit both psychologically and physically, and of course, with no interference of the doctor's protocols. This is good news for patients who believe that alternative or complementary medicine will help them. It is especially welcome to those who have tried conventional medicine with no relief but find that an array of complementary therapies may and do, in some cases, help. Many people believe in complementary therapies, for in the United States alone, Americans shell out some $10 billion a year on alternative therapies, mostly in the form of supplements.

There is a muchness about the whole field of healing. Both pharmaceutical and supplement companies continue to offer new products, many of which are "me too" items. Bookstores now devote entire sections to self-healing books ranging from a single substance to a collection of vitamin products— to body work such as yoga, Chi gong, karate, Tai Chi and various types of massage therapies, acupressure, acupuncture, etc.—to diet, exercise and the like. Some of these therapies have entered into the conventional doctor's recommendation who find no problem with diet, exercise, some of the martial arts and other healing modalities such as meditation, relaxation, biofeedback, visualization and so on. But many conventional doctors cast a wary eye on claims made by the manufacturers of vitamins and other products promising cure for a number of ailments.

The time may be ripening, especially with the ongoing research in the neuroplasticity of the brain, for the two camps to join in an enlightened search for a combination of therapies that will do the most good. Some well-designed studies may persuade some physicians to recommend supplements. Witness the study of a formula based on zinc and other products that slow down the effects of *macular degeneration* (the AREDS formula). A study is now underway to include lutein, zeaxanthin and fish oil in the formula.

What binds together the wide range of therapies designated as complementary is your part in the process. You choose what works for you. Below are some suggestions that may help to formulate a plan of action. We have selected only those of the many self-healing therapies that we have found best foster the mind-body connection. These include meditation, exercise, diet and nutrition, yoga, chiropractic, biofeedback, self massage, self hypnosis, and psychotherapy. Other modalities may also be worth considering should they be more appropriate to your lifestyle. These include *Ayurveda,* faith healing, homeopathy, naturopathy, macrobiotics, psychic surgery, and so on. Therapies and claims for healing methods crop up regularly and the sheer number of choices can be daunting. For guidance, choose a practitioner you trust or consult a publication by a respected author. Whatever your choice, be wary. Like entering a cold ocean, dangle your toe first, then immerse your foot, leg and then take the plunge. Diving head first into a new therapy can be a disastrous experience.

Don't be afraid to design your own routine. You'll probably notice that certain therapies require a time commitment. Don't drive yourself crazy rigidly adhering to the rules or suggestions. Recently I heard of a couple who devoted two hours in the morning and two hours in the evening to meditation. This practice left so little time to accomplish their daily living tasks that they were always frantic. Do what you can. If you decide to explore alternative therapies, bear in mind that none has a track record for curing glaucoma, but, then again, at this writing, neither does the medical community.

THE CONTROLLING MIND

When I was about eight-years-old, I would tell my friends that I could choose my dreams. I would decide whom I would dream about and sure enough I'd come up with an appropriate dream. Children apparently have a capacity often lost in adulthood to control physical experiences such as being told a wart will vanish, and it does. Spiritual belief might be considered a sophisticated development of mind-control. Lisa Reid who regained eighty percent of her vision in one eye after having been informed that her *optic nerve* was irrevocably damaged, a result of a brain tumor when she was eleven, believes that a miracle occurred. There are many studies documenting how a person's spiritual belief, a connectedness to something greater than everyday events, leads to better heath. There are over one-hundred documented studies attesting to prayer regardless of religious affiliation as effective medicine. One study found that people who attend religious services regularly appear to be healthier and live longer lives. The placebo effect is another well-known phenomenon in medical circles. A person may experience a cure or alleviation of pain when participating in a study of a particular medicine or treatment even if unbeknownst to him or her, the so-called remedy has been a simple sugar pill or a sham operation. Furthermore, a receptive individual told that a drug, an alternative therapy, or a particular exercise will be beneficial, experiences relief from a particular symptom. Many health practitioners believe that a person's mental, emotional, physical and spiritual proclivities interact and influence each other. Technology's ability to view brain activity during interactions confirms many of these theories.

Sally, who studied yoga for ten years and who has now become a teacher of the art, and whose *uveitic* glaucoma has claimed the sight of one eye, still has considerable vision in her other eye. Babs, whose father went blind from glaucoma, practices karate, a practice she finds both fulfilling and sustaining.

STRESS RESOLUTION

Patients are not alone in turning to mind-body methods for lowering stress reactions. Michael Lumpkin, PhD, Professor and Chair of the Department of Physiology and Biophysics, Georgetown University School of Medicine, teaches medical students to use mind-body methods to limit their own stress, and in the process help their patients. Chronic stress elevates blood pressure.

Here are some simple steps to de-stress.

1. Toss away the notion that you must be perfect. Do the best you can and if you err, you will not lose face or love.
2. Discuss your troubles with a friend, a spiritual advisor or your significant other.
3. Say no to a request when it will overburden you.
4. If solutions for de-stressing are not readily apparent seek professional help.
5. Look ahead. Thunderstorms today--sunshine tomorrow.
6. Laugh and the world will laugh with you. Cry and you cry alone.
7. Plant a garden even if it's only on your windowsill.
8. Connect with a pet. Studies confirm that pets relieve anxiety and stress.
9. Drink a cup of chamomile tea.

10. Cultivate an easily attained idealized self-guide such as "I will not let my medications get in the way of my life style." As you achieve this goal then tackle another. Progress step by step consistent to your needs.

MEDITATE CONTROL THE CONTROLLING MIND:

Meditation has been around for a long, long time. It is an integral part of Eastern philosophy and its practice is considered essential to reaching Nirvana, the highest level of achievement in Buddhist philosophy. Once considered an exotic import, meditation, perhaps of all the alternative therapies, is regarded respectfully as a healing modality by the medical community. A small study conducted by a Harvard research team did *magnetic resonance imagery (MRI)* on patients who had meditated for at least five years. The pictures of their brains showed that the regions processing cardio-respiratory function were most active. Other studies have documented meditation's profound healing effects on chronic diseases such as migraine, multiple sclerosis, psoriasis, high blood pressure and a faster recovery from chronic diseases and surgery. At Princeton University, a neuroscientist is studying the effects of medication on attention; at the University of California, Medical School, San Francisco, a researcher is studying how meditation assists school teachers to develop empathy. And Dr. Richard Davidson, a neuroscientist at the University of Wisconsin, has published results from brain-imaging systems. A study of Lamas indicated an increase in the part of the brain that registers happiness.

Meditation opens the way to experience peace and tranquility and tap into the body's own wisdom strengthening the ability to focus, that, in turn, frees the mind to drive forward and into other realms of inquiry. This is not as easy as it sounds, for the mind is always scurrying about--fussing, questioning, examining, reviewing, recapping, judging, seething, seeking revenge—you name it, your mind is doing it. In a meditative state, the unstoppable mind is channeled into an attention mode. The thinking syndrome is shed; the mind is emptied of the, "I don't like, I don't accept, I hate, I want, I don't want, etc." Contemplating and agonizing over our physical conditions does harm. Negative thinking becomes cyclic—worry generates more worry producing escalating tension. We're caught up in a washing machine cycle with our minds agitating our bodies and our bodies agitating our minds. Meditation pushes the stop button. Peace.

Recently, I had an interesting meditation experience. My life situation had taken a turn for the worse and I felt terribly burdened. During one of my meditation exercises I felt a weight slide off my shoulders. It was so physical that it was if a hand had lifted it off. Then I realized the power of the mind.

Can meditation affect eye pressure? I am unaware of double-blind studies on meditation and eye pressure. Yet many members of our group practice some form of meditation and report an increased ability to handle problems associated with glaucoma. Concrete evidence does exist, however, of meditation's effect on stress reduction. Apparently each of us has a set point indexing right and left brain moods. Right brain processes anxiety, depression, anger, distress (signs of stress—agita, if you will) left brain— upbeat, enthusiastic, energetic. Researchers working with the Dalai Lama, the exiled Tibetan religious and political leader, documented that training in mindful medication can move the set point further to the left. People trained in mindful meditation also experience more robust immune systems. Mindfulness training focuses on learning to monitor continuing sensations and thoughts. The practice can be accomplished through sitting meditation and yoga.

Meditation has as many flavors as Ben & Jerry's ice cream, but they all achieve the same results. You can choose from such forms as Transcendental Meditation, walking meditation, chanting and a host of others. A form that I like, mainly because it requires so little time—ten minutes twice a day is *MINDFUL MEDITATION*. Here are steps you can follow on your own.

MINDFUL MEDITATION

Remove your shoes. <u>Put</u> your hands on knees. Sit upright to achieve a balance between your feet solidly on the floor and your back firmly against the chair. Release tension in all parts of your body. Gently close your eyes to avoid distraction. Should you get sleepy open and close your eyes several times.

- <u>Relax</u> your jaw keeping your teeth slightly apart. Be aware of your sitting position.
- <u>Listen</u> to the sounds about you. Notice how they ebb and flow totally independent of you.
- <u>Breathe</u> evenly using your stomach muscles. Follow your breath as you inhale through your nose, as the breath travels up from the abdomen, into the chest and then as you exhale from the chest down to the abdomen.
- <u>Observe</u> your breath entering and leaving your body and how natural and unhurried it is.
- <u>Check</u> the passage of breath by placing your finger against your nostril or placing your hand on your stomach and feeling the expansion and contraction with each breath. Be aware of this sensation of breathing.

- <u>Focus</u> on one object such as your perfect always-present breath.
- <u>Take note</u> when you become distracted (thinking), and without chastening yourself, return to the beginning.
- <u>Corral</u> your mind back to your perfect always-present breath.
- <u>Retain</u> throughout a conscious awareness of the sensation of the breath.
- <u>Meditate</u> in the morning, and if possible for a period of ten minutes or so one or two hours before bedtime.

Mindful Meditation trains the mind to notice when it wanders. Remember that you're fighting a lifetime habit of a scurrying mind. Try to meditate daily. If you can free the mind, ten minutes will do for a start.

You may prefer a more active form of meditation such as Tai chi. With this form participants practice slow, fluid, graceful and continuous movement control of arm, leg, torso and spinal positions for as long as seventy-five minutes. Many Chinese practice this form religiously. Tai Chi is believed to engage the brain chemistry through concentrated breathing. In theory, concentrated breathing shifts primary neurological functions to other parts of the brain. There are various small studies that have documented positive effects of Tai Chi on a number of physical problems. Larger studies need to be undertaken before definitive recommendations can be offered. If you choose to learn the practice of Tai Chi, you'll be amazed at how the slow control of body movements increases flexibility, strength and restores balance.

Obviously, meditation has many streams but they all lead to the same river of inner peace and acceptance of self. You may find that you need more training in the techniques of meditation than the simple exercise we have described, and, fortunately, training is available in many sectors. Post-op treatment for cardiac patients in some hospitals includes meditation as part of the therapeutic routine. Many hospitals now offer a division of alternative or complementary therapy. Healing centers, health clubs, church groups, YMHAs, clubs—just about any social or health organization offer workshops. The choice is yours although, at times, choice becomes a serendipitous event. You may stumble onto a class in session as I once did while walking in Central Park where I came upon a spiritual teacher leading a large group of people seated on the grass. Completing the session she was asked how to control the mind from entertaining extraneous thought. The guru responded that the act of beginning meditation was in itself productive.

Since I have been meditating I have noticed changes. Sure, I still get steamed about certain things and I react angrily when my toes are stepped on, but the need to retain this hurt or slight is considerably weakened and I find I'm able to let it go. Ah, how much energy is available when it's not wrapped in negative thoughts. Furthermore, I find that I feel refreshed and experience a deep sense of feeling good. Do I experience bliss when I meditate? Afraid not. I realize I would have to devote much more time to the practice to rise to that level, but I do experience a positive frame of mind.

BREATHE, BREATHE, BREATHE

All the various methods of mind-body healing tap into the same physical mechanisms. By slowing down breathing, the ratio in the blood of oxygen to carbon dioxide changes for the better, for more oxygen brought into the body produces a favorable effect on the brain. The calming effect of deep breathing shuts down the activity of the sympathetic nervous system boosting the performance of your immune system, quieting your conscious brain (the *cerebral cortex*) and the emotional centers (*amygdale and hippocampus*) that then reduces stress hormone activity in your *hypothalamus*. Slowing down the number of breaths per minute from 14-to-18 to 10 or less, using prolonged exhalation relaxes the small blood vessels and has an effect on lowering blood pressure.

How often do you hold your breath, especially when exerting? One, two? Count them. You're probably holding your breath unconsciously as you go about your activities. Imitate a child's natural breathing. Your autonomic system is designed to perform that same function for you, but in a tension-driven society, natural breathing is often abused. The ancients were well aware of this and stressed breathing as the bedrock of all the self-healing therapies. Breathing channels energy. Activity performed on exhalation is far more productive and less strain on the body than activity performed on the intake of breath.

We are not talking about habitual deep breathing for this practice can lead to hyperventilation. Taking quick shallow breaths from the top of the lungs can create hypoxia (oxygen starvation). This syndrome is called the Bohr Effect. Over-breathing lowers carbon dioxide in the blood that binds oxygen and hemoglobin (the carrier of oxygen in the blood) resulting in a dearth of released oxygen to the cells in the brain, heart, kidneys, blood vessels and other organs. Low carbon dioxide disrupts the work of enzymes (protein catalysts), and decreases the work of the mitochondria in producing energy. Hyperventilation can also render the nervous system vulnerable to a number of stress problems such as sleeplessness and irritability. Inhaled carbon dioxide, however, has been shown to produce vasodilation (widening of arteries). Most beneficial is the natural form of abdominal breathing found in infants. Natural breathing expands the abdomen allowing oxygen to flood the entire pulmonary system, and releases carbon dioxide upon belly contraction. In this process, your organs are gently massaged and intestinal movement, blood and lymph flow are promoted. According to yoga belief, we are allowed a certain number of breaths during our lifetime. Slowing down breathing, therefore, extends longevity.

Try these breathing exercises.

Method 1
1. Inhale through your nose from the bottom of your diaphragm to the top of your lungs. Feel the air traveling up through the lungs to the very corners of the top of the lungs. To test if you're meeting this goal, place your hand on the top of your chest and feel its expansion as the air flows in.
2. Exhale through your nose from the top of your lungs to the bottom of your diaphragm. Try to equalize intake and exhalation. Or better still, make your exhalation longer.
3. Repeat three times maintaining the rhythm.

Method 2
1. Inhale through your nose and count to three before you exhale.
2. Count to three before you inhale again.
3. Repeat three times maintaining the rhythm.

RELAX, MELT, SOFTEN

On a treadmill? Not that machine in your bedroom but the machine in your head. So busy, you barely have time to breathe? Facing impossible deadlines? Too many demands on your time? To moderate the frantic pace of modern living avoid the quick fix and adopt relaxation training exercises.

Seeming a contradiction in terms, release of tension actually helps to release bound-up energy. Tension dissipates energy. When the mind is preoccupied with zillions of things to do, energy that might better accomplish tasks is diverted to worry. Tiger Woods, a phenomenal golfer who led the pack in the 90's, practices Buddhism. His ability to focus, together with his innate gifts, propelled him to the top of his profession. Letting go of tension helps to refocus and regenerate your energy.

In the following exercises every movement described requires coordinated breathing Well, I meditate, you say. Isn't that enough? Perhaps. But a relaxation exercise might also benefit, for meditation and relaxation each have different effects on the body and brain. With meditation you empty your mind of thoughts demanding attention and action. With deep relaxation you use your mind to direct your body parts to release tension. The phrase, "let go, let live," aptly describes the relaxation process. Meditation might be described as a state of active body/passive mind, or passive body/ passive mind; deep relaxation may be described as active mind/active to passive body, for while your mind directs the activity, tension melts away.

Initially, you might want to seek help from an instructor or purchase an instructional tape, or alternately tape your personal instructions as a guide for each session. It's not necessary to have a quiet room, although silence often helps in the beginning of your practice. Once techniques are established, you can practice on a plane, train, long bus ride, or even do "a snatch relaxation" while waiting in line in the grocery store. Below is a sample tension-relieving exercise that should take about fifteen minutes. If pressed for time, concentrate on the part that directly concerns the eyes.

Exercise 1 This exercise is best practiced lying on your back.

1. Inhale. Flex your right foot. Exhale. Point the toe of your right foot. Breathe in and out through your nose as you soften your foot, working one toe at a time. Feel the softness extending up through your ankle, your calf, your knee, your thigh.
2. Inhale. Flex your left foot. Exhale. Point the toe of your left foot. Repeat the process with your left foot and leg breathing naturally.
3. Inhale deeply. Exhale. Feel the air softening your stomach and your internal organs. Rest for a moment to enjoy the feeling of relaxation in your body.
4. Inhale deeply bringing the air to the center of your chest around the heart region. Exhale softening the heart and lungs. Rest for a moment to enjoy the feeling of relaxation of your upper chest.
5. Breathe naturally and soften your throat muscles and lengthen the back of your neck.
6. Breathe naturally and soften your cheek muscles, your chin, extraorbital muscles around your eyes.
7. Breathe. Blink your eyes several times. Feel your eyes soften and sink back into the softness of their sockets.
8. Breathe evenly and regularly. Check your body and soften any part that still feels tense.
9. Lie quietly for several moments, soft and relaxed.

10. Gradually reawaken your body. Wriggle your toes. Move your buttocks. Make soft fists of your hands. Inhale deeply and sigh out your exhalation.

Exercise 2

1. Breathe in and out normally.
2. Imagine you are on your way to a beautiful beach.
3. You are light as air as you float down a lovely softly lit hall.
4. At the end of the hall, notice a door that on your approach opens automatically onto a set of stairs.
5. Descend each step drawn ever forward.
6. At the bottom step is a white sandy empty beach. It is all yours to enjoy.
7. The ocean is calm; small ripples lap the shore.
8. Step into the soothing water and wade out until you are waist high, and then lie on your back on the water, lightly suspended.
9. Close your eyes and listen to the soft ocean sounds, the whisper of the breeze. Your body softens and you become as one with the ocean as all tension falls away and are swallowed up by the water about you.
10. Stay here in the soft state for a few moments.
11. Allow yourself to gradually return to daily awareness.

YOGA YOGA EVERYWHERE

When the cartoonists begin to do "takes" on a practice, you know that it's become a universal phenomenon. Everybody, it seems, is practicing some form of yoga, and loving it. I toyed with yoga for many years but could not find the time, but when I discovered that my husband was interested, I managed to squeeze out an afternoon, and after several years of practice, I find it indispensable. I had thought that my form of exercise and long walks were sufficient to keep my body flexible. To my amazement after taking a few yoga lessons, I discovered a new group of underused muscles. I now walk, sit and stand straighter and as well, I have found an unlimited source of energy. But the practice of yoga goes far beyond strengthening the body. A study of one hundred-forty-nine type 2 diabetic patients found that daily yoga, ninety minutes in the morning and sixty minutes in the afternoon for forty days, decreased average blood glucose levels in seventy percent of the participants from 135-to-101 mg/dl. It is difficult to learn yoga from a manual, for you're unable to determine if you're performing the stretches correctly. Since classes in yoga abound, check one out. Often they're free or inexpensive.

DEALING WITH NEGATIVE EMOTIONS

Negative emotions may weaken the immune system's response to flu vaccine according to a study where researchers found that negative emotions stimulated the brain's right pre-frontal cortex resulting in a lower immune response. This is only one of many studies documenting scientific links to body-mind effects on health.

Dorothy, a psychologist, who has glaucoma, has adopted behavior management theory to reward responses that heal. In this system, both positive and negative reinforcement increase the desired response. For example, your instructor complements you on a job well done. (positive reinforcement); you discard tight-fitting shoes for comfortable ones (negative reinforcement). How does this work for glaucoma? It's how you think through a problem. Using reinforcement you tell yourself, "I can manage my glaucoma." With negative reinforcement you break up old habits such as discouragement, morbid thoughts about going blind, fear of what the future may hold, and replace these with positive thoughts such as your ability to cope with whatever comes your way. By learning to focus on desired behaviors, you can change your outlook and teach your brain to remodel itself more positively.

Here are some of the thoughts that can make you sick:
1. Unresolved emotional, psychological or spiritual stressors.
2. Negative belief patterns that control reality.
3. Inability to give and/or receive love.
4. Humorless—inability to distinguish serious from less serious concerns.
5. Ineffective in making positive choices.
6. Not attending to needs of body—physical, emotional, chemical.
7. Loss of meaning in one's life.
8. Denial, unable or unwilling to face the challenges of life.

LAUGHTER

The healing effects of a good belly laugh cannot be overestimated. Think about how great you feel when you've laughed so hard that your stomach hurts. Children laugh four hundred times a day and adults fourteen. Most people enjoy the gags printed in their local papers and in magazines. Many of us never outgrow cartoons, whether in print or at the movies. Humor lifts depression, a condition that may cause adverse changes in the brain.

So, laugh a little or a lot or whenever you have occasion and enjoy life. Your body will thank you with better health and an improved outlook on life. There are books including one written some time ago by Norman Cousins on the healing properties of humor. He had *ankylosing spondylitis* (chronic progressive disease involving joints) and he devised his own treatment of vitamins and humor. He got better. A study that involved fifty-two healthy men who viewed a humorous video for one hour found increases in natural killer cell activity, activating T cells that strengthened the immune system. It lasted up to twelve hours. Take time out of your busy schedule to enjoy a good laugh.

MYOPIA AND GLAUCOMA

Myopia (nearsightness) is the bane of the civilized world. The remarkable eye is equipped with the mechanism to watch a fly ball travel into the bleachers and in an instant, read a timetable. In a healthy eye, these accommodations are a reflex made possible by the *ciliary muscle* that for near vision contracts increasing the roundness of the lens; that then contracts the pupil promoting convergence of the optic axes. When accommodation fails as it does in myopia, correction is possible with eyeglasses or LASIK surgery (See Chapter 6). People who do not spend hours pouring over material requiring close vision most often do not get nearsighted, but in societies where reading requirement begins early in life, myopia frequently develops. At around eight or nine years of age, children begin to use their eyes for close work four-to-five hours at a stretch setting the condition for the development of myopia. This eye disorder, however, may not necessarily be genetically linked. In a group of Eskimos, the illiterate parents and grandparents were not myopic, but sixty percent of the children attending school became myopic. I took to reading immediately and by the age of ten, I needed glasses. Sally needed them by the age of eight. The nerdy kid is the one most associated with myopia, rather than the sports jock. And there are some studies that do indeed find a relationship between high scholastic achievement and myopia.

With computers, palm pilots, cell phones, Blackberries, Ipods, and whatever new gadget makes the cut added to the mix of close eye encounters, children are more than ever exposed to developing myopia. Not everybody who does close work gets myopia, but for the susceptible, myopia is a risk factor for both glaucoma and *retinal* problems. As the globe of the eye elongates, the *retina* stretches and thins. It's like stretching a rubber band. The overstretched possibly causes holes or *retinal* detachment.

Since the early nineteenth century when education began to be viewed as a right in many countries, scientists have had a lively interest in determining how near-point accommodation maintained for at least a two-hour period, changed the shape of the eyeball. It is now understood that accommodation causes a pressure change in the vitreous chamber that results in the elongation of the eye. The change in the shape of the eyeball poses considerable risk of *retinal* detachment for once the eye has become myopic and stronger glasses are require, the eye continues to elongate.

The knowledge that reading and close work can change the structure of the eye has stimulated scientists to speculate on possibly reversing myopia. Indeed, there appears to be some scattered success stories, but these are mainly anecdotal. Proper focusing may lie at the heart of some myopic conditions. An offshoot of optometry, The Optometric Extension Program Foundation, the College of Optometrists and Vision Development, and a small organization called the Optometric Training Institute specialize in training people to focus their eyes properly and to learn to use better whatever vision they have. Babs has worked with a practitioner, an investigative researcher and author, who uses a variety of methods including a machine he invented that helps the patient to properly focus. Babs found to her delight that with this eye training her eye pressure lowered.

One of the earliest pioneers Dr. W.H. Bates specialized in training for reversal of myopia and other eye problems. In 1920, he published a book entitled *Perfect Sight Without Glasses*. Aldous Huxley, a well-known author who lived during this period, worked with Dr. Bates and published his own book attesting to recovery of vision using the Bates method. Like all alternative therapies, the Bates method requires hours of dedicated effort. In my early twenties, prompted by an optometrist who had mastered the crippling effects of polio to the extent that he completed optometry school, opened his own practice, and rode a bicycle to work, I entered treatment with him in an attempt to reverse my myopia. I did not have the success of Huxley, but I did realize that I did not always need to wear corrected lenses for every activity.

There are others, however, who claim to have changed the shape of their eyeball. Dr. Deborah Banker, a practicing ophthalmologist, asserts success in her own case. She has developed a kit of resource materials to help others do likewise although she cautions that the exercises need to be practiced on a continuing basis or the eye will slip back into its old shape. There are always those exceptional few who, through dint of their own efforts, cure themselves and publish their stories. The bottom line, however, remains that cure requires constant effort and hard work, the very thought of which, the time involved, and the "iffy" possibility of positive results, melts down the steel of dedication, especially now with the availability of *LASIK*.

Nevertheless, attention to perception, one of the foundations of focusing, can be improved through a number of simple exercises that do not require hours of time. These exercises serve well for any eye condition. Think how a baby explores its environment eagerly looking and tracking movement whether of people, animals or objects. Its busy eyes are loading perceptual information necessary for sight and visual memory onto to the brain. With diminished sight, we often stop examining our surroundings, thus starving the brain of important visual information, a vital component that helps to build new connections—synapses that remodel the brain. While we cannot yet replace cells lost, there is evidence in the medical literature that throughout our lifetime, the brain is capable of manufacturing new dendritic connections. This observation has been borne out by *MRI* technology. Scientists observing signals from the *optic nerve* on the *visual cortex* of the brain have documented how cells, with a minimum of clues, stimulate encoded messages. You're probably aware of this phenomenon when you recognize an individual by a familiar tilt of the head, curve of chin, slope of shoulder, stride, or any other distinctive feature. Inanimate objects, too, reveal identity through shape and color. Daily, clues to life around you define your visual world, stimulating your brain to make new connections. Knowledge equates understanding. The baby hungrily devouring visual information has no idea that it is encoding messages, nor do we when we scan the street for oncoming cars. Yet our brains ceaselessly work to furnish our comprehensive visual systems. The wider our view the more defined our world becomes.

When we lose some vision, we may stop trying to see--limit perceiving because siht becomes blurry, fuzzy--requires too much effort. Lorraine Marchi, CEO of the *National Association for the Visually Handicapped* has noted when she encourages visually handicapped individuals to use their eyes, that these people report back that they see better again. Granted, that perceiving is more difficult when cells have been lost, but with most individuals, there are still sufficient cells available. Stimulation is perhaps the most important factor if, although not restoring vision, does produce a continuous stream of signals for synaptic connections.

Here are some activities that can help revitalize your brain and sharpen your perception. Remember to breathe evenly while practicing. Start by taking a few minutes to clear your mind by breathing slowly through your nose. Inhale from the diaphragm right up to the corners of the lungs; exhale from the corners of your lungs right down to the diaphragm. Repeat several times. When following the instructions below, be sure to avoid staring. Perception is enhanced through eye movement. Also, blink a lot to continuously lubricate your eyes.

DETAILS—BECOME A DETAIL SLEUTH

- Pick up a stone. Examine its ridges, indentations, smoothness, roughness, pits, hollows, weight, and shape. If it is a flat stone and you're near water, send it skimming over the water and watch for the splash. If that's too distant to notice, take several small stones and drop them into water. Observe the splash. Or you might want to try this experiment in your kitchen using pebbles dropped into a glass of water. Observe both the splash and the rise in water level.

- This is a good exercise while waiting in line at the grocer's. Run your eye over the counter, follow the movement of the cashier's hand, examine the pattern of the clothing worn by the person ahead of you—count your change or check the print-out receipt if you use a credit card.

- Walk in the park or along a tree-lined street. Give a tree a good once-over. Start with the bark. Is it smooth and shiny? Is it rough and furrowed? Allow your eye to examine the crevices and edges of the bark. Look at the tree's leaves. Hold one in your hand and let your eye trace the skeleton of the leaf, its center spine and its branching.

- Building scrutiny. Here is a good exercise while waiting for a bus. Trace the outline of each window frame in a near building. If the building has embellishments, let your eyes follow each curve, curlicue, shape or form. Take a look at the brickwork, the fretwork, the decorated entrance if there is one. Let your eye travel along these decorative features.

- This is a fun activity to do at a meeting of glaucoma patients. It's also a nice way to get to know the person sitting next to you. Turn to that person and examine the facial features. Take your time to register each feature. Guaranteed, you'll remember that individual the next time you see him or her. Now have your partner examine your features.

- Try blinking one eye at a time. To achieve this, slowly move your head from side to side, opening first one eye and then the other when you are at the center of your movement. The slower you're able to move your head, the more control you will have over opening one eye at a time.

- Make up your own eye chart. On a large piece of paper, draw a large E. Pin it to the wall. Now walk away from it until you can just see the entire form. With your right eye (keep your left eye closed or covered) trace in succession each horizontal line and then the vertical line. Repeat this process several times. If you can do this easily you might want to step back further, or make two smaller letters, like an N and a G. Repeat with left eye with right eye occluded. Work on your peripheral vision. Hold a white piece of paper in each hand and extend your arms. Look straight ahead. Can you see the paper? If not, bring your arms in closer to your line of vision. Wiggle your fingers. Concentrate on looking straight ahead as you become aware of your wiggling fingers.

- Use your nose as a pencil. Close your eyes and visualize a figure eight. With your nose trace the outline of the figure 8. Still with your eyes closed, write your name with your nose; write your partner's or friend's name. This is a good exercise to do if you've been on the computer for a long time or if you've been immersed in reading for a few hours
- Look at a wall calendar, a *Snellen* wall chart if you have one, a photograph on the wall, or a picture. Spend a few seconds observing it, and then return to whatever you have been doing—reading, on the computer, etc. Or gaze out the window and observe the passing scene. When you focus again on your present activity, you'll probably find more clarity of vision. Another method to retain focus is to pause, close your eyes and in your mind trace the contours of the last word you read.

TENSION RELEASE

Sometimes we are unaware of the tension we build up during the day. It's a good idea to stop occasionally in the middle of whatever you're doing to practice tension relieving exercises. Your body will feel better, and your eyes will benefit. Be sure to breathe evenly throughout the following exercises.

1. Your jaw holds a lot of tension. Notice how it tightens up when you are engaged in an activity. Soften your jaw, stretch it wide. Open your mouth wide—you'll probably yawn. Smile. If you are into yoga, do the lion's pose; otherwise, make some funny sounds.

2. The back of your neck holds a lot of tension. By self-massaging this area, you relieve the tightness. You want to loosen the sternocleidomastoid muscle—the muscle that runs from behind your ear, down the side of your neck, and into your shoulders. Place four fingers on the right and left side of this muscle and check for sore spots. Press your fingers into each sore spot and massage gently. Now run your fingers the length of the muscle several times. Do this exercise whenever your neck feels tense.

3. A shoulder rotation is one of the best ways to relieve tension and also to remind you to straighten your spine. Close your eyes. Rotate each shoulder separately--3 rotations forward and 3 rotations backward.

4. Head roll. Close your eyes. Sink your chin down towards your chest and move it the right, back, look up, move to the left and back to center where you sink your chin again. Repeat this rotation three times.

EYE STRETCHES AND EYE GAZES

Often following long sessions at the computer or reading, you may experience eye fatigue. A series of stretches may help to alleviate this condition. Start with one inhalation and exhalation of breath and work up to six breath cycles with each position taking longer and involving deeper breaths. Visualize oxygen flooding your eyes.

1. Stand relaxed and gaze straight ahead.
2.   Place index finger to the outside edge of the right eye socket. Inhale look to the left, stretch the skin; exhale, release the skin bringing the eye to center. Repeat positions at the left of the eyes looking to the right.
3. Look upward, inhale, stretch skin. Exhale while releasing skin.
4. Look ahead, inhale, stretch skin just below eyebrows. Exhale, release. Inhale, gaze upward. Exhale gaze downward. Repeat three times.
5. Inhale, gaze in a semicircle in the upper half of the eyes from right to left. Exhale, gaze from left to right. Repeat three times.
6. Inhale, gaze in a semicircle in the lower half of your eyes from right to left. Exhale, gaze from left to right. Repeat three times.
7. Inhale, gaze on a diagonal from top right to bottom left. Exhale, gaze diagonally from bottom left to top right.
8. Inhale, gaze on a diagonal from top left to bottom right. Exhale, gaze diagonally from bottom right to upper left.
9. Inhale, hold your finger to your nose. Now draw your finger away following it with your eyes. When you reach arm's length, exhale while your draw your finger back in. The slower you do this exercise, the better it is for muscles of your eyes. Repeat three times.

CHINESE HEALING PRACTICES: ACUPUNCTURE/ ACUPRESSURE/SHIATSU

Acupuncture has gained favor among many practitioners of the healing arts and has won a respectful place in the general medical community because of its documented healing power in selected illnesses. It is based on the ancient Chinese philosophical principle of yin and yang. The yin represents the female principle, the earth, and the yang the heavens, completing the universe. Harmony is achieved when the yin and yang are balanced. Each body is considered a universe; when the forces are unbalanced, sickness or disease occurs. Correction of this imbalance is achieved through stimulating the meridians or conduits that permeate the body. This stimulation enables the chi (the vital energy or life force) to flow more freely. Points along these meridians correspond to different parts of the body and different organs. Acupuncture is generally considered safe, since there are no documented side effects from the practice (the insertion of fine needles into the acupuncture points).

There are acupuncturists who believe they can promote benefits to glaucoma patients. And some patients do indeed report that their pressures are reduced and that they see more clearly. No full-scale studies exist, however, documenting lasting positive effects of acupuncture on the eyes. Acupuncture is primarily known for is its ability to exert its effects on the nervous system releasing body chemicals known as endorphins and enkephalins, the body's natural painkillers.

Problems exist when considering acupuncture for eye therapy. Although acupuncture for some illnesses is covered by medical insurance, deficiencies in eyes are generally not included. Without insurance coverage, acupuncture requiring a series of visits can become expensive. Additionally, many practitioners recommend a total Chinese medical approach involving along with acupuncture, moxibustion (application of a heated cone or cylinder of cotton wool to produce a counter-irritation on a part of the body), Chinese herbs, specialized exercise and other Chinese modalities. Even so, the practice of acupuncture, even modified is intriguing. Those practicing Chinese medicine claim the liver is the organ of the body associated with the eyes along with to a lesser degree the kidneys and stomach. On a modified scale, there are things you can do for yourself. The series below follow the Chinese massage methods. Use the pads of your thumb and forefingers to press gently but firmly the indicated areas.

1. Stomach Connections
   a. Brings energy and blood to the eyes. <u>Position</u>: approximately an inch from the outside crest of the shinbone lying in the natural groove of the muscle.
   b. Reduces heat from the eyes: <u>Position</u>: The lateral side of the second toe.
   c. Storage and release of tears. <u>Position</u>: Lower eyelid on orbital rim directly beneath pupil.

2. Liver Connections

 a. Reduces heat in the eyes; <u>Position:</u> The web between first and second toes.

 b. Energizers, brightens, helps resolve physiological and psychology eye problems, <u>Position:</u> Top of foot in the depression between big and second toe.

 c. Supplies nourishing blood to eye. <u>Position:</u> Inside of bent knee where crease ends.

 d. Relaxes mind and balances emotions. <u>Position:</u>   About two inches above crease in middle of wrist.

3, Eye energy enhancers. Positions:

 a. One inch below the end of the eyebrow and outer edge of the eye.

 b. At the depression at the lateral end of the eyebrow.

 c. Midpoint between the two eyebrows.

 d The hollow midpoint in the eyebrow above the pupil of the eye.

A second method combining acupressure and shiatsu acts along some of the main points. Massage frees the energy to flow. These exercises take about ten to fifteen minutes. I do them each morning before I get up, alternating the exercises with instillation of my eyedrops. Remember to breathe evenly and wash your hands before doing these exercises.

1. Place your thumbs on each side of your temple and your index fingers bent against your brow. Massage the center of your eyebrow ten times. If you feel tension or pain in that area, massage until the symptoms are relieved. Now with your thumbs still in place, massage along the length of each brow.

2. Massage the lower eye socket just beneath the pupil ten times. If you feel pain or tension, massage until you feel relief.

3. Move your fingers to upper inner corners of your eyes. Very gently in a rotating motion massage this area ten times. This area will be tender for it is the place which you occlude to avoid having your eyedrop leach into your nose.

4. Locate the tear duct and place your fingers just below it. Massage ten times.

5. Place your fingers on the outer corners of your eyes and massage ten times.

6. With your thumbs, press into the hollows of your temple and rotate the massage ten times.

7. Move your fingers up to your forehead and find the hollows just above your eyebrows. Rotate your massage in these areas ten times.

8. Move your fingers to your hairline and massage this area ten times by rotating your fingers in small circles.

9. Find the spot just under the middle of your cheek bone. Press upward and rotate your fingers ten times.

10. Feel the hollow where your jawbone ends adjacent to your inner earlobe. Do a rotating massage ten times.

11. Feel the soft area at the bottom of the bony structure at the back of your head. Check for hollows. Press your fingers or thumbs into this area and rotate ten times.

12. Find the hollows in the back of your head just below the top of the scalp. These are similar to the soft spots in a baby's head. Do a rotating massage ten times in these areas.

13. To complete the process, do a circular massage beginning at the eye sockets and widening the massage area until you have covered your entire face.

Please note: For the pressure points, apply firm but comfortable pressure for a few seconds, release and apply again. For the rotating massage, gently massage the areas. What you want to do is stimulate the areas so that blood and lymph will flow more easily. You'll also feel enlivened after these exercises.

PALM—QUICK, EASY, EFFECTIVE

The simple act of palming is one of the most important exercises that Dr. Bates shared with his patients and readers. There is no better quick fix to relieve built up tension, especially when engaged in close work. Palming rests your eyes completely. It differs from sleeping for although your eyes are closed in both cases, during sleep, especially in the *REM* cycle, the period of dreaming, your eyes actively follow the sequences of your dreams.

You can palm for a few moments, ten minutes, or hours fitting the practice into your schedule whenever you have some free time or concluding with palming after a series of eye exercises or a yoga session. Some people, me included, combine palming with meditation. Here's how you do it. Rub your hands together briskly to release energy. This energy flows from your hands into your eyes as you palm. Gently cup your palms over your closed eyes. They should not touch your eyes but encircle them with healing warmth.

Visualize darkness, blackness—the deeper the absence of light, the greater the effectiveness of palming.

Journaling

Write about your feelings, your experiences, your disappointments, fears, frustrations—let it all hang out when you put your pen to paper or when you write on the computer. You needn't be an expert writer to journal. You can write about trauma, do autobiographical essays, or just merely let loose creative impulses—anything goes. Very early in my life I discovered when I felt in disarray or when a particular incident or interaction caused distress, I would write down my feelings. This practice not only made me feel better but sometimes helped me to resolve a problem. Diarists have long known the wisdom of discharging their emotions onto to paper and in our modern age onto the computer, possibly in the form of blogging. Samuel Pepys, a diarist in the 17th century, became famous because his jottings, observations actually, contributed greatly to comprehension of that period of history. There are some small studies indicating that journaling alleviates some symptoms, particularly those caused by difficult medical situations such as arthritis and asthma. British researchers found that patients who wrote daily for twenty minutes about emotional events healed faster over a three-day period than those who wrote about trivial events. The researchers theorized that writing about your feelings lowers stress and thus strengthens the immune system promoting faster healing. A former New York City magazine editor, now part of a writer's group comprised of people whose ages range from mid-60's to mid-80's, analyzed the experience as providing a method for paying attention to self in its relationship to past, present and yes, the future. As part of his restorative philosophy, Garry Null, holistic practitioner and author, includes journaling in his protocols for health maintenance.

Spiritual Healing

Mind, body and spirit. Many of us are so actively engrossed in everyday affairs we tend to neglect the powers of spiritual healing. According to an observational study, a group of patients with chronic illness were treated by various methods of distance healing. Their quality of life rose ten points as assessed on a health survey scale. Of course, these subjects may have experienced a placebo effect or positive expectation, but whatever the dynamics, they did benefit from the experience. How often when undergoing a crisis or contemplating surgery or other medical interventions, has a friend or neighbor said they would pray for your recovery? Often, this gesture of intended good will produces positive effects for you. Many of us follow some form of spiritual healing that can be as varied as the Eastern philosophies or attending a religious center.

Sound Healing

A research organization called *Sound Health Alternatives* has been studying the frequencies emitted by the body. This group found that frequencies emitted from the ears are missing from the voice. Frequencies that are missing or out-of-tune in the voice may denote pain, physical symptoms and emotional stress. Notes can be missing from any octave. Different octaves relate to different levels: genetic, environmental, biochemical, nutritional, structural, and emotional/psychological. In *Sound Healing* the missing frequencies are sounded organizing the energy field which helps to heal the conditions. This organization has not performed any studies on glaucoma and most of their work is conducted with doctors. Website: soundhealth@starband.net; or 740-698-9119. This discipline raises a personal question--does my tone-deafness have something to do with my glaucoma?

Magnetic Healing

Holistic practitioners have long prescribed magnetic therapy to help heal soft tissue injury, but magnetic therapy effects are still in the experimental stage. Trans cranial magnetic stimulation (*rTMS*), originally developed as a diagnostic tool for mapping brain function, is now being explored as a means for decreasing or increasing excitability in the cortical area of the brain. Patients with pain from stroke, spinal cord injury, lesions on the spinal nerves supplying the arm, forearm, and hand, trigeminal nerve region that includes the eye, drug-resistant peripheral neuropathy, and generalized nerve pain, all responded to the analgesic effects of *rTMS*. Other patients benefited including those with depression, epilepsy and chronic tinnitus. Glaucoma patients have not been included in the studies and this therapy is not yet approved by the FDA. But it is free from side effects and it may one day find a place in glaucoma treatment.

Oxygen Therapy

Slow deep breathing increases the oxygen supply to the body. Oxygen nourishes cells. An infusion of oxygen is possible through treatment in a hyperbaric chamber. Hyperbaric oxygen is commonly used to treat carbon monoxide poisoning, gas gangrene, decompression sickness (bends), air embolism, and smoke inhalation. There have been a few small studies with glaucoma patients and this treatment is appealing, but it has not caught on as a medical recommendation. Another form of oxygen therapy is intravenous ozone considered by the FDA as toxic, but with alternative practitioners an invaluable tool for detoxifying the body. It is said to dissolve clumping of red blood cells, oxygenate tissues, decrease blood viscosity and oxidation of plaque in the arteries. I have used it and found that it lowered the pressure in one eye, but some months later, pressure returned to its former level. I did feel more invigorated, however, and the therapy did cure a shingles infection.

OFF THE COUCH—EXERCISE

We hope that everybody now has the exercise message ingrained on the brain. Practicing daily exercises are highly recommended whatever your health condition. Holistic practitioners mount a holy trinity of exercise, spirituality and diet as the royal road to health. And you cannot pick up your daily paper, visit a bookstore or even talk to your next door neighbor without coming across a reference to daily exercise. Studies, both anecdotal and peer-reviewed attest to the benefits of exercise. We're not suggesting that you attempt to emulate those on the extreme end who despite their handicaps, like Eric Weihenmayer, blind from glaucoma, who climbs mountains or those visually-handicapped individuals who swim, sail, ride horses, kayak or any other sport you can think of. What we recommend is that if you adopt an exercise routine suited to your health and physical condition, you will be healthier and possibly improve the condition of your eyes. Robert Ritch, MD, a well-known glaucomatologist cites a number of research studies considering the effects of aerobic exercises (bicycling, brisk walking, running, jogging, swimming, gym conditioning) on lowering the *intraocular pressure*. Aerobic exercise particularly is beneficial for reducing IOP by 4 mmHg following three months of aerobic exercise training. This study did raise the caveat that when the exercise program was discontinued, IOPs went back to their original reading. Nevertheless, the study confirms that exercise must be sustained to be effective. If you have *exfoliative* or *pigmentary dispersion* glaucoma aerobic exercise should be limited, for bouncing about may knock more particles loose in your eye that may eventually end up in the trabecular meshwork.

Under no circumstances, however, when practicing yoga, stand on your head. Other ill-advised exercises are bungee jumping and scuba diving. Weight lifting is ill-advised according to a study with healthy individuals. Except for bench pressing at the lowest level, eye pressure increased. While this elevation was not considered harmful for these subjects who had healthy eyes, it is cause for concern in those with glaucoma.

Extensive exercise, especially in warmer climates, can increase need for water. Dr. Ritch also cautions that drinking a large amount of water after an exercise session can raise the IOP. If thirsty, drink water slowly.

Today, there are so many choices for exercise that we hesitate to offer advice on a particular form. You can opt for the Eastern derived exercises of yoga, karate, chi gong, or you join a gym, swim, run, play soccer with your kids or grandkids, bicycle, skate, dance, snorkel, garden, walk (my favorite—I try to put in two to three miles daily) vigorously clean house—anything to keep your body moving. Whatever form you choose, be consistent.

If you choose to use a gym for your exercise routine, you may run into an obstacle. Although the American Disability Act cites equal opportunity, this law has not reached into health clubs. An active woman who lost her vision two decades ago saw no reason to let this deter her from seeking out a health club to stay fit. But she found that the five clubs she visited insisted that she hire a personal trainer to use the gym. This story published in *The New York Times* has a happy ending for this woman found a health club, part of a chain of clubs for women only, where the manager volunteered to coach her for no extra fee. (See resources for more information)

The bald fact that health clubs are ill-prepared to accommodate persons with physical disabilities may soon change. New regulations for enforcing the 1990 Americans with Disabilities Act (ADA) are at this writing under review. They would require that health clubs clear floor space of at least 30-by-48 inches around each type of weight training equipment and that swimming pools, depending upon size, be required to have a ramp or lift. While these steps are praised by some advocates of the disabled, the general consensus appears to be that they do not go far enough. This is an instance where advocacy can take a major role.

BALANCE YOURSELF

Exercise, yoga, karate, tai chi, chi gong all can help to restore and strengthen balance that may have deteriorated. Advancing age often brings with it balance issues. Aging affects the receptor cells found in the skin, muscles, joints and tendons that process information about the body's orientation as it moves through space. Exercises geared to strengthening these receptors include: lunging, walking on a low balance beam, and standing on one leg with or without support. We suggest, however, that if balancing is a problem, work with a professional until you're able to walk a balance beam in smooth strides without teetering. It can be done. An assist to balance may be the use of light energy. An FDA approved device can safely increase local circulation and reduce numbness, tingling, and pain from peripheral neuropathy thereby increasing sensation in the feet. It's called the *Anodyne Therapy System*. This device uses infrared energy to release nitric oxide from blood cells. The nitric oxide improves nerve function and sensation by increasing circulation. It is also helps to make new blood vessels and promotes healing of diabetic foot ulcers and wounds. Treatment is relatively simple. Pads are placed on the affected areas and infrared light is passed through the body stimulating blood flow. Although most of the studies have been conducted with *diabetic neuropathy* patients, the system has also been used in dentistry, podiatry, physical and sports injuries, chiropractic, wound care, and pain relief. If you wish to explore further or to find a center near you, call 1-800-521-6664 or go to the web, www.anodynetherapy.com.

VISUAL HEALING

There are some people who, afflicted with their own eye disease, embark on a concerted effort to find a cure. Grace Halloran is such a person. She has *retinitis pigmentosa* and through her own efforts has been able to stem the effects of the disease. The protocol that she put together along with Erik Peper, PhD, Director of Holistic Health Department at San Francisco State University has been used with a small group of patients diagnosed with *retinitis pigmentosa, macular degeneration, Stargardt's Disease*, and glaucoma. Pre and post-visual fields demonstrated that the protocol worked for these people. The treatment consists of an intensive course of therapy that includes the use of the *Electro-Acuscope 80,* the *Tyro color reeducation* designed by Grace, cervical soft tissue rehabilitation, acupressure, deep tissue massage, foot reflexology, biofeedback, and nutritional supplementation. Thirty-two hours of education also include training and exercise on stress management related specifically to visual impairment, positive goal setting and visualization. Her book is available on Amazon.com.

COMPASSIONATE LIVING

Perhaps one of the most important messages in this chapter is to practice compassionate living. The author, Joanne Stepaniak, *Compassionate Living for Healing, Wholeness and Harmony*, calls it the secret ingredient to solving every disagreement and redeeming relationships.

CHIROPRACTIC

This is a case of one patient, but is well worth noting. It concerns a young woman who had *congenital glaucoma* with advanced optic disc cupping in one eye with nearly complete loss of vision. She had also lost vision in her other eye. She visited her chiropractor for treatment of back pain and migraine. Immediately following treatment, her vision improved in her good eye. Four treatments later, her vision had improved from two percent-to-twenty percent of normal. Independent examinations confirmed the result. Miracle? Well, not really. Visual disturbances have been reported in the scientific literature as early as the mid-nineteenth century, although atrophy of the optic disc improvement has not been previously reported as a result of spinal manipulation. Cases in the literature report other instances where field losses responded to spinal manipulation. The authors speculate that blood flow to the brain and especially to the capillary system may be hampered by problems in the muscular-skeleton system. Neurophysiology research offers a possible explanation for restoration of this patient's vision. At a certain level of reduced blood flow, the electrical activity of the neuron shuts down, but no cellular damage occurs. When blood flow resumes, the neurons come to life again. In other words these neurons are sleeping beauties awakening to the kiss of a prince. Based on this one study, spinal manipulation therapy may prove to be valuable for glaucoma patients and especially for those who have the syndrome of *normal pressure glaucoma*. And if you are plagued with migraines, a condition associated with glaucoma, at the very least, these headaches may be relieved through chiropractic.

NATURAL MEDICINES--HERBS

Herbs have a history that reaches as far back as 1000 B.C. An art historian and a medical researcher have divined this information based on frescoes at Thera, a Greek Island. In this fresco the goddess of medicine is depicted overseeing the production of medicinal saffron. Nature has provided us with plants to heal all manner of illnesses. Whether these plants are synthesized in the laboratory and transformed into powerful medications, or whether they are taken in their pure form, decocted from their leaves, stems and roots, the healing power of plants is as old as human history. Evidence documented through the use of a spectrophotometer found that *keto-carotenoid* pigments (*flavonoids*) in the aloe plant, for example, protected it from excessive sunlight. In other words the plant traps damaging light by developing various carotenoids. These nutrients are passed on to us when we ingest the plants.

The use of herbal remedies is a long tradition in the old world and this practice has reached the US through its diversified immigration. I recall my mother resorting to an herbal treatment to cure my bad case of poison ivy when I was a young child. I have no idea what plant was used, but our next door neighbor, a Polish woman, apparently schooled in folk medicine, went into the woods, not far from where we lived, and returned with a handful of plants. She instructed my mother to simmer them for some time and then bathe my tortured limbs with the decoction. And my father consistently made a brew of skullcap, catnip and several other herbs that he and my mother drank daily. My father swore this brew kept him healthy. He lived to the age of eighty-two, my mother to eighty-seven.

According to the Washington-based Institute of Medicine, a non-profit advisory group on health and science issues, plant-based therapies are gaining momentum around the world, with the exception of the USA, where herbal medicine has taken a back seat to pharmaceutical products that work much faster and incidentally, have many more side effects. But in other parts of the world, herbal medicine, often regarded as gentler on the body, is the first line of approach, followed, if ineffective, by pharmaceutical products. In very poor countries or even in outlying regions of more developed countries, herbal medicine may be all that is available. In Germany, herbal medicine is taught in medical school and many of the controversial herbs in this country are regularly prescribed. Today, knowledge about herbal medicines is gathered from people in indigenous populations, mainly the shamans or healers in these regions. Their knowledge of the healing power of herbs has been filtered from centuries of practice to the present healer. These practices are often quite effective. In the hands of an inexperienced practitioner, however, less than perfect results including death may occur.

Anthropologists, explorers and others working with indigenous peoples stimulated curiosity about the herbal medicines. They brought back to their native countries collections of herbs used by healers. Many of these are still the base for medicines to this day. Pilocarpine, derived from the plant jaborandi was one of the first drugs to treat glaucoma. Brought out of Brazil in 1876, it was found to have therapeutic effects on a number of diseases including lowering the pressure in glaucoma. And although many new drugs for treating glaucoma are now available, there are still those among us who find Pilocarpine effective, despite its many side effects.

Poisonous plants are often the source of medications. Plants of the order of Solanaceae that include nightshade, henbane, jimsonweed, and mandrake when ingested in their natural form can be deadly. These plants, however, contain atropine, a substance that is an antagonist of acetylcholine. The drug Belladonna (synthesized from nightshade) when used as an eyedrop, blocks the action of the pupillary sphincter resulting in dilation of the pupil. Scientists in the nineteenth century, seeking an opposite effect to dilating to that of constricting the pupil, investigated various substances and came up with physostigmine purified from the fruit of the caliber bean. It did cause sedation of the spinal cord but when accidentally overdosed, paralyzed the patient. Not to be daunted in their quest for a constricting agent, scientists refined the drug to reserpine that did indeed constrict the pupil, but, alas, vision suffered. Use of the drug caused short-sightedness.

Be aware that a problem may exist with some herbal preparations that have not have been properly screened for toxic metals. Some bilberry preparations have been found to contain toxic metals. Ginkgo biloba supplements have been found to carry lead. Chinese herbal preparations, in particular, appear to be suspect in some cases. Some supplements do not contain the specified amount of beneficial ingredient, thus rendering them worthless. For information on the quality of your supplements, go to the Consumer Labs for their reviews, *www.ConsumerLab.com*. Supplement manufacturers voluntarily submit their products for analysis to Consumer Labs. The organization also publishes a paperback guide to supplements. (*Guide to Buying Vitamins and Supplements: What's Really in the Bottle?*)

MARIJUANA Seeking an herbal cure to reduce eye pressure stimulated herbalists as well as pharmaceutical companies. What could be more beguiling then to find an herbal approach to both protect the optic nerve and lower eye pressure? Marijuana is such an herb exerting intriguing possibilities. Just about everyone is now familiar with the marijuana story. Yes, it does reduce eye pressure. Yes, it is an illegal drug, except for medical use in the United States. Smoking the leaves of cannabis sativa, (marijuana) does reduce eye pressure as studies have shown (at the expense of becoming high), but it also reduces blood flow, which is not a good idea for glaucoma patients. Perhaps more to the point, this drug provides relief from extreme pain without the devastating side effects of traditional pain-relieving medications. The reason it works so well is that the brain seems to have an affinity for it. Researchers studying marijuana have discovered that molecules naturally occurring in the body known as endocannacarbinoids occur throughout the body and brain affecting appetite, pain and memory. These findings most likely account for the widespread effect of marijuana since its carbinoids are similar to those of the body.

Marijuana is perhaps the most controversial herb in today's pharmacopoeia of substances that may have an effect on glaucoma treatment. The first medically recorded use of this herb dates back to China, 3750 BC. Evidence of its use is found also in the ancient writings of India, in second century Rome, during the European Renaissance and in the 19th century. It is a part of *Ayurvedic* medicine. India is so heavily steeped in the cultural and spiritual use of resinous cannabis that its people won a cultural exception to the UN Single Convention Treaty on Narcotic Drugs. Throughout, marijuana was prescribed for a number of ills ranging from treating earaches, joint pain, malaria, Blackwater fever, dysentery, anthrax and just about any other ailment.

Today, its mellowing effect on the nervous system is well documented. That it produces a hallucinogenic state places it in the realm of narcotics and thus is considered an illegal drug in some countries.

While use of the herb continues to be controversial marijuana can be legally obtained to treat illness in many countries. Widespread use has been reported in Canada for pain relief. In the United States, however, despite the government's firm stance against marijuana use, it is legal at this writing in 11 states, and bills to legalize it are pending in at least 7 more. Nevertheless, research in the United States has been stymied. Other countries not similarly restrictive have reported some interesting findings. The government's barring of dispensing marijuana has created an ambiguous role for physicians as to whether to discuss this substance with patients. Physicians, therefore, remain puzzled about whether they will be found guilty under Federal Drug Enforcement regardless of the fact that free speech in the form of the doctor's discussing this option with the patient has been affirmed by The Supreme Court. The Government counters that *Marisol*, a derivative of marijuana, can be used in place of the weed, but patients report that the effects between the two are not equal. Furthermore, although medical marijuana is legal in some states, growing, selling and using it can come at a price of jail or fines.

People with intractable pain express the need for this herb. Side effects include, first and foremost addiction. Toxicity from the smoke affects brain, heart, lungs and a study at the Jonsson Cancer Center, University of California, reported a 2.5% greater risk of head and neck cancers in marijuana users. Brain spectrometry of chronic marijuana users showed dramatic decreases in cerebral circulation depleting neurotransmitter activity. Marijuana, much as certain factions of the public would like to believe, is not a benign substance, especially for young people. A 2002 study published in the *British Medical Journal* found that New Zealand teenage boys who began smoking marijuana before the age of 15 and continued to use it ran the risk of developing schizophrenia. Older people did not face a similar risk. More recent developments found smoking marijuana delivered equal if not more carcinogenic materials as cigarettes.

As a drop form, *tetra hydra cannibinol (THC)*, marijuana's active ingredient, does not penetrate the eye because it is not soluble in water or in oil. A drug, *Marisol*, approved for sale in the United States, is the active ingredient of *tetra hydra cannabinol, (THC)* the psychoactive component of marijuana. According to the FDA, it can be used as an off-label drug for treating glaucoma but it is very expensive (about $500 a month). In January, 2004, England approved sale of the drug, *Sativex*, developed by GW Pharmaceuticals, a British company. This is a liquid extract that is sprayed under the tongue. It has been primarily developed to help people who have severe pain from the effects of *multiple sclerosis*. Unlike *Marinol,* which is a synthetic version of THC, *Sativex* uses the entire plant, and so may be effective for treatment of other conditions among them schizophrenia, head injuries, epilepsy, and rheumatoid arthritis.

Some people with elevated *intraocular pressure* who are not able to sufficiently lower eye pressures with glaucoma medications have experienced significant reduction of pressure with the use of marijuana as an additive treatment, provided it is taken every two-to-three hours. Marijuana works like nature in the eyes spreading the liquid over the eye so that it is eventually absorbed back into the system; it also dehydrates the eye reducing the volume of fluid in the eye. There are some patients participating in a Federal program, with marijuana cigarettes grown by the government at the University of Mississippi, shipped under FDA approval to a few patients. Dr. Paul Palmberg of Bascom Palmer Center in Miami, FL, reports that sixty percent of the patients in a study with high IOP experienced a significant lowering of pressure when marijuana was used as an additive therapy. He also cites the case of one patient whose pressure dropped from 50 mmHg to 28 mmHg on legal marijuana and then to 15 mmHg on timolol. While short-term use does cause changes in mood and thought, these effects lessen with continual use although the mode of action is still unclear. There is speculation that the pathway may begin in the *ciliary body receptors*. This research indicates that cannabinoids decrease aqueous production along with increasing aqueous outflow. These benefits exist in the presence of smoking marijuana, which in the long run may not be the best option. To reap the benefits of marijuana, a drug may need to be developed. An interesting side note about marijuana--the Marijuana Tax Act of 1937 was created to boost logging and synthetic fiber industries by eliminating hemp from the market. This legislation ultimately banned almost all use of the hemp plant in the USA. The Federal Bureau of Narcotics after post-prohibition needed a new cause and found hemp an easy target, and although the American Medical Association sent lobbyists to Congress to oppose the legislation, it was to no avail and possession of marijuana became cause for criminalization. What is the future of marijuana for glaucoma use? Perhaps a tablet retaining the pressure-lowering qualities and eliminating the toxic and intoxicating effects will be developed, since the effects of marijuana appear to work through the brain.

GINKGO BILOBA One of the first herbal treatments for glaucoma that patients turn to is ginkgo biloba. This herb is derived from the leaves and nuts of the ginkgo tree that is resistant to insects and diseases, and is believed to be one of the oldest species on the planet. The nut acts as an expectorant; that relaxes blood vessels, inhibits platelet clumping, increases cerebral and peripheral blood flow by increasing circulation in both large arteries and capillaries, producing a calming effect and toning of the brain. This improvement in circulation made possible by the dilation of blood vessels also enhances the availability of other nutrients by supplying oxygen to every cell in the body. Ginkgo biloba also possesses antioxidant properties important for repairing free *radical damage*. By binding to superoxide molecules it subverts the action of *free radicals* that oxidize oxygen and the peroxyl molecules that oxidize fats. Ginkgo biloba's protective effect on light-induced *retinal* injury was determined to be positive in an animal study. The authors of this study stated that an extract of gingko biloba had a preventive effect as a *free radical* scavenger. Another of ginkgo's actions decreases blood viscosity by acting on the clotting factor and thus increases circulation to the optic nerve. Patients taking blood thinners such as warfarin or Coumadin are advised to discontinue ginkgo. The herb, because of its circulation of blood reaching the small blood vessels in the brain, may provide some control over excess glutamate release, the amino acid that excites the neurons to perform a death dance (apoptosis.)

While there is anecdotal evidence that ginkgo may be beneficial as a glaucoma therapy, double-blind studies have yet to confirm the positive effects of this herb. Small studies, however, are emerging. The following double-blind test involved twenty-seven normal-tension patients with bilateral visual field damage. They used ginkgo biloba extract (standardized to contain 24% flavonoid glycosides and 6% terpenes), three times a day or placebo for four weeks. A significant improvement in visual fields was found in the ginkgo group. Another small cross-over study in eleven healthy volunteers found that although ginkgo did not alter IOP, 40 mg taken three times a day for two days did significantly increase blood flow to the ophthalmic artery. A number of European studies have confirmed ginkgo's positive effect in improving capillary permeability, an important finding for patients with glaucoma. In Germany, doctors prescribe 240 mg. Blood supply to the ophthalmic artery, according to a small study, did increase when the equivalent of two grams of ginkgo was administered to subjects. Studies demonstrating ginkgo's neuroprotective effects, favorable effects on brain metabolism, antioxidant and anti-inflammatory properties and influence on neurotransmitter function, place it high on the list as a quality herbal additive. There is some controversy over whether ginkgo will increase the possibility of spontaneous hematomas (blood clots) in the brain and there are several reported cases of individuals whose bleeding time was slowed by ingesting the herb. Bleeding time increased when ginkgo was discontinued. To be on the safe side, do not take this herb if you are on any blood-thinning medication.

If you decide to take gingko, buy a standardized product that specifies a 24% of the *heteroside flavonoid* content and a 5-to-7% of *terpinelactones*.

Dosages may be in the 40-to-60 milligram range. If you plan to take more than 120 milligrams a day, consult a health practitioner. If you are allergic to tannin, ginkgo is not for you. In general, however, contraindications have not been reported in using this herb. Non-standardized ginkgo may contain toxic amounts of *ginkgolic* acid. The German E Commission has set world standards for ginkgo products; they must contain less than five parts per million of *ginkgolic* acid.

Ginkgo has been studied for its effects on a number of diseases other than glaucoma. In an open trial, eighty-four percent of the respondents treated for antidepressant induced sexual dysfunction responded favorably to the sexual enhancing effects of ginkgo. It has been found to have positive effects on the treatment of dementia associated with *Alzheimer's*. In this study 40% of the patients on a placebo grew worse, while only 19% of those on a dosage of one hundred twenty mg. suffered more decline in cognitive abilities. A drug derived from ginkgo biloba has been used with some success on patients with Alzheimer's and/or dementia diseases. There is also some evidence that the herb preserves antioxidant activity in brain tissue exposed to radiation from cell phone use. Ginkgo has a good safety record and is well tolerated by most people.

BILBERRY (*Vaccinum myrtillus*), a member of the *Ericaceae* family, is the second most widely used herbal aid for eye problems. It contains high concentrations of the antioxidant *Reserveratrol* (the much touted antioxidant found in red wine). This compound is believed to be useful in maintaining and accelerating rhodopsin, the purple pigment used by the rods in the eye, increasing the eye's sensitivity to ambient light that enables the cells to adapt to dim light, thus improving night vision. Bilberry is actually not an herb but a fruit growing on a shrub that is similar to blueberries. What makes bilberry such an important addition to the diet is its high antioxidant content. The deeper the color found also in dark-colored fruit and vegetables provide greater amounts of available anthocyanidins, which is a type of flavonoid brimming with antioxidant activity. is essential for taming free radicals. Bilberry helps to prevent the breakdown of vitamin C which may, in turn, reduce the pressure in the eye. In a report of fifty patients with senile cataracts, a combination of bilberry standardized to contain 25% *anthocyanosides,* 180 mg twice daily and vitamin E, in the form of *di-tocopheryl acetate,* 100 mg taken twice daily for four months slowed cataract progression by four months. By limiting the damage caused by *free radicals* and thus decreasing the permeability of tiny capillaries, delivery of nutrients to the muscles and nerves of the eye is enhanced. Bilberry protects and strengthens blood vessels that feed the eye when combined with full spectrum vitamin E. People with macula diabetic *retinal* abnormalities may see improvement taking a bilberry supplement. In a study of thirty-seven patients, 79% improved within one month taking 160 mg of bilberry. Bilberry has a blood-thinning effect and if you are taking blood-thinning medications, check with your doctor before adding it to your routine. Even bilberry or blueberry jam will help, but eating jam increases sugar overload. Try to eat plenty of blueberries, cranberries, huckleberries or bilberries either fresh or frozen year round. You'll probably be providing your eyes with a super charge of free radical therapy. But you have to stuff yourself with the fruit to sustain the effect. Many of us, therefore, choose to supplement in addition to eating the fruit. Supplements can be found in any drug or health food store and are also available on line. Look for a product that specifies a content of 25% *anthocyanosides*. Dosages run from 40- to-60 mg. If you plan to take more, consult your health care practitioner.

FORSKOLIN, studied at one time as a possible IOP lowering preparation and ultimately abandoned because of toxic side effects, still remains an intriguing herb for eye health. Some studies indicate that forskolin does reduce *intraocular pressure* but this has been largely confined to healthy subjects. Still lacking are clinical studies on glaucoma patients of the use of forskolin in drop form.

The herb, derived from a species of coleus found only in India, possesses properties that strengthen the heart by lowering blood pressure, increasing energy compounds in cells, reducing inflammation, increasing insulin secretion, increasing thyroid function, and inhibiting blood clotting. It is also said to act on stimulating hormone production and regenerating nerves that have been injured.

Supplements may be labeled *Forskolin* or *Forskolii*. A supplement should contain 18% forskolin.

Other herbal preparations while added in some supplements that are touted to support eye health have not been explored for their effects on glaucoma. But these are herbs that have a long folk history of containing soothing properties and they are worth examining.

EYEBRIGHT (*Euprhasia officinalis*) helps to relieve redness, swelling, visual disturbances, inflammation, conjunctivitis, and blepharitis. It is an astringent and is anti-bacterial. If your eyes feel irritated, a compress of eyebright may help. A rinse can be made by boiling the herb in water for ten minutes. Let the water cool and apply to each eye five times. It can also be purchased in tablet or liquid form or drunk as a tea. As previously stated it is often included in vitamin preparations for the eye, but its mode of action has not been documented to the extent of ginkgo biloba and bilberry. Do not put the liquid form directly into the eye.

Two other herbs, PASQUE FLOWER (*Anemone pulsatilla*) and BARBERRY (*Berberis vulgaris*), have been used in Europe and other countries for eye problems. Pasque flower used as supplement helps such eye conditions as iritis, *retinal* problems and is said to help glaucoma and retard cataract development. Barberry contains an alkaloid, *berberine* that aids in overcoming inflammatory conditions and chronic allergic conjunctivitis. Berberine constricts the blood vessels helping to decrease the bloodshot appearance of strained eyes. It possesses a slight anesthetic effect that helps relieve pain. Other herbs containing berberine compounds are (*Hydrastis canadensis)* and *Oregon graperoot (Berberis aquifolium*).

The Chinese have been using herbal products for over 5,000 years, and while they have embraced western medicine, they have not discarded their traditional healing methods, choosing instead a practice combining both. Their interest in herbal medicine, however, has in no way abated and one of their products, an herbal remedy, has been rigorously tested in double-blind studies in China. It is still under review and not generally available in the United States. This product is a combination of herbs that act to protect the optic nerve provided *intraocular pressure* is under control. This formula, ERIGERON BRIMSCOPUS (VANT) HAND-MAZZ, is patented and produced by Xiang Ya Pharmaceutical Co. The SDA (comparable to the FDA in the U.S.) based on double-blind studies has approved this product for glaucoma. You can order these capsules directly from the company. Dosage is two capsules three times a day and should be taken for six months for a demonstrable effect to become apparent.

Other Chinese herbal preparations that have not received rigorous studies but are still said to be helpful for controlling glaucoma include: *Fructus ligustri lucidi (FLL); Rhizoma ligustict: Chuanxiong*; and *Radix astragali* seu *hedysari (RASH*, the root of a species of astragalus known as milk vetch). The mode of action is said to increase microstimulation, possibly improving the blood supply to the optic nerve. Another herb, the root of salvia (*dan shen*) also improves microcirculation, slows blood clotting and dilates blood vessels. Reported improvement in visual acuity and visual field exams warrant further study of these herbs. A study in China using a combination of herbs including salvia showed improvement in the visual field after thirty days. *Schisandra (Schisandra chinensis)* is a Chinese herb that is valued by practitioners of Chinese medicine for its effects on improving work capacity, mental efficiency and toning the nervous system. Its antioxidant properties that protect the liver make this a valuable herb for eye health. Typical dosage is up to a 580 mg capsule per day or 15-to-25 drops of tincture in water, or you can make a tea of it, drinking two cups per day. Should you wish to use any of the herbs described, however, we suggest you consult a herbalist and make sure that the herbs you use are free of toxic metals.

LYCIUM BARBARUM is generating some interest in both China and other countries as a possible neuroprotectant. It is a common traditional Chinese medicine. The entire plant is used, its red seeds, its leaf for tea or in cooking. Studies are underway to investigate its medicinal effectiveness for glaucoma.

HUPERZINE A (*Huperzia serrata*) is derived from a small plant commonly known as club moss. Used for centuries in China to treat inflammation and fever, it has gained favor in this country for its action on brain chemicals. It increases the levels of acetylcholine by blocking the enzyme *acetylcholinerase*, a compound that decreases nerve transmission. Important for glaucoma patients, it also has been found to decrease neuronal cell death caused by the amino acid glutamate. Improvement of memory function in people with memory impairment is another of its positive effects. Typical dosage is 20-to-50 micrograms two-to-four times a day. Should surgery be prescribed, advise your doctor that you are taking this compound.

GOTA KULA (**Centella asiatica**) used in India for centuries contains phytosterols that reduce inflammatory processes. It improves capillary permeability through increasing venous blood flow and seals leaky veins. It rejuvenates the nervous system. Many practitioners use it for wound healing and skin problems. It has an effect on connective tissue by strengthening the perivascular sheath that provides the vein with support. Some studies suggest that mental functions such as memory are improved. It is considered one of the herbal remedies for coping with stress and fatigue, gently relieving anxiety. Drink it as tea, two to three cups daily, or take a supplement of up to eight, 4- to- 5 hundred mg capsules or 20-to 40-drops of a tincture twice a day.

BROMELAIN is a proteolytic enzyme found in the fruit and stem of the pineapple plant. People with damaged blood vessels, a common problem with chronic glaucoma and other eye diseases, often have increased fibrin (clots) circulating in their blood. Bromelain helps to dissolve these clots and also to decrease inflammation.

BAIKAL SKULLCAP This herb is recommended by George Dever, O.D, who is also an herbalist and a doctor of optometry for more than fifty years. He leads a clinic in Seattle, Washington. One of the herbs he recommends is a Chinese liver remedy, and according to Dever, it has an effect on *intraocular pressure*.

AYURVEDA--India, another country noted for its reliance on herbal treatments, has promoted the practice of *Ayurvedic* medicine, a formalized method of treatment that that was consolidated 2,500 years ago. An Ayurveda program includes diet, spirituality and herbal treatment. The use of medicinal herbs is only one branch of the Ayurveda. Yet some of these herbs consistent with the practice are now available in health food stores and by mail order and are used routinely by nutritionists and the public at large. These include *ashwaganda*, a plant from the nightshade family that contains compounds that stimulate the immune system by increasing the number of white cells to fight bacteria, viruses and fungi. It has an effect of regulating the release of cortisol, the stress hormone. Studies have shown that it reduces anxiety and relieves pain and swelling associated with inflammation. It is sometimes called the Indian *ginseng*, and like all *ginsengs*, it enhances the body's ability to cope with stress, and increases mental acuity, reaction time and physical performance. *Guggal (commiphora mukal)* is a resin, an extract of which is called *gugulipid*. It has been shown to lower LDL cholesterol and triglycerides while raising HDL and it has a protective effect from *free radical* activity that is important for eye health. It also may be beneficial for arteriosclerosis by reducing the fat in the blood. *Gugilipid* is sold as a standardized extract containing five to ten percent *gugilsterones*. This herb can be taken long term. *Schisandra* is considered an energy tonic by improving general health, through increasing liver function (has been used to cure hepatitis), stimulating the brain and spinal cord, and improving respiration. When purchasing herbs manufactured in India, be sure the herb has been certified as free of contaminants. Lead and arsenic have been found in some products.

In *Ayurvedic medicine* topical treatments with herb decoctions or oils are commonly used. These are administered with an eyedropper or eye cup. Solutions of chamomile flowers, chrysanthemum flowers and rose petals reduce inflammation. Honey is used in early glaucoma and two drops applied daily. The eye should remain closed for five minutes. Honey acts as a vasodilator and lymph circulator enhancer in non-inflammatory conditions. Use only pure honey.

DETOXIFICATION should be taken into consideration when planning your healthy lifestyle. Our modern society spews thousands of pounds of chemicals onto the foods we eat, into the air we breathe and the water we drink. Many medical and dental procedures incorporate toxic metals as part of the therapeutic practice. Toxins in the body cause inflammation and may be responsible for some of the inflammatory conditions that plague so many of us. In particular inflammation (swelling) of the optic disc may be a result of toxic exposure. And there is no shortage of parasites and bacteria present in the water we drink and the soils we use for agriculture that are also toxic.

Surprisingly some of these substances do good as well as harm. Isn't that the way of life? The bacteria, *helicobacter pylori*, a major risk factor for stomach ulcers, may be beneficial in preventing gastro-esophageal reflux and esophageal cancer. Intestinal worms may be beneficial in treating autoimmune diseases such as inflammatory bowel disease.

There are many ways to detoxify heavy metals. Diet, herbal therapies and chelation are among those most commonly used. Omega-3 fatty acids found in flaxseed and salmon, herring and sardines have been found to reduce fibrinogen and have anti-inflammatory, vasodilative (enlarging the blood vessels), and blood thinning effects. It is important, however, not to overdose on the omega-3s for the brain needs a balance of all fats to function properly. Arachidonic acid, often given a bad rap, is the most prominent essential fatty acid in the red blood cells and comprises twelve percent of the total brain. The brain is sixty percent lipid, and the dendrites and synapses so important for neuron connections are eighty percent lipid. Fluid membranes will kick off oxidized cholesterol and neurotoxins. Note that while the blood-thinning effects of heparin may seem like a good idea, low-dose heparin according to a finding can turn a benign fungal infection into a toxic shock-like reaction.

Maintaining your health is your responsibility. You rely on your doctor to attend to the medical and surgical aspects of retaining your vision, but your doctor relies on you to take proper care of your body. In the next chapter we will examine how healthy eating can help you to attain and retain eye and body health.

CHAPTER 11

Nutrition—Its Contents and Discontents

○ ○

"Very simply, good food keeps us healthy and it is obtained without permanently destroying our natural resources or exploiting other people."

Roberta Maria Atti, Nutrition,
Immunity and Spiritual Growth, 1996

"Foods must be in the condition in which they are found in nature,
or at least in a condition as close as possible to that found in nature,"
Hippocrates, 460?-377? BC

What is more splendid than a great dish of food eaten in the company of good friends and loved ones? In societies where food is plentiful this has always been a given. Where food is scarce, a handful of rice may seem a blessing. Food is central to our existence, essential for the maintenance of health and a constant source of pleasure.

Without food and water we cannot survive. Simple, yes? Then why has food become such a football tossed from one diet to another; why has it generated countless books on nutrition, created a division between small and industrial farming, spawned a vast industry of junk food? Why is it more difficult in our present civilization to find food that is clean and uncontaminated with pesticides, herbicides, additives, pathogens and genetic tinkering? Evidently, this is the price exacted in industrial societies for the privilege of easy access to food. But, rather than falling into the trap of accepting all that is put out there, with due respect tothe industrial giants who claim that production of food requires countless additives from start to finish, there are those of us who value our health enough to seek out sources of quality food.

Eating healthfully is not a new concept. Ancient cultures have considered diet essential to health. *Ayurveda*, as described in the above chapter advocates a diet based on a person's body type. The Chinese cook special meals containing combinations of proteins, herbs and vegetables to cure specific diseases. Traditional diets in Japan, India and other cultures that have not been contaminated with Western prepared foods, appear to prevent diseases such as cancer and heart disease. Even the diets in the USA before World War II were considerably healthier since packaged and fast foods were not as prevalent as today.

Can diet make a difference in coping with glaucoma? We have good evidence that diet does indeed cast both shadows and light on some forms of cancers, colon especially, certainly in control of diabetes, and most probably in cases of atherosclerosis, high cholesterol, macular degeneration, and cataract development. Studies at The Schepens Eye Research Institute confirm findings that a diet high in dark green vegetables and orange fruits and vegetables do make a difference in eye health. In the *Blue Mountain Study* people eating more fruits and vegetables had less cataract and macular degeneration. In the Harvard School of Public Health's ongoing study of some 70,000 physicians, two groups of foods were found effective for preventing heart and other diseases. Longitudinal studies are beginning to reveal that diet does, indeed, have an effect on the eyes. An ongoing study in Beaver Dam, Colorado found that those who ate foods containing fat and cholesterol were more likely to develop macular degeneration than those who limited their intake of these foods. A comprehensive review published in the *Review of Ophthalmology* of analyzing data from 1,584 women revealed that eating fresh fruits and dark greens (collards and kale) were protective of glaucoma. The studies are still considered exploratory but the trend is evident. Fresh fruits and vegetables do make a difference.

As people age, many of them experience along with eye problems and heart disease. Eating fresh, not canned, fruit provided the greatest protection for heart-disease. Oatmeal and whole grain cereals cooked in water without added sugar also significantly prevented heart disease. Oatmeal, usually cooked at relatively low temperatures, was found to be the most protective of the whole grain cereals. Shredded Wheat and Cheerios also worked. But because these two cereals, like most cold cereals, are baked at high temperatures, the protein intrinsic to cereals becomes glycated (bound) with the starch component of these grains and produces acrylamides also found in fried foods such as French fries, potato chips, potato wedges, etc. Acrylamides are potent carcinogens and possibly neurotoxins. A large order of innocuous French fries contains at least 300 times more acrylamides than the US Environmental Protection Agency allows. Acrylamides are not only a United States issue, but worldwide, for these toxins are found wherever food is cooked and where pesticides such as Roundup, which contains acrylamides, are used. One of the thrusts of glaucoma treatment involves providing neuroprotective measures. Doesn't it make sense then that eliminating dietary neurotoxins in the diet would help to control some of the effects of glaucoma?

Raw foods are considered by some nutritionists to be the answer for providing perfect health. And, indeed, there are now a few restaurants specializing in raw foods that have gained in popularity. Raw foods are life-giving for they provide the full spectrum of enzymes, catalysts that maintain tissues and general body functions and are essential for proper digestion. During cooking, enzymes become degraded and, therefore, less effective. Furthermore, cooking produces *free radicals*; the higher the heat, the more *free radicals*. Cooking also transforms fats changing them into the damaging trans-fatty acids. Enzymes cannot be synthetically produced. Most of those found on the shelves are derived from pigs' pancreas. The body makes its own enzymes. When not enough enzymes are introduced with food, the body must work harder. Digestion is a two-step process. Food sits in the upper stomach for 30-to-45 minutes where the exogenous enzymes (those that are part of the food) do their thing; then when the food travels to the lower stomach, endogenous enzymes step in.

Fermented foods, sprouts and juices, chock full of enzymes, aid digestion. Benjamin Lane, OD, who practices nutrition along with eye care, claims that a raw or barely cooked food diet does help those with glaucoma. He has also suggested that raw foods may help to reverse or prevent myopia, a risk factor in open-angle glaucoma. Aside from Lane's anecdotal evidence, there are no studies on diet and glaucoma comparable to the well-documented Harvard study of physicians on heart health and other diseases. A vegetarian diet, nevertheless, eliminates most of the arachidonic acid produced by meat and dairy products. Excess arachidonic acid elevates inflammation that not only affects the health of the eyes but is held in some part responsible for joint disease. A study suggests also that benzene may harm the bone marrow, the site of blood cell manufacture, possibly causing leukemia and other blood ailments. Dioxin, although long banned as a pesticide in the US, is still ubiquitous in the world's environment. Vegetarians who eat organic foods are most likely to have the lowest dioxin levels in their tissues. An important amino acid, glutamine, found abundantly in the blood, is derived from high protein foods such as meat, fish, legumes and dairy. Glutamine is an essential amino acid and plays a major role in the immune function. It is also converted to glutamate. Should you, therefore, cut down on the amount of animal protein ingested to prevent excess glutamate activity in the eye? Without research evidence, it's hard to say but the guidelines for protein ingestion of a three-ounce serving at a sitting makes eminent good sense in the light of glutamine's prevalence in the blood.

It is well known that as people age, visual sensitivity is lost due to the loss of neurons. The bid for retaining and protecting the remaining neurons is abetted by a diet high in carotenoids, the vitamins found in fruits and vegetables. Measurement of visual sensitivity in older people who ate a diet high in carotenoids compared favorably with younger individuals. Eating a high-carotenoid diet maintained the thickness of the macula pigment, the part of the eye that is implicated in macular degeneration and visual sensitivity. Now that's food for thought—can diet reverse accepted theories on the aging process? It is certainly a non-invasive way to promote a healthier environment for your eyes. Your doctors are available to treat conditions that require various medical and surgical interventions that will hopefully enhance the quality of life, but you have a part in your health maintenance as well, for when in good health you seek treatment for a particular condition, chances are that medical therapy and surgical outcomes will be more successful. When a disease manifests, it is worthwhile to examine your entire routine and make changes where needed. While it is difficult to ascertain exactly why you suddenly have a certain condition, the onset of this condition is a signal to explore the reasons that your system has broken down. This may be the ideal time to embark in a journey heeding your body's needs.

IMMUNE SYSTEM IMPLICATIONS

A healthy diet helps to build a strong immune system. Nearly every cell, organ and tissue is involved in the immune process. The immune system contains two main components. Innate immunity, the oldest part, dates back millions of years. Learned or acquired immunity is a continuous interaction between the body and the environment. Innate immunity possesses many functions. The skin and mucous membranes offer nearly impenetrable shields against most microorganisms. Dead cells cover the live cells in the skin protecting the live cells from damage. It is nonspecific and includes barriers such as intact skin, and healthy mucous membranes that in the nasal passages, trap pathogens. In the body the white cells mount a magnificent defense system against invading pathogens. The macrophages, neutrophils, eosinophils recognize a bacteria and work to rid the body of it. The presence of the lymphocytes, the T and the B cells communicate between an innate acquired immunity via immune messenger chemicals that are called cytokines-- messenger peptides that are small peptides modulating all facets of the immune response. They are manufactured as needed. Acquired immunity includes the T helper cells that are differentiated into TH1 and TH2 that fight intracellular organisms, TH2 produces antibodies.

Five major types of white cells, the lymphocytes, monocytes, polymorphonuclear cells or neutrophils, basophils and eosinophils play their roles. Innate immunity includes the neutrophils, basophils, eosinophils, monocytes and a subset of monocytes called macrophages. Each cell in the body has a self-marker that identifies it as a part of the body. If it lacks that self-marker, the cell is destroyed by one of the above sentries.

The learned part of the immune system reacts to the environment. The white blood cells involved in this process are the B and T lymphocytes. Each is in charge of different aspects of learned protection. B-lymphocytes are in charge of humeral immunity, mainly the immunoglobulin, proteins that act against foreign bodies. These proteins are known as antibodies (antigens) and are divided into five major classes, each of which has a different function. The T-lymphocytes are the immune arm referred to as cellular immunity. These are responsible for defense against deeper bacterial infections, strong viruses, most fungi, cancer and parasitic infections. They are responsible for protecting the body against most chronic, disabling and fatal diseases. A sub-group of T-lymphocytes, the T-helper cells (CD4's) issue commands in chemical codes and are known as cytokines. The T-helpers essentially keep the body healthy by swiftly responding to an insult. The T-helpers along with other T-lymphocytes are educated in the thymus gland, necessitating an active and vigorous thymus.

The thymus is slightly larger than the heart at birth. It takes about two years to mature, reaches its maximum output in the mid-teens and then slowly decreases in size, efficiency and output. By the age of seventy, the average person has less than ten percent thymus output as was present at the age of fifteen. How is the thymus related to glaucoma? A lowered output of thymus may indeed affect the eyes. And some researchers have taken note. Dr. Michal Schwartz, in Israel, has been working on using T-lymphocytes as a treatment for glaucoma. Other researchers have recommended the use of thymus extracts, (used in Europe for the past fifty years) to treat deeper, more protracted illnesses. Should you want to explore restoring your thymus function and, by extension, investigate the impact of the endocrine glands such as the adrenals or thyroid that also may have an effect of glaucoma, do work with an endocrinologist.

Low thyroid (hypothyroid) function may be a problem associated with glaucoma although the evidence is anecdotal. The conversion of T4 to T3, the most active form of the thyroid hormone, is controlled by the pituitary and hypothalamus glands. In the conversion process, about ninety percent of T4 and ten percent of T3 is produced. This process takes place in the liver producing oxidative stress. The main components of the thyroid system include: hypothalamus, pituitary, thyroid gland and its enzymes, adrenal glands and glucocorticoids, cytokines (hormone-like substances that play a role in modulating physiological function and are also part of the immune function as described above), cellular membranes, mitochondria, and cell nuclear receptors. A malfunctioning thyroid can play host to a large number of diseases, among them Raynaud's syndrome, a peripheral vascular disease that has been associated with glaucoma. Thyroid problems have been approached by targeting underlying causes. In an article entitled "The Thyroid Gland: Cures, Fallacies and Fixes," Dr. D. Yurokovsky cites a book called *Wilson's Syndrome* in which Dr. Wilson states that a dysfunction of the bioenergy systems of the body account for thyroid conditions. Dr. Wilson has used low-dose cortisone, and notes successful treatment outcomes.

Again, as we have stated above, should you want to explore whether your hormones are involved in your glaucoma condition, do work with a physician who can offer the proper support. That said there is a need for more research to determine whether hormones do have an effect on glaucoma conditions. Women, especially, appear (observation on my part) to be especially vulnerable during peri-menopause or menopause to develop glaucoma.

INFLAMMATION

Can allergies affect glaucoma? Yes, possibly an allergic response to food can trigger an inflammatory response in the entire body and that includes the eyes. According to Jeffrey Morrison, MD, who presented a lecture to our Group, allergies to certain foods may cause low-level chronic inflammation resulting in elevated IOPs. Most of us become aware of allergic reactions when we eat foods that produce a rash or a skin eruption. But invisible allergies may cause inflammatory responses within the body not readily apparent. These are the dangerous ones, for hidden inflammation is responsible for worsening of many diseases. By identifying and avoiding food(s) to which you may be allergic, you may possibly reduce and prevent vision loss. Milk, wheat, soy, tomatoes, and oranges cause the most common allergic reactions, but all foods eaten on a daily basis, however healthy, can end up triggering allergic symptoms. Generally, people tend to eat an unvaried diet that invites the build-up of allergies. Should you wish to know if you are allergic or sensitive to foods, test it. A drop of a food essence is pricked into your arm and if a reaction occurs, you've developed sensitivity to that food. In this case, remove the food from your daily routine for a period of time. It's not forever. Within months, you can resume eating the food, but remember variety is the spice of life. You've probably noticed, although most hospital food is blandly prepared, that should you be staying for several days, different fruits and vegetables are offered each day.

Allergic reactions to food occur less frequently with a rotating diet. Variety can exist within the spectrum of a single vegetable such as potatoes where the russet no longer rules as the only available spud. True variety may be hard to come by, however, for although the supermarket shelves are brimming with produce, in truth, just nine crops now account for over three-quarters of the plants consumed by humans. Fortunately, in many parts of the country, farmers' markets offer a greater variety.

Many people are lactose intolerant and find they cannot drink milk or eat milk products. These people lack sufficient lactase, an enzyme necessary to digest milk sugar. If you are lactose intolerant, skip the dairy products and seek other dietary sources of calcium such as dark green leafy vegetables, sardines or canned salmon with the bones. To moisten your cereal or for use in cooking, any of the processed milks—soy, rice, almond, grains—are good substitutes. Early in my glaucoma history, I explored food allergies and discovered that wheat, milk and eggs primarily caused my allergic reactions. When I eliminated these foods, my health improved to the extent that my headaches vanished and my energy increased. I've had glaucoma for more than thirty years, and while the sight in one eye is not what it used to be, the sight in the other gives me good near and far vision and is holding its own. Miriam, a vegan (with fish) at the age of 86 with a genetic disposition for the exfoliation syndrome, shows no signs of glaucoma, although her mother was blinded from the disease.

Achieving a healthy body is an investment. Evidence of diet and exercise for continued good health was documented in a study that over a seven-year period monitored seniors. Those healthy at the beginning remained healthy. Health predictors included high HDL (the good cholesterol), non-diabetic, thinner carotid arteries, lower blood pressure, lower C-reactive protein (an inflammatory process in the blood), regular exercise, not taking aspirin or smoking.

A good diet, free of preservatives (the body cannot digest or breakdown preserved foods) maintains healthy tissues. Studies have documented a good diet's effects on other eye diseases such as retinitis pigmentosa and age-related macular degeneration (ARMD), which has also yielded to a diet rich in deep green vegetables. Additionally, a healthy diet promotes better blood flow. While large double-blind studies have not yet confirmed this theory, I feel I have profited from a wholesome diet as have some of my compatriots in the glaucoma group. Taking charge of what and how you eat is but another rung on the ladder of assuming responsibility for your own health and the course of your treatment. Furthermore, a well-balanced diet strengthens your immune system, an important factor for the maintenance of health, as noted above.

THE CHOICE IS YOURS

You're in charge of what you put into your body, what article of clothing you choose to wear, your particular lifestyle. You're the manager of your body, your mind, your spirit. You're also responsible for what makes you feel good. Within reason, if you choose a particular diet, one you've become accustomed to, changing it might feel like deprivation. Your brain has come to expect what you put into your mouth. This is especially evident on a weigh-loss diet. As you shed weight, your brain becomes alarmed at the starvation messages it's receiving, and signals restoration of lost weight.

The best form of diet is simple--eat whole foods and as much raw fruits and vegetables that you can tolerate. This suggestion is based on credible research. Diets rich in herbs, fruits and vegetables play a significant role in preventing disease, particularly neurodegeneration that is caused by excess *free radicals*. Whole foods provide vitamins, enzymes, amino acids (the building blocks of protein), and fiber necessary for healthy body functions. For example, eggs, once considered cholesterol producing, have been reevaluated by some nutritionists to be a perfect food, provided they are cooked properly. Oxidation is the key here. Frying and hot scrambling exposes eggs to form oxysterols (*free radicals*). Soft, poached, over-easy, hard-boiled do not oxidize the cholesterol in eggs which is harmless in ninety-nine percent of the cases. Properly cooked, eggs are beneficial for they help avoid many of the degenerative diseases such as asthma, arthritis, allergies, cancer, and heart attacks. Furthermore, eggs also assist in the detoxification process, for the egg white contains a bactericidal character that fights infections. Most important, the yolk is rich in quality lutein and zeaxanthin, important for nourishing the *retina*. Spray drying, a process used to make powdered egg yolk, powdered milk, and one and two percent milk, generates oxysterols and should be avoided.

When planning a diet you will want to include a hefty supply of immune-enhancing foods. These are the vegetables and fruits that contain carotenoids of which more than six hundred are known. The flavonoid complex or polyphenols in fruits and vegetables are broken down into five classes--flavones, flavanones, catechins, flavonols, and anthocyanidins. Diets high in carotenoids and flavonoids may offer reduced risk of some cancers, cataracts and heart disease. They enhance immune function and promote anti-inflammatory action. Antioxidant protection from *free radical* damage in both the lipid portions of cells and tissues and water portions inside and outside the cells and tissues are most effective when consumed as families (the total fruit or vegetable). Produce of varying colorings provide a variety of carotenoids. For example, a purple carrot is rich in anthocyanidins; a red one possesses more lycopene; orange, beta carotene; yellow, xanthophylls. The same holds true for lettuce and cauliflower that can be had in several beautiful shades. Phytochemicals and the flavonoids found in select whole unprocessed foods such as spinach, strawberries, grapes, kale, carrots, broccoli, blueberries, cayenne, peppers and buckwheat possess many properties that produce positive reactions that are antioxidant, antiallergenic, anti-inflammatory, antiviral, antiproliferative, and anticarcinogenic. Spinach, for example, has been found to be more effective in reducing neuronal vulnerability to oxidative stress than vitamin E of equal antioxidant capacity. Quality anthocyanidins found in beets, blackberries, blueberries, cherries, red grapes and purple cabbage protect capillaries, blood vessels and collagen formation from oxidative damage. Blueberries, especially, are highly recommended. Here's a wonderful tasting fruit that can affect the brain. A study of rats fed blueberry extract learned faster and improved their motor skills. Figs contain more antioxidants than cherries, grapes or strawberries and more fiber and minerals than most other fruits and vegetables. Five to six small dried figs pack 244 mg of potassium, 1.2 mg of iron, and 5 grams of fiber, while delivering only 108 calories. The sulfur compounds found in garlic, onions, shallots, leeks, scallions, broccoli, nettles, Brussels sprouts, cabbage, cauliflower, sprouts, mustard greens, radishes and turnips improve estrogen balance and fight tumors. Vegetables that contain chlorophyll found in beet greens, bok choy, collards, nettles, greens, and blue green algae enhance the immune system. Caution–don't overcook your vegetables, raw is better since no enzymes are lost, but seniors may need to lightly steam such vegetables as broccoli, cabbage, cauliflower, etc. to promote digestion.

Some nutritionists claim that sprouts are superfoods and should be included in the diet. While sprouts are indeed valuable foods providing high concentrations of antioxidant nutrients such as vitamins A, C, E, and B, minerals (selenium and zinc), bioflavonoids, superoxide dismutase, chlorophyll and fiber, they must be kept fresh and free of fungus. But raw sprouts do contain eighty-five percent more bioavailability nutrients than cooked foods and are worth adding to your diet.

Scientists using advanced fluorescent microscopy have formed a clearer image of developmental plant processes, which provides an interesting insight on why plant foods are protective. In the presence of light, the plant develops flavonoids as protective mechanisms. These are the important *free radical* scavengers that are passed on to us when we eat quality plant-based foods. Ninety-nine percent of the intake of fruits and vegetable juices are absorbed efficiently and a steady diet of these insures optimum nutrition.

Wonderful and healthy flavor enhancers include the entire allium family. All of the alliums (garlic, onions, leeks, shallots, and scallions) have antibacterial and antifungal properties, but garlic tops the list. To use garlic most effectively chop, mash or mince and add to your dish just before serving. High heat destroys its beneficial properties. Ginger is another terrific flavoring. It aids digestion and it too, should be added just before serving.

Vegetarians and persons who rely heavily on soy as a protein in their diet might want to consider findings on this food. Tofu is said to be high in the amino acid glutamate that is implicated in *retinal* cell death and may be linked to a finding of mental decline in Japanese-American men living in Hawaii. Researchers Sally Fallon and March G. Enig, Ph.D, claim that soy does more harm than good, while Bill Sardi, health reporter, refutes all counts. On the other hand, the isoflavones found in soy and lecithin (a soy product) increase the action of the antioxidant enzymes catalase, superoxide dismutase and glutathione peroxidase, important for eye health. There is evidence that soy lowers lead levels in the blood. The calcium in soy-based foods may keep the body from absorbing and retaining lead. Because of the controversy about soy, I've cut down but not eliminated my intake. Another consideration for limiting soy foods is the processing-- using heat to manufacture soy-substitute foods such as burgers, cheeses, spreads, meats, etc. Some nutritionists, however, especially those committed to vegetarianism, still claim soy is a good food, but suggest that it be used as in Asia, as an accompaniment to the main dish, not a sole source of protein.

Diet, especially among the more affluent who can afford choice seems to be on everyone's mind. Book shelves in bookstores on the diet and nutrition groan under the burden of diet books. Take your pick. You can go with the New Diet Revolution by Dr. Atkins, The South Beach Diet, The Zone, or any of the other books touting that adhering to a particular diet will melt off excess poundage and improve health. Or you might want to consider following the glycemic index and eat only foods that deliver a minimum amount of carbohydrates to your diet. Some diets advocate eating only fruits in the morning, others stress starting off with a breakfast that is the main meal of the day and tapering off to less food as the day progresses. Still others suggest eating six or more small meals throughout the day. And there are those claiming that body type is destiny and split humans into two categories--high and low food metabolizers. And then there are some that hark back to imitating the primitive diet of hunters and gatherers.

Some diets do seem to work. The Atkin's diet and others that followed this same vein called attention to excess carbohydrate intake, measured in some part by the glycemic index. Given the explosion of obesity in the United Stated and other western civilizations, this theory bears consideration. Over-consumption of high-glycemic foods can cause excessive production of insulin even in healthy people especially with increasing age. The blood glucose response after eating a high-glycemic diet can be twice as high as after eating a low one. In addition to adding pounds, this insulin surge contributes to chronic inflammation (as discussed above) and glycation, a binding of a protein molecule to an insulin molecule. This condition leads to formation of damaging non-functional structures in the body contributing to such manifestations as cataract, neurological impairment and arterial stiffening. The glycemic index measures how quickly fifty grams of a given carbohydrate are digested. Food that is digested more rapidly may raise blood sugar, prompting the pancreas to deliver insulin in an attempt to restore blood sugar levels. A high glycemic index, resulting from eating foods that are rapidly digested, taxes the insulin system and may lead to insulin resistance and diabetes. Foods high on the list of the glycemic index include white bread, food made from refined starches, baked potatoes, peas, prepared foods, sugary foods and drinks. Foods lower down the scale include legumes, whole grains and nuts, fruits, vegetables especially the deep green ones. The American Diabetes Association, the American Heart Association and experts who determine the federal government's dietary guidelines, however, consider the science on the glycemic index to be incomplete, and do not recommend following it too rigidly. Shunning carbohydrates for all members of the population loses sight of individual differences, such as those who are lean and healthy and who do not put on weight eating carbohydrates. I'm one of them. For years I could eat anything without adding a pound of weight. I still weigh what I did when in high school.

Should white potatoes or pasta never pass your lips? Not at all. Actually the denseness of pasta lowers the glycemic value, and fat, usually part of a pasta preparation, slows absorption reducing glycemic indications. It's best not to drive yourself crazy looking at figures. As the ancient Greeks said, live your life in moderation.

Grains, once considered the staff of life, unfortunately in western societies, have taken a back seat due to the high carbohydrate content. The problem lies not with the grain itself, but from the refining process, a method for removing the important bran and hull layers to render the grain more "palatable" read more easily digested. But rapid digestion quickly metabolizes the grain into sugar, a process that overloads the system with excess glucose. Whole, unrefined grains take longer to digest and therefore, the release of sugar is slowed down allowing the body to assimilate and effectively use the glucose produced. Whole grains are a good food. They brim with fiber, the B-vitamins--thiamine, riboflavin, niacin, B6, the minerals--magnesium, zinc, copper and iron and other plant constituents that nourish the body and protect against disease. Grains, the seeds or fruits of grasses (except buckwheat and amaranth that comes from plants) are composed of three layers, the inner germ, the surrounding packet of starch and the layer of bran--all encased in a hull and all of these components are healthy to eat. Grains receiving the highest score according to Nutrition Action Newsletter are quinoa, amaranth, buckwheat groats, bulgar, barley, wild rice, brown rice, triticale and wheat berries.

The Europeans, Asians and other cultures, who do not struggle as much as the Americans with obesity are in many cases, especially among the non-city dwellers, interested in food as a major enjoyment in life. For example, in Tuscany, a province of Italy (the Italian or Mediterranean diet is touted for its health-giving properties), eating is considered one of the major activities of the day. The midday meal, for which five or six dishes are prepared, may take well over two hours. Wine accompanies the meal. It is a social gathering looked forward to with great pleasure. After the meal light exercise and a nap sets one up for the rest of the day. Compare this manner of eating to a sandwich at your desk for lunch and a take-out dinner at night possibly eaten in front of the television set. Unfortunately, fast food is making an inroad in Europe and this wonderful way of eating may go the way of the Edsel (a car that flunked the market.)

PLANNING YOUR DIET

Planning your meals should not be a complicated affair. There are now so many cookbooks devoted to the long and short of it that by consulting one or two, you can probably find nutritious recipes that fit into your agenda. Simply follow a few rules. Servings of breads, cereals and pasta (whole grain please) should be limited to two or three servings. Increase the servings of vegetables and fruits to seven or eight. Two to three servings of milk, yogurt, enriched soy or rice milk or cheese should be adequate. Two to three servings of protein foods such as meat, poultry, fish, or legumes should round out your meal intake for the day.

Eat fresh foods wherever possible. Fresh fruit is better than canned. Fresh-squeezed juices have somewhat higher vitamin content and taste better than pasteurized or reconstituted juices, but the whole fruit is even better. Purple, red and blue fruits highest in anthocyanidins; include fruits in the melon family. When not in season substitute frozen organic berries (raspberries, blueberries, blackberries in your diet). Make a smoohie. Cut up one frozen banana. Add ½ cup of any of the frozen berries. Process in your food proceesor. Serves two.

Surprisingly, some foods considered high in calories belie this premise. Three ounces of lobster minus the dipping sauce has eighty calories, one tablespoon of whipped cream has eight. Two ounces of smoked salmon, sixty-six, twelve large shrimp, sixty; one-half cup of water chestnuts, thirty-five; three and a half ounces Portobello mushrooms, grilled or roasted with a brush of olive oil, twenty-five.

Some people may be in a quandary as to whether to include dairy products. There are some nutritionists who believe that dairy products are not suitable for adults since nature intended milk to be fed primarily to infants and toddlers. Furthermore, because these nutritionists claim that adults do not need this food, they have suggested that dairy products contribute to various physical ailments such as arthritis and inflammation. Justification for these theories has not been proven, albeit that some societies have existed thousands of years without eating dairy products and have been found to be generally healthy and less prone to disease. They, as with people from other cultures such as Africans, Asians in general and some people of Mediterranean ancestry, may be genetically lactose intolerant. But like so many foods we were told to avoid, there is a movement now to again include dairy products in the diet.

Vegetables providing the most bang for the buck are the dark green leafy ones such as spinach (high in folate, iron, lutein and zeaxanthin), kale (high in calcium, potassium, phytochemicals and B vitamins), collards (high in calcium, beta-carotene, phyto-chemicals) and dandelion greens (a superb liver cleanser—high in potassium). Also good liver cleansers include celery, lettuce and cucumber. Parsley, a wonderful diuretic, included daily, may ease bloating and is a great source of iron, potassium and vitamin C and A. Parsley also contains the essential oil, *apiole* that is a kidney stimulant. Dried is less nutritious than fresh raw parsley. Other foods high in carotenoids and flavonoids include apricots, broccoli, butternut squash, yams, sweet potatoes, pumpkin, cantaloupe, carrots, dark leafy greens, endive, Swiss chard, mangoes, papaya, peaches, pink grapefruit, red bell peppers, strawberries, tomatoes (high in lycopene), apples, beets, berries, and cherries. Nettles are one of the few vegetables high in amino acids and also are a good source of calcium. All members of the allium family (onions, garlic, shallots, leeks, scallions) should also be included.

Lightly steam vegetables or eat raw or pureed to get the biggest antioxidant boost. Eat fruits in season. These appear to be better absorbed. If imported fruits are not organic they may contain pesticides and other chemicals. Even if organic, imported fruits have most likely been picked green and will be lacking in flavor and texture and possibly nutritive value.

For protein and minerals, eat one or two servings daily of fish, chicken, or turkey. (Note that the standard serving size is three ounces.) Chicken or turkey should be skinned and the fat trimmed away. Red meat and pork--if you must have them at all--can be used to diversify your diet, if they are trimmed of all fat. A word about pork. Both Muslims and religious Jews because of religious dictums do not eat it. This ancient wisdom may have some dietetic merit. It is known that pigs are scavengers. They have a pus build-up instead of sweat glands making their flesh acidic and toxic. It is believed by some nutritionists that pork cannot be physiologically metabolized and assimilated by humans like beef, venison, lamb or chicken.

Lane, an optometrist-nutritionist, advises against eating both a heavy protein diet and the use of trans-fatty acids. In a small study he conducted, hydrogenated fats called trans-fatty acids (hardened fats such as margarine and shortening) and a heavy protein intake was associated with *pigmentary-dispersion* and *exfoliative* glaucomas. It's easy to eat lots of protein because restaurants, including fast food outlets, serve huge helpings of meat, poultry and fish. Well-cooked protein, according to Lane, prevents transaminase enzymes in the gut from converting the denatured amino acids from the diet to make the amino acids required for special proteins into "original-equipment" quality proteins to assure non-leaking "tight" junctions in the continual remodeling of *Bruch's membrane*, the tissue that separates the *retinal* from the choroid in the eye.

As the body remodels *Bruch's membrane* with the surrogate proteins, with time the membrane begins increasingly to leak, producing the appearance of so-called "age-related" "wet" or "leaking" *Exudative Macular Degeneration*. Then, as persons consume excessive damaged fats and oils, the risk for leakage is increased through the leaky junctions. The risk of acquiring more leaky junctions is mitigated by the fact that a person eating 100 grams of food is also recycling about 60 grams of his own uncooked bodily protein as the body remodels key tissues.

Lane posits that most people eat too much protein and that even the recommended Dietary Allowance (RDA) for protein is too high for people in their forties, fifties, and sixties. People in their seventies and beyond may be ingesting the right amount of protein but may still turn up with *macular degeneration* and Lane attributes this to a lifetime of eating well-done protein with its subsequent accumulating damage to *Bruch's membrane*.

Eat fish. When purchasing fish, the smaller, the better. Fresh sardines are good. Big fish should be eaten rarely because toxic chemicals such as mercury may accumulate in their tissues. Is fish a brain food as grandma used to say?

Possibly, and as you are probably aware, the eye is a part of the brain. The sight-saving benefits of eating cold water fish such as salmon, mackerel and herring together with vitamins A and DHA capsules has been demonstrated in several studies of *retinitis pigmentosa* patients. A New Zealand study involving over 4,000 adults fifteen years or older compared fish eaters with abstainers. The fish eaters had higher mental health status. The researchers attribute this finding to the presence of higher omega 3 fatty acids--eicosapentaenoic acid (EPA) and docosahexaenoic acid (DHA). Fish high in the omega 3's include Pacific herring, 2.4 grams, Atlantic herring, 2.3 grams, Pacific or jack mackerel, 2.1 grams, Atlantic salmon 1.1 grams, sablefish 2.0 grams. Fish containing 1-2 grams include canned pink salmon, whitefish, Pacific oysters, Atlantic mackerel, sockeye or red salmon, Coho salmon, bluefish, trout, Eastern oysters, rainbow smelt, whiting, and hake. Tuna has only 0.3 grams. Imitation crab made from pollock has none. Of course, you need to bear in mind that you may be weighing nutritional fats against fish that are contaminated with organic mercury.

But is fish safe given the pollution of the rivers, lakes and oceans? According to the Maine's Natural Resources Council, the safest fish are haddock, cod, hake, flounder, Atlanta salmon, herring, smelts, clams, shrimp, scallops, lobster (don't eat the tomalley which can contain dioxin), and canned light tuna although other studies find tuna high in mercury. Shell fish once considered high in cholesterol are actually lower than found in chicken or beef. The safest fresh water fish are brook trout, yellow perch, and land-locked salmon. Vegetarians are advised to include fish. Three to six ounces of cooked fish is considered a good serving.

People who are concerned with the environment may find themselves in a quandary in choosing which fish are environmentally harvested. The choice narrows considerably when this is taken into account. Farmed shrimp displace mangroves and wetlands and are treated intensively with antibiotics and the waste from the operation pollutes surrounding waters. "Wild caught" seafood usually means that trawl nets dragging the bottom are destroying the ocean floor and, furthermore, fishermen discard pounds and pounds of other creatures caught in the nets. Scallops are preserved by soaking in phosphates and then sitting in a pool of water (use dry scallops). Farmed salmon have a high level of sea lice that are now infecting wild salmon. Disregard of the environment ends up hurting all of us, for such blinkered behavior which may for a short time sustain a fishing industry, in the long run, results in poisoning the waters and increasing the toxic levels found in seafood.

A CUP OF--Some of us who can't get through the day without a morning cup of coffee. And that's fine, for coffee like tea has its share of anxioxidants. One or two cups of coffee are not a problem. If the coffee intake, however, averages out to ten or more cups a day, serious health problems may occur. Coffee can acidify your system which should be on the alkaline side. Furthermore, the caffeine in coffee reduces blood flow to the brain. And a recent finding indicated that brain scans are thrown off by ingesting a few cups of coffee previous to the scan. A more profound problem may occur with some people who are allergic to caffeine. Such an allergy decreases blood flow to the brain and may cause obsessive-compulsive disorder (persistent thoughts, ideas or impulses.

TEA Although pound for pound, tea contains more caffeine than coffee, a pound of tea yields several hundred cups while a pound of coffee beans less than one-hundred cups. An eight-ounce cup of coffee may contain from 60-to-180 mg of caffeine; a similar serving of tea 20-to-90 mg. Decaffeinated versions of both have less than five milligrams of caffeine, about the same as an ounce of milk chocolate.

A study published in the Proceedings of the National Academy of Sciences offered direct evidence of the potent antioxidant properties of tea. Five cups a day has been shown to boost the activity of the immune system by stimulating the production of the antigen, alkylamine, an amino acid in tea that acts as a precursor to other important antigens. Antigens are immune-system components prompting the body to form antibodies that provide the immune system with disease-fighting abilities. Drinking tea (black, green, and oolong) spurs the liver to process L-theanine into the alkylamine antigen which in turn, prompts certain immune cells (gamma delta T cells) to mount a memory response. Green tea (*Camellia sinensis*) has become a hot item in the health food industry. It contains the highest amount of antioxidants--one cup delivers 30-to-40 mg of *epigallocatechin galate*. Several polyphenols, *EGCG,* found in tea enhance glutathione peroxidase and catalase and are potent free-radical scavengers. Other benefits from drinking tea include protection of arteries from plaque, protective effects from cancer, possibly an increase in bone density, decrease of the severity of arthritis and reduction of cataract formation. An animal study proved positive in inhibiting oxygen-induced neovascularization (runaway blood vessels). In young women, however, green tea may impair ability to absorb iron from vegetables.

SALT Excess sodium has been implicated in the development of high blood pressure, strokes, calcium deficiency, osteoporosis, fluid retention, weight gain, stomach ulcers, and stomach cancer. The average American's salt intake is two to three teaspoons per day, providing 4,000-to-6,000 mg of sodium, far more than what the body needs. Since we evolved in a low-sodium environment, our body is designed to hang on to whatever sodium it receives. According to the Institute of Medicine, under normal circumstance, daily intake of sodium should not exceed one teaspoon in total—that includes also the salt added to prepared foods. We absorb salt from food, the salt softened water we drink and bathe in and from clothes washed in the water because it is efficiently absorbed through the skin. Use sea salt and go the natural way.

WATER is a nutrient. The faithful drink eight or more glasses of water a day. There are those who may feel that they can't possibly ingest that much water. Some nutritionists suggest dividing your weight in half and imbibing that many ounces—half of one hundred fifty pounds would be seventy-five ounces. Recent research adds up all beverages as part of your liquid intake. A report from the Institute of Medicine found that a total consumption of liquids equivalent to ninety-one ounces of fluids for women and one hundred twenty-five ounces for men was adequate. Of course, the need for additional water increases with strenuous exercise and in hot weather. I appreciated this information for I found it difficult to drink eight cups of water in addition to other beverages.

The benefits of hydrating your system are manifold, for water flushes toxins from your system while hydrating the cells and tissues. Water is the principal chemical component of the body. It comprises sixty-five percent of the body weight for males and fifty-five percent for females. Metabolic activity requires water, and it is the medium in which chemical reactions take place in your body. Surrounding the cells, it provides a medium for substances to be transported throughout the body. Do not wait to feel thirsty. Drink up--it's important for your health.

Quality of water, however, may be an issue. Long ago the purity of water was a given right. Today, this assumption may be questionable. Controversy swirls over whether the additives such as chlorine to kill organisms and fluoride to protect children's teeth against cavities cause more harm than good. While some may consider chlorine a necessity given the deadly contaminants present in the water supply, a small but vocal group opposes widespread fluoridation. Over the thirty years of water purification, children ingesting fluoridated water had an increase in dental fluorosis (mottled and brittle teeth.) Persons taking fluoride for osteoporosis may find their symptoms worsening and contrary to some reports, fluoride does little to prevent fractures, for while it increases bone density, bone strength and bone quality is decreased. Of interest to glaucoma patients is fluoride's effect on the arteries. It promotes calcification and in some people, visual disturbances. Earlier in the twentieth century fluoride was prescribed for persons suffering from hyperthyroidism. Drinking fluoridated water can, therefore, have an unwanted effect on the thyroid. Many seniors suffer from hypothyroidism. There are also reports linking fluoride to cancer and to *Alzheimer's*. Fluoride is a direct byproduct of aluminum production and is an extremely toxic agent. It is registered as a pesticide for killing rodents. In undiluted form it is corrosive and eats through metal. The industry involved in manufacturing aluminum and other products such as fertilizers would be forced to dispose of fluoride at great expense, a disposal that would require a class-one landfill. It was reasoned, therefore, that an ideal vehicle for fluoride disposal would be the so-called purification of water.

Another problem exists with the addition of aluminum to the drinking water. This is an agent used to gather together small particles. Aluminum and fluoride form a number of complexes, the most deadly being aluminum tetrachloride. Most of Western Europe and some cities and counties in the United States have rejected the use of fluoride in the water supply.

Aside from fluoride contamination of water, the substance is present in toothpaste, aluminum and non-stick kitchenware. Conventially-grown apples and grapes are commonly treated with high fluoride pesticides.

Many people interested in the purity of their water choose to either filter or distill their drinking water. Bottled water considered by many to be free of contaminants may not live up to its promise. Some waters are merely purified tap water (coded P.W.S.). One study found that thirty-three percent of more than one hundred brands tested were contaminated with bacteria, excess fluoride, arsenic and other synthetic chemicals. Unlike the pure water requirements of The Clean Water Act of 1972, bottled water suppliers are not required to meet these standards. Furthermore, discarding the used bottles has become an environmental hazard.

But water is also exposed to medicines. Drugs of all kinds—antibiotics, antidepressants and hormones have been found in our water supplies. They cause genetic mutations in small fish and amphibians, and unfortunately, filtration methods do not always remove these microcontaminants.

You've probably heard about the relationship of drinking lots of water causing a rise in IOP. Yes, this can occur if you drink a quart of water at one sitting. Your pressure does not rise, however, if you sip water throughout the day. So, please do not give up on water. Just be sure that it's pure. For further information on clean water call the EPA Safe Drinking Water Hotline, 1-800-426-4791.

IN GENERAL-- Convenience foods while saving time are in the long run detrimental to health. These foods may contain questionable additives and other unwholesome substances and may be deficient in essential vitamins and nutrients. Try to avoid popping a prepared meal into the microwave, eating at the desk, or ordering in and eating in front of the television to name a few mind-numbing activities associated with eating. Simply doing things with others may be one of the best therapies you can incorporate into your life style. Debra Keston in *The Healing Secrets of Food*, New World Library, 14 Pamaron Way, Novato, CA, 94949 writes that socializing and connecting with others during mealtime is the best health secret. She cites an experiment conducted at the University of Texas where rabbits were fed artery clogging food. Those rabbits that were cuddled and received interaction from their caretaker had sixty percent less plaque in their arteries. Keston also suggests that mindfulness including the cook's preparation and the consequent eating of the food produces better digestion. Consider cooking and eating as a meditative and healing practice.

Not everything grown in nature is good for the body. A new look at capsaicin found in Chili peppers, a staple in many indigenous cultures and in the Southwest of the United States, questions its use as a condiment. Harvard researchers have found hot Chili peppers may cause some forms of arthritis. The chemicals in these peppers are called *capsaicinoids*, which are strong irritants acting on the pain receptors in the skin and mucous membranes. Ongoing research has confirmed *capsaicin* to be a primary cause of the burning pain associated with inflammation, tissue damage and arthritis. These peppers are cousins of the tobacco plant family (*Solanaceae*) and they contain as many toxins as tobacco, placing these peppers in the same league as the dangerous toxin (nicotine) found in tobacco smoke. *Capsaicinoids*, used commercially as a pesticide on fruits and vegetables, are considered by the researchers in this study to be one of the most toxic used today. Glaucoma conditions often carry with them a low inflammatory component and shunning hot peppers may help with this condition.

For those of us who long for a magic bullet, the pace of health changes conferred by diet can be maddeningly slow. Do not despair. It took a long time for that diet lacking the proper nutrients and containing toxic substances to rob your body of its vital energy. Repairing the body is an ongoing process, and results are achieved in extremely small increments. But you will probably find, as I did, that by eliminating foods that you are sensitive to, decreasing the amount of processed foods you eat, avoiding white flour and sugar, and eating the freshest vegetables you can find-- in essence, following the newest guidelines recommended by the U.S. Department of Agriculture--you will provide your body with the nourishment necessary to rebuild and maintain itself.

In general, following a few simple rules requiring more preparation may pay off in better health. For example, to prepare breakfast, instead of using packaged breakfast foods that in many cases are high in empty carbohydrates, cook up a cereal from steel cut oats, raw buckwheat groats, teff, barley, or brown rice. Add honey as a sweetener.

Feeling deprived? There's no reason not to indulge occasionally in the foods you love. You can eat salad dressing, condiments, ice milk, ice cream, sour cream, cream cheese, peanut butter, various chips, potato salad, fried potatoes, cookies, cake, white rice, and fast foods sometimes. They won't hurt you provided you follow the "occasional" rule. But do be careful about potato chips—there's some evidence linking this seemingly benign snack to stomach cancer.

And there's always cocoa. Yes, cocoa. Who can resist a good chocolate bar? Its perfume entices as does its luxurious velvetiness mouthfeel inducing good feelings and a calming of the spirit. The chocolate bar, unfortunately, may contain only twenty percent cocoa along with undesirable sugar, corn syrup, milk fats, dairy products, and hydrogenated oils. Chocolate, however, has gained respect as a healthy food provided that it's made mainly with cocoa, limited sugar and fats. It contains the flavonoid, *theobromine* that incidentally, is toxic to horses and many other animals affecting their kidneys, heart and central nervous system. Healthy for humans in addition to the flavonoids, it contains folic acid, copper, and magnesium. It does have relatively high copper content and should be avoided if eating high-copper foods. Fresh cocoa beans give about ten thousand flavonoids per one hundred grams (about seven tablespoons). Processed, the flavonoids drop to about half. Yet, there is some research that states that the polyphenol amount in one dark chocolate bar is equivalent to two days' worth of fruits and vegetables rivaling Concord grape juice, blueberries and black and green teas. And cocoa powder may be more powerful than green tea as a protective antioxidant food; also cocoa may have an aspirin-like effect on blood clotting. Studies reveal that people who ate a diet rich in cocoa powder and dark chocolate had lower oxidation levels of the bad (LDL) cholesterol, higher blood antioxidant levels, and four percent higher levels of good HDL. Possibly, cocoa can also reduce blood platelets from clumping together and some of the proanthrocyanindins in cocoa trigger production of nitric oxide that helps keep arteries flexible and increases blood flow. Hello. Could chocolate help get blood into the eye? No studies on that score, but the possibility is intriguing. A very small study (twenty male and female patients, mean age forty-three and seven-tenths years) found that untreated hypertension patients with 100 grams daily for 15 days of flavonal-rich dark chocolate significantly decreased blood pressure and serum LDL cholesterol, improved dilation of the brachial artery (main artery of the arm,) and decreased insulin resistance in patients with essential hypertension.

In the meantime, tread carefully. Please do not replace your leafy green vegetables with a large bar of chocolate. Chocolate is high in fat, thirty percent of which is stearic acid that may increase the risk of heart disease. The oxalates in chocolate may contribute to kidney disease. Sweeteners in general are to be avoided and some people are just simply allergic, suffering headaches, eczema, asthma and other ailments. Want to eat chocolate? Make it dark, organic if possible, bitter-sweet and eat it sparingly. A good way to start the day or to give you a lift is to have a cup of chocolate chai. Place a heaping teaspoon of cocoa, a bit of honey, and a teabag in a cup. Pour boiling water and add some soy creamer. Enjoy.

Much of the research on chocolate has been conducted by Mars (the manufacturer of the Mars candy bars). The authors of the research cite that the papers produced have been published in peer-review journals.

Nuts, walnuts in particular, are another beneficial delicious food to include in your daily food intake. They are high in protein and rich in unsaturated fats, vitamin E, fiber, folic acid and other B vitamins, and heart-healthy omega 3 fatty acids. A small study of hypertensive men found a lowering of blood pressure on a walnut-rich diet.

The Bottom Line:

- Have a decent breakfast at home, preferably a hot cereal cooked in water.
- Eat at least three meals a day or four to five combinations of snack and small meals.
- Consume a plant-rich diet with at least sixty-five percent in vegetables and fruits.
- Use foods made from whole grains.
- Snack on fresh nuts (1/2 cup daily.)
- Include wild-caught fish preferably salmon, herring, sardines, mackerel, etc. several times a week.
- Buy poultry or meat from 100 percent grass-fed animals if meat is a part of your diet.
- Minimize dairy products.
- Limit cooking oils; switch to cold-pressed organic olive oil.
- Treat yourself to limited amounts of dark chocolate.
- Drink green tea.

FOOD ABSORPTION & DIGESTION

One of the downsides of the aging process for some of us involves a lessening of our innate ability to absorb all the nutrients from the food we eat. A common problem, *hypochlorhydria* (low stomach acid) may lead to many different diseases. Low stomach acid diminishes electrolyte activity in the body as well as depriving those electrolytes already present of their ionic qualities. The health of the eyes depends upon an adequate supply of B vitamins that in turn needs the soluble electrolyte forms of zinc, magnesium, selenium, sulfur, and manganese. Absorption of vitamin A and B complex depend upon zinc absorption. Increasing the absorption of minerals and vitamins may produce a positive effect on some eye conditions. An adequate amount of the minerals calcium and magnesium are needed to utilize vitamin C that is protective of the lens of the eyes; sufficient absorption of zinc, selenium, vitamin E and taurine are necessary to guard against macular degeneration, and excess nitric acid found in chronic open-angle glaucoma; *blepharitis*, a bacterial infection caused by deficiencies of vitamin A, B complex, C and zinc--all may benefit from stepping up the absorption of foods. Betaine hydrochloride will reestablish stomach acid as do fermented foods, for these are rich in active enzymes. A plentiful supply can be found in such foods as yogurt and kefir, sauerkraut, soy sauce, miso, tempeh (fermented soybean cake), kimchee (a Korean pickled vegetable dish), and cheeses such as Roquefort, Gorgonzola and others with a pungent smell.

Organic apple cider sipped through a straw (to protect your teeth) will stimulate digestive juices. A good diet is meaningless if you are not digesting your food properly. Eating raw foods, especially fruits, vegetables, and sprouts, provide your body with the enzymes necessary to break down foods. Chewing your food thoroughly mixes in saliva that is programmed to jump-start the digestive process. Supplemental enzymes may also be taken to assure proper digestion. Normally, your gut should contain a full quota of beneficial micro-flora necessary for proper digestion, but our modern life style depletes the body of its resources. Antibiotic treatment, chlorinated water, food preservatives, junk foods and pollution all take their toll. You may have heard of probiotics as an aid to digestion. In the presence of a yeast infection, probiotics are almost always lacking. Probiotics are a form of healthy bacteria needed by the body. These are found in foods such as yogurt and cultured milk products. If you decide to take a supplement, be prudent in your choice. Although lactic acid bacteria has a long history of safety in dairy products (the various yogurts using live cultures), probiotics in pill form may be problematic. Any bacterial culture that has no history of prior safe use in humans should be questioned as to whether it has been subjected to toxicological studies. A superior probiotic should play a role in: colonization of the intestinal, respiratory, and urogenital tracts; cholesterol metabolism; inhibiting carcinogenesis by stimulating the immune system; the metabolism of lactose; the absorption of calcium and synthesis of vitamins; reduction of yeast and vaginal infections, constipation, and diarrhea diseases; gastritis and ulcers, and acne and other skin problems. Furthermore, the probiotic strain should produce natural antibiotics, lactic acid and hydrogen peroxide, inhibit bad bacteria, and be able to survive stomach acids. It's a tall order for a supplement. All probiotics degenerate quickly at room temperature, so should be refrigerated immediately.

Minimally-processed foods provide the best quality of amino acids, vitamins E, A, chromium, and magnesium for nourishing the body. Foods especially beneficial include: sprouted or pre-soaked whole grains and legumes, almonds, Brazil nuts, walnuts, sunflower seeds, raw milk cheeses, seed cheeses from sunflower seeds and wheat berries, buttermilk, home-made yogurt or yogurt that contains beneficial bacteria--(*Lactobacillus bulgaricus, Streptococcus thermophilus, L. yugurti, L. acidophilus or L. bifidus* P). These helpful bacteria repopulate the intestines playing an important part in the digestive processes.

DO I HAVE TO BE A PURIST TO PROTECT MY EYES?

Possibly. While a highly-industrialized society has brought us extraordinary medical developments, an incredible technological connectedness through computers, palm pilots, I-Pods, etc., the ability to visit every corner of the globe, the world we live in also has produced excessive pollution, excessive emission of ultraviolet rays, toxic foods, a contaminated environment, ocean depletion, etc.,etc. The list is, unfortunately, lengthy. And although convenience foods appear to be a boon for people too busy to shop and cook, there is a troublesome trade-off in consuming empty calories, such as the breakfast of coffee and donuts. We need to be steadfast to resist the bombardment of ads touting processed foods. What the manufacturers don't tell us is that as soon as food is processed, it loses essential nutrients and even if nutrients are still present after processing, a long shelf life or degradation from the preservatives, which renders the body incapable of digesting the food, the promised nutrients may be lost. So what do you do? Squint at the tiny printed labels spending valuable time or choose instead to prepare fresh food? People who are diabetic who cheat with a sweet roll, possibly raising blood sugar, may be courting diabetic retinopathy. We don't suggest that you become obsessive—that would present other problems affecting your health, but we do submit that an awareness of what you ingest, that if you treat your body (you have no other) as a cherished friend, you will be rewarded with good health.

Optimally, we should not have to wait for the body's distress signals. By building up the habits of sensible nutrition and exercise, many health problems may be averted or at least tempered. Once you take responsibility for your own health you will increase your digestive juices according to a study at Temple University. There is also something to be said for the interaction between the cook and the diners. I find that when I've spent a long happy time in the kitchen preparing food for guests who then do not praise my food, but simple chew away at it, I feel diminished and yes, angry. Incidentally, I don't invite them again. In my experience, confirmed by professional chefs, food tastes better when savored and enjoyed in the presence of good friends and relatives. Even if you live alone, enjoy preparing food and make eating it a high point in your day.

WHY EAT ORGANIC?

Steer Clear of the pesticide, herbicide, fungicide trap.

Exposure to the vast array of chemicals that are now part and parcel of food production and delivery can be easily solved by growing your own or buying organically-produced food. Prices are higher, but if more people buy these products, organic farming will grow and prices may drop. The investment in organic food not only serves to make us healthier, but improves the health of the soil that has been degraded of many of its life-giving minerals. Here are the Federal guidelines for production of organic foods:

- Prohibits use of irradiation, sewage sludge or genetic engineering.
- Requires notification of "drift" of a prohibited substance from a neighborhood property of other source.
- Prohibits use of antibiotics in livestock production.
- Disallows use of pesticides for at least 3 years prior on land to be used for organic farming.
- Sets specific intervals between application of raw manure to crops and their harvest.

These are important guidelines, but because of the widespread use of pesticides, organically-grown foods are not totally free of pesticide. They do, however, contain a much lower dose. For example, these differences have been found in a sample of foods between the levels of pesticide present.

	Organic	Conventional
Grapes	25%	78%
Peaches	50%	93%
Pears	25%	95%
Strawberries	25%	91%
All Fruit	23%	82%
Lettuce	33%	50%
Spinach	47%	84%
Bell Peppers	9%	69%
All vegetables	23%	65%

Environmentalists would, if they could turn back the clock to a time when food was free of dyes, added chemicals, radiation, and dubious enhancements such as the growth hormone given to dairy cows to increase the production of milk. Outbreaks of "mad cow disease" in England, large-scale food-poisoning from salmonella that has infected foods from hamburgers to lettuce to peanut products to cheeses and more, plus bacterial contamination of the water supply in some large cities, are only a few examples of the dangers consumers face daily. In 1994, according to the U.S. Centers for Disease Control and Prevention, some seven million Americans became ill and nine thousand died from acute food poisoning. Clean food may well become a consumer battle against industrial contaminants, as people worldwide become more aware that they are eating coli-poisoned meat, salmonella-infected chicken and eggs, chemically-contaminated seafood, pesticide-laden fruits and vegetables, and a new wave of genetically-altered foods.

Taken into consideration the differences in climate, soil, fertilization and farming practices, many studies point in that direction, although in some cases, claims that organic food is more nutritious are difficult to evaluate, given the variables in food production. Nevertheless, evidence is mounting that food grown organically is of higher quality. A study published in *The Journal of Agriculture and Food Chemistry* that measured the effect of pesticides on certain levels of phytochemicals, found that organic produce measured out to fifty percent more antioxidants. Apparently, when a plant is attacked by insects, and/or shields itself from the sun's rays, it naturally produces phytochemicals such as flavonoids to protect itself. By applying pesticide the pressure is removed from the plant to make more antioxidants. Sustainable farming, without pesticide but with some herbicides and fertilizers, produced the highest levels of disease-fighting compounds. In the above study, corn, strawberries, and a type of blackberry called marion berries were measured. Furthermore, other studies show a greater diversity of plants, bacteria, fungi, nematodes, earthworms, butterflies, spiders, beetles, insects, mammals and birds in organic farmland. Enlightened countries, such as the United Kingdom and those in the European Union, reward farmers with monetary subsidies for careful stewardship of farmland. Another article published in *The Journal of Applied Nutrition* found that organically-grown foods contained higher levels of selenium, a mineral that acts as an antioxidant. In a review of 41 studies and 1,400 comparisons of nutrients, the authors found that organic crops contained significantly more nutrients—vitamin C, iron, magnesium, and phosphorus and significantly less nitrates. The differences were attributed to soil fertility management and its effects on soil ecology and plant metabolism. Faster spoilage of organic foods may be a problem. The level of bacteria remaining on the plant determines the rate of spoilage. Pesticide does kill most of the bacteria and that is one plus. Organic foods harboring a greater amount of bacteria need to be refrigerated immediately to retard spoilage.

Eating food grown on rich top soil aids dentition. An analysis of seventy thousand sailors' dental records indicated that those who ate produce from rich topsoil had fewer cavities than those eating food from depleted soils. A two-year study comparing organic and conventionally-grown apples, peas, potatoes and corn from Chicago markets found twice the nutritional content and far less of the dangerous metal residues of aluminum, lead and mercury when compared with conventional crops.

Growers of conventionally-grown produce counter the claims of organic growers that their foods are healthier claiming that the addition of nitrogen, phosphorus and potassium are the only minerals needed to produce healthy plants. And, indeed, the plants do flourish, but depending upon the quality of the soil may be deficient in manganese, zinc and iron and at least sixty other trace minerals. Both zinc and manganese have been associated with eye health. When these minerals are missing from the soil, the plants take up dangerous metals. A literature review in 1996, found organic fruits and vegetables to have four times more trace elements including more than thirteen times selenium, twenty times calcium and manganese and forty percent less aluminum, twenty-five less lead, twenty-nine percent less rubidium (a soft metallic metal that combusts spontaneously in air). Controversially, Bruce N. Ames, Ph.D., a well-known researcher claims that because of the natural toxins in plants, it should make no difference whether or not one eats organic or conventionally-grown plants. Yet, the RDA's for dog foods are upgraded every three years and farm animals are given a super diet six months before slaughter.

Pesticide accumulated in the body can be measured. A study conducted by the University of Washington of forty households concluded that those children fed on an organic diet had six-to-nine times less toxic pesticides than children fed a conventional diet. Many countries now issue standards for organic farming. Read labels carefully on foods before purchasing. Also, be alert to petitions to the government to weaken the standards in place. Occasionally, industry, searching for waste disposal sites, kites a proposal. One that raised a storm of protest was to use the sludge from waste-disposal plants as fertilizer in organic farming. Consumer outrage beat back this proposal.

Unfortunately, the solution offered by the US government to protect food from contamination by various pathogens lies not in cleaning up at the source of contamination as in Sweden but by irradiating it--a profitable solution for industries' nuclear waste disposal. Effects of radiation exposure include increase of the aflatoxin mold found on peanuts, botulism, and chromosomal damage—a situation that occurred in India where starving children showed signs of radiation poisoning after two months of eating irradiated wheat.

FOOD LABELING

Numbers on the stickers placed on your apples, pears, etc. are codes advising how the food is grown.
- 4011--Conventionally-grown foods carry the numerals 3 or 4
- Genetically-engineered foods carry the numeral 8.
- Organic reads organic on label. Processed organic foods must contain at least ninety-five percent organic content. Made with organic ingredients must contain at least seventy-nine percent organic ingredients.
- Natural is not synonymous for organic.

FREE RADICALS

A free radical is a loose molecule, or a highly-reactive fragment of a molecule, that has an unpaired electron spinning in its orbit. It needs a counterbalance and like a thief, it snatches an electron from an adjacent molecule or donates one of its own to the molecule; either way the molecule is destabilized. This process is called oxidation, hence the term antioxidant—substances to quell *free radicals* or the oxidation of tissues. One of the most feared transactions occurs in the oxygen molecule that, when oxidized, is quite damaging. About five percent of inhaled oxygen becomes oxidized. *Free radicals* multiply. One can generate hundreds of *free radical* reactions damaging cells leading to aging, cataracts, heart disease and other disorders.

Not all reactions are disastrous. Nature seldom imposes a reaction of a substance that has only a negative effect and *free radicals* are no exception. *Free radicals* assist the immune system to squelch pathogens, aid the digestive system to break down the food eaten and fire up the muscles, thoughts and feelings. Observable *free radical* action can be seen on the rusting of metal, the browning of an apple, toasting of foods and the searing action of barbecue to name a few examples. If, however, there is an overload of *free radicals*, the body becomes overwhelmed.

There are many *free radical* stimulators--radiation from electronic equipment, power lines, the sun {ultraviolet A (UVA) and ultraviolet B (UVB) rays}, pollution (ozone, carbon monoxide, nitrogen oxide and particulates), pesticides, and organic solvents—all add to the mix, as do fats—the cooking oils, both saturated and unsaturated when heated to high temperatures. Should the oils be rancid, peroxidizing occurs. Oxidized fats are likely to accumulate in blood vessels and are the source of arterial damage. Other sources include alcohol, tobacco smoke, chlorine, aluminum and fluoride found in drinking water. Aluminum pots should not be used. Shallow breathing reducing oxygen stimulates *free radical* activity. Also, naturally occurring metals such as iron, copper, etc. react with oxygen to form *free radical* activity.

In nature, plants are exposed to a heavy load of oxidizing UV light rays from the sun that generates *free radicals* in plant tissues. Reactive or singlet oxygen is also generated in the chloroplasts (green bodies in the cells of leaves important for photosynthesis). To protect itself, the plant generates a large array of antioxidant chemicals and enzymes, the benefits of which pass on to people eating the plants. Fresh whole foods are the richest in these antioxidant properties. Your body, too, has developed means for protection. In the case of iron, for example, it is safely stored in the red blood cells or is provided with a protein to ferry it where needed.

Should the system be corrupted or if an influx of certain metals overwhelms the body's systems, a chain reaction occurs that generates *free radicals*. It's possible to view *free radical* activity through digital infrared microscopy and scientists have found them in the *retinal* of rats. Possibly, also, many diseases are caused wholly or in part from *free-radical* activity. Among them, cataract formation, macular degeneration, type II adult-onset diabetes, *Alzheimer's*, and *Parkinson's* are suspect. Also, cardiovascular disease may be partially a product of *free radical* activity. In the brain, *free radical* chemical reactions reduce blood flow, a major concern in glaucoma patients. Reactions between *free radicals* and DNA may cause certain types of cancer. And *free radical* activity has been linked to diminished lubricant found in the joints and/or interference with the cells that provide elasticity of the tendons. *Free-radical* activity can also occur during a corrective procedure in the operating room. A study of oxidative stress following laser treatment concluded that antioxidant supplementation should be a part of the treatment.

A *free radical* is an opportunist. It is ready to move into any unprotected organ, and the eyes, exposed to the elements, may be a likely target. As stated above, cataract may be partially caused by *free radicals* damaging the lens of the eye, and the vital nerve tissue in the *retinal* may be subject to oxidation. Is there a way to halt this destructive process? Possibly. Those of us with glaucoma may need to expend extra effort to nourish our bodies.

HEALTHY EATING AS MEDICINE

Enzymes tackle the *free radical* problems--superoxide dismutase (superoxide at low levels plays a role in the signaling pathways); catalase and glutathione peroxidase scavenge and destroy free *radicals*. Another set of enzymes, endonuclease, exonuclease, and polymerase, repair DNA that has suffered *free-radical* damage. Those of us working with computers protected with an anti-viral system trust the system to defend our computers against worms, viruses and other invasive species. Your body, however, needs outside instruction to repair the some ten thousand daily assaults on its DNA from *free radical* activity. Most of the damage is repaired almost immediately. But the job is abetted by antioxidant enzymes extracted from healthy eating, for embedded in that leaf of kale, that spinach salad, a whole orange, an array of fruits, yellow and green vegetables are vitamins and minerals that bolster the antioxidant activity of the enzymes. Dried blueberries can actually serve a medicinal purpose. Pop 3 tablespoons into your mouth when you're suffering from upset stomach or diarrhea.

Extracted from the food we eat, especially high-quality whole foods, vitamins and minerals troop up to the front lines to do their part. Want to know how much lutein and zeaxanthin is contained in one-half cup of cooked foods? Kale tops the list with 10,270 units followed by collard greens at 7,690, spinach 6,340, turnip greens, 6,080, broccoli, 1,740, corn, 1,480, Brussels sprouts, 1,480, peas, 1,150, green beans, 1,010, okra, 440. Raw foods: spinach, 3,580, romaine lettuce, 1,480, carrots (8 baby), 290, one orange 240, orange juice (one cup), 340.

Oxygen Radical Absorbance Capacity (*ORAC*) is a test to measure the antioxidant activity in foods and natural supplements. As measured by ORAC, high levels of antioxidant activity have been found in blueberries, blackberries, and raspberries. The wild blueberry scored higher than the cultivated; pomegranate, black raspberry and high-desert bee pollen scored among the highest. Certain laboratories now screen for levels of polyphenols, aromatic compounds, and a class of nutrients that includes bioflavonoids, organic acids and phenolic acids. Most of the antioxidant activity of a food is created by polyphenols. Generally speaking the more polyphenols the healthier the food. Whole foods give the most for the buck.

By the same token, whole food vitamins should also score high. In general vitamin formulas are based, as in conventional medicine, on a single isolated element, i.e., vitamin C, or beta carotene. Furthermore, these elements are synthesized chemically in the laboratory and are often called "miracle foods" because of the purported belief that this single vitamin will cure or help this or that condition.

Vitamins are complex organic substances necessary for human life and metabolic processes—growth, maintenance and health. Vitamins must be obtained from the food we eat for the body is not capable of manufacturing them. Each vitamin is a complex of chemically-related compounds. When the vitamin group is separated into single portions, the vitamin is converted from an active micronutrient into a debilitated chemical with little value to the living cells. The body is smart and it can select exactly what it needs from whole foods or a whole food complex. This is why vitamins should be taken with meals. They are co-factors and need food to work.

That said, there is apparently a place for supplementation in the human diet. But realize that antioxidant nutrients are a supplement. In no way does a supplement replace the combination of vitamins and minerals found in say, an apple, or a serving of spinach. The most active antioxidant vitamins include A, E and C, the carotenoids, coenzyme Q10, alpha lipoic acid, the bioflavonoids and phenolics (found in dark fruits and vegetables), plus fiber. Some of the important minerals are selenium, zinc, calcium and magnesium.

SUPPLEMENTING A LESS THAN PERFECT DIET

Ideally, the food you eat should supply all the antioxidants and nutrients necessary for a well-nourished body and healthy eyes. But when time is limited, job and home pressures mount, shopping for and preparation of foods may move from front to back burner and swallowing a handful of vitamins may be regarded as the next best thing. According to a small study of twenty active men and twenty active women (24-to-50 years), their diets were below the RDI'S (*Referenced Daily Intakes*) and both males and females recorded 138 micronutrient deficiency out of the possible 340 studied. Bear in mind that these standards, set by the Food and Drug Administration, are considered below what is actually needed for health by many nutritionists. A lead article in *Review of Ophthalmology*, February, 2004, asked *"Can Nutritional Supplements Benefit Ocular Health?* The article cites that despite conflicting evidence on the efficacy of supplements, the public's love affair with these products has not dampened. In 2002, $18.7 billion was spent in sales of nutritional products. The vitamins and minerals studied included: vitamins A, D, E, K, B-1, B-2, B-3, B-6, B-12, folate, iodine, potassium, calcium, magnesium, phosphorus, zinc, and selenium. Further studies across a broader spectrum of both age group and physical activity would shed more informative light on this very important topic.

So far, research has confirmed that antioxidant formulas, along with supplemental carotenoids for macular degeneration, do have an effect on eye health. Vitamin C has been documented to have an effect on lowering the risk of nuclear cataract. Ginkgo biloba, which increases microcirculation, and bilberry fruit, which has anti-angiogenic properties, may help to decrease blood vessel leakage and can possibly help glaucoma patients. Both of these substances also have antioxidant properties. Research has shown that the essential fatty acid (EFA), omega-3 in the form of docosahexanaenoic acid may help in rebuilding photoreceptor cells. The essential fatty acids have also been found to help maintain nerve fiber function. Dry eye syndrome may benefit from EFA's that may be depleted in the lens. The EFA's block inflammation associated with this syndrome.

Antioxidants do help sweep *free radicals* out of the body, and furthermore, there is good evidence that a synergy exists among antioxidants according to Lester Packer, PhD, a top antioxidant researcher. For example, alpha lipoic acid helps recycle vitamin C, E, glutathione and CoQ10. Vitamin C and other antioxidants enhance absorption of iron; zinc interacts with every nutrient and is especially important for the absorption of the fat- soluble vitamins A and E. The essential fatty acids increase calcium absorption from the gut by enhancing the effects of vitamin D, thereby reducing the excretion of calcium through urination. Gamma linolenic acid together with alpha lipoic acid has been shown to have significant benefits in treatment of diabetic neuropathy.

One of the causes of cataract formation cites deficient glutathione levels that contribute to a faulty antioxidant defense system in the lens of the eye. Precursors to glutathione include glutamic acid, cysteine and glycine. Nutrients that increase glutathione levels include alpha lipoic acid, vitamins E and C and selenium; decreased glutathione results in part from a deficiency in vitamin A levels, carotenoids, lutein and zeaxanthin. Riboflavin, one of the B vitamins plays an essential role for it is a co-factor of glutathione. Folic acid, melatonin, and bilberry may help to prevent cataract formation.

High IOPs may be related to faulty glycosaminoglycans (GAGs)--a complex form of sugar synthesis. This syndrome involves the breakdown of the trabecular meshwork associated with the outflow of fluid. Nutrients that can impact GAGs such as vitamin C and glucosomine sulphate may help with outflow activity. Other nutrients include lipoic acid, vitamin B12, magnesium, and melatonin. Helpful botanicals that include ginkgo biloba, forskallin and intramuscular injections of *salvia miltiorrhiza* may improve visual acuity and peripheral vision.

Epigenetic science has revealed that the kind of food ingested by pregnant mothers, whether human, animal or insect, can change gene function without altering the DNA sequence. Genes function in a number of different ways, one of which is called methylation, which acts like a brake, turning gene expression up or down. Methyl groups have many functions including relaxing or tightening certain spots on chromosomes, inactivating past viral infections, and playing a role in prenatal and postnatal development. These imprinted genes must first be methylated to function and are, therefore, vulnerable to diet and other environmental factors. Methylation is nature's way to tweak gene expression without making permanent mutations. Methyl groups are entirely derived from the foods we eat. Is it possible that a mother who has glaucoma may, by eating a whole food diet, alter the course of one of the risk factors—family history—of passing along glaucoma? That said, isolated substances do work and work quite well to heal many diseases. It makes sense, therefore, not to "throw the baby out with the bathwater," but to judiciously examine how well-chosen supplements can help to boost the immune system and alleviate various medical conditions.

There are presently three large studies assessing the effects of vitamins: The *Women's Antioxidant and Cardiovascular Study* (8000 women with cardiovascular disease); is assessing 600 IU vitamin E and 500 mg C, daily or beta-carotene, 83,000 mg. every other day; *Women's Health Study* (40,000 healthy women) 600 IU Vitamin E, 100 mg. aspirin, both or a placebo on alternate days; and The *Physicians Health Study II,* (15,000 male physicians), 500 mg vitamin C every day, 500 IU vitamin E, every other day and/or beta-carotene, 83,000 IU every other day. These studies did not indicate whether the vitamin E used was the complex form, but the newest research recommends that vitamin E supplementation should be in this form.

VITAMIN C (ascorbic acid) holds top place in the pantheon of vitamins.

For that reason countless research studies have been devoted to proving or challenging vitamin C's effectiveness in scourging *free radical* activity. The following is a partial list of what we know about vitamin's C's activity. It helps support the cells against damage caused by *free radicals*, enhances the immune system and is essential for the formation and maintenance of collagen, a protein forming the basis for connective tissue. It strengthens all connective tissues, promotes wound healing, helps to promote capillary integrity, fights inflammatory processes and aids in preventing permeability. Concentrated at high levels in the aqueous humor and the trabecular meshwork, it may play a role in cell metabolism. Its high level in the aqueous humor, more so than in blood circulation, is required because the eye's transparency subjects it to ultraviolet radiation. High levels of vitamin C prevent cataracts—but a lot is needed, much more than is required to prevent scurvy, the observation made by a doctor of the British Navy who in 1747 conducted a small study of sailors and determined that the juice of lemons (high in vitamin C) prevented the disease. It took the British, however, forty-one years to accept this finding and another two-hundred years or so (1932) for vitamin C to be isolated as a cure for scurvy. Long before any of these findings, native healers knew that an extraction of pine needles (think pycogenol) would heal scurvy. Another study of 492 non-diabetic women between the ages of 53 and 73 found that those who were less than 60 years of age and consumed 362 mg/day of vitamin C had a fifty-seven percent lower risk of developing cortical cataracts and those who took the vitamin for ten years decreased the odds to sixty percent. A large study of 50,000 women found that those women who consumed the highest amount of vitamins C, E, and the carotenoids were forty percent less like to develop cataracts than those women with low amounts of these antioxidants. And in the *Nurses Health Study*, supplemental vitamin C over a period of ten years was associated with a seventy-seven percent lower incidence of early lens opacity and an eighty-eight percent lower incidence of moderate lens opacities. In this study, no significant protection was noted for those below ten years of use. Yet there are studies that point in the opposite direction. A recent study of 4,600 participants who took 500 mg of vitamin C, 400 mg. of vitamin E, and 25,000 mg of beta-carotene daily for six years showed no difference in cataract rates as those persons not taking the supplements. In Europe and Asia, vitamin C has been used as an adjunctive therapy, and there are studies indicating that high doses of the vitamin have shown promising results for glaucoma patients, but these doses run the risk of gastrointestinal symptoms.

The mode of action is believed to cause acidosis (over-acidity of the tissues), but only if nonbuffered ascorbic acid is taken. Should you be interested in a high-dose routine of vitamin C, divide the dose into three to five buffered doses. When subjects followed this routine, acidosis became less of a problem. Persons with sickle cell disease, however, need to be cautious, especially if on *Diamox* (acetazolamide, a carbonic anhydrase inhibitor). Although this medication is rarely used today to lower glaucoma pressure, those persons still on it should be warned that *Diamox* raises the level of vitamin C in the aqueous humor, and this action increases the sickling of cells. *Neptazane*, another drug in the carbonic anhydrase inhibitor family, does not present this difficulty. Several studies bear noting. A three-year multicenter randomized clinical study (Europe and America) of 445 early cataract patients found that a combination of 750 mg of vitamin C, 18 mg of beta carotene, and 600 mg of vitamin E produced a small deceleration in cataract progression. An observational study from Harvard Medical School, Boston found that women who consumed the highest levels of vitamin C had a sixty percent lower risk of developing nuclear cataracts as did those who took it for ten or more years.

Vitamin C also improves the dilation of blood vessels, increasing the flow of nourishing blood. In a small study, vitamin C reduced the constriction of arteries in both heart-disease and healthy patients, and it has been found to be useful in preventing fibroblast activity following surgery. In concentrations normally found in the immune system, vitamin C acts to interfere with the efficiency of the fibroblasts.

What many glaucoma patients would hope for is a lowering of IOP pressure by taking vitamin C, but this effect has not been documented. An alternative approach, however, is advocated by some complementary physicians and nutritionists, who claim that vitamin C administrated intravenously in high units does lower IOP. These results are based on anecdotal evidence.

Obviously, there are many studies, more than can be mentioned here, in the literature on the effects of vitamin C on the health of the eye. Unquestionably, it is a powerful antioxidant. According to Dolores Perri, nutritionist, vitamin C works beneficially by increasing blood osmolarity, a process that draws blood from the eyes and into the blood stream. In some people, this process may lower inner eye pressure. Vitamin C also provides structural strength to the eyes and is involved in the production and flow of the eye's fluid. Notwithstanding the protective effect of vitamin C for glaucoma patients, the amount necessary for health maintenance varies among complementary nutritionists and physicians, as well as the FDA (see below). Some nutritionists claim intake of vitamin C doses should be up to bowel tolerance, possibly as high as 10,000 mg daily. Others, including Ben Lane, an optometrist and director of the Nutritional Optometry Associates, recommends no more than 2,500 mg daily, taken preferably in the morning and evening, or as a 2-time a day schedule, allowing an interval to absorb copper, chromium, calcium and other minerals which vitamin C may block. To be most effective, vitamin C should be taken along with bioflavonoids and most formulas do contain them.

There is no limit on the foods containing high levels of vitamin C. Good sources include citrus fruits, red peppers, beets, broccoli, cauliflower, papaya, kale, strawberries, asparagus, cantaloupe, spinach, tomato, nettles, and mangoes. Almost all the fresh fruits and vegetables contain some amount of vitamin C. High heat destroys the vitamin content. Most of these foods are best eaten raw or lightly steamed especially with the cruciferous vegetables (broccoli, cauliflowers, etc) which older people cannot break down when eaten raw. (DRI—women 75 mg. men 90 mg)

BIOFLAVONOIDS, FLAVONOIDS, POLYPHENOLS

This group of pigments rounding out the vitamin C complex is reported to have pharmacological properties as well as being powerful antioxidants. They pack a wallop in terms of health benefits. Brightly colored, jewel-like fruit and vegetables found in the natural world have attracted humans and animals and have been known and venerated throughout history as life-giving. Several thousand flavonoids have been identified which provide much of the flavor and color in fruits and vegetables. As a result, these substances now form an impressive taxonomy. Deeply-pigmented fruits such as purple grapes, plums, bilberries, blueberries, cherries, raspberries, cranberries, and strawberries, rich in flavonoids, provide impressive amounts of antioxidants. These pigments often possess medical actions that keep the body healthy. Flavonoids are workhorses. In the body, they decrease capillary fragility by strengthening capillary walls, prevent venous connective tissue breakdown, prevent red blood cell clumping, tone up the vascular smooth muscles and stabilize cardiovascular support structure. The flavonoids extracted from grape seed especially rich in these compounds, have been found to inhibit the activity of proteolytic enzymes responsible for breakdown of connective tissues, thereby slowing down the destruction of venous structures. Based on several clinical trials by researchers in ophthalmology, grape seed extract has been found to reduce glare sensitivity, improve contrast sensitivity, *retinal* function, and myopia sensitivity. The scientists believe these positive results are due to the increased microcirculation resulting in better nutritional delivery to the *retina*. Both bilberry and blueberry have been shown to decrease the progression of pathologic blood vessel proliferation, lipid and calcium deposits of damaged blood vessels. Bioflavonoids may help build resistance to colds. They also decrease oxidized low-density lipoprotein (LDL).

Rutin and/or hesperidin, another class of bioflavonoids acts to strengthen blood vessel walls. A very early study on rutin claimed a reduction in IOP, but since this study has not been replicated, the evidence is unclear. Quercetin found in buckwheat is a compound similar to rutin and it produces the same protective effects. Rutin should not be taken as a supplement since in vitro it has shown to mutate genes. Nevertheless, rutin is an important nutrient and it is perfectly safe ingested <u>only</u> from food sources, for the body has erected a protective gastrointestinal barrier for this form. Since it is found in a wide variety of fruits and vegetables, its benefits of fighting diabetic retinopathy, free radicals and platelet aggregation can be appreciated. When low, there is a greater risk for vascular degeneration, bruising, capillary fragility, periodontal bleeding, varicose veins, hemorrhoids and aneurysm. Copper is an inhibitor of hesperidin and vitamin C and should copper levels be high, no amount of supplemental vitamin C will increase levels in the body. Vanadium and selenium support rutin uptake and molybdenum and sulfur support hesperidin. Both rutin and hesperidin, like calcium and magnesium. support each other and should be equally present in the body.

Anthocyanidins are another class of flavonoids that are also powerful antioxidants. These are found in tea, beets, cherries, plums, red grapes, Hawthorne berries, pear, grape seed, pine bark, beer, cranberry, red beans.

Isoflavones found in soy products, yet another class, also provide antioxidant action. As well, these substances possess phytoestrogenic properties that are said to promote bone density in post-menopausal women and may possibly be beneficial in preventing cardiovascular diseases.

Reserveratrol found in red wine is a powerful antioxidant and may help to explain the benefits of the Mediterranean diet. These polyphenols also those found in green tea inhibit xanthine oxidase, an enzyme responsible for free radicals. These substances also increase intracellular vitamin C, strengthen veins and capillaries and inhibit the destruction of collagen—all important for maintenance of eye health.

VITAMIN A AND THE CAROTENOIDS

VITAMIN A, one of the essential nutrients, is vital for the functioning of most organs of the body. It is a generic descriptor for the retinoids that include *retinal*, retinoic acid, 11-cis retino-and *retinal palmitate*. Vitamin A is available in a number of different forms, including preformed vitamin A and beta-carotene, which the body converts into vitamin A as needed. Unless you suffer from diabetes and/or anorexia, use beta-carotene as a source of vitamin A because it also acts as an antioxidant.

Reproductive processes for both sexes depend on this nutrient. It also maintains the outer layers of many tissues and organs and builds up resistance to infections, especially in the respiratory tract. Night vision is enhanced, for vitamin A promotes the formation of visual purple (rhodopsin) in the rods of the eye helping the eye adjust to low-level light. In third world countries, deficiency of this vitamin is the leading cause of blindness in children, the first signs of which are dry eyes (*xeropthalmia*). Vitamin A is converted to the fat-soluble compound retinol that is stored in the liver for use as needed. Zinc, required for its release from the liver, transports it to the eyes in particular and to other parts of the body as well. Sources of vitamin A include fish, fish liver oil, eggs, nettles and liver. Not everybody has the ability for the above conversion process. Diabetics, in some cases, may lose this essential action and need to take vitamin A in its fat-soluble form. Moderate vitamin A intake increases immune function.

There is some evidence that taking supplemental vitamin A palmitate in combination with manganese may be helpful for people who have glaucoma. Ocular health in general may benefit from this vitamin. Symptoms of a deficiency include dry, itchy, or inflamed eyes and night blindness.

According to an Institute of Medicine report, strict vegetarians need to increase consumption of dark green leafy vegetables to provide adequate vitamin A and iron. Carrots, broccoli and sweet potatoes may provide only half of the needed amount. Most supplements contain adequate levels of both vitamin A and iron.

An exciting development for those with retinitis pigmentosa cited that 15,000 units of vitamin A palmitate did benefit patients and that the addition of DHA (docosahexaenoic acid) shortened the time for vitamin A to become effective in new patients, but, the addition of DHA on patients already using vitamin A, had no effect. The study also found that vitamin E was not effective and may, in fact, be detrimental. Yet eating fish with high fat content resulting in a high blood level of DHA did demonstrate protection of vision. A study following a cohort of 50,823 nurses for eight years, found that those in the highest quartile of vitamin A consumption had a thirty-nine percent lower risk of cataracts. There is a retrospective study of nurses linking higher intake of vitamin A to hip fracture in post-menopausal women. This finding may be flawed because the intake of vitamin D was not considered.

Like all natural substances, vitamin A does not easily mount a defense system against air pollution, nitrates, nitrites (used as fertilizers), cooking and canning, but when consumed as a whole food, eaten raw and organic wherever possible, you at least know that you're providing your body with essential nutrients.

(FDA--DRI women, 5,000 IU, men 7,000 IU, top level-- l0, 000 UL)

Since a high intake of supplemental vitamin A is toxic, beta-carotene, one of the carotenoids, a precursor of vitamin A, is usually recommended. Beta-carotene converts to vitamin A in the liver and then travels to the *retina* where it is converted into rhodopsin, the night-vision chemical. Beta-carotene has taken a number of hits since it was first identified as an important nutrient. In one large randomized trial of US physicians, followed over a period of thirteen years, some 2,000 cataracts were confirmed, but those physicians taking beta-carotene reported 998 cataracts while those on placebo, 1,019 cataracts. This poor result may lie in isolating beta-carotene from the other carotenoids found in fruits and vegetables where the compounds work synergistically. Importantly, carotenoids protect vitamin E from the action of *free radicals*. Supplemental beta-carotene should not be taken alone. Vitamins E and C are necessary to prevent the oxidation of beta-carotene.

Beta carotene is only one of the carotenoids. Others include alpha carotene, zeta carotene, cryptoxanthin, lycopene, lutein, zeaxanthin. Isolating all six hundred or more of the carotenoids will take some years. The carotenoids are important for eye health. Two isolated carotenoids, lutein and zeaxanthin, are especially essential for those people who have macular degeneration. Did you know that edible flowers can be a major source of nutrients? When lutein was first identified, it was extracted from marigolds. So throw a few marigolds into your salad and enjoy. Of course, supplements are available and lutein is a vital part of the formula for any supplement designed for the eyes. Lutein and beta-carotene compete for the same sight on the cells, and although nature knows little of this distinction, this information should be considered when taking supplements to be sure that each vitamin is fully assimilated. A few vitamin manufacturers concede this possibility and provide these supplements in a separate capsule to take at a different time of the day. Blue-eyed individuals need greater amounts of these nutrients. Both lutein and beta-carotene are more readily absorbed with a bit of fat such as a salad dressed with olive oil. A supplement of at least 6 mg daily of lutein has received the highest correlation with disease prevention.

The body cannot make lutein on its own but can manufacture it from zeaxanthin. These vitamins are especially critical for the health of the *retinal* for they act to filter out the destructive UBV rays. They do not convert to preformed vitamin A, as do the other carotenoids. Thus, it is important to eat adequate amounts of foods containing them. A small study out of Chicago found that five ounces of sautéed spinach four to seven times a week improved, or in some cases resolved, scotomas associated with macular degeneration. A study in the Netherlands found that dietary lutein and zeaxanthin increased the density of the macular pigment. Apparently one of the functions of lutein according to a study conducted in Texas is the reduction of the effects of oxidation over time. A study evaluating 356 case subjects diagnosed with advanced macular degeneration and 560 controls aged 55-to-80 found that a high intake of foods rich in lutein and zeaxanthin protected the macular tissue from photo-oxidation by filtering and blocking blue light and absorbing and dissipating damaging ultra-violet light (UV). A study of persons over 60 showed an increase in the macular density. The *Nurses Health Study*, an ongoing analysis of the dietary intake of a large cohort of nurses (77,466 female nurses, aged 45-to-71 found that those who had the highest levels of lutein and zeaxanthin had a twenty-two percent decrease in the risk of cataract development. A study comparing subjects ingesting foods rich in antioxidants compared to subjects eating low amounts found after fifteen weeks an increase of the nutrients in the blood plasma level. A study of 36,644 male professionals, those in the highest quartile for intake of lutein and zeaxanthin, established a nineteen percent decreased risk of cataracts. The *Beaver Dam Eye Study* examined risk for developing nuclear cataracts and showed only a trend in cataract development with ingestion of carotenoids. While there appears to be no hard evidence that these nutrients make a difference for glaucoma patients, the improvement in health cannot be ignored.

The adage "you are what you eat" cannot be better demonstrated. Foods containing lutein can be lightly cooked and still retain the full quota of nutrients. If your diet is varied, chances are you will not be lacking in the lutein and zeaxanthin, as well as the other carotenoids. The most important foods are kale, spinach, collard greens, broccoli, Brussels sprouts, leaf lettuce, green peas, and summer squash. The foods containing carotenoids are often ranked by the amount found in each. The yellow vegetables especially high in lutein and zeaxanthin include sweet potatoes, carrots and the squashes. Leafy green vegetables such as Swiss chard, Brussels sprouts, bok choy, broccoli, asparagus, romaine lettuce, green peas, Savoy cabbage, endive, collard greens, kale, turnip greens, beet greens, and purslane, a common weed now highly regarded as an excellent source of vitamin A and essential fatty acids. In our community garden, I zealously search out the purslane sprawling amid the flower beds happily combining weeding with food gathering. Other vegetables include red pepper and tomatoes. A particularly important carotenoid, lycopene, found in tomatoes (better absorbed in cooked form), fights against cell damage, especially in the prostate. Fruits provide their share of these nutrients. Mangoes, cantaloupe, fresh or dried apricots, nectarines, prunes, tangerines, and bananas are good sources. Eating at least seven–to-ten servings of the above fruits and vegetables assure that you receive your full complement of the carotenoids.

Warning: megadoses of beta carotene can cause hypercarotenemia—peripheral corneal rings or a yellowish orange deposition on the peripheral cornea (DRA 1000 ul)

VITAMIN E

Best known for its positive effects in delaying or protecting against cataracts, Vitamin E is the third in this trio of important antioxidants. It consists of eight closely- related fat-soluble compounds: four tocopheryls and four tocotrienols, designated as alpha-beta, gamma-beta and delta-tocopherols, and alpha-, beta-, gamma- and delta-tocotrienols. Both synthetic and natural forms are available. Preferred are the natural forms and these are listed as d such as d-alpha. Research has indicated that d-alpha is transported through the body on a protein made in the liver. Synthetic alpha, however, is degraded and excreted. While these forms work synergistically, each has its own special role. Alpha-tocopheryl, the most common form and considered the star of the group, is found in the membranes. Both alpha- and gamma-tocopherols activate enzyme function in anti-oxidation and anti-inflammatory conditions. Gamma tocopheryl steps in only when alpha-tocopheryl stores are depleted. Like alpha-tocopheryl, it appears to work in a different manner, trapping and neutralizing *free radicals*. Neuroprotection factors have been documented in a number of studies with moderate benefits to patients with *Alzheimer's* and amyotrophic lateral sclerosis (*Lou Gehrig Disease*). Researchers have found that gamma-tocopheryl can protect brain cells against free radicals and may have a role in delaying blood clot formation. It partners with vitamin C, selenium and beta-carotene to eliminate waste materials in the eye. Studies have confirmed vitamin E's positive effects on the eye. A joint study by researchers at Johns Hopkins University and the National Institute of Aging found that those with a moderate to high intake of vitamin E developed fewer cataracts than the controls. An ongoing study by researchers in Australia has enrolled 1,204 volunteers aged 55-to-80 years to explore whether 500 IU of vitamin E versus placebo can prevent the incidence and/or progression of cataract and age-related macular degeneration. The *Beaver Dam Study* that tracked eye health in 252 patients found that fifty-seven percent of those with a low level of vitamin E developed cataracts five years later. Turkish researchers have reported that tocopherol may protect the *retina* from glaucomatous damage. A positive effect of a combination of good diet and supplementary vitamin E on helping to decrease cataract formation has been noted in a number of other well-designed studies. Vitamin E, by protecting phagocytes (immune cells) from free radical damage, and enhancing T cell production, also boosts the immune system. It also plays a role in diabetic patients by improving the glucose tolerance factor.

Dr. Rick Wilson in a Glaucoma Chat Group sponsored by Wills Eye Hospital suggested taking 400 I.U. of vitamin E for neuroprotection. Taking 800-1,000 units before strenuous workouts might eliminate the aftermath of sore muscles. Vigorous exercise stimulates free radicals generating inflammation. Vitamin E reduces inflammation and also enhances immune function.

It's hard to eat enough fresh green leafy vegetables to assure sufficient vitamin E. For example, to get the value of 151 IU's of this nutrient you would need to eat 240 slices of whole wheat bread, 16 eggs and 20 pounds of bacon. But a goodly amount can be still be obtained from essential fatty acids, oil-rich fish such as salmon, mackerel, trout, and sardines, fortified cereals, poultry, and seafood. The oil of wheat germ has one of the highest; other oils, such as cold-pressed corn, soy, and cottonseed and products made from these oils do supply some of this nutrient but these oils should be used, if at all, only in moderation.

Because of the difficulty of ingesting enough vitamin E from food sources, supplementation may be necessary, especially since it plays such an important role in protecting against age-related degenerative diseases including cataracts, arthritis, heart diseases, and some types of cancer, atherosclerosis, possibly *tardive dyskenesia*, *diabetes*, and *Parkinson's* disease. When choosing a supplement, select the natural form of vitamin E and a formula containing all of the tocopheryls. Be particularly careful of the supplement you buy to be sure that the oil has not turned rancid. Dry forms of vitamin E are also available. The natural form d-alpha as stated above is the way to go. (DVD 30 IU, 22 mg)

THE ANTIOXIDANT FAMILY GROWS

COENZYME Q10 (ubiquinone*)* is one of twelve types of ubiquinones but the body manufactures only one type coenzyme Q10 (CoQ10*).* This enzyme is named for its molecular structure that resembles a head with a tail consisting of ten repeated units. A coenzyme is a compound that must combine with another substance for a chemical reaction to occur. CoQ10, high on the list for antioxidant activity, is a catalyst for metabolism—that complex chain of chemical reactions that breaks down food into packets of energy. The body uses this energy to digest food, heal wounds, maintain healthy muscles and perform countless other functions. This substance is found in the mitochondria of every cell in the body and is especially abundant in the heart. It is essential for the production of cellular energy in all organisms utilizing oxygen.

Energy production consists of two cycles, the citric acid cycle that converts carbohydrates and fats to fuel called adenosine triphosphate (ATP) and oxidative phosphorylation (OXYPHOS) that combines hydrogen with oxygen. OXYPHOS is seventy percent efficient as an energy producer. Compare it with the ten percent produced by internal combustion used in car engines and forty percent percent for hydrogen-fuel cells used in spacecraft. During the process of energy transport it neutralizes *free radicals.* Dysfunction of the mitochondria produces the *free radicals* that interact with oxygen to produce superoxide, a potent *free radical* found in the eyes. Lower levels of CoQ10 have been found in patients with congestive heart failure, renal failure and periodontal disease. Research indicates that CoQ10 may lessen the symptoms of Raynaud's disease (poor circulation in the extremities), protect against blood clots, lower high blood pressure, strengthen the heart, slow aging, increase cellular vitamin E and boost immunity. Some health practitioners believe the presence of this substance is vital to warding off many diseases. Patients taking the cholesterol-reducing statin drugs need to be aware that these drugs drive CoQ10 from the body. Supplementation can correct this situation.

Does the compound have an effect on glaucoma? We don't know yet since studies are scarce, but we do know that both its powerful antioxidant and increased circulation activity should help glaucomatous conditions. The efficiency of mitochondrial energy production declines with age and may account in part for age-related diseases such as *Parkinson's, Alzheimer's,* heart disease and others. It may prevent side effects from beta blockers. A study of sixteen patients on timolol, who were given ninety mg of CoQ10 for six weeks, registered a decrease of bradycardia (slow heartbeat) and other cardiac effects. The possibility exists also that supplementation of CoQ10 and vitamin E may have an effect against *Creutzfeldt-Jacob Disease* (CJD-- mad cow disease), the symptoms of which include memory loss, impaired judgment and ability to reason, visual disturbances, strange behavior, and irritability. Other symptoms may include spasticity, *Parkinson's*, muscular atrophy, and dementia. Significantly, patients with a high incidence of brain and eye operations have been found to have a form of CJD. Inadequately sterilized instruments, grafts and transplants and injections of human neural tissues from cadavers may be implicated.

Foods rich in this nutrient include bran and wheat germ, soybeans and other legumes, meat, fish and unrefined vegetable oils. Refining robs the oil of its CoQ10 properties. Supplements are also available. If you take a supplement, either take it with food in which a small amount of oil is present or dissolve it in hot water to which you add a little bit of oil. I take it with my dose of cod liver oil. Supplements are also available packaged in oil.

GLUTATHIONE is a compound composed of the amino acids cysteine, glutamic acid, and glycine. This is a powerful antioxidant and *free-radical* scavenger and it is important for eye health. Another important function of glutathione is its support of the mechanisms by which vitamins C and E detoxify *free radicals* found in the eye. Glutathione degrades hydrogen peroxide to water, renders oxidative stress impotent by reducing bad fats to innocuous fatty acids and helps to restore the liver by recycling vitamin E.

Studies have indicated that glutathione can protect the *retinal* and the lens from *free radical* injury. A small double-blind study of three months' duration by researchers in Italy found that thirty-one percent of patients had improved vision and fifty percent did not experience any further deterioration. Those on placebo got worse. Research indicates that glutathione also plays a role in preventing cell death, an important consideration for glaucoma patients.

Glutathione and its constituent amino acids lower with age. Levels in people over the age of sixty-five were lower than in younger people. It is hard for the body to absorb glutathione in supplement form, although some supplements do indeed contain it. But its precursors, cysteine, glutamic acid and glycine readily enter the system and there are a number of supplements that contain these three ingredients. Plant foods are a good source of these amino acids.

N-ACETYL CYSTEINE (NAC) approved by the FDA as a prescription medicine to treat acetaminophen injury (from pain killers such as Tylenol), in supplement form is an antioxidant helpful in combating viruses, toxins and pollutants and is considered a potent liver and lung protectant. It is derived from the amino acid cysteine. NAC scavenges *free radicals* and enhances the production of glutathione, for while glycine and glutamic acid are plentiful in the body, cysteine is more limited. Degenerative diseases such as *multiple sclerosis, Lou Gehrig's disease, Alzheimer's, diabetic neuropathy* and others have been treated with this supplement and the researchers document some improvement. Double-blind studies with a pharmaceutical-grade dose, however, might be necessary to validate the claims. Meanwhile, its effectiveness in detoxifying the body and delivering antioxidants has been documented. NAC is usually included in a quality vitamin formula, but the amount may not be sufficient to make a difference and you might want to add an additional supplement. Because of its effect on glutathione and its positive antioxidant properties, it should be useful for those with eye conditions. Be sure to include vitamin C and zinc for they act synergistically with NAC.

MELATONIN The hormone melatonin is a *retinal* neuro-hormone produced by photoreceptors in darkness and suppressed by light. It is synchronized with the twenty-four day-night cycle—the diurnal curve. It is the principle hormone secreted by the pineal gland and it helps regulate the body's clock. This hormone declines with age and may contribute to sleep-pattern difficulties found in seniors as well as in blind people who may find difficulty in establishing the circadian regulation cycle. Researchers at the Sleep and Mood Disorders Laboratory, Oregon, have found that a 10 mg dose of melatonin can correct the situation.

Melatonin is an important antioxidant and as a result this hormone has been studied for eye conditions. A non-placebo study of one-hundred individuals, mean age seventy-one, with either the wet or dry forms of age-related macular degeneration received three mg/day of melatonin at bedtime. After six months, the majority were found to have a reduction in the pathological changes of ARMD. In animal studies, melatonin has been found to inhibit both chemically-induced and UVB cataract formation. The researchers speculate that its protective action may result from the quenching of lipid peroxides and thus enhancing glutathione.

Worldwide, scientists are studying the effects of melatonin on the body. Japanese scientists using a mouse model found that melatonin reverses age-related changes in brain tissue and reduces brain-cell vulnerability by scavenging *free radicals*. Similar results by researchers in India found that melatonin inhibits age-related decline in glutathione. They speculated that the hormone acts as an anti-aging agent. Scientists at the University of California, Irvine, also found that supplemental melatonin restored activity in aged rats to the level of younger animals. In sum, melatonin scavengers a variety of toxic oxygen-and nitrogen-based reactants, stimulates antioxidant enzymes, increases the efficiency of the electron-transport and enhances the mitochondria, releasing more energy. Melatonin is not recommended for people under the age of thirty-five. Dosage should be regulated on how easy it is to fall asleep. If you use it, start with one mg and add a higher dose if necessary, or consult with your doctor. Melatonin in walnuts protects against cancer and heart disease.

ALPHA LIPOIC ACID **(ALA***)* (thiotic acid) is now considered one of the most important antioxidants.   Like Co-Q10, it is found primarily in the mitochondria and is, therefore, involved in the production of energy by working synergistically with thiamine and niacin. It is absorbed from the gut and readily passes through the blood-brain barrier penetrating into the tissues of the brain and the eye. Because it is both water and fat soluble, it is a supreme scavenger of a wide variety of reactive oxygen molecules including superoxide and lipid peroxides. It regenerates vitamin C and E and raises glutathione levels. Animal studies have shown a lowering of oxidative stress resulting in protection of the *retinal* ganglion cells. Human trials are underway.

Combined with GLA (gamma linolenic acid), it becomes synergistically more powerful. This nutrient is especially beneficial for control of diabetes and it is approved as a drug for diabetic neuropathy in Germany. Four randomized double-blind, placebo-controlled studies have indicated that supplementation with alpha lipoic acid reduces neuropathological deficits and symptoms. While short-term IV injections appear to be more effective, some clinical trials have indicated improvement in nerve conduction over a two-year period using oral doses. Other conditions possibly benefiting from this supplement include liver cirrhosis, cataracts, heavy metal toxicity, radiation damage, atherosclerosis, and AIDS. Researchers in a study of open-angle patients treated with 150 mg of alpha lipoic acid reported 45%-to-47% enhancement of color visual fields. There is also some evidence that this vitamin is neuroprotective. A small study found that it helped to prevent LDL (the bad cholesterol) from oxidizing. Because it improves the blood flow to the peripheral nerves, it may in some cases stimulate these nerve fibers or at least protect them. As a detoxifier, ALA helps to prevent poisoning from arsenic, cadmium, mercury, lead, and some of the pesticides. It also boosts glutathione levels into the cells and it is soluble in both fat and water. Spinach and red meat are good sources of this vitamin.

CARNITINE AND ACYTL-L-CARNITINE While this supplement has been typically associated with weight loss it does have other benefits that may promote better eye health. These are its energy-enhancing and immune system function effects. Acetyl-L-Carnitine, a natural antioxidant, found in every cell, benefits mitochondrial efficiency, protects the cholinergic neurons, helps to increase levels of choline acytltransferase which makes the valuable neurotransmitter acetylcholine and increases nerve growth factor and most important for persons with glaucoma, it enhances the cerebral and cardiovascular blood flow protecting the neurons in a wide range of disease processes. Aging reduces the amount of this substance in the body.

CARNOSINE composed of two amino acids, histidine and alanine, declines with age by sixty percent or more. It has antioxidant properties, acts as a chelating agent, strengthens the immune system and also has been found to be a blood thinner through its action of dissolving blood clots. This nutrient may be effective in reversing some forms of senile cataracts according to a Russian study. It also appears to help heal corneal erosion, inflammation, swelling and dry eye. Carnosine has been found to restore proteins in the lens by removing *free radicals* and is thought to function as a "molecular water pump" that may explain its positive effects on the cornea. L-carnosine and N-acetyl carnosine are considered equally effective; although N-acetyl is not as potent, it lasts longer.

PHOSPHATIDYLSERINE is a nutrient located in all cells but is highly concentrated in the brain cells, comprising about seventy percent of its nerve tissue mass. It stimulates release of dopamine (a mood regulator), increases production of acetylcholine necessary for learning and memory, enhances the glucose metabolism (the brain's fuel), reduces cortisol levels which, if elevated, can be damaging to the nervous system, and boosts activity of the nerve growth factor that superintends the health of cholinergic neurons. This compound is derived either as bovine or soy extract. It does have a side effect for persons on Coumadin or Heparin (blood thinners) at the recommended 300 mg dose.

RESERVERATROL Most of the benefits are linked to studies with mice and the French Paradox. People in France eat a high fat diet and drink red wine derived from grapes. The wine possesses a high percentage of the polyphenol, reservatrol. Yet the French have fewer heart attacks and live longer. Researchers working with mice have increased the activity and aging in the animals. Possibly this effect is a result of stimulating an enzyme called SIRT1 which helps to spur the growth of new mitochondria in cells. (Mitochondria are the organelles of a cell that convert fuel to energy). Another group of researchers reported that reservatrol eradiated plaque and might increase the ability to chelate (remove) copper. This action may be helpful for patients with *Alzheimer's*. While there is not yet any evidence that this nutrient has a direct effect on the eyes, the research does suggest that as a supplement it may increase bodily health.

GRAPE SEED EXTRACT is an excellent source of proanthocyanidans and its antioxidant activity is considered superior to the antioxidants found in vitamin C and E. It protects the strength and flexibility of collagen found within the blood vessels, teeth, bone and skin.

HAWTHORNE BERRY (*Crataegus oxyacanatha*) is an antioxidant that stabilizes collagen, the most abundant protein in the body, enhances blood supply to the heart and has been found to stimulate the activity of superoxide dismutase. It is also helpful in reducing hypertension.

Herbs found on your kitchen shelf possess antioxidant and other beneficial properties.

CILANTRO, a common herb increases the excretion of mercury, lead and aluminum. Researchers have found that cilantro in pill form taken with the antibiotic *Doxycycline* cured both heavy metal deposits and herpes.

CINNAMON improves sugar metabolism, keeps fats in check.

GINGER (Zingiber officinale) is an antioxidant and can work as an immune enhancer. It also relieves osteoarthritis for it blocks an enzyme that triggers joint inflammation.

ROSEMARY, a culinary herb, does wonderful things in addition to flavoring foods. Its antibacterial effects retard food spoilage. But more important, it also stimulates blood circulation especially to the capillaries, thereby increasing the flow of blood to the brain and eyes. Drink rosemary tea. And if you have a ghost lurking in your dwelling, sprinkle a few rosemary sprigs on the floor and the spirits will vanish in twenty-four hours.

TURMERIC (**curcuma longa**) is a powerful antioxidant that aids in detoxification and guards against harmful bacteria and fungi. It also reduces inflammation. Researchers have noted that people living in India do not have as high a rate of *Alzheimer's* which they attribute to the high turmeric intake added to the cooking of foods.

THESE VITAMINS ROUND OUT THE PICTURE

Along with the antioxidants, vitamin D and the family of B's are essential for eye health and in general the health of the body

VITAMIN D3 and SUNLIGHT

Oxidative Effects of Sunlight

Without question, light from the sun does induce *retinal* damage especially in the photoreceptive cells. We do need sunlight, however, for the manufacture of vitamin D3. Some early researchers felt sunlight taken in small doses would have a healing effect on the eyes. Researchers now claim that unfettered exposure to sunshine or its equivalent several times a week can help ward off a host of debilitative and sometimes deadly diseases. This means twenty minutes of sun exposure daily While the younger person in the presence of sunlight usually produces all vitamin D needs for the most part, older adults, especially in winter, who both venture out less often and avoid the sun altogether because of fears of skin cancer and wrinkles, do suffer the consequences of insufficient vitamin D. In 2003, at a *National Institutes of Health Conference*, a study found an "alarming prevalence" of vitamin D deficiency in the United States and according to Michael F. Horlick, Director of the vitamin D Skin and Bone Research Lab, Boston University Medical Center, a silent epidemic of vitamin D deficiency exists in people. You don't need a lot of sunshine and you should take care that you don't get sunburn, but exposure, especially in the summertime, of one-fourth of your body five-to-ten minutes between 11 a.m. and 3 p. m. is advisable. Some researchers believe that sun screen may actually contribute to the rise of skin cancer despite the claims made that sunscreen protects against overexposure to sun. *Oxybenzone*, a principle ingredient in most sun screens absorbs UV rays. Scientists reporting on studies contraindicated sun screen application and suggested limiting time in the sun or donning protective clothing and brimmed hats.

A judicious amount of sunlight may actually stave off osteoporosis, hypertension, diabetes, multiple sclerosis, rheumatoid arthritis, depression and cancers of the colon, prostate and breast. The latest research implies that vitamin D may be a significant factor in protecting you from colds and flu. Sunlight ranks as good medicine. It produces vitamin D that, when exposed to the ultraviolet B (UVB) rays, manufactures vitamin D3, a vitamin that performs a myriad of biochemical roles in the cells. Along with the well- known fact that vitamin D is essential to bone health, this vitamin also has profound effects on other organs in the body. Vitamin D regulates the absorption of calcium and phosphorus from the intestinal tract. A deficiency of vitamin D results in rickets in young children, irritability, weakness, and softening of the bones in adults, and underutilization of calcium and phosphorus in bone and tooth formation in people of all ages. Vitamin D may have a direct effect on the eyes, and it is vital for maintaining overall good health and balance. A study of one hundred forty-eight women with a mean age of seventy-four found the addition of vitamin D to the calcium supplement lessened falls.

Since vitamin D deficiency is linked to less calcium being absorbed, more fractures mainly in menopausal women and men after the age of fifty may occur. *Osteomalacia*, a mineralization defect sometimes called adult rickets, is one of the painful symptoms of vitamin D deficiency. Vitamin D may also have a role in lowering blood pressure. High blood pressure can cause reduced blood flow to the optic nerve. But studies have not yet determined the ideal level of supplementation to achieve the blood pressure lowering effect. Massive doses of supplemental vitamin D can result in *hypercalcemia,* too much calcium in the blood, and such doses should be avoided.

While the health-giving effects of sunlight are abundantly clear, heavy sunlight exposure is not a good thing for the eyes. Reactive oxygen species (ROS) produced by the sun's rays, UV-A and UV-B, damage the delicate tissues of the eyes. The lens and the *retinal* are particularly sensitive to the sun's rays on the photoreceptors and the lens by producing ROS, a molecule that kills healthy cells. Young people absorbing UV radiation may account for the cumulative effect that in the later years develops into macular degeneration and cataract formation. Fortunately, the majority of cataract operations using the newest lens technology now provide protection from most dangers of the UV rays. Sunglasses also should be considered from cradle to the grave to screen out the harmful UV rays. .

Along with vitamin D3 from the sun, good food sources include fortified milk, butter, egg yolks, liver, fish liver oils, oysters, fatty fish such as salmon, tuna, herring, and sardines. Supplements are available and most multivitamins include a sufficient amount for persons under seventy, although more recent findings show an alarmingly low level of vitamin D3 in all people. To achieve the proper dosage, some scientists are now recommending testing for vitamin D and then prescribing accordingly. One thousand IU's are usually recommended for older individuals. Intake should be a mix of foods and supplements. The blood test, 25-hydroxy-vitamin D determines whether this nutrient is readily available in your body.

(DRA ages 51-70 400 IU, 70+ 600 IU, 2,000 UL).

THE VITAL B'S

B vitamins work as a team and for best results should be taken together, but each of the B vitamins has its own agenda. The B family is extensive and although the major B vitamins have been known for many years, new B vitamins are still being discovered. These vitamins support the body in many of its functions and are essential for good health. They act as coenzymes combining with enzymes to insure that oxidative reactions essential for cell growth and carbohydrate metabolism occur. Persons on oral contraceptives may suffer a depletion of the B vitamins 1, 2, 3, 12, and folic acid, along with vitamin C. The B vitamins 1, 6, and 12 have been found to reduce post-operative immunosuppressant—prevention of the formation of the immune response. Before the advent of white flour, produced through the removal of the bran portion of the wheat, insufficient B vitamin intake did not exist, for these important nutrients are readily available in breads and other products made from whole grains.

Vitamin B1 (*Thiamine*)

Thiamine plays a major role in the metabolism of carbohydrates, energy production, *RNA* synthesis, niacin, fatty acids, and the transmission of nerve impulses. As well, it is involved in detoxification. The body uses thiamine to produce an enzyme called cocathoxylase that is a natural cholinesterase inhibitor (cholinesterase inhibitors lower IOP).

Thiamine deficiency can lead to impaired vision and damaged nerves. A Guyana study found that people who ate a diet deficient in the B vitamins suffered a preponderance of open-angle glaucoma as compared with those whose diets contained sufficient amounts of this vitamin. Thiamine, along with methylcobalamin and nicotine, appear to be antagonists of the amino acid glutamate implicated in cell death in glaucoma. Some glaucoma patients may be deficient in thiamine, not because of deficient intake, but rather from an impaired absorption of this vitamin. Thiamine deficiency has been associated with a degeneration of the ganglionic cells in the brain and spinal cord and possibly in the optic nerve, although more research is needed to confirm the latter. Diabetics are especially affected by thiamine dysfunction. High glucose or blood sugars corrupt the natural process of converting thiamine to its energy-producing stage and has been found to have a detrimental effect on blood vessel health in the eye leading eventually to diabetic neuropathy. Thiamine is found in brewer's yeast, peas, wheat germ, pasta, peanuts, whole grains, beans, liver, and pork. (DRA 1.5 mg.)

A vitamin called *Benfotiamine* that has been used in Europe and now found in US health food stores purports to have several properties that may help alleviate diabetic retinopathy. *Benfotiamine* is fat soluble and thus more bioavailable than thiamine. It normalizes cellular processes fueled by glucose metabolites and helps to maintain healthy cells in the presence of blood glucose.

VITAMIN K This fat soluble vitamin works synergistically with vitamin D to enhance bone health. It is necessary for blood clotting and for the uptake of calcium. This is another vitamin synthesized by friendly bacteria in the gut. People with healthy flora in the gut usually produce sufficient vitamin K, especially if the diet consists of dark green leafy vegetables. As with other vitamins synthesized in the gut, long-term use of antibiotics diminishes vitamin K. As an antidote, yogurt and other cultures containing friendly bacteria can help to alleviate this situation. (DRA, 45 mg.)

Vitamin B2 *(Riboflavin)*

This multitasker breaks down dietary fat, synthesizes fatty acids, activates vitamin B6 and folic acid, acts on the neurotransmitters, synthesizes corticosteroids, red blood cells and glycogen, the form in which energy-supplying glucose is stored. Riboflavin plays a major role in the metabolism of muscles and liver. A deficiency can affect the moist tissues of the eyes and nose. In the lens of the eye, it maintains a level of glutathione, a major antioxidant which may help prevent cataract formation. Riboflavin is a precursor to *flavin adenine dinucleotide*, which is a co-enzyme to glutathione reductase. For glutathione to protect against *free radical* activity, it needs this chemical reaction stimulated by riboflavin. An amazing case study of twenty-four patients with lens opacities treated with 15 mg of riboflavin daily, reported the disappearance of lens opacities, but such results would need confirmation through a large, double-blind study. In China, an intervention trial of multivitamin supplementation involving 12,141 participants, found a thirty percent reduction in nuclear cataract, and another trial involving 23,249 participants, involving four different vitamin combinations (retinol/zinc, riboflavin/niacin, ascorbic/molybdenum, and selenium/beta carotene/alpha- tocopheryl), revealed that only the group taking the *riboflavin* combination had a significant decrease in nuclear cataract. Excessive intake of this supplementation may be toxic because riboflavin reacts with light, producing toxic peroxides that can damage the liver and cells. It has been found to play a pivotal role in some of the damaging effects of UV light exposure, including damage to the *retinal* cells in experimental animals. These findings are confusing, for deficient riboflavin is linked to cataracts, while the combination of riboflavin with light is used by scientists to induce cataracts in animals. The problem appears to be with dosage. The human requirement is less than 2 mg a day, but many vitamin supplements contain much more. Dietary sources of riboflavin include Brewer's yeast, broccoli, wheat germ, almonds, milk, cottage cheese, yogurt, pasta, kidney, liver, and heart. Processing foods destroys this vitamin, and pasteurization of milk products depletes it. (DRA 1.7 mg.)

Vitamin B3 *(Niacin, Niacinamide)*

This vitamin occurs in two forms—niacin and niacinamide. It aids in the breakdown of protein and fats. Because it dilates blood vessels, it is often used to lower blood pressure and is used to lower blood cholesterol as well. Large doses of niacin are best taken with equal amounts of vitamin C for greater tolerability. A coenzyme, *nicotinamide adenine dinucleotide (NADH)*, provides the spark for the production of energy we get from food. NADH is in every one of our cells. As people age, their levels of NADH may decline. There may be a role for NADH in combating *Alzheimer's* disease, *Parkinson's* and depression, but further studies are required. The use of niacin, itself, however, can lead to ocular problems including decreased vision, periorbital edema (excess fluid around the eyeball), loss of eyebrows or eyelashes and corneal distress. Other problems range from flushing, GI complaints, weakness, to liver toxicity. A safer alternative to niacin appears to be *Inositol Hexancinate*. A number of studies in managing cholesterol, blood pressure, peripheral vascular disorders such as *Raynaud's Disease*, and diabetes, have indicated superior control with minus side effects with this substance as compared with niacin. The body can make niacin from the amino acid tryptophan, but thiamine, riboflavin, and vitamin B6 are also necessary for this synthesis to occur.

Food sources of niacin include brewer's yeast, peanuts, soybeans, and whole grains, as well as high-quality protein foods such as eggs, milk, poultry, fish, meat, and liver. Cooking depletes foods of niacin, and alcohol destroys it. If taken in supplement form in heavy amounts, the vitamin may produce a temporary flush following ingestion, and if taken in excess doses over prolonged periods of time, it may cause liver damage. Although *niacinamide* is not believed to have these effects, it is not considered as effective at lowering cholesterol or increasing circulation. (DRA 20 mg 35 UL)

Vitamin B5 *(Pantothenic Acid)*

This is your brain chemical. *Pantothenic acid* plays a role in the production of neurotransmitters. It is converted to co-enzyme A, catalyzing the breakdown of fats, carbohydrates and proteins as well as the synthesis of red blood cells, cholesterol, and corticosteroids. Energy production is one of its many features, but it also stimulates antibodies and intestinal absorption. A deficiency can produce a profound effect on the eyes resulting in nerve and optic degeneration. In animal studies, this vitamin has been found to be protective of chemically-induced cataracts provided that it is administered within eight hours of exposure.

Deficiencies of this vitamin were uncommon before modern food processing. In addition to the depletion of *pantothenic acid* from food processing, modern food production, especially as practiced in factory farms, contributes to the loss of this nutrient in foods, as do sterilized soils, and fumigation of stored foods with methyl bromide. We do pay a price for the abundance of inexpensive food.

Major food sources include liver, kidney, heart, Brewer's yeast, sunflower seeds, peanuts, buckwheat, royal bee jelly, egg yolks, bran, fish and whole grain cereals. (DRA 10 mg)

Vitamin B6 (*Pyroxidine*)

This busy vitamin is involved in many metabolic processes, including the breakdown of amino acids (important for protean formation), manufacture of hormones and enzymes, and breakdown of fats and carbohydrates necessary for the production of lecithin, release of glycogen from the liver to supply energy, and the synthesis of antibodies, red blood cells, DNA, and elastin. As well, indications from one study revealed that *pyroxidine* promoted Co Q10 production, a compound necessary to produce cell energy in the mitochondria. Most importantly, it lowers the incidence of heart disease and plays a role in brain function and it is crucial to maintenance of the immune system. It is also an antioxidant. Pyroxidine has been found to help women combat morning sickness during pregnancy, reduce swelling in the hands and feet and aid carpal tunnel syndrome. Deficiency of this vitamin is most often found among senior citizens. Oral contraceptives and other drugs may deplete this vitamin.

Food sources include lima beans, legumes in general, avocados, bananas, walnuts, filberts, buckwheat, peanuts, chicken, steak, tuna, kidney, beef, pork, veal, and salmon. (DRA 2 mg)

Vitamin B12 (*Cyanocobalamin and methylcobalamin*)

A synthesizer of RNA and DNA B12 is active in glucose metabolism. It should be taken along with folic acid. Most importantly for people with glaucoma, it helps maintain nerve tissue. An early study of its effects on the eye found increased tissue strength in new cases of glaucoma, but in long-standing cases, however, these results were not apparent. A later study confirmed the first findings mentioned and suggested a protocol to produce the effect. In a study of laboratory monkeys, deprivation of vitamin B12 showed gross visual deterioration but when supplemental B12 was started within six months of degeneration of the peripheral visual pathways, no abnormalities were found in the treated monkeys. There is also good evidence to support a role in general cognitive functioning with sufficient B12. People who consume alcohol, women taking birth control pills and those who have problems absorbing this vitamin from food sources may be deficient in B12. Also, older people may have difficulty absorbing this vitamin resulting in loss of energy, weakness and numbness in the extremities. In young people, this vitamin has been shown to help with diabetic retinopathy. This effect was not found in older patients. Nevertheless, the results of some important longitudinal studies indicate that a deficiency of B12 exists among older people, contributing to degenerative illnesses such as heart disease, *Alzheimer's* dementia, frailty, depression, osteoporosis, and in some cases cancer. Some experts are advising those over fifty to take supplements and/or eat more of the foods rich in B12.

A variety of foods including liver, sea food, poultry, fish, clams, salmon, Brewer's yeast, sea vegetables, and eggs provide this vitamin. But because it is found mainly in animal foods, vegans may need to include supplements in their diets. It's best to take B12 sublingually and in the methylcobalamin form which is purported to be more easily absorbed by the body. Suggested doses for maintaining health—100-to-250 micrograms daily. (DRA 6 mg)

FOLIC ACID

Folic acid prevents anemia, regulates cell division and transfer of inherited traits from one cell to another. A deficiency (common among people who do not eat fruits and vegetables) may cause chromosome breaks in human genes. Inadequate folate along with vitamin B-12 has been linked to cognitive defects and neurotoxicity in children. This vitamin supports the health of gums, red blood cells, skin, gastrointestinal tract and the immune system. A deficiency in folate in pregnancy may have a profound effect on the fetus resulting in *spina bifida* (defect in the spinal canal). Doctors now routinely advise pregnant women to take a folate supplement to prevent this disastrous birth defect. Yet, even if you eat a wonderful diet, you may not be absorbing sufficient folate should you have a high homocysteine level, a condition associated with ischemic heart disease. A study found that 8 mg of folic acid daily reduced homocysteine levels and that food fortification did not equal this amount. Like vitamin B12, a sufficient intake of folic acid may also help with eye problems. Some people can't break down folic acid. The form *Tetrahydrofolate* which is already broken down may be a better choice of this supplement.

Cooking destroys folic acid. Regular use of aspirin can lower levels of folic acid. Twenty-eight arthritis sufferers who took a combination of 400 mg folate together with 20 mcg vitamin B12 had less tender hand joints than a comparable group who used NSAIDS (over-the-counter pain-relieving drugs). Folic acid is present in a large variety of foods. Raw green leafy vegetables (where have we heard that recommendation before–to eat these vegetables?) and ripe raw fruit provide a plentiful supply. It is also found in liver, eggs, asparagus, endive, bean sprouts, garbanzo beans, whole wheat, barley, brown rice, cheese, beef, and salmon). (DRA 400 mcg1000 mcg UL)

BIOTIN metabolizes energy and synthesizes antibodies, niacin and digested enzymes. It is a helpful substance for diabetics by lowering blood sugar and may have some effect in lowering IOP in glaucoma patients. Because this vitamin is normally produced by the bacteria in the gut, heavy doses of antibiotics deplete it. Should you wish to experiment on IOP control using biotin, seek your doctor's cooperation.

Foods that contain biotin include liver, kidney, egg yolk, milk, yeast, whole grains, cauliflower, active culture yogurt, nuts, legumes, and fish. (DRA 30-to-100 mcg).

CHOLINE is another of the brain chemicals. Synthesized with the aid of *pantothenic* acid and *acetylcholine* it is one of the chemicals functioning in nerve transmission so important in the management of glaucoma. As a major component of lecithin (its companion is inositol), choline is essential in normal fat and carbohydrate metabolism and is also involved in protein metabolism. It plays a role in managing plaque formation in the arteries by aiding production and transportation of fats from the liver where a deficiency of choline can cause a problem. Healthy individuals normally produce their own supply of choline provided, of course, that their diets consist of foods rich in this compound such as unprocessed foods, egg yolks, soybeans, fish, cereal, legumes, lecithin, nettles and liver. Most fatty foods contain choline, but because of rampaging obesity, eating these foods cannot be recommended.

PARA-AMINOBENZOIC ACID (*PABA*) is more than a sun-blocking agent. In the body, it is involved in protein metabolism and the synthesis of folic acid. As well, it plays a role in vitamin B metabolism as an enzyme co-factor. It is also known to inhibit the effectiveness of sulfur drugs, so it is wise to discontinue its use should you be on sulfur drug therapy.

TAURINE. You will probably find taurine listed among the ingredients in any good supplement for eye health. Although taurine is considered an amino acid, it possesses a set of properties that places it apart from the amino acid family. It counters oxidative stress and preserves oxidative health. The liver requires taurine for detoxification. A derivative of cysteine it accumulates in the *retina*, platelets and nerve cells. According to a researcher at Texas Tech University in Lubbock, animals made deficient in taurine suffer damage to their *retinas*, possibly because taurine also functions as a protective antioxidant.

THE SALTS THAT HEAL

From ancient to modern times hot springs loaded with minerals have been considered beneficial for healing the body. By attracting large numbers of people to these natural treasures, cities such as Saratoga Springs in New York established spas. And in Europe, spas in Germany particularly, are integral to an array of healing modalities. Just about every country in the world takes advantage of the natural minerals bubbling out of the ground for healing purposes.

Minerals influence virtually all the chemical reactions in the body, including some of the vital processes necessary for eye health, and are vital for proper electrolyte balancing and crucial for maintaining the body's homeostatic mechanisms.

Generally, salts or minerals required by the body may be divided into three sections--structural (framework of the body), lesser, not quite so vital but important, and trace (needed only in micro amounts) but still essential. Once the possibility existed that these minerals were ingested as part of the daily diet, for they accumulate naturally in food and water. But food grown in depleted soils and quality of water compromised by pollutants may not provide a full spectrum. Moreover, acid blockers such as *Zantag*, *Tagamet* and *Prilosec* can diminish levels of iron, zinc and calcium over a period of time.

THE STRUCTURAL MINERALS

This family of minerals includes calcium, methyl sulfonyl methane, phosphorus, magnesium, potassium, sodium, chlorine, and sulfur.

CALCIUM We cannot exist without calcium. Stored in the skeleton and teeth where it is essential, it is the most abundant mineral in the body. It is also involved in growth, blood-clotting, muscle contraction, nerve impulse transmission, adaptation to the cold, and cell permeability, and is a catalyst in many physical reactions. When calcium in the blood plasma drops too low, it is drawn from the bone reservoir that, unfortunately, weakens the bones. Calcium is dependent on the absorption of vitamin D3 obtained through exposure to the UV-B rays from the sun on the skin or from dietary calcium. It is absorbed through the intestines and regulated by the kidneys. The three hormones involved are: calcitriol; calcitonin, and parathyroid hormone. Calcium is an element that cannot be produced synthetically.

Milk products, enriched calcium beverages, and leafy dark green vegetables, mustard greens, broccoli, sardines with bones are sources. Wheat bran and other unrefined flours and a varied diet should balance out calcium absorption. Foods containing oxalic acid such as rhubarb and, to a lesser degree, spinach deplete absorption of calcium, but added lemon juice retains the calcium. The best supplement according to the publication, "Worst Pills, Best Pills" is calcium carbonate that delivers the most elemental form of calcium. This group does not recommend either calcium derived from coral or dolomite as it may contain heavy metals. (DRA 1,000 mg. 19-to-70, 4,000 mg, 70+3000 mg.)

MAGNESIUM often listed as a companion of calcium plays its own important role in the body. It is a catalyst in many reactions, including the transmission of nerve impulses, muscle relaxation, cellular energy production, and adaptation to cold. Tooth enamel and bone structure involve magnesium. Studies have found a severe deficiency of magnesium in adults, a factor that may be attributed to the deficient soils in which crops are grown. A deficiency also associated with a loss of calcium and potassium may aggravate diabetic cataracts. In one study, a magnesium supplement twice a day benefited open-angle and normal-tension patients with improvement of the visual field and reduction of peripheral vasospasms after four weeks of treatment. Some health professionals advise a one-to-one ratio of magnesium to calcium and suggest that as a supplement it be taken at different times of the day.

METHYL SULFONYL METHANE *(MSM)* is a natural sulfur compound that inhibits cross-linking (faulty construction of tissues) of collagen and proteins and builds and maintains supple, permeable cell walls. This substance becomes depleted with aging. It opens up circulation softening leathery eye membranes allowing the penetration of nutrients that are capable of removing waste products in the eye. Found throughout the cells, it is an important nutrient required by the B vitamins, antioxidants, minerals and the enzymes to function. MSM occurs naturally in fresh fruits and vegetables, milk, coffee, tea, fish and grains. It is absorbed well in both supplemental oral and topical forms and is one of the first line palliatives for arthritic pain.

POTASSIUM The macro-minerals, especially potassium and salt, are involved in electrolyte activity. The balance between potassium and salt is crucial for the regulation of the body's fluid balance, nerve-impulse transmission, muscle relaxation, and insulin release. Medicines containing diuretic effects may deplete potassium. Some people with glaucoma who still need to take certain systemic drugs such as Diamox and Neptazane may need to supplement since these drugs may drive too much potassium out of the body. Supplementation, however, should be done under the advice of a general practitioner.

Although the potassium intake recommended is 4.7 grams, American women from 31-to-50 years of age consume about half this amount and men don't do much better. It's easy to keep your potassium levels normal. One cup of baked butternut squash or a cup of cooked lima beans will each provide 1,200 mg, one cup of spinach, 1,160 mg. and a cup of cooked black beans, 1,000 mg. Foods such as banana, cantaloupe, mango, potato, avocado, nettles, broccoli, apricot, fig, date, liver, milk, peanuts, and citrus fruit and juice are especially good sources. Green juices are particularly rich in potassium.

Sodium Once a rare commodity and sought after as an important spice ingredient, sodium, essential to life, is now linked to various ailments. Yet it is so important, that humans have a specific sensor on the tongue to detect salt, developed thousands of years ago as a survival mechanism to balance their rich potassium intake. It is found in every cell in the human system, and it permeates the fluid between cells (extracellular fluid). It is necessary for survival and is involved in electrical potential, fluid balance and pH balance. Potassium and salt must be in a constant dynamic balance to facilitate the movement of nutrients and waste across cell membranes. It is also necessary for the blood and lymphatic fluid and for the production of hydrochloric acid, the digestive enzyme in the stomach. Along with potassium, sodium is required for proper nerve function and muscle contractions. About twenty-five percent of salt intake is stored in the bones, a reservoir for blood needs, making bones hard. What's the problem then in consuming salt? Well, we consume too much of the wrong kind of salt. Industrial (table) salt production leaches all the minerals from the product. It falls into the category of "white foods" for its snowy look is the result of stripping away its minerals and its salt content is increased by the addition of the anti-caking agents. It is a denatured product that has no nutritional value.

Consider using unrefined sea salt to flavor your foods. It is balanced with naturally-occurring minerals to help rid the body of toxins. Unrefined salt has the fluidity to move in and out of cells, unlike refined salt that does not exit the cell easily, thus disturbing osmotic pressures and fluid imbalances.

Too much sodium, however, can cause high blood pressure, which has been linked to blood flow in the eyes in susceptible individuals, but too little also poses problems, leading to spasms, weakness, nerve disorders, weight loss, poor heart health and disturbed digestion. Yes, it is possible to have a deficiency even in this day and age, especially for those people who practice a salt-free diet and/or take diuretics. A balance between sodium and potassium must be maintained.

The recommended sodium intake daily is 2,400 mg about 1 teaspoon. It's easy to exceed this amount if you eat out a lot and rely on prepared foods to stock your shelves. You even get a sizable amount from sodium-softened water when you bathe.

THE LESSER MINERALS

The body uses tiny amounts of these minerals daily, but they are vitally important for health maintenance. These include copper, iron, manganese, zinc. When foods are grown in mineral-deficient soil, increasingly common in factory farms, the chances of an adequate supply of these important minerals diminishes.

COPPER aids in the absorption of iron, a combination involved in red blood cell formation. In the body, copper is found mainly in the liver, bones, and muscles, with traces in all other tissues of the body. It is a component of many enzymes in the body. It is also found in the hormone epinephrine (related to expressions of fear and anxiety), and in antioxidants providing a boost of protection from *free radical* activity. It is essential for the synthesis of collagen, elastin, and melanin.

Most people do get enough copper because of its wide distribution in foods and especially, drinking water that may be enriched by flowing through copper pipes. Lotions containing copper can also enter the skin. Major sources of this mineral include shellfish, liver, cherries, nuts, cocoa, whole grains, green leafy vegetables, and gelatin.

Take copper supplements with caution, since an excess can result in *free radical* activity and can also cause nausea and vomiting. As well, excess copper inhibits the uptake of vitamin C and the flavonoid hesperidin. Some multi-formulas do not include copper while others do. Where copper is included, check to be sure that the copper is not derived from cupric acid, for then your body can't absorb it. The level of copper in the body must be carefully balanced, for an overload is toxic, while a deficiency may cause hypothyroidism, a condition that may affect *intraocular pressure*. The total body content of copper is from 100-to-150 mg; normal ingestion each day is less than 2 mg. (DRA 2 mg, 10 mg)

Iron essential to life is found in all living things. Plants require it to manufacture chlorophyll, other living things for the formation of hemoglobin, the protein responsible for delivering oxygen to the tissues via the bloodstream. Our needs for iron are tiny, but this mineral is poorly absorbed from food intake, and we require foods rich in iron to meet at least the 15-to-30 milligrams daily to assure adequate function. Higher numbers are usually required for menstruating women, lower for seniors. Additional iron may be needed for those recovering from injury or surgery. High iron levels, however, have been associated with heart disease, and an excess can cause explosions of *free radical* activity. Older people, especially meat eaters, may harbor excess iron. A socially acceptable method for reducing excess iron is to donate blood once or twice a year.

Some people may need to increase absorption. Acidic foods—vitamin C, citrus fruit, and food cooked in iron pots help. Foods rich in iron are apricot, peach, prune, raisins, fig, Brewer's yeast, turnip and beet greens, spinach, nettles, alfalfa, liver, clams, meat, chicken, fish, asparagus, and cream of wheat. (DRA 18 mg)

Manganese This is an important mineral for those with glaucoma. It plays a role in the formation of connective tissue and bone, supports healthy brain function and reproduction, is necessary for glucose metabolism, and also plays a role in energy production. It acts in conjunction with vitamin C and is also a major element in the enzyme superoxide dismutase that is a scavenger of the toxic oxygen radical. Lowered manganese may manifest in flabby muscle tone, diabetes and heart disease.

Found in rice and wheat bran, corn germ, whole grain cereals, green vegetables, nuts, dried legumes, tea, ginger, clover, blueberries, citrus fruits and juices, seaweed, and alfalfa, it's hard to imagine deficiencies but they do occur. Be careful about supplements. They should not be over 20 milligrams daily except under the direction of your doctor. (DRA 11 mg.)

Zinc This vital mineral plays many roles in the body as a cofactor in some twenty different enzymes including the important superoxide dismutase, the enzyme vital to combat oxygen *free-radical* activity in the eyes. It stabilizes cell membranes, assists in protein synthesis, and is essential for the development and maintenance of the immune system. It also activates vitamin A and is essential for a healthy immune system.

It is known for its widespread effect on fertility, skin growth, healing, taste, protein digestion, carbon dioxide removal, disease resistance, brain function and the processing of alcohol, and it has gained additional purchase as a supplement especially for use in combating macular degeneration. The epithelial cells lying under the *retina* have the highest concentration of zinc, with the exception of the prostrate gland, of any tissue of the body. A study (AREDS—Age Related Early Diagnosis Study) found that a vitamin formula consisting of 80 mg of zinc, the antioxidants vitamins C, E, beta-carotene and copper documented a twenty-five percent decrease of advancing severe macular degeneration. Cataract formation may also be delayed using zinc. And this supplement helps to fight colds. Over the past twenty years, some dozen studies have cited that people taking zinc aspartate or zinc gluconate lozenges have shorter and milder colds.

The highest dietary source of zinc is found in fresh oysters (3.5 oz. provides 148.7 mg). Other sources include eggs, oatmeal, buckwheat, liver, nuts, beef, lamb, peas, carrots, milk, herring, clams, wheat germ, bran, and green leafy vegetables. As with so many minerals, food grown in factory farms may not contain zinc unless it is added to the soil. Zinc is also diminished in the presence of mercury that leaches it from the body. Fish, especially the big fish, may contain substantial amounts of mercury. If you are taking an immunosuppressant drug like cyclosporine, zinc, an immune system booster, may counteract the effects of the drug.

The preferred forms of zinc supplements are picolinate, orotate, gluconate, or chelated zinc. (DRA 15 mg)

TRACE ELEMENTS—MICROGRAMS WITH POWER

These trace elements are essential for the functioning of the bodily processes, among them iodine, for maintaining a healthy thyroid gland, chromium to regulate insulin production and molybdenum for carbohydrate metabolism.

CHROMIUM supplementation used in weight-loss and strength-producing programs has been considered by some nutritionists to be effective, but there is little scientific evidence for this premise. A high intake of sugar and refined carbohydrates is associated with chromium depletion. Diabetics are particularly vulnerable and they may respond to chromium supplementation. Several studies have produced encouraging results, citing that chromium supplementation interacts with insulin. Diabetics taking 200 micrograms a day normalized blood sugar. The control group on placebo did not experience the same effect. Blood sugar or glycemic control is the cornerstone of diabetic management. Diabetic retinopathy is one of the three leading causes of blindness. Even in non-diabetics, low chromium can affect patients with glaucoma. The association between glaucoma and chromium levels has been studied by a few researchers. There is apparently a disparity in those with healthy eyes who averaged a blood chromium level of 279.25 mg/ml, and those with open-angle glaucoma who averaged only 118.05 mg/ml. Dr. Lane, a nutritional optometrist associated with the Nutritional Optometry Institute who has studied the effects of chromium depletion, suggests that chromium's interaction with insulin may be one of the factors that sustain strong ciliary-muscle eye-focusing activity--the ability to read fine print. More study is required to establish this linkage. A small study comparing the effects of chromium with and without the addition of nicotinic acid found that chromium does not work effectively in the absence of niacin for both lowering cholesterol and decreasing fasting glucose. This study confirms the theory that none of these nutrients works in isolation.

Chromium is present in a number of foods. Highest sources include beef and calf's liver, baked potato, oysters, parsnips and Brewer's yeast. Other sources include sweet fruits, starchy vegetables, whole grains, egg yolk, molasses, cheese, butterfat, legumes, peas, broccoli (one of the best-absorbed sources), black pepper, and even red wine. Refined sugar leaches chromium from the blood and the mineral vanadium may counteract the action of chromium. Therefore, sea vegetables and/or large quantities of mushrooms, which are rich in vanadium, should be somewhat restricted in the diet.

If you choose to supplement, take chromium at a different time than vitamin C, which drives chromium from the body. (DRA 120 mcg.).

IODINE Think iodine and its association with thyroid comes to mind. As well it should. Iodine is a regulator of the body's energy by acting on thyroxin, the hormone produced by the thyroid gland. The medical community has yet to explore the relationship between the thyroid and glaucoma despite the evidence that many menopausal women display low thyroid function. Yet, it is known that on average a person's diet is not likely to be deficient in iodine. Nettles are a good source of iodine as are sea vegetables. People living close to the oceans are said to have less severe arthritis because of the iodine in the air. (DRA 1,100 mg)

MOLYBDENUM This mineral sees to it that stored iron in the liver is mobilized, and it also plays a role in the excretion of uric acid and carbohydrate metabolism. Along with sulfur, it supports the flavonoid, hesperidin. Whole foods such as whole grain cereals, brown rice, millet, buckwheat, legumes, alfalfa, and Brewer's yeast provide minimum requirements. (DRA 2mg)

SELENIUM deficiency may increase mortality and ozone damage. It affects the lungs and other body organs according to a small animal study. This important antioxidant works in conjunction with vitamin E by vacuuming up *free radicals*. It protects against heavy metals such as cadmium, mercury, and arsenic. It is a component of the powerful enzyme glutathione peroxidase. It appears to be less active in persons who develop cataracts. This mineral may be deficient in whole grains, especially if they are grown on selenium-depleted soils.

Highest sources include smoked herring, a cup of cooked oats, 3.5 ounces of smelts, a cup of whole milk, 10 Brazil nuts. Other sources include cooked red chard, brown rice, scallops, lobster, shrimp, clams, king crab, oysters, wheat germ, and orange juice. (DRA 70 mcg)

SILICON stimulates the growth of collagen vital for the health of connective tissues, including those found in the eye. It is highly concentrated in the cornea, *sclera*, and vitreous. While this nutrient has not been studied with relationship to glaucoma, it is evident that it is involved in the health of the eye.

Eat whole grains, vegetables, and fruits to be sure that you receive an adequate supply of this important nutrient.

SULFUR is one of the ingredients in the medications dorzolamide (*Trupsopt*) and brinzolamide (*Azopt*), the action of which is to decrease the production of aqueous fluid. It plays a part in the synthesis of proteins such as collagen, essential for healthy hair, skin, and nails. It aids in blood clotting and acts as a detoxifier. It also may play a role in depressed thyroid function. Should this be a problem, it might be wise to limit sulfur- containing foods such as garlic, onion and the cabbage family. Otherwise, if thyroid function is adequate, the above-mentioned, as well as radishes, turnips, celery, horseradish, string beans, watercress, nettles, soybeans, asparagus, egg yolk, and meat are good sources of sulfur. Hyperthyroidism may be aggravated or induced, however, by eating kelp.

AMINO ACIDS

Amino acids are the building blocks of proteins that govern growth and maintenance of bodyweight, heat, energy, and repair of tissue. There are over twenty different amino acids important for body function. They are primarily derived from a wide variety of quality foods.

Some amino acids, however, when excessive can create serious problems, especially for people with glaucoma. The amino acid glutamate, also called glutamic acid and glutamine, the only amino acid synthesized in the brain, is primarily involved in neurotransmission, a necessary brain activity that conducts information from cell-to-cell. Excessive amounts of glutamate, however, produce an over-excitation of the neurotransmitters (neurotoxicity), causing important neuron cells to die.

HYALURNON

This substance also known as hyaluronic acid is high in water solubility that primarily relieves inflammation and pain. It is also involved in maintenance of cellular and extracellular homeostasis. Its lubricating properties far exceed those found in the finest motor oil. This substance, comparable to chondroitin sulphate (a large molecule that gives cartilage elasticity), is a naturally-occurring glycosaminoglycan (GAG's, a type of amino sugar). The level of hyaluronic acid appears to have an effect on glaucoma. Morphological changes in collagen structure may precede increased IOP. In a small study, a decrease in the level of hyaluronic acid and an increase in chondroitin sulfate were found in the eyes of patients with glaucoma. Another study found a seventy-seven percent lower level of hyaluronic acid with higher levels of chondroitin sulfate in the trabecular meshwork, *iris*, ciliary body and *sclera* in donor glaucomatous eyes as compared to normal donor eyes. The researchers speculated that normal aqueous outflow is regulated by the content of GAG's ability to form a highly viscous, elastic gel-like substance that is the hallmark of hyaluronic acid.

Researchers from Ohtsuma University, Tokyo, found that 45 days of treatment using a capsule containing 40 mg hyaluronon improved skin conditions and improved eyesight. Some ophthalmologists use viscoelastic or hyaluronic acid when conducting eye operations.

Essential Fatty Acids (EFA's) And Other Vegetable Oils

Much as some nutritionists would have us believe that we can live without fat to avoid cholesterol overload, cutting fat out of our diet can result in serious deficiencies of the essential fatty acids (EFA's). We need fat for the formation of cell walls, brain tissue, hormones, and enzymes, and for the utilization of vitamins A, D, E, and K. Fat protects our internal organs and keeps skin healthy, and it functions as a building block in the membranes of every cell in our bodies--including the cells of the eye. EFA's found in the lens may help to maintain transparency.

That we ingest too much of the wrong kind of fat is indisputable. That many of us are lacking in essential fatty acids is also indisputable. According to data from The *Blue Mountain Study*, a higher intake of polyunsaturated fats was associated with reduced prevalence of cortical cataract. No nutrients, however, were associated with posterior subcapsular cataract. Longitudinal studies are still ongoing. Researchers in Boston, Massachusetts, linked fat bellies in middle-aged men to cataract development. The Schepens Eye Research Institute has conducted studies that demonstrate a clear relationship between the amounts and kind of fat we eat and the risk of dry-eye syndrome (Sjogren's syndrome and other dry eye conditions). *Sjogren's syndrome* is believed to be an autoimmune disease and may be associated with rheumatoid arthritis, xerostemia (dryness of the mouth), and dryness of the conjunctiva. It occurs mostly in menopausal women. Some nutritionists claim that an underactive thyroid may account for this syndrome. When it occurs in the eye, it affects tear production, the natural lubricant that keeps eyes healthy. In another small study of persons with dry-eye syndrome, gamma linoleic acid (GLA) was found to be helpful in reducing inflammation. Although a number of eye conditions may produce this syndrome, the inclusion of essential fatty acids in the diet appears to ameliorate the symptoms.

EFA's are found in breast milk and are critical to the formation and function of the *retina* in infancy, and evidence from epidemiological studies suggest that absence of EFA's may account, in some degree, for retinitis pigmentosa. DHA supplementation to a small group of patients with retinitis pigmentosa demonstrated that oral supplements could improve *retinal* function. Research has shown that a high intake level of omega 3's is associated with a lower risk of macular degeneration. A 2003 study published in the journal *European Neuropsychopharmacology* cited benefits from EPA and DHA supplements. Thirty-two patients received either placebo or a supplement containing 440 mg of EPA and 220 mg of DHA. After only eight weeks, significant benefits were reported in the omega 3 patients compared to those on placebo.

WHAT ARE ESSENTIAL FATTY ACIDS?

These are the fats labeled Omega 3's and 6's. They must be obtained through nutritional sources. The Omega 3's, alpha linolenic acid (ALA) in a well-functioning body, will be converted into hormone-like compounds known as eicosapentaenoic acid (EPA), and later into docosahexaenoic acid (DHA), which aids in many bodily functions, including vital organ function. *Rescular,* a pressure lowering glaucoma drop, is based on the properties of DHA.

Omega 3's make cell walls supple and flexible, improve circulation and oxygen uptake. When deficient, mental abilities, learning problems, and decreased memory, a tingling sensation of the nerves, poor vision, possibly blood clots, increased triglycerides, higher LDL, hypertension, irregular heartbeat, and decreased immune function may be present. Along with preventing or lessening many of the above mentioned ailments, Omega 3's have been found to increase the levels of serotonin and in several studies have shown more improvement than *Prozac* in alleviating depression. Omega 3's may play a role in irritable bowel syndrome, bi-polar syndrome, and rheumatoid arthritis. Fish oils have a mild anti-clumping effect on blood platelets that may account for fish's reputation for reducing incidence of stroke.

The Omega 3 long chain fatty acid is one of the primary structural components of the brain, which is composed of two-thirds fat and each neuron is encased in a layer of fat. Cell communication requires journeying through two layers of fat and Omega 3's are more flexible than Omega 6's and better able to this. Proper DHA levels are essential for optimum functioning of neurotransmitters. DHA makes up sixty percent of the photoreceptor cells and cell membranes in the *retina* and may, therefore, help to rebuild these cells. Memory loss and depression have been linked to deficiencies of this essential fatty acid. Chain length determines the inherent characteristics of a particular fat. Shorter chains are more water-soluble and are easier to digest. In longer chain lengths, Omega 3's tend to aggregate or stick together, a process that protects the fat from oxidation.

The Omega 6's, linolenic acid, is the primary one. In a healthy human, it will be converted from linoleic acid into gamma linolenic acid (GLA), which later is synthesized, with EPA from the Omega-3 group, into eicosapentaenoids. Some of the Omega 6's improve treatment in diabetic neuropathy, rheumatoid arthritis, PMS, skin disorders (e.g. psoriasis and eczema), and cancer.

In the body, the Omega 6's are metabolized into arachidonic acid (AA). This fatty acid serves as the raw material for a whole family of chemicals including the good guys—some of the prostaglandins that regulate blood pressure, inflammation, fluid balance, digestion, blood flow and steroids. Arachidonic acid can be synthesized from linoleic acid and, therefore, does not need to be supplied as a supplement. It can become problematic, however, when ingested from food. It is found largely in meat and while it produces a prostaglandin-like substance that increases platelet aggregation, important for clotting of wounds. It is detrimental when blood thinning is required. Some prostaglandins also have a down-side promoting tumor growth, immune responses and inflammation. The Omega 6's have been associated with an increase in blood pressure, inflammation, platelet aggregation, allergic reactions, and some of the newest research to glaucoma, and cell proliferation (cancer). The Omega 3's have the opposite effect.

Most Americans obtain an excess of linoleic acid, for it is not often converted to GLA because of metabolic problems caused by diets rich in sugar, alcohol, or trans fats from processed foods, as well as smoking, pollution, stress, aging, viral infections, and other illnesses.

FOOD SOURCES

EFA's, primarily the Omega 3's, are present in Boston mackerel, lake trout, herring, anchovies, salmon (wild, if possible), cod fish oil, nuts and flaxseed and in plant oils such as hemp seed, evening primrose, borage, and black currant. These may come in liquid or capsule form. Some nutritionists claim that evening primrose oil is the best of the lot. Flaxseed is an excellent choice since it contains both soluble and insoluble fiber—grind the seeds or if using the oil--keep it refrigerated. Danish researchers suggest that fish oil may help to reduce IOP. The researchers suggest taking six grams of fish oil daily. The study indicated that eating fish or taking a fish oil supplement lowered IOP by as much as eleven percent. Other sources include walnuts, eggs, purslane, green leafy vegetables and some legumes. Milk fat and meat fat can be eaten if derived from grass-fed cows.

Persons with bleeding problems or those on anticoagulants such as warfarin and aspirin, taking vitamin E, garlic, and ginkgo biloba, may increase risk of bleeding when fish oil is added as a supplement.

The Omega 6's referred to as the polyunsaturated oils are primarily present in oils used for cooking—corn, soybean, cotton seed, safflower, sunflower, and olive oil which is a monounsaturated oil and in a different class. Cold-pressed virgin olive oil is good for you (the Mediterranean Diet). It lowers heart attack risk and arteriosclerosis, and aids in cancer prevention.

The benefits of cold-pressed virgin olive oil (based on research) continue to confirm what the Italians have known for centuries. One of the more recent studies attributed reduction of inflammatory processes to ingestion of olive oil. The researchers found the oil to be as effective as drugs such as ibuprofen at taming inflammation. The substance in olive oil, oleocanthal, produces the same effect as low-dose cox inhibitors commonly used to treat various forms of inflammation. The researchers recommend that extra virgin olive oil be used liberally instead of butter. To know if the olive oil you purchased has an adequate supply of oleocanthal, taste it, and if it leaves a good throat sting, you've purchased the right brand.

The American diet is over the top in 6s with a ratio of 20-1. A diet high in polyunsaturated fats has adverse effects on the thyroid gland, causing hypothyroid symptoms such as fatigue, weight gain and edema (swelling). An ideal diet should be balanced -- Omega 6's/Omega 3's--1-1 or at least 2-1 with a top of 3-1.

BE ON GUARD

The transformation of liquid oils into solids to produce items such as shortenings and margarines, transform the oils to trans-fatty acids. These food items raise LDL cholesterol which, when oxidized, clogs the arteries. Soft margarines are somewhat less destructive. Fortunately, food manufacturers have developed margarines and solid fats free of trans-fatty acids, but read the labels on all prepared foods, especially baked goods. Labels, however, do not always carry accurate information on fat content. For example 2 percent low-fat milk has more fat than the FDA allows, lean ground beef has 21 percent fat, extra-lean 17 percent. When cooking with fats, contrary to what you have heard, virgin olive oil is best used warmed rather than highly-heated that turns it into trans-fat. Under high heat, certain oils become carcinogenic. A better choice might be grape seed oil or, even despite warnings about the use of saturated fats, palm kernel, coconut oil or even butter. Coconut oil is a medium chain fatty acid and, therefore, more readily digested and absorbed. Some nutritionists believe it can reduce the risk of arteriosclerosis, heart disease, cancer and other degenerative diseases. It produces more energy and less body fat than other fats. It also has been shown to produce less weight gain than the polyunsaturated fats. Coconut oil is antiviral, antifungal, antibacterial and anti-protozoa. Studies have also shown that these fats are more protective against carcinogenic compounds

It is, of course, preferable to get your essential fatty acids from foods and cold water fish listed above. Although pesticides are found in wild salmon as a result of run-off from fields into the streams where salmon breed, farmed salmon have consistently higher levels of several toxins and PCB levels are reported to be as much as ten times higher. Color is also added, for farmed salmon unable to feed on sea creatures such as krill, which contain a carotenoid pigment (astaxanthin) that turns the flesh pink, are fed a synthetic version of astaxanthin derived from a number of sources--red dye #33, chemically synthesized astaxanthin or originating from yeast or microalgae. The most persistent contaminant found in fish, however, is mercury. Those fish highest in mercury are the larger fish such as king mackerel, sword fish, shark, tuna and tilefish.

The Manufacture Of Oils

Commercially-extracted oils rely on huge, continuous-feed, screw-type (expeller), heat-producing oil presses that remove natural substances that keep the oil from spoiling and add synthetic antioxidants, producing, in the end, tasteless, denatured oil. Quality oil manufacturers, on the other hand use organic seeds whenever possible, presses that prevent light and air from contaminating the oil, and gravity rather than filtering, to extract impurities. Flaxseed oil is considered to be vunerable to rancidity. It should be stored in black polyethylene or dark bottles to prevent deterioration from light and it must always be refrigerated. Taste for rancidity. Flaxseed oil has a sweet nutty flavor. A bitter aftertaste indicates rancidity. Pearled oil capsules are more stable but like flaxseed, oils are best kept in the refrigerator.

Supplementation In General

Complementary care has taken on a Cinderella aspect. Once dismissed as a fad, vitamins are often recommended by doctors to their patients. In the late 90's, nutritional supplements constituted over a $4-billion industry and this figure grows each year as people seek complementary therapies to manage their health. According to an article in the *Journal for the American Medical Association,* adults should take daily supplements to help prevent illness. Researchers in Boston, Massachusetts, reported, based on studies involving more than 120,000 men and women that taking a daily supplement of 100 or more units of vitamin E reduced the risk of coronary disease.

Our Stone Age ancestors certainly did not supplement, but they also had short life spans. No doubt, supplementation is a modern phenomenon--a quest for the elixir of health, a promise of a long and healthy life. Underlying this need for supplementation is the assumption that our foods do not contain their full quota of necessary elements. Yet there is also growing alarm that supplements are replacing a good diet. It is impossible to nutritionally substitute a supplement for an apple, for example. Some people who eat a variety of foods grown in healthy soil appear to do quite well without supplementation. Nevertheless, for many of us, supplementation adds another layer of protecting health. One noted ongoing study at Beaver Dam, Colorado, found that people who took multiple vitamin supplements had a forty percent lower chance of developing cataracts than those not taking supplements, even taking into account such factors as drinking and smoking.

Furthermore, thanks to modern medicine, we are living longer and as we age, our digestive processes may not sufficiently extract the vitamins and minerals necessary for maintenance of health. Studies have confirmed that aging decreases the ability to absorb nutrients from food. Research has indicated that those over sicty need greater supplementation than their younger compatriots, and furthermore, seniors, most likely taking increased medications, decrease the ability to absorb nutrients. Add the fact that seniors who live alone often pay little attention to what they eat. Even old dogs suffer. Yes, dogs. According to a study, 48 beagles ranging in age from 9–to-14 years that were fed antioxidant-enriched food and given cognitive enrichment scored significantly higher than the controls fed ordinary dog food without enrichment. Vegetarians are also advised to supplement with vitamins. A strict vegetarian eschewing all sources of animal protein for thirteen years became legally blind (vision 20/400 in both eyes). Doctors found deficiencies in vitamins and minerals and that the vitamins B12 and B1 probably accounted for his vision problems.

The Age-Related Eye Disease Study (AREDS) involved 4,757 individuals ranging in age from 55-to-80. Researchers found benefits from vitamin supplementation. People at high risk of developing advanced stages of macular degeneration lowered their risk by approximately twenty-five percent. In the same high-risk group, those with intermediate ARMD in only one eye lowered the risk by nineteen percent. The vitamin formula that can be bought over the counter contains 500 mg. vitamin, C, 400 international units, vitamin E, 15 mg beta-carotene, 80 mg zinc oxide and 2 mg. copper oxide. Some nutritionists suggest that this formula needs to be adjusted and some supplement manufacturers have added the missing vitamin B6, as well as lutein and zeaxanthin, important nutrients for eye health. Also, the large amount of zinc may be toxic; furthermore, zinc and copper are antagonistic and should be taken separately. Researchers have found that a Chinese herb, *Fructose Lycii* (Gou Qi Zi), increased the levels of zeaxanthin in the macular pigment's optical density.

ABSORPTION

Yes, absorption may be a problem. Just about everyone is familiar with the findings that tablets may pass intact through the digestive system. Small highly- compressed tablets that have been heavily coated (some manufacturers use shellac), may not easily break down and dissolve in the digestive system. Give your stomach a break and choose a tablet that disintegrates easily. Also buy supplements that state expiration dates. The fresher the better, especially with herbal products. Liquid or sub-lingual vitamins are most easily absorbed. Capsules are the next best choice. I open capsules and mix with juice or water.

Some nutritionists claim that taking vitamins on an empty stomach increases absorption; others feel that vitamins are best absorbed taken with food, but in any case, avoid taking your pill with a cold or iced drink. For that matter, it's also best to avoid cold drinks when eating. Many of us who decide to start a program of nutritional supplementation are put off by the need to take pills or capsules, because of difficulty in swallowing. If so, try this. Place a tablet on your tongue and take two successive gulps of liquid without pausing. On the first gulp, swallow some liquid. This action causes the epiglottis to fold down and cover your larynx. On the second gulp, swallow the pill with some liquid. It will slide down your throat before the distracted epiglottis can resume its sentry position.

HOW ARE SUPPLEMENTS MANUFACTURED?

Contrary to the claims of vitamin manufacturers, just about all the basic ingredients of a vitamin are produced by pharmaceutical companies. For example, Hoffman-La Roche makes most ascorbate (vitamin C). The raw product to which an additive may be used to preserve it against oxidation is bought by a wholesaler who maintains an inventory of the purified nutrients from the various manufacturers and sells these to supplement companies that then label and package the product. This assemblage involves several steps. Most of the assemblers add various substances to aid in the tableting or capsuling process. Agents such as silicates prevent clumping, and stearites and fats keep the nutrient from sticking to the machine in the manufacture of tablets. Additionally, fillers may be added if room still remains in the capsule or tablet after the proper amount of nutrient has been placed. These fillers, called inert materials, such as cornstarch or milk sugars, may ignite allergic reactions in people sensitive to corn or dairy products.

Supplements should contain grade10 ingredients and be free from solvents, glues, lubricants, asbestos, binders, fillers and other toxic chemicals.

Some manufacturers take a different approach to manufacturing vitamins based on the findings that foods contain hundreds of physiological important factors such as phytochemicals and bioactive amines (life-giving compounds) and use food-based fillers that, while generally superior to the inert substances mentioned above, might trouble people with food sensitivities. Lastly, binders for tablets (honey is sometimes used) keep the product from crumbling. Tablets which are very stable do contain excipients. Commonly used are microcrystalline cellulose lubricants such as silica gel and magnesium stearate.

ARE HERBAL AND VITAMIN SUPPLEMEMENTS SAFE?

Although there have been claims that supplements derived from synthetics may be carcinogenic, they are certainly safer than prescription medicines that cause over 100,000 reported deaths yearly. Complaints about supplements are far fewer and most of them can be attributed to misuse, such as taking ephedra for weight loss. But although standardization does exist, especially in herbal products, it is still up to the consumer to sleuth out the best of the lot. Self-education or working with a nutritionist is generally a good idea. Continued use of herbs, for example, changes the body's response to these products lessening their effectiveness. There are supplements readily available that do cause harm. Some of those known to have dangerous side effects include aristolochic acid, a Chinese ingredient toxic to the kidneys; chaparral can cause hepatitis, comfrey can cause chronic liver disease, ephedra has been linked to high blood pressure, strokes, heart attacks and is two-hundred times more likely to cause an adverse reaction than all other herbs combined, and kava is a suspect for liver damage. PC, SPES, and SPES supplements promising prostate-cancer fighting, work like hormones only because they are spiked with hormones, a blood thinner, an anti-inflammatory, and several other drugs. The supplement itself is a fraud. Tiratricol, a weight loss supplement can cause strokes and heart attacks; usnic acid, found in lichen, appears to be toxic to the liver.

Supplements, as with any other substance, should be taken judiciously. Certain conditions may preclude their use. For example, regular use of cranberry concentrate tablets might increase risk of kidney stones. Echinacea is not recommended for people with auto-immune disease; ginkgo biloba and saw palmetto possess, as one of their properties, blood thinning, and should not be taken by hemophiliacs, or before or directly after surgery; ginseng may have an adverse effect on women with breast cancer and raise blood pressure in people not on blood pressure medication; soy isoflavones may affect thyroid function; St. John's Wort should not taken by people sensitive in sunlight or taking UV treatment. Sometimes an idiosyncratic response to an herb-drug combination is reported. A 70-year-old man developed blurred vision five days after he started taking 80 mg of a concentrated ginkgo leaf extract daily. According to his physicians, blood had built up in the layers inside the eye. The doctors speculate that the condition may have resulted from combining aspirin and ginkgo biloba, both potent inhibitors of platelet buildup. After the man stopped ginkgo biloba, his vision cleared. Another case revealed a heart patient who experienced an increased risk of blood clots after adding ginseng to his daily dose of pharmaceutical drugs. Apparently ginseng interfered with the warfarin's anticoagulation function. The author of this article, respected for his knowledge and dedication to herbal therapy, suggests that as herbs reach mainstream, more research is needed on interactions between the herbal supplement and pharmaceuticals.

Quality control of herbs should be an important factor in choice of a supplement. Extracts can be classified into two main groups--total and purified. Purified and/or standardized denotes that substances considered useless have been removed. As a rule, purified are in the dry state and they are a mixture of chemically-related substances endowed with a particular activity. While purification may seem preferable, material removed may, indeed, add to the herb's activity. These herbs containing all parts of the plant are considered total. Liquid abstracts are manufactured by processing the plant parts with either water or alcohol or a combination of both. Dry forms of the herb are usually stable. Liquid forms, more difficult to produce, are fortified with methyl, ethyl or propyl esters to prevent fermentation if that is considered a problem. The bottom line--try to purchase your supplements from a reputable manufacturer, one willing to publish the quality of the herb used and the extraction process.

Of the thousands of herbal and vitamin preparations on the market, the above represents only a small example of both benefits and adverse reactions. There are many volumes devoted to the science of using herbs to treat illness. It is best to work with a herpetologist or nutritionist when deciding on supplementation.

Supplement Myths

- **MYTH:** Supplements are unregulated. **FACT:** The Dietary Supplemental Health and Education Act (DSHEA) of 1994 allows the FDA the authority to insure safety of dietary supplements and the accuracy of their claims and labeling.
- **MYTH:** FDA has limited authority over ingredients used in dietary supplements. **FACT:** Manufacturers must notify the

FDA if they wish to use an ingredient not previously used commercially and provide safety records.

- **MYTH:** Dietary supplement manufacturers need not follow the same guidelines as do other consumer product firms. **FACT:** The dietary supplement manufacturers follow the same guidelines in effect for the food industry.
- **MYTH:** Scientific data is lacking to support the safety and efficacy of dietary supplements. **FACT:** Numerous studies in major scientific journals cite findings about how dietary supplements reduce or enhance specific medical conditions.

Further information can be had from The Dietary Supplement Information Bureau. Website: *www.supplementinfo.org.*

Consumer Lab routinely checks supplements for quality and potency. If you want to find out if the supplement you take has the standardized potency, check out *ConsumerLab.com*

REVIEW YOUR SUPPLEMENTATION PROGRAM

In November, 2001, the USP (United States Protection Agency) created a dietary supplement certification program. Based on quality and identity of USP-BF standards, a seal reading"Dietary Supplement USP verified" can be found on products that qualify. This seal helps assure consumers that the product they purchase contains what the label states and meets the USP stringent criteria. The USP has taken its place as the watchdog over dietary supplements. In February, 2003, they announced that new safety criteria would be applied to dietary supplements before allowing their admission in the USP-NF, which publishes standards, articles and monographs on botanicals as well as regulations, safety issues and agricultural practices. More information on the program can be found at www.usp-dsvp.org.

That said, choosing supplements from the displays at health food and drug stores can still be overwhelming. Some people prefer to take organic vitamin supplements. Organic may refer to only the fillers (see above) or in the case of an herb, the whole product. Others feel that synthetics are equally effective. Claims can be confusing. If you decide to take nutritional supplements, refer to the information above or choose a brand recommended by your doctor, nutritionist, or other health care provider. Additionally, below are a few general tips taken in some part from Guidelines from the *Center for Science in the Public Interest* on buying quality supplements.

- Ask for a list of all substances contained in any product.

- Ask about the dissolution rate of tablets.
- Ask how long it takes for the raw ingredients to make it from assembly to the retailer's shelf.
- Check your supplement for an expiration date.
- Keep the supplements out of light and heat.
- Choose a multivitamin that contains the minerals chromium, copper, magnesium, zinc.
- Check out whether an item is listed in micrograms. It takes a thousand micrograms to make one milligram. High potency should mean at least as much, if not greater, than the amounts of the DVD (daily vitamin allowance) of all the items listed.
- Check that specially formulated supplements such as for men and women contain at least the DVD amounts.
- Evaluate claims for structure or function to be sure that at least DVD requirements are met.
- For a specific remedy, check with your doctor, the web, a nutritionist or library research. Check that the recommended DVD doses be present, realizing that miniscule quantities of dehydrated foods such as broccoli, spinach, parsley, bell pepper add little value to the supplement.

Last word—The *Nutrition Action Newsletter,* published by the nonprofit *Center for Science in the Public Interest,* regularly runs columns on supplements. While their views may not take into account the many studies on supplements, they cast a cold eye on claims made by manufacturers. Published is a supplement guide, *Supplements: Latest Research on Vitamins and Herbs.* (See Resources for address information.)

CLINICAL TRIALS

There is no doubt that many clinical trials lead to major breakthroughs in treatment, both for allopathic and complementary medicine. In the year 2002, an estimated 80,000 clinical trials designed to assess the safety and effectiveness of new drugs, devices, and medical procedures were conducted. The National Institutes of Health sponsored over 7,000 clinical trials.

Daily, people with various medical conditions are advised of clinical trials being conducted that may impact on their particular health conditions, and   although these trials are generally considered safe for the participants, tragedies can and do occur resulting in adverse effects and even death. Also, not all clinical trials are valid. Unscrupulous researchers may falsify data and may conduct sloppy trials.

In the past, only young, healthy people were recruited for clinical trials. This situation, thankfully, is in the process of being remedied. Older people, once considered as undesirable subjects, are now being courted to participate in clinical trials especially if the medicine or procedure is slated for a particular illness mainly affecting this population. This makes eminent good sense, for age-related differences in how drugs are absorbed, metabolized and excreted need to be taken into account. In 1989, the FDA issued guidelines for including people over 65 and now about 15-to-30 percent are also included, although those 75 or older are usually eliminated from trials, despite the fact that this is the age group with the majority of disease conditions. Is anybody watching how these trials are performed with respect to safety of the participants? Yes; in addition to the FDA that appears to act only when a trial goes wrong, a Washington-based watch dog organization, *Center Watch* keeps tabs on clinical trials. The Group estimates that one of every thirty patients in clinical trials experiences a serious side effect. Should you participate in a clinical trial? If you feel it will promote cure or protect the optic nerve in the case of glaucoma, you may benefit. But first thoroughly inform yourself of the process. Ask these questions:

- What is the purpose?
- Will the trial have an effect on my condition?
- What advantages can I expect from my participation?
- Who is funding this project? Do the investigator and doctor have a financial stake should the trial be effective?
- Is this experiment being compared to a standard treatment?
- Who pays for medical procedures if something goes wrong?
- Can I opt out of the trial if I cannot continue for various reasons?
- If the treatment is helping me, is there a way I can continue to receive the medication? Who pays in this case?
- When will I know if I received the medicine or a placebo?

SMOKING

We do know that smoking is positively associated with cancer, heart disease and other physical problems. As if the statistics relating smoking to cancer are not convincing enough, there is now documented evidence from *The Blue Mountains Eye Study*, *The Beaver Dam Eye Study* and one from researchers in Australia, linking smoking to lesions in age-related macular degeneration and an increased risk of early-onset macular degeneration. In another study, defective visual field tests were found in healthy, heavy chronic smokers, although central vision was unaffected. The authors speculate that heavy smoking has a cumulative effect on the *retina* and/or optic nerve functions even when there is no evidence of eye disease. Another study found nicotine a risk factor in glaucoma because the substance reduces choroidal blood flow. The association between smoking and cataract formation has been studied in a number of populations and it appears indisputable that among other physical ailments caused by this noxious weed, eye problems can be added. A study by researchers in India stated that "consistent with other studies, tobacco smoking was strongly associated with a higher prevalence of nuclear and cortical cataracts and history of prior cataract surgery."

A DRINK OR TWO A DAY CAN'T HARM OR CAN IT?

There is a common belief that liquor lowers *intraocular pressure*. It certainly does and it can be used therapeutically when eye pressure is abnormally high, which will occur during an acute angle-closure attack. But the effects wear off and the IOP reverts back to its original pressure. By and large, alcohol is really not good for you. It is toxic and it breaks down into formaldehyde that generates harmful *free radicals*. Although there is some evidence that moderate drinkers live longer than non-drinkers, the choice is yours if you have glaucoma—extend your life or extend your sight. That said, the case for drinking red wine cannot be disputed, for *Reserveratrol* found in red wine protects the cardio-vascular system. The molecule, which is concentrated in the skins of grapes, is highly insoluble. Red wine processed from the whole grape protects the molecule from light and air because the wine is stored in dark, light-proof bottles and the alcohol helps to   extract it. According to a researcher at Harvard University, Cambridge, Massachusetts, supplements are useless because of the short shelf life of this molecule.

THE IMPACT OF TOXIC CHEMICALS AND HEAVY METALS

A 1998 report in the United States documented 33,000 food-borne illnesses and 9,000 related deaths. Bio-monitoring has come of age. In 2005, the Centers for Disease Control and Prevention completed screening for the presence of 145 toxic chemicals in the blood of a broad cross-section of Americans and found the presence of them in the vast majority. Another study tested for 210 industrial compounds, pesticides, and other chemicals, and in that study, a total of 167 chemicals were found in the participants. These people did not work with chemicals or live near an industrial facility. The substances found are known to cause cancer, be toxic to the brain and nervous system and cause birth defects or abnormal development.

Similar screenings in European countries have produced comparable results. Given the widespread agribusiness use of high levels of pesticide, fungicide and herbicide products, and the vast output of chemicals spewed into the air from all manner of industries including the Pentagon, there is every reason to believe that we are living in an untenable toxic environment. Industry releases a staggering amount of pounds of toxic chemicals into the environment each year. In the United States alone, some 600 million pounds of hydrochloric acid, 500 million of zinc compounds, 400 million arsenic, 400 million lead, 300 million copper, 2,500 million nitrates, 200 million manganese, 1,700 million barium, 1,600 million methanol, 1,500 million ammonia, 1,400 million sulfuric acid acid, 78 million hydrofluoric acid, 64 million,toluene, 47 million styrene, and so on. And the problem is worldwide. In reaction to the havoc caused by the PCBs and DDT, the United States government passed in 1976 the Toxic Substances Control Act. While this piece of legislation marked an awareness of unsafe substances, it grandfathered in 62.000 industerial chemicals already in use. Eighty percent of these chemicals are still in use today. Furthemore, the EPA (Environmental Protection Agency), which administers the Act, and which is dependent on inudustries' volunteer information on chemical risk, has not attempted to ban a chemical since 1989.

Daily, there are stories of pesticide poisoning, some serious enough to promote death. A story in *The New York Times* cites examples of inadequately trained exterminators causing harm to themselves and others. One couple lost a thriving exotic bird business when pesticide fumes seeped into their facility from a neighboring MacDonald's. Subsequently, the 44-year-old owner died of heart omplications. Another couple lost their 23-year-old son, training in forestry, who died after spending a full day spraying. Chemical poisoning was the cause. Although the EPA is charged with collecting and reporting on the impact of pesticide use on the population in the US, its efforts have been hobbled both by lack of funding, inadequate reporting from states (it's voluntary), a backlog of entering reports on hand into the system and inability to enter reports because of confidentiality.

There is a polarity between environmentalists and industry on chemical use with industry lobbying for less stringent laws and environmentalists lobbying in the opposite direction. While some of the older chemicals such as dioxin may no longer be used in the United States, it still remains one of the chemicals used extensively in other parts of the world. Unfortunately, when one chemical is banned, other chemicals fill in the breach. Mercury, for example, is now found at increasingly higher levels in people. Many glaucoma patients complain of burning, itching, excessive tearing, a feeling of heaviness and pressure within the eyes. While these complaints may be related to food sensitivities, they may also be caused by toxic chemicals in the environment. In the United States, regulation of chemicals is still hard-won, but in European countries, positive action has ccurred. Chemicals submitted to the European Union require manufacturers to complete a scientific catalogue of the chemical makeup of the global economy. Burden of the proof will be on the manufacturers who have ten years to complete the process. There may be a link between persistent organic pollution (pesticides) and the incidence of Type II diabetes and the scientists who discovered this link suggest that more study is necessary.

For a comprehensive list of chemicals released into the environment, click on *www.scorecard.org/chemical-profiles/rank-chemicals.tcl?h.*

CHLORINE, renowned for its germ and bacteria-killing properties, should be used judiciously. It enters the water system mainly from industries' solution for disposal of the industrial highly-reactive chlorine waste and the nation's prolific use of chlorine to purify water. In the water, chlorine oxidizes lipid contaminants to form *free radicals* and destroys the antioxidant vitamin E. Although the body uses *free radicals* for metabolic processes, an excess damages the arteries. Some studies have found an accumulation of arterial plaque in animals after drinking chlorinated water. Water-borne chlorine also destroys protective acidophilus, which nourishes and cooperates with three-to-three and a half pounds of immune-strengthening friendly organisms lining the gut as well as destroying essential fatty acids necessary for the brain and central nervous system. Hydrogen peroxide provides a healthful simple solution to the chlorine problem. This compound has been found to be 4,000 times better than chlorine in destroying organisms in the water. It is also an excellent household cleaner.

PESTICIDES lace our foods and while organic food is not totally free of pesticides, they do not carry as much. Below are some of the chemicals that may still be present in the foods that reach your table:

- *Daminozide (Alar)* regulates the growth of apples, nuts, cherries, peaches, grapes, tomatoes and pears.
- *Alachlior (Lasso)* is used on corn and peanuts. Residues contaminate crops, animal products, ground water, and soil.
- *Kwell* and *Scabene,* a miticide used in the medicines to quell lice, is absorbed through upbraided skin and is a neurotoxic agent.
- *Diazinon,* a leading cause of neurotoxicity. Found in garden products is considered by the EPA to be highly toxic. Thirty percent of the uses were restricted in 2003, but seventy percent still remains available.
- *Imidacloprid* used in agriculture, turf, and for controlling fleas in household pets, can produce uncoordinated movements, labored breathing, convulsions and thyroid lesions.

- *Atrazine*, a herbicide, banned in Germany, Austria, The Netherlands, and France, causes eye injury, disrupts the immune system, causes mammary tumors in lab rats and exerts a toxic reaction on the nervous system. It decreases electrical activity of cells governing motor function, muscle tone and balance.
- *Rotenone* has been linked to Parkinson's disease, a neurodegenerative disease. Glaucoma is considered a neurodegenerative disease.
- *Acetone,* found in many products, may cause allergy problems. Exposure results mostly from air, drinking water or with products that contain it. Moderate to high exposure can irritate the eyes, cause dizziness; in susceptible people, cause loss of consciousness.

INERTS are another problem. These substances are found in many products. Of the over 2,000 substances labeled "inerts" over 1,700 are of unknown toxicity; 209 are hazardous air and water pollutants; 127 are listed as occupationally hazardous, and 21 are listed as known or suspected carcinogens.

Inert Ingredients according to a booklet published by Eliot Spitzer, former New York State Attorney General, include suspected carcinogens and neurotoxins that are linked to kidney and liver diseases and birth defects. Some inerts cause short-term health effects such as eye irritation. Problems are compounded when   more than one pesticide is used causing a synergistic effect.

CLEAN UP YOUR FOOD

Given that you may not be able to purchase organic food, incorporate these simple procedures below in your daily food preparation.

- Wash bananas, corn, grapefruit, melons, lemons, and oranges before peeling them. Avoid using orange or lemon peel unless organically grown.
- Thoroughly wash cabbage, cucumbers, eggplants, peppers, and tomatoes. Discard the outer leaves of lettuce and cabbage.
- To preserve and improve appearance, wax is often found on cucumbers, eggplants, peppers. This coating is hard to remove. Scrub any suspect produce well or use a wax remover, obtainable in health food stores. Alternatively, peel fruits and vegetables. Apples especially carry a heavy load of pesticide. Peaches, too, have residues of pesticide and it's best to peel them. Pears and carrots as well should be peeled.
- Wash cauliflower, cherries, grapes, green beans, lettuce, potatoes, and strawberries very well in either a gallon of water laced with a few

drops of hydrogen peroxide or kosher soap, a pure product made from coconut oil. You can find kosher soap in supermarkets.

- Peel potatoes, cut away any green areas, and scoop out the eyes before boiling or steaming them. Baking is acceptable, since dry heat inhibits some of the migration of the toxins.
- Place conventionally-raised broccoli or spinach in a bowl of water with a drop of liquid dishwashing detergent (or swish kosher soap into the water).
- Lower concentrations of pesticide residues are found on canned tomatoes or tomato sauces from the United States. Imported produce is more likely to have larger amounts of pesticide residues. About one-third of the fresh and frozen foods are derived from imported vegetables and fruits. It is not always possible to tell the origin of produce. It is fair to assume, therefore, that out-of-season fruits and vegetables are imported.
- Beans and peas register low levels of pesticide residues.
- Buy cold-pressed vegetable oils processed without chemicals and without preservatives, and store them in dark bottles in your refrigerator. Virgin olive oil is one of the better choices. In Tuscany, a part of Italy, noted for the healthfulness of its Mediterranean Diet, the natives do not cook with the oil but use it on their food after the cooking process. High heating of oils renders them carcinogenic.

BEAUTIFY AND DETOXIFY

Hazardous chemicals or pesticides commonly found in household products include: acetone, aluminum, asbestos, copper, fluoride, fluorine, formaldehyde, lead, mercury, nickel, radon, tin and zinc. Profiles of these substances can be found at *http://allergies.about.com/es/chemica*

Detoxify your living quarters by adding greenery to your living quarters and breathe cleaner air. Some of the plants that are the most efficient detoxifiers include: *Aloe Vera*, (Medicine Plant), *Chlorophytum* (Spider plant,) the *Dracaenas* (Corn Plant and Dragon Tree), *Hedera helix* (English Ivy), *Pepperomia Philodendron cordatum* (Heart-leaf *Philodendron,*) *Sanservia* (Snake Plant), *Spathiphylum* (Peace Lily), *Schefflera* (Umbrella Plant). Have at least three plants in every room.

GENETICALLY-MODIFIED FOODS (GMOS)

Of course, it had to come. Scientific discoveries and possible advances are unstoppable. Although Europeans may resist buying genetically-grown soybeans and corn, these and other foods are creeping into the food chain and according to some reports, it is estimated that seventy percent of the foods on the supermarket shelves now contain some GMOs. Banned in Canada and Europe, but in the United States, thirty percent of the dairy farmers, interested in increasing the volume of milk from their cows, use BGH (bovine growth hormone) despite its ill effect on the dairy cows and humans. Milk carrying BGH also contains elevated levels of IGF-1. This is an endocrine growth regulator that has been known to accelerate cancer growth, and indeed, a study did find an increased risk of breast cancer among pre-menopausal women carrying the highest levels of IGF-1 in their blood. More than fifty percent of the soybeans, thirty-five percent of the corn, and five percent of the potatoes are GMO products. New GMO foods are constantly being introduced. It is estimated that sixty percent of all processed foods have a GMO ingredient and they may even be found in vitamins such as E extracted from soybeans. Those siding with their European cousins whose long history of growing wholesome foods decrying the GMO stampede worry about possible undesirable effects resulting from the introduction of genes from one species to another. Still unknown, is the effect upon the environment when genetic materials escape and contaminate wild plants and perhaps, most important, contribute to the loss of the diversity of plant species, not to mention effects on human health down the road.

British researchers have discovered DNA material in human gut bacteria raising the specter of antibiotic-resistant genes compromising a person's ability over time to fight off infections. The supporters claim the benefits outweigh the risks, citing that GMOs will be instrumental in reducing world hunger, lowering pesticide use through growing pesticide resistant plants, and enhancing the taste, nutritive value, and shelf life of foods. Where the GMO revolution will take the food industry is anybody's guess, but despite the rumble of concerned parties, GMO researchers continue to mix and match species. They have developed altering grapefruit with genes taken from cattle. Citrus meat? What's next? GMOs do not enter into the cultivation of organic foods.

FOOD ENHANCERS AND FLAVORINGS

In the last fifty years or so, producers of packaged foods began to tinker with natural products by adding dyes, waxes and other substances to enhance the attractiveness of the product. Somehow, the food producers believed that pale or natural color of many foods would not attract customers. So food became eye candy and lost its wholesomeness. Additionally, there are flavorings, emulsifiers, stabilizers, and numerous "substitute" ingredients, some of which are considered safe as approved by GRAS, the European standard. Others—well there are questions about their value as a substitute foodstuff. Notwithstanding dubious claims, our food industry is ingenious in attempting to solve problems caused by unhealthy eating. Eating too much fat? Use a non-fat alternative. Find food bland? Wake up the taste buds. Gain too much weight? Use the sugar-free drinks now dominating the marketplace. Additives do raise safety issues and questions. Can the food we eat cause illness? Will these additives have subtle effects on vision? Below is a brief summary of some findings.

FAT SUBSTITUTES

Simplesse, a fat substitute made from whey (a byproduct of cheese) is dried and broken down into microparticles with the same texture and particle size of fat. It can be used in any food product that requires fat, although baking recipes need to be adjusted to maintain the proper balance between liquid and dry ingredients. *Simplesse* is generally considered safe because it is a food product.

Olestra is a questionable synthetic fat substitute. It can be used at high temperatures. The Center for Science in the Public Interest, among others opposes its use, for it may deplete the fat-soluble vitamins (A, E, D, and K) dissolving them and thus eliminating them from the body. Possibly, because it is not digested or assimilated by the body, digestive problems may result. This is reflected in the manufacturer's own studies, where a third of the volunteers experienced diarrhea after eating twenty grams of *Olestra* a day--about the amount in a single two-ounce serving of potato chips. It can also cause anal leakage resulting in greasy feces and stained underwear and may cause liver problems.

THE FLAVOR ENHANCES

Monosodium glutamate (MSG) is the sodium salt of glutamic acid. Although this protein has the amazing attribute of jazzing up the taste of food, it is not a benign additive. It has been associated with more than sixty symptoms among them--migraines, nausea, diarrhea, change in heart rate, chest pain, mood swings, a sensation of facial pressure, headaches, extreme allergic reactions such as burning sensation along the forearms or in the back of the neck and excessive sweating. Studies with lab animals have found brain damage and reproduction dysfunction. There are some studies in the literature indicating that an excess of glutamates may be responsible for the death of cells in the eye. While no direct connection has been established between MSG and eye damage, for glaucoma patients, the possibility exists that MSG may, in some way, be a factor in the overproduction of glutamate in the *retina*. This can result in the death of *retinal* cells, for this product is a free glutamic acid, not to be confused with glutamate naturally occurring in the body which is a bound glutamic acid. It probably is a good idea to limit or avoid foods containing MSG.

In addition to enhancing the flavor of Chinese food, MSG is found in many other foods such as canned soups, dry soup mixes, canned meats, prepared meals, flavored potato chips, prepared snacks, frozen dinners, salad dressings, cured and luncheon meats, poultry injected with broth, soy sauce, soy extract, gravy and seasoning mixes, spices, ketchup, chili, chicken, pork, beef and smoke flavorings, seasoning salts, breading mix, carrageen or vegetable gum, canned tuna, ice cream, frozen yogurt, low-fat foods, crackers, candy, chewing gum, whey protein concentrate, protease, protease enzymes, and, unfortunately, in baby foods. Read labels carefully. When it is part of another food such as hydrolyzed vegetable protein, bouillon cubes, autolyzed yeast extract, natural flavorings and potassium gluconate. It may not appear on the label. Food found in health food stores is not exempt from some of these additives. Over 120,000 pounds are used annually in the United States.

SWEETENERS

We seem to be addicted to sweetening our foods and as a result, sugar or artificial sweeteners are found in just about every product including coated vitamin tablets. At the same time, we have been told that sugar is bad for us, promoting tooth decay, weight gain, and diabetes. The industry, of course, has stepped in with an array of artificial sweeteners that, for many people, satisfy sugar cravings. But are these sweeteners safe? Do they benefit or impair human health? Here are some thoughts worth considering when you pour that packet of sweetener into your coffee or tea.

Acesulfame-K, sold under the brand names Sunette or Sweet One, is synthesized from ketones and oxocarbonic acid. Each serving contains less than 4 calories and is equal in sweetness to two teaspoons of sugar. *Acesulfame-K* is found in confections, canned fruit, gelatins, puddings, custards, chewing gum, dry beverage mixes. It can be used in baking, The FDA does not report any toxic effect but the safety of *acesulfame-K* rests on three animal studies conducted in the mid 1970's. The Center for Science in the Public Interest reported that in two separate animal studies, those animals fed *acesulfame-K* were more likely to develop tumors than those in a control group. On the basis of their research, The Center for Science in the Public Interest advises that it should be avoided.

Aspartame (NutraSweet or Equal) is derived from two amino acids, forty percent aspartic acid and fifty percent phenylalanine and ten percent of a methyl ester that promptly becomes free methanol after entering the stomach. Each component leaves a toxic trail. The body attempts to detoxify methyl alcohol by oxidizing it to formaldehyde (a deadly neurotoxin) and then to formic acid or formate. Free methyl alcohol may remain in the system for three days before it is oxidized into harmless carbon dioxide. Persons with phenylketonuria (PKU) must avoid this product, as they lack the enzyme necessary to break down phenylalanine. The accumulation of phenylalanine in the brain can cause mental retardation in children, along with other adverse effects. As well, phenylalanine through the action of breaking down into dopamine, norepinephrine, and epinephrine, can cause pulmonary hypertension and cardiac arrhythmias.

Ocular and other manifestations of aspartame dramatically improved when patients no longer ate products containing this additive in sweetened foods. Visual fields improved. It has also been implicated in dry eye syndrome and other more serious visual problems such as toxic amblyopia, and transient blindness diagnosed as optic neuritis that may be partly due to the breakdown of methanol.

Neurological manifestations include headache, dizziness, unsteadiness, confusion, memory loss, severe drowsiness and sleepiness, convulsions, severe slurring of speech, severe tremors, hyperactivity, restless legs, atypical facial pain, aggravation of diabetic neuropathy, birth defects, and aggravation of *Parkinson's Disease*. In other reports, fibromyalgia, multiple sclerosis, systemic lupus, and *Graves' disease* (associated with hyperthyroidism) have been traced to extensive *aspartame* use. Sleep apnea in *aspartame* users may reflect neurotransmitter dysfunction in the respiratory center. Carpal tunnel syndrome, both unilateral and bilateral, has occurred in five patients who consumed considerable amounts of *aspartame*.

This substance, according to some reports, can cause serious cardiovascular, neuropsychiatric, metabolic and other adverse effects. Also, reports of headaches, asthma, allergies, fatigue, irritability, hair loss, heavy menstrual bleeding, abdominal pain, weight gain, dryness of skin, epileptic-like episodes, and deaths have been linked to the ingestion of *aspartame*. The Palm Beach Institute for Medical Research reports that of 2,300 *aspartame* reactors in their data base, 103 had symptomatic arrhythmia, 85 atypical chest pains and 64 with aggravated hypertension. Of this group, one hypertensive patient developed heart block, another underwent unsuccessful radiofrequency ablations in the heart—symptoms related to *aspartame* consumption. Diabetic patients should consult with their physicians before using this product.

Aspartame is found in over 6,000 products, including soft drinks, desserts, baked goods, gelatins, gum, frozen desserts, juices, cereals, vitamins, and pharmaceuticals, and of course, as a table sweetener. Unfortunately, for some who ingest large amounts of *aspartame,* addiction becomes a problem. While these people may strive to eliminate *aspartame* sweetened products, they are foiled by their own cravings.

The consultant to The NutraSweet Company takes exception to the above by citing the following: "Since its approval, *aspartame* has undergone further investigation through clinical and laboratory research, intake studies and postmarketing surveillance of anecdotal reports of adverse health effects…the Committee (the Scientific Committee on Food of the European Commission) concluded on the basis of its review of all the data in animals and humans available to date to suggest…earlier risk assessment…(confirming) …the safety of *aspartame.*"

SACCARIN (Sweet 'N Low, Sugar Twin) in use since 1879 is another problem sweetener. In 1977, the FDA announced it would ban the use of *saccharin* in foods, based on Canadian studies that linked it to bladder cancer in laboratory animals. At the time, Americans consumed a whopping five million pounds of *saccharin* yearly, seventy-four percent in diet soda, fourteen percent in dietetic food, and twelve percent as a tablet or sweetener. The Calorie Control Council, an organization comprising commercial producers and users of *saccharin,* howled in protest, and the FDA, urged by Congress, caved in, delaying the ban, although warning labels were instituted. Yet the National Cancer Institute in one of its own studies found some evidence that heavy *saccharin* use (six or more servings of sugar substitute) was linked to bladder cancer. Britain banned *saccharin* in 1979 for uses other than as a tabletop sweetener. France has outlawed its use except in nonprescription drugs, and Germany restricts its use in certain foods and beverage. We are still waiting for the US to act.

SWITCH BACK TO SUGAR?

No, no, no. Sugar is implicated in many diseases including cataracts. Although fructose is sometimes touted as a safe alternative for sucrose, the opposite is true. The ingestion of large amounts of fructose (a large soft drink) has been shown to accelerate the aging process. Large amounts overwhelm the body's fructose-metabolizing capacity and when this occurs there can be a possible adverse effect on autoimmune disease resulting in inflammation. For sweeteners, try xylitol or stevia, both naturally sweet substances. They can also be used for baking. Mashed bananas also add a nice touch of both of sweetness and moisture to baked desserts.

Subversive Substances—Mycotoxins/molds/yeasts/fungi

Moldy foods are toxic. Yeast infections can infect the eyes. Some researchers claim that mycotoxins causing inflammation are responsible for a number of the diseases. *Candida Albicans,* found in just about all of us, is kept in check by friendly bacteria in the gut. When out of bounds, however, in the presence of a weakened immune system, it can invade all major organs including the brain. *Candida* presents a problem of infection found in people of all ages from infants to seniors. *Candida* growth in the gut is abetted by a diet high in sugars and refined foods (the *candida* family gorges on these nutrients). Medical interventions such as chemotherapy, joint replacements, catheter implantation and other invasive therapies become unwilling hosts to Candida. There are possibly hundreds of species of mold that infect our bodies and our food. Some are found in USFD&C Indogene #3 and Fast Green (FCF). These dyes, which should be avoided according to Center for Science in the Public Interest, are found in such foods as gelatins, puddings, dairy products, medicines, ice cream, sherbet, baked goods, lollypops, and confections. Today, colorings and dies, many of which are carcinogenic, are found in cereal products, baked goods, snack foods, meat, fish, poultry, cheese, butter, alcoholic and soft drinks.

Antibiotics destroy both the good and the bad fungi in the gut and should be replaced immediately with friendly bacteria found in such foods as yogurt and probiotic supplements. The body's successful ability to fight off *Candida* is seen in the laboratory where antibodies to heat shock proteins are present.

Preserved Foods

In ancient times, people devised means for preserving foods through a variety of methods. These techniques actually enhanced the nutritious value of the foods. Pickling cabbage, onions and cucumbers produces probiotics that help to digest food. Cheeses like Stilton, Gorgonzola other strong-smelling cheeses and those made from raw milk contain probiotics as do kimchi, a Korean preserved vegetable, sauerkraut (the German version), soy sauce and other Japanese preserved products. These methods of preserving foods actually transformed them to an equally healthful alternative.

Modern methods for preserving foods aim to keep the food intact by adding chemicals. *Butylated hydroxyanisole (BHA)* and *butylated hydroxytoluene (BHT)* prevent oxidation and retard rancidity when added to foods containing oil. Animal studies, however, suggest the possibility of carcinogenic action although it is unclear whether BHA is the cause, since some studies say the chemical prevents cancers. BHT is classified as GRAS which means that it is considered safe, but in England, they are taking no chances, for it has been prohibited as a food additive.

Potassium nitrate is the chemical responsible for that lovely red color in corned beef, ham, bacon, and hot dogs. It inhibits the growth of botulism-causing bacteria and it is in itself harmless, but when it is ingested, bacteria found in foods and in the blood easily convert it to nitrite, which, when combining with natural stomach and food chemicals, forms nitrosamine, a cancer-causing substance. The high temperatures at which many of these foods, especially bacon, are cooked also promote this transformation. Bacon and other meats cured with ascorbic acid or erythorbic acid, which inhibits the formation of nitrosamines, are safer--but they still contain dangerous saturated fats.

Sulfites. What can be more attractive than a box of artfully arranged dried fruit? The glowing colors immediately tempt the appetite. Left to dry naturally, fruits such as apricots or figs simply darken, considered by food purveyors to be unattractive. Enter sulfites. There are six sulfites currently classified as GRAS: sulfur dioxide, sodium sulfate, sodium and potassium bisulfate, and sodium and potassium metabisulfite. They are used in many processed foods, but since they can cause allergic problems including acute asthma attacks, loss of consciousness, anaphylactic shock, diarrhea and nausea in susceptible individuals, the use of sulfites must be placed on the label. They should not, however, be used in fresh foods, but sulfite dioxide fumigation may still be used in products such as table grapes, and some restaurants and foods stores use them to keep their display of fresh vegetables from wilting. Wines, soy sauce, and balsamic vinegar have natural and added sulfites.

Carrageen is a carbohydrate derived from seaweed that is used as a stabilizer and emulsifier in oils, cosmetics, and foods. You will probably find it listed as one of the ingredients in chocolate flavored drinks, pressure-dispensed whipped cream, ice cream, frozen custard, sherbets, ices, cheese spreads, salad dressings, artificially sweetened jam, and jellies. It is considered safe.

Plastic Is it possible to live today without encountering the ubiquitous plastic wrap? Not likely. Yet this seemingly benign material is host to some serious health and environmental problems. Plastics do not biologically degrade, causing environmental damage. Phthalates, plasticizers used to make plastic wrap, migrate into fatty foods such as cheese and meat. Phthalates are also found in Barbie dolls, children's toys, baby foods, bottles and teethers. The Bisphenol-A (BPA) component of plastic products found in products such as metal food cans, polycarbonate water jugs and the sealant on children's teeth has been under study as to its effects on humans. Women of child-bearing age had fifty percent higher phthalates than average. These substances have been shown to increase the risk of miscarriage in women. Animal studies have shown BPA to alter male reproductive organs. They mimic estrogen, possibly inducing cancer. Nevertheless, there is controversy over whether these substances do indeed cause harm. Research gathered in England has found that it does not harm humans, stating that the major research studies have been in rodents and cannot be translated to the human. The main problem may be the environmental impact of millions of plastic bottle filling land-fills, polluting oceans, and endangering fish and sea turtles that ingest the bottles.

But you may still want to protect yourself when buying plastic-wrapped items by immediately storing them more safely in rigid containers, wax paper or glass. When purchasing plastic wrap, choose America's Choice, Duane Reade, Foodtown, Glad, or White Rose. We do not recommend microwaving but if you must, use glass or ceramic containers. There is a drive on to encourage food chain stores to stock only items that do not contain phthalates. Make your voice heard. *TANNING AGENTS*

Either oral or external, used in excess can cause canthaxanthin retinopathy—crystalline deposits in the *retina* and visual acuity loss.

ELECTROMAGNETIC ENERGY

The revolutionary benefits of harnessing electromagnetic energy to power our homes, the spread of microwave equipment, the world of digital technomics and of course, the ubiquitous cell phones and I phones, etc. cannot be underestimated in its impact on the environment we live in. Even toddlers attending nursery school possess their own cell phones providing parents instant access to the child's needs. Unfortunately, this almost constant flow of radioactive energy may produce detrimental effects upon the body. Industry denies linkages between radiation and cancer, the disease most often linked to environmental changes. Microwaves emit radioactive energy. Cell phones held against the ears have been implicated in the rise of brain cancer although the industry assumes since tissue is not heated, use of cell phones in moderation does no harm. But with the addiction to cell phone use that has swept around the world, moderation appears unlikely. Fortunately, newer versions do not require ear contact. Nevertheless, it is instructive to note that the brain's cells respond to the low-frequency magnetic fields produced by cell phones.

Longitudinal studies may yet reveal what some health practitioners intuit to be the cause of increased *free radical* activity in the brain.

Cell phones are not the only instruments increasing exposure to electromagnetic energy. Electric blankets, toasters, digital clocks, television sets, computers, the electrified kitchen—these marvelous products that reduce drudgery—all emit radiation that may be harmful. There is a small movement among a group of people who preach SIMPLIFY. Perhaps some resistance to the newest electrical "gadget" might also benefit health.

A WORD ABOUT COOKWARE

Stay away from aluminum. It may be carcinogenic. Use copper pots only if lined. Cast iron and steel are good. Ceramic manufactured in China, Hong Kong, India and Mexico may contain lead that can leach into foods. Non-stick is problematical. Left on high heat, Teflon and similar coatings can create unhealthy fumes. Microwaving is considered by some health experts to be unsafe. Nuked food introduces unaccustomed molecules and energies to the body. Microwave energy from the sun and stars is direct current but microwave ovens use alternating current that forces a billion or more of polarity reversals (from north to south and vice-versa), an agitation that heats up the food. This molecular friction damages surrounding molecules, often deforming them and impairing quality. The electrical potentials between the inner and outer sides of the cell membranes, the very life of the cell, are neutralized. The process destroys nutrients and transforms some amino acids into carcinogenic compounds. A small study in Germany found that after two months of eating microwaved foods, subjects showed pathological changes as compared with controls who cooked their food the old-fashioned way. Microwaved food, therefore, contains unknowns and there are cases in the literature where eating these foods has caused harm. If you feel you must microwave, then at least do not use the plastic container or plastic wrap despite the manufacturer's claim that the material is microwaveable. Carcinogens and xenoestrogens (combining form containing strange or foreign material) reach the food at four million times the FDA standard when cooked in plastic. Use ceramic or Pyrex containers.

Aside from health concerns, taste and texture are altered in microwaved foods and some purists complain that even water boiled in the microwave alters the taste of coffee and tea.

FOOD AND DRUGS THAT DON'T MIX

Some of us take other medications in addition to our glaucoma therapies. As we learned, foods contain a multitude of compounds and some of these interfere or are contraindicated when taking specific medications. Alcoholic beverages may increase drowsiness when taking seasonal allergy medications or antidepressants (*Prozac, Zoloft, Paxil*) and *Ambien* for insomnia. Taking Glucophage or Glucotrol XI may prolong the risk of abnormally low blood sugar. *Lanoxin* for congestive heart failure should be taken separately from meals high in bran fiber. Avoid gingko biloba, bilberry, foods high in vitamin K such as turnip greens, broccoli and deep-green leafy vegetables and alcohol if taking the blood thinner *Coumadin* or *warfarin*. High-fat meals slow the rate on absorption of *Viagra*. Grapefruit can slow the absorption of *Propulsid, Norvasc, Cardizem, Procardia* or *Adalat*. It also acts in the same manner with the statin drugs—*Lipitor, Zocor, Pravachol*. Potassium-rich foods, including salt substitutes containing potassium, are contraindicated when taking *Zestril, Vasobac, Acupril, Lotensin or Prinivil*. High fiber and soy diets may decrease the amount of absorption. Take *Fosomax* on an empty stomach, for mineral water, orange juice, coffee and tea, high-fiber diets, and soy products can decrease the drug's availability.

NUTRITIONAL CONSEQUENCES OF COMMON DRUGS:

Coumadin	Blocks enzyme that synthesizes vitamin K
Iron	Competes with chromium and other minerals for iabsorption
Calcium	Competes with magnesium if taken together
Antibiotics	Destroys good bacteria in intestine
Corticosteroids	Reduces vitamin D, decreases absorption of calcium, chromium loss
Diuretics	Increases urinary losses of zinc, magnesium, water
B Blockers	Reduces coenzyme Q10
NSAIDS	Affects folate synthesis

CHAPTER 12

Take Charge

○ ○

Now I know the things I know
And do the things I do,
And if you do not like me so,
To hell, my love, with you!
Dorothy Parker, "Indian Summer,"
Enough Rope, (1926)2

We carry our homes within us which enables us to fly,"
John Cage,"45' for a speaker,"
Silence (1961)

Like Pearl Harbor, 9/11 is a day that will live in infamy in the history of the United States and the world. Its disastrous consequences still echo in the hearts and minds of many who were involved, some of whom courageously rescued and saved themselves and others. One incredible escape that emerged from the inferno of that day touches glaucoma patients most poignantly. Omer E. Rivera, a systems analyst, working at the World Trade Center had lost his sight to glaucoma. With his dog Salty, he pushed forward down the stairs to emerge on the ground floor an hour and fifteen minutes later. Then although both he and his dog were exhausted they managed to run from the scene, narrowly escaping the collapse of the tower. Taking charge comes naturally to Rivera. Although he lost his computer containing thirteen years of files, he began to immediately reconstruct his life.

For some of us, it is not a sudden catastrophic event that disrupts our lives, but rather a steady erosion of our faculties in the presence of a debilitating disease. Richard M. Cohen, a journalist and former television producer has written a book, *Blindsided: Living a Life Above Illness* is according to a review by *The New York Times* an "extended treatise on the psychology of coping," for not only has Cohen lost the use of his legs, but his voice is weakened and he is legally blind. The onset of the illness, *multiple sclerosis*, did not keep Cohen from completing graduate school, traveling and reporting from war zones and talking his way into a job with CBS. In Cohen's case, denial of his limitations left him free to pursue his dream.

That quality of life diminishes with any disease is a given and loss of vision falls into this unfortunate syndrome. More worrisome, however, are reports that when vision diminishes, mortality increases. A study by researchers in Melbourne, Australia found that of 3,271 patients participating, 231 had died in the intervening five years. Decreased visual acuity was significantly related to an increased risk of mortality with increasing age. Since the publication of this study, other studies have claimed no difference in death rates of the visually impaired as compared with the general population. Noted in a study of 2,107 participants aged 60-to-87, the visually impaired may also experience hearing loss leading to increased disability. Those participants with both hearing and vision loss scored thirty percent lower than those with only vision loss on a scale measuring the impact of these losses on physical disability.

Another phenomenon, an upwelling of hallucinations, occurs at times with patients who experience severe vision loss. Many of these patients, especially those over the age of seventy, are reluctant to share this experience with their doctors fearful of being evaluated as mentally deficient. Nothing to fear should you experience hallucinations. This phenomenon is called *Charles Bonnet Disease*. Researchers estimate that ten-to-fifteen percent of those whose eyesight is worse than 20/60 develop this condition. The range of hallucinations varies with each patient--some report monsters, others nice little geometric figures. Medications do not help, for manifestation of the disease lies in the loss of neurons in the brain, and the tendency of the visual cortex to fill in the gap left vacant by this loss. Apparently, the primary visual cortex is programmed to both receive information and to remember images. Normal vision requires a fusion of incoming sensory information with internally-generated sensory input. In the case of hallucinations, expectations of what you think you see confounds with what you actually see.

YOU AND YOUR DOCTOR

According to a survey conducted by the Glaucoma Research Foundation, patients did not fully understand the implications of being diagnosed with glaucoma. More than 49% (the cohort included 4,300 responses) did not realize that glaucoma could lead to blindness, while 87% of the patients expect that their doctors will educate them about glaucoma. When patients do not comply with the medication prescribed, it's primarily because, given glaucoma's silent footprint, they lack understanding of the nature of the disease. Although the majority of the respondents (70%) remained loyal to their physicians, those who switched mentioned lack of communication as the major cause. When diagnosing glaucoma, doctors need to be sensitive to a patient's emotional reactions to the bad news. Subconsciously, patients often deny the gravity of this disease as a defense. Should a doctor takes a few minutes to explain the nature of glaucoma, they have found that patients are more willing to comply with the medical protocols and, if necessary, to laser and filtration procedures.

Nevertheless, the quality of health care is an important issue that bedevils patients and has some bearing on patient education. Whatever solutions are proposed, the results often fall short. Patients complain that they are not getting the service they need. The requirements of the HMO's (Health Maintenance Organizations) that doctors see X number of patients in X minutes of time leaves very little breathing space for discussion and establishing confident doctor-patient relationships. With Internet access, patients are better informed about their particular afflictions, including possible alternative or complementary approaches. They often desire to discuss these approaches with their doctors, only to find their doctors either reluctant to talk about them or simply dismiss them as irrelevant. That is not to say that everyone is dissatisfied with their medical care. Patients who have long-standing relationships with their doctors are extremely loyal, as noted in the survey and trust their doctors to make the right decisions about their care.

A problem arises when the primary physician retires or needs to relinquish practice because of illness. As competent as the new doctor is, only with time will a new relationship blossom into mutual respect and trust. Recently, I had to find both a new primary care and a glaucoma doctor, for both my doctors retired. With these doctors, I had established a fulfilling relationship, and although they did not entirely agree with some of my views, especially relating to complementary medicine and my resistance to certain common procedures, nevertheless, they granted me that autonomy. Subsequently, I found a primary care doctor and aired my views with him, confidant that he, too, would respect my active role in my own health care. To my surprise and shock, a year later when I needed to have a physical because of an upcoming eye operation, I found him to be dismissive of my philosophy considering it to be in defiance of his recommendations. He no longer wished to be my doctor. Fortunately, I had better luck with my glaucoma doctor, who is intrigued by my views and open to my attempts to maintain optimum health, provided I follow his recommendations for eye care. I subsequently found a new primary care doctor who respects my views. There is an emotional component that cannot be ignored in a good doctor-patient relationship. Above and beyond efficient and sustainable medical practice is the mutual respect and yes, love. Losing a doctor either from illness, new location or for any other reason for the patient is like losing a lover. I can attest to this as can Bill, also a glaucoma patient, that loss of a beloved doctor can leave an empty space in the heart.

GETTING THE NEWS

Doctors are trained to detect glaucoma conditions and in the words of George L. Spaeth, MD, Wills Eye Hospital, "we may ignore the forest for the trees… Because we concentrate on indirect measures of disability and because we rarely attempt seriously to develop quantitative estimates of rate of change, we may allow real disability to develop unnecessarily and make patients ill with medications unnecessarily, as we try to prevent projected disabilities that do not exist and will actually materialize…when the primary outcome measures should be quality of life and activities of daily living." One member of our Group reported that when she received a diagnosis of glaucoma, she immediately switched from the doctor she had been seeing to a glaucoma specialist, reasoning that she now needed a doctor who would "impart a sense of understanding and empathy for what it's like to have this disease." She considered a doctor to be a partner in maintaining the health of her eyes, one who listened and respected her concerns. Another member described receiving the news as being punched so hard in the stomach, it took her breath away. That glaucoma would imperil her carefree lifestyle particularly troubled her. And still another member of the group described receiving a diagnosis of ocular hypertension at age 28! This gentleman, puzzled, after seeking a second opinion, learned that he had angle-recession glaucoma. Fortunately, years later, with continued care, he has lost very little vision. Patients are extremely sensitive and alert to a doctor's reactions. One ARMD patient was shocked to hear a doctor say "wow" when he examined her eyes. Although she knew she had ARMD, this doctor's reaction disturbed and frightened her. Earlier in her medical history, she was told she had drusen but was given no further explanation of her condition and what might lie ahead. She finally found a doctor who discussed her condition and recommended in addition to treatment a dietary change along with particular supplements.

Treatment options follow hard on the heels of diagnosis. Before my glaucoma diagnosis I had little idea of the meaning of chronic illness—yes, I had been exposed to my mother's neurasthenia, but my life style and attitude was far different from hers. Yet, here I was with this label of chronic illness pasted on my consciousness. Many persons like me who develop glaucoma relatively early have never experienced much more illness than a severe cold.

To be suddenly told that their condition requires consistent surveillance is shocking news. Here is where early patient education pays off. Not fully understanding the implication of high *intraocular pressure*, the patient may not consider his/her condition seriously and/or may be delinquent in following the doctor's recommendations. It's like a diabetic saying, "I have little bit of sugar," or a teenager saying, "I'm a little pregnant." Some patients deny the diagnosis, and others, totally at sea, obsessively seek other opinions among friends, other doctors, allied patients, the internet, indulging in a pseudo-scientific numbers game of comparing their IOP's with other glaucoma patients. In the early stages of glaucoma and where significant damage is not apparent, patients may balk at taking drops. Some patients experience difficulty in understanding that precautions taken when the risk seems minimal will pay off in the future.

COMMUNICATION—LET'S TALK

Today, the glaucoma doctor possesses many tools backed by evidence-based research to treat glaucoma patients. Throughout this book we have cited numerous studies justifying doctor-recommendations. Perhaps the most significant has been the conclusion that lowering *intraocular pressure* to the low teens is of benefit in managing glaucoma. In fact, there are some patients with advanced glaucoma who may do better with IOP's in the high single digits. Patient resistance to taking additional medication may evaporate should the doctor share this information with them. If a procedure does not turn out as predicted, patients want to know possible reasons and other options. I recently had an almost daily exchange of E-mails with a daughter distraught because a cataract operation on her mother's glaucomatous eye left the mother in worse shape than before the operation. The doctor would not discuss the situation with the mother or daughter. Instead he recommended other procedures failing to explain clearly why the recommendation or the possible outcomes. Both mother and daughter were hysterical from anxiety and fear. There are times when hand-holding and thoroughly explaining a procedure can mean the difference between success and failure. Hysterical reactions lead to stress, a condition that bodes poorly for a successful outcome following a procedure.

Naturally, there are two sides to this coin. There are those patients who can try the patience of a saint. Everyone knows at least one. These are the people so beset by anxiety that they never cease lobbing questions and/or challenges to the doctor at every step along the treatment path. Often they repeat the same question again and again cornering doctor, technician, other patients, and so on. They summon up outdated information as justification for not following their doctor's recommendations. Understandably, these patients tax the doctor, who after all has comparable need—an affirming relationship, a knowledge that the recommended treatment is working, and that the patient is being helped.

Between these two extremes, we've arrived at a sort of consensus of what patients and doctors want from each other. We've drawn from material published over thirty years ago where one of the speakers described three basic types of doctor-patient relationships at an annual meeting of the Pacific Coast Ophthalmological Society in California.

1. **Active–passive.** The doctor makes all the decisions. Usually, this relationship is found in treatment of infants, those with severe injuries or who are comatose.

2. **Guidance–cooperative**. Many doctors might find this the ideal relationship. The patient seeks help and faithfully follows the doctor's instructions to the letter. This most common relationship resembles the parent-child interaction.

3. **Mutual participation**. This is an adult-adult cooperative relationship, one worth achieving if possible especially for those with a chronic disease such as glaucoma. Management of chronic diseases requires the full cooperation of both patient and doctor.

4. **The difficult patient**. A quite different category taken from the doctor's viewpoint may be added to the above. These are patients who are antagonistic to the system, who may take matters in their own hands without consulting their doctor, who threaten to sue, or who simply ignore the doctor's instructions while complaining loudly that they are not being helped.

Let's review what happens in the doctor's office today. Have relationships between doctor and patient evolved into Mutual Participation? Do we now have more democratic, adult-adult relationships with our doctors? Observationally, it appears that although the authority figure—doctor, teacher, boss, political leader is challenged more frequently, the doctor, tightly holding the health reins, is often timorously approached. Some members of the support group express a love-hate relationship with their doctors. When their visual fields appear to be stable, they love and praise their physicians. When various tests indicate vision loss, they may revile the care they receive and seek out other opinions or options. They recount how they followed their doctors' instructions and yet their glaucoma worsened. Some members complain of being rebuffed when they attempt to establish more mature, equal relationships with their physicians.

The limited time a doctor spends with a patient is at times frustrating. Doctors pressed for time often cut to the chase, but the patient faced with the threat of losing sight (or any other life-changing medical condition) may need a reassuring climate--hand-holding, per se. Time-constraints often take place in a teaching hospital where the patient's preliminary workup has been completed by a technician, resident fellow, or assistant before being seen by the primary doctor. If all goes well, the patient grimly accepts whatever the situation appears to be, but when further intervention is needed, patients often grumble about the lack of time spent with their primary glaucoma doctor.

We humans have an insatiable desire to categorize—black-white, good-bad, great-awful, caring-uncaring, and so on. Can we classify doctors as uncaring, unfeeling and out of touch with emotional needs? Should we expect the doctor to be sensitive to our feelings as well as attendant to our treatment? Should doctors trained in medicine, diagnostics and surgical procedures also be required to study human relations?

Well, apparently, yes. Teaching hospitals have introduced courses to sensitize medical students on the importance of understanding the emotional and physical components of having a chronic disease. Nationwide, hospitals are incorporating sensitivity training sessions into their residency programs. In these programs, medical students and residents assume the role of patient. They may wear blurred contact lenses, walk around with joint-restricting splints, listen to actors impersonating elderly and/or ill persons, and/or spend the night in a hospital bed in traction or with IVs in their arms, to name but a few of the techniques (and indignities) thrust upon the patient. Reports from the institutions that have used this type of training are encouraging. Many of the doctors who have completed such programs say that the experience changed their attitudes towards their patients. Yet, only recently, a series of articles in *The New York Times* reported on the indignities that patients still experience when hospitalized. In the long run, despite such reports, the fact that the training institutions are attending to the emotional component of patients' needs is good news. We do need, however, to understand that professionally, a doctor would be emotionally destroyed if he or she were to beat up on him or herself when a condition worsens or even fails after recommended treatment. Our expectation, therefore, of the perfect doctor-patient relationship may be unrealistic. Ultimately, it is up to each of us to choose to remain with or to seek another doctor.

Whatever the choice, it's as much up the patient as the doctor to establish a responsible adult-adult relationship. This may be difficult if you are one of those patients who regard the doctor as an authority figure. To get some insight into your own attitude, try the following. Draw a picture of yourself and your doctor. Did you draw both you and your doctor of equal size? This little test may give you some idea of how you regard yourself in relationship to your doctor. If you drew yourself as tiny in comparison to your doctor, your innate perceptions may interfere with establishing a mature relationship with your physician.

WHICH DOCTOR IS BEST FOR ME?

Here, you're in the driver's seat. The doctor does not choose you—choice of doctor is up to you. This is your first step in developing a satisfactory relationship. For your condition, you want to select a doctor with adequate experience in treating glaucoma. Consider also location. Difficulty in reaching your doctor may both compromise scheduling and exhaust you given traffic and transportation conditions. If you're hassled getting to your doctor, you may be stressed out, a condition that may impact on your treatment.

Perhaps one of the most difficult problems once the above has been resolved is the choice. A primary physician or a support group for members can help. The primary physician will usually be familiar with experts in the field and members of the support group can share their experiences and offer suggestions. You might want to contact the American Optometric Association or American Academy of Ophthalmology (see Resources) for a list of doctors in your vicinity. Should there be a teaching hospital in your area, you will have a wide selection of doctors.

If you have been assiduous in your search for a doctor, you may find yourself in a quandary as to which doctor will be right for you. In this case, you might make appointments with several doctors and check out the vibes during your first visit. Usually, this seat of the pants method works well. Intuitively, you know whether this is the doctor for you. You may be one of those people particularly sensitive to office set-up including décor and staff attitudes. Are the seating arrangements comfortable? Is the temperature in the office comfortable? Is the lighting adequate for reading? Glaucoma patients are very sensitive to light conditions. Many patients like to read while waiting to see their doctors. Are there flowers or plants to calm your spirit? Are there pictures on the walls? Is the staff (one or many) courteous and willing to listen to your needs such as appointment preferences? Is the staff helpful in setting up an emergency appointment if needed? Will the staff help you wade through the insurance documents? Will insurance cover the costs of treatment? A comforting secretary or technician can set the tone for a stress-free experience. When you've chosen a doctor, you are as responsible as is the doctor to enact a positive and instructive tone. Avoid passivity. Some doctors believe that passivity is a risk factor in managing a chronic disease.

Here's how you can take charge of your treatment.

- Bring along your medical history. By law, you have the legal right to all your medical documents. Keep this information in a medical packet readily available for all your physician appointments. This is especially helpful should you elect to change doctors.

- Inform your doctor if there's a genetic history of glaucoma in your family.
- Keep your doctor informed of current health problems and required medications. Some of these medications may be contraindicated for glaucoma patients.
- Write down all your questions. Often during a visit questions evaporate from your mind, and re-emerge after you've left the premises.

Write down your doctor's instructions. Memory plays tricks. Although you're certain that you'll recall exactly what the doctor said, the mind often interweaves prior information with what you have been told reconfiguring your doctor's message. As an aside, my husband and I, when relating trips we've taken together, speak of completely different versions of the same experience.

- Be sure to write down instructions you need to follow if you are slated to have a procedure. Note common questions in Chapters 6 and 7 to ask your doctor.
- Bring along, a friend, spouse or partner if you have trouble remembering or record the session
- Find out how best to contact your doctor in case of an emergency.
- Establish a follow-up plan. Ascertain your doctor's hospital affiliation, for should you have an emergency, you will want to be treated by your own physician.
- When traveling prepare a "medical passport" containing information on your medications, doses, supplements and homeopathic therapies.

REASONABLE EXPECTATIONS BETWEEN YOU AND YOUR DOCTOR

Patients, according to a series of interviews conducted a few years back, want their doctors to be confident, humane, empathetic, personal, respectful, outright and thorough. These ideals may fall short when on a first visit, the doctor may ask, "What brought you here?" You launch into an explanation, perhaps tendentious, but in your mind, necessary. Eighteen seconds later, your doctor interrupts. If you are not intimidated, you may (chances are you won't) respond, "let me finish." This common patient-doctor interaction is considered by some researchers to have an effect on the outcome of treatment. Furthermore, the researchers advanced the possibility that a satisfactory relationship limits the possibility that a patient will sue for malpractice should the outcome of treatment result in loss of function. A good bedside manner, once an integral ingredient of the doctor-patient relationship, is making a slow comeback based on research findings that good communication between doctor and patient has an effect on patient outcomes. Researchers have demonstrated reduction of pain in cancer patients, improved emotional and physical health, reduced stress and anxiety, lower blood sugar levels in diabetic patients, and lower blood pressure in hypertensive patients.

When I joined the support group, the coordinator at that time told me about a particular doctor whose patients appeared to do well under his treatment. Subsequently, I became his patient and I understood why he had gained his reputation. He spent as much time as needed (often more than an hour) with each patient. In my case, he thoroughly explored my unique requirements and responded to all my questions. Managed care administrators intent on containing costs have frowned on this extravagant use of time, but they, too, heeding research findings citing hard evidence for stretching doctor-patient time, are reexamining time constraints

Treating a chronic disease such as glaucoma requires both art and skill. Patients who are confident of their doctor's judgment often accept interventions willingly, realizing various procedures to be part of the inevitable continuum of treatment. Yet there are those patients who balk at any intervention other than the use of eye drops. These patients may need to seek out corroborating information from a variety of sources. One of the members of the group balked at the suggestion of filtration surgery offered by her doctor who abruptly told her she was losing sight but did not fully explain the consequences. Not until she explored *trabeculectomies* on the internet and learned the consequences of uncontrolled pressure did she decide to proceed with the filtration operation, but first, she wanted to talk about it more fully with her doctor. She called and asked to speak to him and requested he call her at his convenience. After three attempts when the doctor failed to respond, she transferred to a more accommodating physician willing to spend time with her and who then successfully performed the filtration operation.

Trust in the doctor's judgment is essential to glaucoma treatment. That trust is formed first and foremost by the doctor's acceptance of the patient's qualms, and secondly, from the patient's perception of the doctor's experience and ability. Even so, the patient may want to seek a second opinion and appreciates a doctor's acceptance of this common practice.

For a positive doctor-patient relationship, you can expect your doctor to:
- Provide information on the condition of your eye(s)—*intraocular pressure, optic nerve evaluation, visual field* results and prognosis, if that is relevant.

- Unequivocally respond to all your questions.
- Describe the action of the medication. If additive medications are recommended, explain why. Help the patient set up a schedule for taking the medications. Explain how to instill a drop.
- Describe procedures to follow should an *angle closure glaucoma* attack occur with patients who have not had prophylactive surgery
- Explain the common outcomes in detail of *laser* or *filtration* surgery, the pre-and post-op treatment should these procedures be required, and to be available following surgery to trouble-shoot should there be complications.
- Should your sight worsen, referral should be made to a low-vision specialist along with assistance of the required paperwork for referral to the State Office for the Visually Impaired.

As a patient, you need to do your part to assure that the doctor-patient relationship works for you

- Be responsible. Follow your doctor's instructions. Take your drops, keep your appointments or give a day's notice if you must cancel.
- Let your doctor know about allergic reactions to the medication such as red eye(s), persistent head or eye pain, sudden loss of sight, swollen eye(s), etc.
- Trust your doctor's judgment call with regard to your care.

A good relationship between you and your doctor is an important consideration in your quest for care. Many patients who have been with their doctors over a period of time consider the doctor as friend, while at the same time retaining the patient-doctor relationship. In choosing a doctor in whom you trust, you will find the freedom to express your own views and desires. Optimally, your doctor will consider your role essential to the therapy. At the beginning of the relationship, you might simply write down a few thoughts, perhaps as a credo that you can share with your doctor. Most physicians truly want to help their patients and will not dismiss your concerns. If you practice any number of self-help therapies such as spirituality, special diets, supplementation, yoga, karate or other forms of activity, you might want to compose something comparable to the statement below. Even if you are too shy to show your credo to your physician, just writing down what you feel is beneficial reinforces your focus and perspective.

MY CREDO

I believe in self-empowerment. Stories of people who have fought back when they received a diagnosis of disease and claim they've been able to protect and in some cases change their diagnosis inspires me to continue activities that include: supplementations, exercise, Buddhist practices, meditation, etc. I believe that what I do for myself helps my condition. When I discuss these practices with you then, please don't dismiss them as irrelevant, for I feel I must do everything I can to retain my vision.

Despite your attempts to come to terms with your doctor's recommendations and your own beliefs, you may find that your doctor feels stymied by your resistance to the recommended treatment. Yes, your doctor has every right to fire you as a patient. Obviously, you and your doctor do not see eye-to-eye (excuse the pun) and the relationship is best terminated. You can, however, ask your doctor for a referral to another doctor who may be more tolerant of your requirements as a patient. A physician wrote in the *New York Times* of various instances when he found it necessary to discharge a patient who refused various medications and to follow instructions and furthermore, was abusive to staff.

MEDICATION IS NOT AN ENEMY INVADER

Many of us resist taking any kind of drug, even an aspirin. I'm one of them. If you fall into this cataegory, needing to take drops to lower your eye pressure may present a conflict until you realize that the prescribed eyedrops may save your vision and help to avoid more invasive surgeries further down the line. Or you may not mind using medications provided that you do not experience difficult side-effects. Whatever your view on medication, it is important that you realize that your prescription is not an instrument of torture but with the wide choice of eye medications available, provides a good possibility that glaucoma progression will be slowed if not halted.

Bear in mind that your physician's primary consideration for prescribing a particular medication is based on the protocols established by the medical community. Certainly you are free to question why a particular medication is prescribed, but faith in your physician's judgment strengthens both the doctor-patient relationship and treatment options.

When filling your prescription, use the same pharmacist if possible, for should you be on multiple medications, a pharmacist possessing knowledge of your medical history can alert you to adverse drug interactions including those drugs purchased over-the-counter that may interact with your new prescription. If you are uncertain whether to attribute a particular side-effect to your medication, check first with your pharmacist. Do share with your primary practitioner specialists a list of all the medications you are taking. In this age of specialization and because there are now so many drugs on the market targeted for specific illnesses, you may find your prescription pantry growing. You're on a two-way street. Your glaucoma doctor needs to know about your other prescriptions and your primary doctor and/or other specialists need to know about your glaucoma medications. Information also on how each medication affects you is useful in establishing a medical routine that works best for you. It's also a good idea to check out the possible medical interactions that may occur. Some of these interactions may be relevant to your treatment. Also, if you have what is considered an idiosyncratic side-effect, please report this to your doctor. Likewise, if you are using supplements and herbs, please check with your doctor for possible interactions with the medication you now take, especially if you are scheduled for surgery. Antioxident herbs such as bilberry, garlic supplements and ginkgo biloba that affect blood clotting should be suspended several days or a week before surgery to avoid excess bleeding. Other herbs that affect blood clotting include ginseng, eleuthero (*Eleutherococcus senticosus*), evening primrose oil (*Oenothera biennis*), grape seed extract, ginger, andrographis (*Andrographis paniculata*), celery, dong quai (also known as Chinese *Angelica*), feverfew (*Tanacetum parthenium*), green tea, horse chestnut (*Aesculus hippocastanum*), kava (*Piper methysticum*), pau d'arco (*Tabebuia spp.*), and turmeric (*Curcuma longo*).

Aside from the perils of bleeding after surgery, merely mixing any of the above herbs with aspirin or other blood-thinning agents such as warfarin might result in slower healing response and greater bruising should you bump into something or injure yourself. Likewise, if you notice blood clots forming under the skin this might be a sign that you're taking an excessive amount of blood thinning agents. You may need to cut back on your herbs or supplements.

Glaucoma patients are often anxious, and in some cases, take anti-anxiety medications. If you fall into this category, avoid taking large doses of herbs and foods that stimulate the system such as products containing caffeine. Herbs that help to boost the immune system response such as Echinacea (*Echinacea spp.) astragalus (Astragalus membranaceus*), garlic and ginseng, are better not taken if you've had an organ transplant. Younger patients on birth control pills may find that St. John's Wort and even garlic interferes with the action of certain medications. Garlic may also interfere with the action of some allergy medications (*Allegra*), some antifungal drugs (*Nizoral*), some pain medication (*Sublimaze, Alfenta*), calcium channel blocker blood pressure medications (*Cardizem*), and some cancer chemotherapy (*Taxol*).

Ginkgo can interfere with *Tylenol, Valiuim,* some antidepressants (*Prozac, Desyrel*), estrogen, some asthma medications (*theophylline*), some antifungal drugs (*Nizoral, Sporanox*), some blood pressure medications (*Inderal, Lopressor*), some cholesterol lowering drugs (*Mevacor*), and some narcotic pain relievers (*Demerol, Ultram*). Asian ginseng can interfere with the action of antidepressants (*Prozac, Desyrl*), narcotics, (*codeine, Demerol, Siblimaze, Ultram*), and some blood pressure medications (*Lopressor*). St. John's Wort can interfere with the effectiveness of some antidepressants (*Prozac*), some allergy medications (*Allegra*), some antifungal medications (*Nizoral*), some pain medications (*Sublimaze. Alfenta*), and some chemotherapy drugs (*Taxol*). Valerian might increase blood levels of many medications among them the antihistamine *Allegra,* the antifungal *Nizoral,* the cholesterol lowering drug *Mevacor,* and the chemotherapy drug *Taxol.*

What's the bottom line? These interactions, while possibly present, are nowhere near as hazardous as pharmaceutical drug side-effects. To be on the safe side, however, refrain from taking anticoagulant herbs and supplements two weeks before surgery; don't take herbs or supplements that have the opposite effect of a prescribed drug, and if you use garlic, ginkgo, ginseng, St. John's Wort or valerian, check with your physician about drug-herb interactions.

HANDLING GLAUCOMA THERAPY EFFECTIVELY

Until the day arrives, and it will, when medications for lowering *intraocular pressure* morph from drops to various microdelivery systems, you will be faced with instilling drops in your eyes, inevitably from the day of glaucoma diagnosis, and in many cases throughout your lifetime. Side-effects from medication are common. If on multiple drugs, schedules are complicated. If you are still employed, you may find administering drops during the workday, especially should you not wish to advertise your condition, particularly galling. I never found it so, but Marylou would take a bathroom break whenever she needed to instill a drop.

There are some of us who do not take a diagnosis of glaucoma seriously and fail to take medications on a regular basis. The National Eye Institute found that some patients use up to twenty-five percent less of their prescribed doses. You're cheating your eyes if you fool around with your medication. Scheduling your medication is important for both maintaining your vision and for your peace of mind. When you establish a workable schedule, you will no longer be anxious over whether or not you've instilled a particular drop. Some people set up a daily check list. Others time the medication to breakfast, lunch, dinner and bedtime. Most important to remember is the correct timing between drops. Twice a day, therefore, means a 12-hour span between the first and second drop; three times a day, every eight hours, and four times a day, every six hours. Should you be on additional medications, develop a workable schedule.

When an eyedrop is prescriped, ask a professional in your doctor's office for a demonstration of the instillation technique. For written instructions please refer to Chspter 5.

Traveling long distances by plane, especially when crossing time zones, may present a problem for timing instillation of eyedrops. In my case, I don't change my watch until I arrive at my destination, keeping to my schedule as closely as possible. Just to be sure you're covered, you may need to take a medication before its allotted time, if the difference is less than an hour, rather than expose your eyes to three-or-four hours of no protection. Keep the medications with you when you board the plane rather than leaving them in your suitcase. If you drive long distances, keep your medications in the car with you. Do not store them in your suitcase that is then stored in the trunk or boot of the car. A hot sun beating down on the car can instantly destroy eye medications.

Usually diet does not affect topical eye medications, but if you are on *Diamox*, a systemic medication, be sure that your potassium intake is adequate by eating foods rich in potassium. Diet, however, may affect medications other than those prescribed for glaucoma. Certain foods, especially grapefruit and other citrus fruits, may be contraindicated with certain classes of medications. Check with your primary care physician if you are in doubt as to food-drug interactions.

KEEP RECORDS-- ESPECIALLY IF YOU TAKE MORE THAN ONE MEDICATION.

Write down:

- Name of medication; name, address, and phone number of doctor prescribing the medication; pharmacy filling the prescription, interactive precautions with food or other medications, directions for administration, date of refills. Paste it to the refrigerator door.
- Let someone else in your household know where you've stored this information. If you live alone, advise a friend, relative or neighbor.
- Develop a chart, especially if you are on multiple medications. Many clinics have preprinted charts that may suit your purpose, or you can develop a simple chart from the sample below. Post the chart inside

your bathroom or kitchen cabinet door where it will be in plain view. Be sure to check off each time you take your dose.

- Keep an adequate supply of medication on hand. You can lose some vision if you run out of medication and are at the end of your refills, especially if this situation occurs on a weekend when you might not be able to reach your doctor. Of course, if you are taking *Xalatan,* it's best not to keep a second bottle on hand because this medication is dated.

SUGGESTED CHART

Medication	Time of day	#of times	comments
Timoptic XE	AM	1	Reorder in 2 wks

Should you be pursuing complementary therapies and believe that you've been able to control your glaucoma and also believe you can dispense with the prescribed medication, DO NOT, I repeat, DO NOT stop your prescribed medication until your physician has checked your pressure, not once, but over a period of time. Touching your eyeball, although practiced in some regions where tonometers are not available, is not a substitute for the use of a tonometer in your doctor's office. Even if you use a home tonometer and you find your pressure reduced, please double check with your physician before taking it upon yourself to reduce your dosage.

HANDLE YOUR MEDICATIONS CAREFULLY

Shun the bathroom medicine cabinet as storage for your medications. The warm, steamy environment of a bathroom can cause subtle chemical changes in medication such as loss of strength or produce toxicity. Choose a cool storage area. Extremes of heat can destroy the effectiveness of a medication and in some cases, render it toxic. As an example, timolol (*Timoptic*) loses twenty percent of its potency at 212°F, and at approximately 250°F, its shelf life is shortened to thirty-five weeks. It can be frozen, however, and thawed and not lose its effectiveness. After being heated to 219°F and with a temperature rise to 250°F, *dorzolamide (Trusopt)* will remain useful for only one week. Check the insert accompanying your eye prescription for a range of temperatures suitable for maintaining the viability of the medication.

Needless to say, build-up of heat should be avoided for any medication. If you order medications by mail, especially *Xalatan*, be sure that the company packs the medication with cooling materials and watch for its delivery so that you can immediately refrigerate it. Some mail-order companies claim that *Xalatan* can remain viable for three-to-eight days of shipping and the manufacturer is attempting to change the protocol for refrigeration necessity. It is a good idea to check your medication for signs of deterioration. *Epinephrine,* for example, oxidizes in warm temperatures and needs to be refrigerated. Discoloration is a sign of oxidation. Check for odor. Glaucoma medications do not smell. Consult your pharmacist if you have doubts.

Do not transfer eye medications to other containers.

Liquids would be difficult but tablets not. If you're taking a variety of tablets that are timed to different periods of the day, mark each dosage and time carefully on the container and use a chart such as suggested above. This system can limit confusion when traveling. Alternately, you can use old containers and simply count out the tablets needed for the length of the trip. But be sure to include a few extra for you may be required or elect to stay a few more days.

Do not use medications in a darkened room especially if you are on multiple ones. This includes your eye drops. Mistakes happen, and you may find you've taken a medication at the wrong time and thrown off your schedule. Practically all eye medications come in different sized bottles and each cap is color-coded. Use these clues for identification.

At six-month intervals, discard all expired medications including the over-the-counter ones. Should you have sample medications with no expiration date, check with either your doctor or pharmacist as to whether the medication is still viable. The pharmacist can check this out by the lot number found on all medication containers.

Avoid using someone else's medication or allow another person to use yours. While it may be tempting to test out a medication prescribed for someone else, quell this impulse. It's not like trying on someone's jacket. If you are on multiple medications, be sure to advise your primary care physician as well as the specialists you visit. When Bob's primary care physician prescribed a new medication, Bob was a nervous wreck until both his primary care physician and his ophthalmologist assured him that the new medication would not interfere with his glaucoma medication or cause adverse side-effects.

Another problem lies in prescribing unsafe drugs to those over sixty-five. Our bodies change as we age and we may not be able to metabolize certain drugs. Yet doctors routinely prescribe unsafe medications to seniors.

Researchers at Duke University found, after comparing a list of unsafe medications with a data base of over 700,000 patients over sixty-five, that 21% received an unsafe drug and 15% received two unsafe drugs. We need to be alert to polypharmacy and not be cowed but to ask questions of the medical professionals as to their recommendations. Recently, one of my friends who had just turned ninety, fell in her apartment and hurt her arm. Since the severe pain did not diminish after a week, she visited a neurologist who discovered that she had an infection in her lungs. The pulmonary doctor she next visited prescribed an antibiotic, a drug that raised her blood pressure. Alarmed, her cardiologist increased her dosage of blood pressure medication and judged her arm pain to be a result of arthritis. She could not eat, was in constant pain, so her doctor prescribed pain medication that also raised her blood pressure. She was than put on stronger blood pressure medication, but she deteriorated into such a poor state of health that she felt she would soon die. But being a feisty individual, she took matters into her own hands and demanded that her various specialists consult with each other and determine the minimum amount of medication they could safely prescribe for her.

Unfortunately, this scenario is not unique. The multiple ailments of the elderly often require extensive medical therapy, but treatment needs to be coordinated between specialists in order to minimize adverse effects. Since seniors comprise thirteen percent of the population but ingest thirty percent of prescription drugs and experience more adverse affects than younger people, this is a problem that needs to be addressed.

UNSAFE DRUGS

Daily it seems a particular drug touted as superior to similar drugs already on the market is recalled following alarming statistics of deaths and harmful effects. We need to bear in mind that drugs are toxic substances, albeit that if used judiciously, will provide medical benefits. Nevertheless, there is severe competition for market share among pharmaceutical manufacturers, and some drugs may reach the market prematurely or may be more limited in application than what is believed from the hype about the drug. You can find out which drugs are considered most dangerous by taking a look at the publication *Worst Pills, Best Pills* published by Public Citizen, 1600 20th Street, NW, Washington, DC 20009. One issue lists as "DO NOT USE" the drugs *Indapamide (Lozol)* prescribed for high blood pressure and *Valdecoxib (Bextra)* for arthritis.

For the narrow-angle or *angle-closure* glaucoma patients, certain medications can cause an *angle-closure* glaucoma attack that if not caught in time can destroy all or a part of the optic nerve. These medications include those in the sulfa family of drugs causing the eyes to swell, a condition that narrows the angle through which the fluid leaves the eye, possibly causing a back-up of fluid that presses against the optic nerve, damaging the ganglion nerves. Other pharmaceuticals that can dilate the pupil causing the *iris* to block the outflow channel include certain antidepressants, antispasmodics, antihistamines and anti-*Parkinson* agents. A small glaucomatous eye (nanophthalmos) because the real estate in that eye is limited in space, may be especially vulnerable to a glaucoma attack should the eye be dilated.

Here are some drugs to avoid if possible should you have narrow-angle glaucoma.

- *Cataract Surgery--Alpha-chymotrypsin.* This is an enzyme that is sometimes used during surgery extraction to lyse (cut) the zonules (ligaments) that secure the lens. The medication may cause a rise in IOP, but perhaps more seriously, the debris may float into the trabecular meshwork where it can clog the drainage passages. *Hyaluronic acid* and *sodium sulfate,* used to protect the cornea increases the viscosity of fluid in the eye, and if not washed out thoroughly after surgery can impede the passage of fluid through the trabecular meshwork.

- *Analgesics.* These over-the-counter medications carry FDA warning of contraindication for glaucoma. In most cases this warning applies to those with *narrow-angle* glaucoma; nevertheless, confirm this information with your doctor.

- *Orphenadrine citrate* (Norgesic) has been reported to cause problems.

- Aspirin may be dangerous for *narrow-angle* patients. Aspirin may cause lens swelling along with a shallowing of the anterior chamber producing a rise in pressure. Aspirin may worsen myopia. Contrarily, aspirin may save your vision if you are diabetic according to a report from the Schepens Eye Institute citing that aspirin taken in the early stages of *diabetic retinopathy* may save sight. Aspirin helps prevent the formation of tiny blood clots in the eyes. And aspirin taken along with statin drugs according to research reduced the risk of developing the wet form of *macular degeneration.*

- *Anesthetic agents.* Generally, anesthetic drugs lower *intraocular pressure,* although with the anesthetic agents, *succinylcholine, ketamine,* nitrous oxide, and *choral hydrate,* a rise in pressure has been documented. Do have your anesthesiologist check with your ophthalmologist should you be undergoing an operation that may require the use of one or more of these drugs.

- *Anti-arthritis drugs.* The drug *Chloroquine* (Aralen) may cause *retina* changes.

- Antidepressants. These drugs *Amitriptyline (Elavil), phenelzine (Nardil),* and *tranylcypromine (Parnate)* can all aggravate glaucoma.
- *Antihypertensive agents.* Controlling blood pressure is not debatable. But some of the drugs prescribed for that purpose may be dangerous for persons with *narrow-angle* glaucoma. *Clonidine (Catapress)* may precipitate an *angle-closure* attack. Lens swelling may occur with *chlorothiazide (Diuril),* hydrochlorothiazide *(Esidrix, Hydro-Diuril, Oretic,* and others), *polythiazide (Renese* and others), *chlorthalidone (Biogroton, Hygroton,* and others), *hydralazine (Apresoline), spironolactone (Aldactone* and others), and *trichlormethiazide.*
- *Antinausea drugs. Scopolamine (Donnagel, Transderm)* may cause a rise in *intraocular pressure.* Preferred is *dimenhydrinate (Dramamine)* for motion sickness.
- *Anti-Parkinsonian agents. Trihexyphenidyl (Artane)* is an anticholinergic agent, and may precipitate an attack of *angle-closure* glaucoma.
- *Antipsychotic agents. Perphenazine (Trilafon)* and *fluphenazine (Prolixin),* treat psychological disorders, but are in a class of drugs associated with pigment deposits in the eye, and they are also known to have anticholinergic effects.
- *Antispasmodic agents. Propantheline (Pro-Banthine)* and *dicyclomine (Bentyl),* treat peptic ulcers and irritable bowel syndrome, but are contraindicated for people with glaucoma.
- *Cardiac agents. Disopyramide (Norpace)* an arrhythmia regulator (irregular heart rhythm) is an anticholinergic agent.
- *Cocaine.* In addition to its many other harmful effects, this drug dilates the pupils and can cause *angle-closure.* But patients with *open-angle* glaucoma may not be exempt. Avoid if possible.
- *Hormones.* A paper written by Ivan Goldberg, MD, Sydney, Australia, discusses a thyroid-related eye disease linked to glaucoma. An under or over thyroid activity can be associated with "thyroid-associated ophthalmology." When this occurs, inflammation in the socket of the eye can result. White blood cells and fluid can then collect in the tissues behind and along the sides pushing the eye forward. The eye may look angry and red, may not close properly and the IOP may rise to dramatic levels leading to nerve damage. This is a case where the endocrinologists and eye doctor need to work together to treat both conditions. Thyroid associated glaucoma is a self–limiting condition, but make take years to abate. The effect of the diminishing supply of the hormones estrogen and progesterone that marks the menopause passage in women also appears to be linked to glaucoma although studies in this area are scarce. Nevertheless, those of us who were

diagnosed with glaucoma shortly after menopause cannot help but associate the depletion of these hormones to the onset of glaucoma. A small study appears to confirm this observation. Women taking oral HRT (hormone replacement therapy) had greater blood flow to the ophthalmic artery than women not taking the hormone. HRT is now considered unsafe, but it may still be prescribed in certain situations. It is possible to use natural estrogen derivatives, but these should be prescribed by a gynecologist, endocrinologist or holistic physician. There is a need for a multi-factorial study in this important area.

- *Parasympatholytic agents.* Dilating drops, *Cyclopentolate (Cyologyl)*, *tropicamide (Mydriacyl)*, *hydroxyamphetamine (Paredrine)*, atropine (*Atropisol, Homatro, Hydrobromide)*, and *scopolamine (Hyoscine)*, used to widen the pupil before certain diagnostic procedures, may produce adverse effects in patients with both *closed-angle* and *open-angle* glaucoma since the dilation may push the *iris* into the drainage channel. At greatest risk are those who do not know they have glaucoma.

- *Parasympathomimetic agents.* Old standbys, pilocarpine and *carbacohl* that are still used by some glaucoma patients can precipitate *angle-closure* in patients with narrow angles. Pilocarpine has also been found to aggravate the conditions of *uveitis*, malignant glaucoma, neovascular *glaucoma*, or *pupillary block glaucoma*. Additionally, some practitioners advise against using these agents along with certain other glaucoma drugs, including *phospholine iodide (Echothiophate)*, *Demecarium (Humorsol)*, and *diisopropyl fluorophosphate (DPF, or Floropryl)* for certain glaucomatous conditions.

- *Sulfa drugs.* The drugs in this family, a class of antibiotics have been associated with swelling of the lens in some people.

- *Sympathomimetic agents.* The drugs, in the epinephrine family, are pressure-lowering agents that dilate the pupil and may in people with narrow-angle glaucoma cause a rise in pressure and precipitate an acute angle-closure attack. Repeated usage of inhalers for asthma or treatment of hemorrhoids in the *phenylepinephrine* family can worsen or even precipitate a glaucoma attack in sensitive patients.

- *Tobacco.* Of course, everyone should know by now that smoking is a no-no. Evidence of smoking-related eye disease also poses a risk. In a study of 100 glaucoma patients, twenty-five who stopped smoking experienced an average drop in pressure of two- to-seven mmHg after they quit. Seventy-five diehards showed no change. Another study involving cataract development found, through statistical analysis of a large group of American male physicians and female nurses, that those who smoked twenty or more cigarettes a day had twice the risk of developing cataracts than those who had never smoked.

- *Vasodilators. Nitroglycerin*, a treatment for angina (a type of cardiovascular disease that causes chest pain as the primary symptom) and which is sold under many brand names, has produced transient partial blackout of vision, but this may be related to a dip in blood pressure. This substance, however, does cause dilation of the pupils, although no cases of glaucoma have been reported. Because of the dearth of reported negative effects, vasodilators are considered safe for patients with either narrow-angle or open-angle glaucoma.

Herb and drug interaction

Many of us believe that herbs are safe and can be taken with impunity. But with the wide access to an ever-growing variety of nutritional supplements including herbal preparations along with the use of prescription medicine, the possibility arises that uninvited interactions may occur. A guide to scientific literature and clinical implications is available on the internet. This guide lists interactions between prescription drugs and herbs, vitamins and other nutritional supplements. For example, licorice root is contraindicated for people with hypertension. Topics are listed under: Drugs, Herbs, Nutritional Supplements, Drug Classes, or Herb Groups. Drugs are listed by both brand name and generics. Entries are formatted for quick review and written in a thorough, practical style designed for sharing with patients. To access, the company *Integrative Medical Arts* has a website: *choicesforhealth.com* and IBIS consumer health service. More information can be found at *interactions@ IBISmedical.com.* Or, if you want to talk to someone, the phone number is 503-526-1972,

Be drug smart

We must admit it. Drugs much as some of us may abhor taking them do fight certain diseases and improve selective health conditions. Unfortunately, along with the benefits of drugs, negative interactions may occur. These can be mostly averted by taking an active role in both your supplemental and medical prescriptions. Speak up whenever a professional in the health field hands you a prescription. Here are some useful tips.

- Ask your doctor when you visit --How will this drug help my condition? What are the numbers we hope to achieve (cholesterol, diabetes, blood pressure, eye pressure)? What are the side-effects? Will this drug interact with drugs I'm already taking?

- Take only the prescribed amount of drug and at the scheduled time.
- Don't be shy. Tell your doctor about all your symptoms and your medical history.
- Certain drugs are effective taken during specific times of the day. Also determine before you leave your doctor's office to check whether the drug should be taken on an empty stomach, with or after a meal. Keep to the recommended schedule.
- Alert your dentist of your prescribed medications. Some of the medications your dentist may recommend including antibiotics, anesthesia, and painkillers may not mix well with your prescriptions. For example, if your medications cause dry mouth, your dentist may want to prescribe a saliva-inducing medication, since saliva is your best defense against tooth decay.
- Talk to your pharmacist about interactions if you're taking more than one medication.
- Review your medications and supplements with both your eye doctor and your GP at least once a year.
- Ask your doctor if ethnicity might affect your dosage.
- If you watch your diet, exercise and improve your life style, be sure to advise your doctor. Perhaps your condition will be positively affected and you might possibly be able to lower the amount of your prescription.
- If you are of small stature, weighing in the neighborhood of 100 pounds, your dosage may be too high. This may be a problem that is seldom addressed.
- Senior citizens may not be able to metabolize certain drugs. You have the right to say no if a drug is recommended that you would rather not take.
- Don't pulverize a medication unless your pharmacist or doctor approves.
- Don't transfer your pills to another bottle. You may forget which is which.
- Follow recommendations for driving when taking certain medications.
- Forgetful? Set up reminders—notes, pager, electronic pill containers.
- Be ingenious. You know what works for you.
- Do not use expired medications, even in a pinch.
- Take the entire prescription if it's a one-time remedy such as an antibiotic.

- Don't attribute some negative symptoms to age. Your medications may be the cause. Check with your doctor.
- Try a home remedy for some of the effects of medication, such as prune juice for constipation caused by narcotic and other medications.
- Replace with vitamins when taking certain drugs that deplete nutrients. Ask your doctor when prescribing a medication if the medication drives out certain vitamins.
- Drugs too expensive? Shop around. Drug prices can vary widely. Also consider getting drugs over the border, but choose a reliable source. Check into a generic form. Alternatively, depending upon your income, you may take advantage of the charity prescription drug programs sponsored by drug companies.
- Trying out a new medication? Ask your doctor for free samples to see if it works for you.
- Check for drug-drug interactions, especially if you go to a number of different doctors.
- Be aware of drug-food interactions. Vegetables containing vitamin K may neutralize anti-coagulating medicines; grapefruit and citrus fruits should not be eaten with most drugs for lowering cholesterol.
- Drug interactions, such as taking a sleeping pill, can complicate breathing problems and cause nasal decongestion. These are dangerous when taken by people with heart problems; decongestants are dangerous when taken by people with urinary problems.

Want to know what the abbreviations mean on your prescription? Here's the code

ac—before meals,
bid—twice a day
gt—drop
hs—at bedtime
od—right eye
os   left eye
po—by mouth
pc—after meals
prrn—as needed
q3h—every three hours
qd—every day
qid—four times a day
tid—three times a day

The above material has been extracted from a pullout guide published by AARP (American Association of Retired Persons). Copies may be ordered by calling 800-424-3410 or from the website, www.aarp.org. Refer to stock number D17608.

WHEN SURGERY BECOMES NECESSARY

If medication fails to control your glaucoma, your doctor may recommend a filtering operation (See chapter 7). You have a right to seek a second opinion. You may ask, "Won't I risk antagonizing my doctor by questioning his or her judgment?" Yes and no. Some physicians welcome a patient's involvement. Other physicians argue that they themselves seek second opinions from colleagues in particularly challenging cases. What is most important, however, is your confidence in your physician's recommendation. Faith in your doctor's ability increases the chances for a successful procedure.

Filtration surgeries take place in the hospital. But surgical techniques are now so advanced, especially with eye surgeries, that they rarely require an overnight stay, at least in the United States. Some people, however, do want to stay overnight and usually this wish can be accommodated. In other countries, overnight or even a stay of several days still remains routine. As an outpatient, you're home the same day but you are required to return the next day for a pressure check and possible complications.

WHAT YOU SHOULD KNOW TO PREVENT HOSPITAL ERROR

Although you may be entering a hospital for a procedure other than for your eyes, and although your eye care physician may have left instructions for the timing of your drops, take a moment during the admission procedure to review the routine for your eye medications with the nurse supervisor. See to it that these instructions are clearly listed on your chart. Some hospitals prefer to provide all medications and insist that hospital staff administer them, while others have a more relaxed attitude and allow the patient to self-medicate and use medications brought from home. If a nurse insists on administering your eyedrops and if you're using more than one eyedrop, be sure to inform the practitioner to space the eyedrops at least ten minutes apart. Nurses not trained in ophthalmology may not realize the value of this procedure, and when harried by other patient's demands, may dispense with this chore as soon as possible.

Admittedly, although you're entering the hospital because of an illness that may be severe, should you be able to take an active role in your care you will probably feel better. When presented with medication other than that which you use for your eyes, check with the staff to be sure that it will not cause a rise in pressure. If you are in the hospital for eye surgery and have arranged with a specific doctor to perform this surgery, gain assurance that the doctor you have chosen will perform the procedure. In a teaching hospital particularly, when a case is considered routine, Clinical Fellows may be assigned the surgery under the supervision of your doctor. In the majority of cases, this common practice should not be a problem, but it can also lead to medical error. A complication is usually a result of a medical error.

Don't assume an operation that is considered routine, as with most cataract extractions, for example, will pass muster in your case. Should you have a condition called *exfoliation* (See Chapter 2), where the ligaments holding the lens in place may have become weakened from exfoliated debris, you need a surgeon, in all likelihood, a glaucoma specialist experienced with this particular condition.

RIGHTS AND RESPONSIBILITIES

Whether your hospital is paid by private insurance, Medicare, an HMO plan, or some form of government insurance, you still have rights. If you feel that your care is being short-changed, speak up. Should you receive less than adequate care from the hospital staff, ask to speak to a patient advocate or to a hospital administrator. You should also receive a written discharge plan along with instructions from a staff person who will explain what you need to do at home. Try to have someone with you when you are discharged from the hospital. After having undergone a procedure, you may not be able to fully absorb your after-care instructions.

SAMPLE OF PATIENTS' RIGHTS AND RESPONSIBILITIES

- If you do not understand your rights the hospital MUST provide assistance including an interpreter.
- Receive treatment without discrimination as to color, religion, sex, national origin, disability, sexual orientation, or payment source.
- Receive care in a clean and safe environment.
- Receive emergency care if needed.

- Be informed of the position and name of the doctor in charge of your care while in the hospital.
- Be informed of the names, positions and functions of staff involved in your case and reserve the right to refuse treatment, examination, or observation.
- Access to a no-smoking room.
- Receive complete information about your diagnosis, treatment and prognosis.
- Receive information on informed consent for any proposed procedure that shall include possible risks and benefits.
- Receive all information (proxy) you need to give informed consent for an order not to resuscitate, including your right to designate an individual to give this consent if you are too ill to do so.
- Right to refuse treatment and be told the effect of your refusal on your condition.
- Right to refuse to participate in a research project.
- Privacy and confidentiality regarding your records.
- Participation in all decisions about your treatment in the hospital; discharge with a written discharge plan.
- Review without charge your medical records; receive for a small fee a copy of your records.
- Receive an itemized bill and explanation of all charges.
- Complain without fear of reprisal. If hospital refuses to cooperate you may take your case to the State's Health Department.
- Make known your wishes with regard to anatomical gifts. You may designate your wishes on a donor card or in the health care proxy.

MEDICAL RECORDS

Why Do I Need My Medical Records? Knowledge is power. In the United States, federal law requires that doctors, clinics, and hospitals provide patients with access to their records on demand. One exception is psychotherapy notes. Access to your medical records is an excellent means for establishing a partnership with your present physician. Records also provide important information not readily available, such as vaccinations, immunizations, various physical work-ups, conditions you may not even remember having. Continuity of care is another factor. Should you move to a new location or should your doctor no longer be available, you will be in a better position to inform your new physician of the details of your condition including dates and records of procedures. As an example, evidence of a *trabeculoplasty* (a laser procedure) performed several years back, may not be apparent upon examination. Medical records provide better access for seeking medical care that best serves you.

Personally, while it may be shocking at times to discover the extent of your illness, this knowledge can make it easier to accept the treatment offered and determine if, in addition, there are steps you can take to help heal yourself. I recall a sinking feeling when I first read my glaucoma record, but these emotions spurred me to do everything in my power to help myself, such as seeking out every possible treatment, examining all the available literature, and preparing myself for any eventuality my condition might throw my way.

Lastly, you also have the opportunity to assess the accuracy of your record and check for errors and misinformation. Privacy is, of course, uppermost, but organizations such as insurance companies and employers who have insurance plans do have access to your records and errors may be embedded in your medical history. Most states have laws protecting patient-physician privilege and limit access to outside groups through special rules, laws or exceptions to laws, but you are not guaranteed that these laws will be in effect in your case.

You may run into reluctance on the part of the hospital and/or physician treating you to release your medical records. You may not be able to understand the medical terminology but you will be in a better position to ask for an explanation of your condition. Medical errors do occur. Doctors worry about disclosing them to patients and are fearful of lawsuits, so often the patient is the last to know. Each State has its own regulations for access. A helpful guide as to your State's position is Medical Records published by Public Citizen, 1600 20th Street NW, Washington, DC 20009.

PROTECT YOUR IRREPLACEABLE EYES

Take a page from Prevent Blindness America's guidelines for eye safety and follow their rules faithfully. A cardinal rule implies that however adept you are at wielding tools and other equipment, practicing eye protection is a necessity. Safety glasses should be worn by all who work in factories to protect against flying objects and chemical exposure. Activities such as mowing the lawn, using chemicals and harsh cleaning agents around the house, operating hand tools or working on the car are not harmless. Consider: a flying object or a chemical drip or mist can be damaging, if not blinding, to the eyes. Safety glasses should have the monogram "Z87" on the bridge of the glasses, and should include the manufacturer's logo on each temple. Like the helmets that children now routinely wear when skating or bicycling, safety glasses should also be included under hazardous conditions. Glasses can be purchased in hardware stores, home care centers, and safety equipment suppliers. Safety glasses can be quite stylish so you needn't feel self-conscious or odd if you choose to wear them.

Shop and science classes and sports account for much emergency room treatment of eye injuries. Baseball, particularly, is associated with the largest number of eye injuries, especially for batters and catchers. Of the 2.4 million eye injuries in the US alone, 43,000 are related to sports. Worldwide, eye injuries continue to be a problem. A youthful eye injury can lead to a glaucomatous condition later in life and is one of the risk factors.

ACCIDENT-PROOF YOUR LIVING QUARTERS— WAYS TO COPE WITH YOUR VISUAL LIMITATIONS

Longevity, while bringing with it many rewards, also imposes a variety of health burdens such as deterioration of posture affecting balance, and visual problems that include a narrowing of peripheral vision and declining contrast sensitivity. A small study comparing glaucoma patients with controls found glaucoma patients were over three times as likely to fall as the controls. You've probably noticed how *contrast sensitivity* affects your ability to perform household tasks and if you're still employed, dampens your efficiency on the job. Yolanda, a real estate agent, found *contrast sensitivity* interfering with her ability to show apartments because of badly lit hallways and stairs. Poor lighting can cause accidents in the most inopportune circumstances. Just recently, my yoga instructor, a woman with superb balance, but who also has glaucoma was walking quickly through a room and failed to notice the leg of a coffee table jutting out in her pathway. She tripped over it and broke a toe. There is a *contrast sensitivity* gradient which your doctor can administer to assess your level—good information, but while providing you with a number, hardly corrects your situation. You may be able to improve *contrast sensitivity* with the use of various tinted glasses. Work with a vision specialist and choose the pair that is most comfortable for you. Also, when you can control it, use good lighting.

There are steps you can take, whatever the state of your vision to help improve your quality of life and protect your limbs from disastrous falls. Review your home environment. Is it well organized? Do you stack your groceries in an order that requires minimum searching and reaching for items? Are your spices and condiments clearly labeled? Do you have clear pathways between rooms? Chances are that you no longer need to deal with scattered toys (except when your grandchildren visit) but other objects may obstruct your path, especially if you're in the throes of redecoration. Nothing is more hazardous than a paint job where the furniture and rugs are displaced. I found that out when I tripped over a floor fan that injured my knee. If your vision is severely compromised, ask those who live with you and who may have better vision, to close cabinet doors after use, restock shelves in the patterns you have established and not leave stuff lying around. If you have lost most of your sight and someone in your household decides to rearrange the furniture, be sure to be walked through the new configuration several times until you are comfortable with it. For more strategies to help you cope, read on or have this material read to you. Some forty percent of accidents occur right in the home. Each room has its particular hazards. In the bathroom, slippery tubs and floors, in the kitchen burns, knife cuts and falling pottery and glassware, in the living quarters, rugs and sagging furniture to name only the most obvious possibly dangerous situations. If you have been a parent, child-proofing your home was a necessity. Now it's your turn. Here are some ways to proof your home against household accidents.

- **Floor coverings.** Juanita loves rugs. All her rooms are nicely carpeted and she has lived in the same apartment for many years. But Juanita is aging and she no longer sees as well as she once did. She didn't notice that her entry rug had curled up in one corner, and one day, hurrying to answer the phone, her foot snagged on the rug and she fell in such a way that she knocked a large picture off the wall that landed on her arm, injuring it. Falls on insecure carpeting can be especially dangerous and at times responsible for an otherwise healthy individual to develop a chronic condition. Floral patterned rugs can be confusing. Choose single-color carpeting and secure scatter rugs. Avoid slippery waxes on the floors and immediately clean up spills.
- **Light it up** It is a fact of life. With advancing years, the clarity of vision diminishes. I recently gave myself a fat lip by not lighting up my way from room to room. I stumbled and my mouth hit the corner of a bookshelf. To see an object that a teenager sees, a senior needs two-to-three times the amount of light. Also, glaucoma patients are particularly sensitive to the quality of light. Brilliant sunlight for some patients wipes out vision, and for others, provides beautiful contrast. While you can't control outside lighting except by using sunglasses, or change the lighting in restaurants, department and grocery stores, you can still make the lighting in your home comfortable. Fluorescent bulbs provide a wide range of possibilities including full-spectrum light at minimal wattage. Full-spectrum light is most closely associated with natural light. There are some people, however, who find fluorescent lighting uncomfortable. One of the

members of the group has solved this problem by placing a yellow acetate cover over her fluorescent desk lamp that softens the light and increases contrast. Should this strategy prove inadequate, be assured that a full-spectrum incandescent light bulb is still available. It does burn hot, especially if you use a wattage higher than 60, but if this is the most comfortable light for reading or close work, do use it. For more information on visual aids, see Chapter 13.

- **Stairs**. To use stairs safely, you need to distinguish between brightness levels. The flat part of the stair is often brighter than the vertical and to view the entire stair, you need to able to make this distinction. The eye can no longer feed size and height information to the brain. Light stairwells adequately. Use color coding to improve contrast sensitivity. Climbing is often easier than descending for the vertical view may be completely obscured. At home, the problems of stairs and height variations between hardwood floors can be lessened by using yellow strips on the edges of the stairs. Use tightly woven solid color carpeting for stairs and be sure it is fitted carefully. You may need to sacrifice elegance for safety, but isn't it worth it to avoid a fall?

  If the edges of stairs in public places are not clearly marked, they may present a hazard to you and others. If you frequent buildings and facilities such as hospitals, cafeterias, subways, etc. that require movement from one level to another, and the stairs are not clearly marked, pester the authorities to correct this dangerous situation. A good argument that personnel in charge will heed is that modifying an architectural feature is far cheaper than a lawsuit.

- **Safe Eating out**. Traditionally, restaurants are more interested in décor than in following safety measures. Some restaurants are housed in converted town houses with washrooms located in the basement requiring negotiating a narrow flight of stairs. Please hold on to the handrails. If a restaurant has several levels and no handrail is available, ask staff to assist you. Insurance of your safety is as important to the restaurant owner as it is to you. Sturdy handrails should be a part of all stairs even on as few as a set of two to three stairs. Stair accidents can happen anyplace. At an open picnic in the community garden to which I belong, in waning light, several people arrived, two of them young and agile who easily maneuvered two short steps; the third, a woman in her 70's, missed the bottom stair and fell wrenching her shoulder. We immediately installed railings to prevent further falls.

- **Bathroom sense**. Install grab rails. If your bathtub is slippery, use a rubber mat on the bottom. Use a rug that does not slip and bunch up on the floor. Keep the medicine cabinet doors closed. Anna, forgetting to close her medicine cabinet door, bumped into the sharp edge in the middle of the night when she rose to void. She got a nasty bruise on her temple just inches away from her eye.

- **Steady Yourself.** After years of efficiently running our homes, we may be reluctant to avoid some activities such as hopping on a step ladder, hanging curtains or retrieving an item from the top shelf. To avoid accidents, be sure that your step ladder is solidly constructed. Always open a three-step ladder completely. A half-opened ladder, even if propped against a cabinet, can slip. Alternatively, use a step stool.

- **Enhance Your Table Settings.** In the kitchen and dining room, eschew the floral patterned dishware and tablecloths. Choose instead solid light colors. Fashionable dark colored plates, tablecloths and place mats swallow light and diminish contrast. Food is more enjoyable if seen properly. Don't know what to do with your exquisite set of china? Check among your relatives as Barbara did. She discovered that her niece, about to be married, had long envied her aunt's décor and welcomed the unexpected gift of china and other kitchen furnishings. If you're still a do-it-your-selfer, as is Clarence, you can repaint everything in the kitchen white, and replace the counter tops with white ceramic tile; helps also to see invasive insects.

- **Pamper Your Feet and Save Your Bones**: Falls may also occur because of insecure footwear. Do choose sensible footwear especially when you shop or take a recreational walk. Low-heeled, non-skid soles, laced shoes are usually the most comfortable and provide the best balance. And there's nothing like a good sneaker. If you cannot find a shoe in which you feel securely balanced, you may need a special molded shoe. Medicare will pay for it. Problems with feet most often occur with diabetic patients, but should your toes deform because of arthritis, you may also qualify.

- **Rise and Shine**: Keep the height of your bed reasonable. When arising, don't leap from bed immediately, but sit on the edge of the bed for a minute or two to allow your body to readjust to the postural difference and avoid becoming dizzy if you rise too rapidly. For more information on safety measures, write to The American Academy of Orthopedic Surgeons, PO Box 1998, Des Plaines, IL 60017 and send a self-addressed stamped envelope with your letter. Call 800-824-2663

Someone To Watch Over You

Those of us gifted with long life and an equally long and fruitful marriage may suddenly find ourselves cast into the role of widow or widower. Alternatively, we may find ourselves in the role of caregiver at a period when our own resources have diminished. It becomes especially frightening if the lost partner had good sight and assisted with general accommodation. Fortunately, services exist in most developed countries to provide assistance to those in need. Diana, who has minimal sight left in one eye and whose husband is blind, is enrolled in a program that provides full-time assistance. In most cases, this level of care extends only to those whose income is below the poverty level. If you do not need services in the home, but continue to live alone, you can sign up with a medical alert system such as Medic Alert. These organizations are on 24/7 alert. By wearing a bracelet provided by the organization, you are protected from medical error should an accident occur while away from your home. A call into the organization will provide those coming to your aid with your important health information. If you prefer, you may carry a wallet card providing medical information along with an 800 phone number that a medical emergency team can check should you not be able to provide this information yourself. Alternatively, you may elect to sign up with a monitoring alert system that with a press of a button will summon help. We urge that if you live alone and have a chronic medical condition—glaucoma is not exempt—to enroll in one of these services.

Limitations need not be limiting—vacations and such

Sure, with diminished sight, approaching unfamiliar places can be threatening to your safety, equilibrium and sense of confidence. And you do risk falls. I've had my share, I'm sorry to say, both because of balancing confounded by sight problems and lack of conditioning and my own determination not to miss out on exploration and adventure. One of my more disastrous mishaps occurred on a trip to the Galapagos Islands. My husband I were the oldest members of our group, and we were told that one side trip was not advisable for either of us. Naturally, I insisted I could handle it and both my husband and I went along. I soon discovered why the guide had tried to dissuade us, for we had to follow a narrow, tortuous, tufa ridged path under a hot sun. Of course, I fell and fractured a wrist. Fortunately, there were two medics along on the trip who patched me up and I was able to finish the visit. I don't advise, however, that you tempt the fates as I foolishly did. Here are some saner methods for adapting to a new environment.

On a vacation, walk around your hotel area with a guide, friend or mate to familiarize yourself with the walkways. When walking alone, be on the alert for sidewalk depressions, cracks and curbs. You may want to carry a folding cane and use it when you walk around alone. Try to cross the street where the curbs have been eliminated for wheelchair access. In crossing a street, be on the alert for potholes. Always wear solid walking shoes or sneakers.

EXERCISE, STRENGTH, BALANCE

Studies have indicated that aerobic exercise does lower eye pressure and should you be able exercise vigorously, your IOP may lower and your balance improve. Balance problems are prevalent among the aging population for as people age, they tend to slow down and to walk less. This diminished action results in loss of strength and flexibility. I've found that yoga and other Eastern practices of exercise that require slow steady movement help to restore lost balance. Strength training using weights may also be helpful, but weight lifting   needs to be moderate. Intensive effort raises *intraocular pressure.* A simple exercise routine with or without aerobic activity can take as little as fifteen minutes a day and the benefits can be rewarding for the body has the capacity to regain some of its lost flexibility. You can design your own exercise routine but in the beginning, to achieve maximum results, work with a professional. Here are a few exercises that will help achieve better balance.

- Stand barefoot, if possible, and try to stand with all four corners of your feet solidly on the floor. Engage your legs until they feel firm. Your trunk should be steady as a tree. Raise your arms slowly with palms meeting overhead. If you are firmly rooted, your arms should be feather-light. Do this exercise everyday.
- Remember as a kid you walked a balance beam without a problem? Do a version of this exercise by placing one foot directly in front of the other for ten steps. Increase the activity to twenty or thirty steps.
- Stand on one foot. You may need to steady yourself by holding onto a solid object. It's not cheating to do this. As you practice, you may find that you can eliminate the support.
- Strengthen your thighs. Lie on the floor on your back and lift one leg at time a foot off the floor. Hold for ten seconds. Do this ten times. Gradually build up to ten repetitions with each leg.

JUST WALKING AROUND

Accidents are most likely to occur under ordinary circumstances such as going to the corner store for milk. You may have learned your pathway well and traverse the same route safely innumerable times, only to be ambushed by an unexpected impediment or a careless bystander who forgetfully leaves an object in your pathway. Happily trotting down the street one day, I narrowly avoided a collision with a rolling suitcase. On another occasion, a leash attached to a dog almost tripped me up. And numerous times, uneven sidewalks, unsuspecting protuberances such as tree enclosures and sidewalk dips have caused falls, some of these resulting in broken bones. Do not despair. Practice a few of these tips and you'll be safer.

- Walk in a relaxed fashion. When your body is rigid, it loses flexibility to recover from an inadvertent shove from a passerby.
- Take note of the postures of people around you. An extended arm may be holding a dog leash, a shopping cart or rolling suitcase.
- Educate your sense of hearing to determine whether a sound means that something is rolling towards you.
- Be especially sensitive to bicyclists when you cross the street. They often ride against traffic, so be sure to look both ways.
- Watch for kids on roller blades, scooters or skateboards. Step aside and let them pass.
- Carry a flashlight—an LED light sheds a focused bright light or use one of those nifty lighted magnifiers.
- Avoid squinting. It decreases peripheral vision.
- Practice side-stepping at home by creating a pathway strewn with objects. This will help you to move easily through crowded spaces.

BE VIGILANT IN CARING FOR YOUR EYES

Viewing television can be hard on the eyes. Children and seniors seem to want to narrow the distance between themselves and their television sets. Closeness to the screen should be avoided. For the healthiest distance sit away at least five times the width of the screen.

Inclement weather, especially strong winds, may dry your eyes and/or throw grit into your eyes. Use protective goggles on windy days. Wrap-around sunglasses help in this situation.

Contact Lenses: Tempting as it is to wear extended contact lens, glaucoma patients are safer using daily-care lenses mainly to protect against the possibility of infection. Caution is especially recommended for those who have had *trabeculectomies*, for the eye is more vulnerable to infection after this operation. You can certainly continue wearing contact lenses if you use prescription eyedrops. Simply instill the drop before putting your lens in or after you've taken your lens out. Unless recommended by your doctor, it's best to avoid over-the-counter medications to eliminate redness for these drops do have preservatives and cause eye irritations. Furthermore, they may interact with other medications. Your eye doctor can advise you of the best over-the-counter drop for you.

LOOKING GREAT!

Boost your spirits by beautifying. Looking into the mirror and seeing a well-groomed reflection is uplifting as opposed to the gloom of viewing a worried face and messy hair. Three stories come to mind--a 94-year-old friend would not greet me until she had applied make-up and was properly dressed; a 92-year-old woman would not wear her glasses because she had heard glasses aged one (the spirit is there for this lady although her reasoning is invalid); a 93-year-old woman, while in the hospital recovering from a cardiac episode, asked her daughter to order a prescription retinol cream. Yes, these women have made physical appearance a part of their living experience. While only one of these women had visual problems, limited vision should in no way limit application of make-up and attractive hair-styling. Here are a few tricks for looking your best.

- Use a super-magnifying mirror (3X) when applying makeup, provided you can see. Otherwise, keep your rouge, blushes and lipsticks in the refrigerator. The coolness of the cosmetics guides you in applying these cosmetics to the proper areas.
- Apply foundation with your sensitive fingers. It's superior to a sponge for you can feel your entire face.
- Blot your face with a tissue following the application to mop up any foundation that might have been applied too thickly.
- Feel your cheekbones—the apple nearest the nose--apply cooled rouge or blush. As you touch the cosmetic to your cheek, smooth it towards the near ear.
- When darkening your eyebrows, run your index finger along your eyebrow and follow that pathway with either an eyebrow brush or eyebrow pencil.
- Eye liner, eye shadow or mascara not generally recommended for glaucoma patients, but if these cosmetics have been a way of life, carefully use your finger or a short brush to apply eye shadow under

the brow bone. For mascara, rest your hand against your chin and, very slowly, apply mascara to your lashes. Be careful not to leave mascara on for a long time for old eye makeup can cause serious eye infections. Eyelashes naturally contain bacteria. Eye lash brushes become easily contaminated after just one use. Over time bacteria builds up increasing both the risk of eye infection and an allergic reaction.

- Should you use multiple lipsticks, distinguish one from the other by wrapping the inner tube in transparent (not cellophane) tape, and applying a number of different glue drops for each color. To remember the numbers, always use the same numbers for colors. Chill your lipsticks so that you can more easily sense the contour of your lips.

- Please note. All cosmetics should be replaced every four to six months to avoid bacterial contamination, especially those used for the eyes.

- Skin Cleansing. Do your eyes first. Saturate a sterile cotton ball with a water-based makeup remover if you have used makeup, or simply use water if you have not. Gently draw the pad under the lashes, first with eyes closed, and then eyes open. Use fresh pads or balls when doing your second eye. Follow with a gentle cleansing of your entire face. Should you use a toner, be sure to keep this substance away from the eyes. Thoroughly rinse your face following this application. For masks and scrubs, avoid the area around the eyes and rinse thoroughly when finished. Should you use a variety of creams and have trouble distinguishing one jar or bottle from another, try coding the tops of the jars with a drop of glue that you can feel or you can glue raised letters to the tops. When sight diminishes altogether, you may find that your sense of touch becomes exquisitely selective and that you soon embed in your memory the feel of each of the products you use. Even if you still have decent sight, try closing your eyes and see how many different products you can differentiate by touch; you'll be surprised at how accurate you are.

In previous chapters, we have discussed the addition of additives to foods that may be harmful to the body. Cosmetics are not exempt from the harmful drug syndrome. All cosmetic products contain some bacteria. Manufacturers, therefore, add a preservative, although some manufacturers claim the preservative extends shelf life. Toxic metals can be found in moisturizers, lotion, sun block, sunscreen, mascara, eye shadow, rouge, face powder, lipstick, and theatrical and clown makeup. It's possible to suffer a variety of health effects from the use of these products. The most toxic are mercury compounds permitted by the FDA for use in eye makeup of concentrations up to 65 parts per million. *Bronopol,* used in mascara and other cosmetics, has caused blindness and death in laboratory animals; formaldehyde-releasing ingredients are found in brands of skin and hair products. Other toxic chemicals, which may cause a number of health problems include lanolin (may be contaminated with DDT), mineral oil, *1-naphthol* and *2-naphthol, nitrosamines, p-hydroxybenzole acid benzyl ester (PHB esters, petrolatum, propylene glycol, quarternium-15,* talc. These chemicals in some cases may be more efficient at entering the body through the skin than through foods and medicine that contain toxic materials, for the chemical is absorbed by fat and doesn't pass through the liver. Scientists state they can get the same effect of a vaccine in a laboratory by rubbing it on the skin of a mouse as by injection. Cosmetics contain synthetic chemical preservatives known as *parabens* that are readily absorbed through the skin where they can enter the bloodstream. These are not always listed and manufacturers may hide it under "fragrance," a collective term that covers over 2,000 different chemicals including carcinogens and other toxins. *Parabens* are also found in foaming cleansers, body mists, body lotions, lipsticks, skin creams, shower gels, hand lotions, moisturizers and lip glosses. Shampoos, soaps, and other personal products may contain a detergent known as *sodium lauryl sulfate (SLS).* This substance is rapidly taken up in the eye and can be retained in eye tissues for up to five days. It is capable of changing proteins of the eye tissues and retards corneal healing. Younger eyes are more susceptible to this effect. Hair dyes, especially the permanent ones have been linked to bladder cancer.

The safest cosmetics are: Aubrey Organics, Avalon Natural Products, Burt's Bees, Inc., Chica Bella, Clearly Natural, LLC, Dr. Bronner's Magic Soaps, Ecco Bella Botanicals, Farmaesthetics, Kiss My Face, Lily of Colorado, Logana Nature de France, Natural Glycerin Bar, Pure Approach and Weleda. But don't be misled by the term "organic". In 2003, the Executive Director of the Organic Consumers Association complained that companies claiming products to be organic may, because of lack of government oversight, market items containing petroleum-derived and other synthetic ingredients. In some cases, the list of ingredients is similar between organic and non-organic products, but the amount of ingredients in organic products is less and might, therefore, be less irritating.

If you cannot find any products listed above since they are mostly carried in health food stores, use swimmer's goggles when you shampoo and incidentally, when you swim in a chlorinated pool. Apply cosmetics judiciously.

The top ten makeup brands claimed "brands of concern" are: Chanel, Sally Hansen, Ultima II, Revlon, Gillette (men's skin care), Estee Lauder, Clarins, Ulta, Cover Girl, and Elizabeth Arden.

DRIVING SAFELY

Researchers found in a small study that glaucoma patients were more than six times more likely to be involved in a car accident than the controls. The strongest risk factor was impaired selective attention. *Contrast sensitivity* may be one of the problems drivers face, for they must be able to instantly assimilate roadside features and obstacles. Sunglasses help to improve *contrast sensitivity* in these occasions.

You can drive with limited vision, provided you follow the rules of your state, as they vary from state to state. If your vision falls between 20/40 and 20/70 and you have a visual field of not less than 104 degrees, you may be able to obtain a restricted license. This special license involves restrictions such as a shorter than normal renewal period, permission to drive only in daytime, special mirror requirements, or limitations on highway driving.

Should your visual acuity be less than 20/70 but better than 20/100, and if you are equipped with bioptic telescopes (See Chapter 14) augmenting your vision to 20/40, have a 140-degree angle and have participated in special training, you may be issued a restricted license.

An unrestricted license generally requires corrected acuity in your good eye of at least 20/40.

Most at risk are drivers who have a blood relative with glaucoma, have diabetes or blood pressure problems, have myopia or hyperopia (long-sighted), have suffered a previous eye injury, have used steroids over an extensive period of time, or who suffer from migraine and poor circulation. These drivers may be unaware of diminished acuity.

Even though glaucoma may not have dramatically affected your visual acuity, you still need to be especially alert when behind the wheel. Glaucoma reduces the number of rod cells affecting your peripheral vision. This condition requires religious use of side mirrors to enhance the quality of sight. To drive safely, you must be able to see cars moving up alongside especially if you intend to change lanes. Mirrors also expand vision to include seeing pedestrians or animals on the side of the road and who may be close to the path of your car. Other factors to consider are the effects of multiple medications that may blur eyesight and nighttime glare from other drivers' headlights. You may also find that tracking an object in low light to be difficult, if not impossible. Twilight is the worst time for clear vision.

Relinquishing the wheel turns out to be, for some people, not as traumatic as expected. Results of a study revealed that before participants stopped driving, they worried about being a burden to others, losing the ability to travel about, and loss of independence. But on giving up driving, they discovered that their relationships at home remained the same or even became closer, that they reduced stress, lowered costs, and learned to appreciate others' attributes.

Alternatively, giving up driving may bring on depression. If so, try practicing a few simple safety precautions recommended by American Optometric Association. Consider, however, that by 2020 more than 40 million Americans seventy years or older will have driving licenses. Compared to middle-age drivers, these older folk will be three times as likely to be involved in an automobile accident and more likely to die or be seriously injured as a result. People over 70 are more likely to experience decline in physical and mental abilities. Nevertheless, if you are serenty or older and feel you must continue to drive, do--

1. Select proper glasses for both day and night driving.
2. For nighttime driving do not wear tinted glasses.
3. Use UV protected good quality sunglasses in sunlight.
4. Try not to drive during dusk especially and at night.
5. Keep your glasses clean.
6. Narrow–temple eye frames are better than wide-temple which can interfere with side vision.
7. Be alert. Keep eyes on the road ahead but check each side of the car for vehicles, children, animals, or other hazards. Move your head and eyes frequently from side to side and glance often at the rear view, side mirror and instrument panel
8. Keep pace with the flow of traffic.
9. Choose a clear windshield when you purchase a car.
10. Keep your headlights and tail lights maintained.
11. Clean your windshield often.
12. Belt in at all times. Air bags should be adjusted for short persons.

For free booklets offering tips for safe driving-- *"Old and Wise Driver,* *"Managing Disabilities, Time and Space for Safe Driving"* and others as well as a *CD that can be purchased "Road Wise Review",* write to The American Automobile Association (AAA) at AAA Corporate Communications, 1000 AAA Drive, Heathrow, FL

TRAVEL TIPS

Taking a trip? Here are a few tips to keep you anxiety-free if you are using medication for your eyes. Make a list of all your medications. Include the generic name, strength and dosage. I ran into a problem on one of my trips. Arriving in our hotel, I looked for and couldn't find my medication (found it later when my anxiety abated). Nevertheless, in a state of panic, I went to a drugstore and told the pharmacist my problem. Obligingly, the pharmacist allowed me to purchase the medication without a prescription. Bring enough medication to last the trip. Store the medication in a cool dark place. Some patients purchase a small thermos for storage. Take only unopened medications with you. That way, you'll not run out of your prescription or run into a problem at airport security. Ask your doctor for advice on administering your drops if you plan to cross several time zones.

Plane travel will not affect your IOP, but the air on a plane is very dry and you may need moisturizing drops. Take along an extra pair of prescription *GLASSES* and also an extra pair of sunglasses.

PUBLIC TRANSPORTATION

The American Disabilities Act provides that transportation be made available to persons who are disabled. Across the United States, you should be able to find accommodative transportation from specially-equipped buses or vans that will take you to important appointments. Fern, who lives about twenty miles out of Boston, but whose glaucoma specialist practices in Boston, uses such a van to transport her back and forth for her appointments. She's thrilled with the service, for although she still drives, she doesn't feel safe making the trip and additionally, she need not ask family and friends to take her. All public transportation is required to provide disability access.

CHAPTER 13

How To Make Your Workplace Vision-Friendly

o o o o o o o o o o o o o o o o o o o o o o o o o o o o o o o o o o o o o o o

"Far and away the best prize that life offers is the chance to work hard at work worth doing."
                    Theodore Roosevelt, Labor Day Address,
                                        Syracuse, NY, 1903.

"Whether our work is art or science or the daily work of society, it is only the form in which we explore our experience which is different."
                    Jacob Bronowski, "The Sense of Human Dignity."
                                Science and Human Values, (1956)

Irrational barriers and ancient prejudices fall quickly when the question of survival itself is at stake.
                                    John F. Kennedy, address,
                        United Negro College Fund Convocation,
                            Indianapolis, Ind., April 12, 1959

TO TELL OR NOT TO TELL

Cathy, an attractive and personable woman in her forties had no problem preparing her resume. She had an excellent job history and could provide good references. But she left out a vital element—her visual handicap. Cathy has "low vision." She does not perceive written material as rapidly as others, is sensitive to glare and needs special lighting. Unlike legal blindness and more obvious physical disabilities, limited vision is not readily discernable to others and Cathy, considering her eminent ability to handle job assignments within her training and experience, shrank from revealing her visual condition. She is not alone. Many visually impaired individuals in the workplace struggle over whether to tell or not to tell.

In our high-powered society, jobs can be demanding and highly pressured. Notwithstanding the advances in technology that have revolutionized the workplace, the complexities accompanying them requiring rapid visual assessment often challenge even those with healthy eyes. People with visual problems may find certain forms of work to be excruciatingly taxing on the eyes, especially if various accommodative facilities are not available.

On the job and facing difficulties, Cathy obsessed as to whether to reveal her condition immediately or postpone it until she was able to assess the bare minimum requirements she needed to do her job well. Cathy chose to bide her time and after several weeks on her new job, embracing the advice of a job counselor "to think simple", she was able to come up with a short list of requirements. Cathy requested that her colleagues provide her with hard copy of important documents preferably in 14 point bold type. To her surprise, hard copy also increased the efficiency of other staff members. Cathy's second request--for increased time to shift focus from one item to another instead of desperately attempting to accommodate to "instant read"--added to her work comfort and output. Also, a gentle suggestion that notes be written in black magic marker completed this modest but important list of Cathy's needs. She managed her own glare problems by installing a lamp in her workspace that shed light without glare.

Telling, in this instance, proved to be both beneficial for Cathy and also provided a new route of access for her associates. People with visual problems appear normal, capable and in control of their environment. They take in stride most situations and develop superb accommodative skills. But these skills often need to be bolstered in a busy office where everybody is involved in the business of the day that moves at lightning speed. If we expect a sympathetic colleague to infer our needs, we are being overly optimistic. Successful integration into the workplace requires that we take the helm, analyze the extent of our needs and determine how they can be filled at minimum expense to the employer. A first step might be to discuss our needs with colleagues with whom we are in close contact, either in a business or social relationship. Cathy found to her surprise and gratification that her gentle hints or reminders established a positive working relationship and that her co-workers expressed eagerness to assist her wherever possible. Informed, Cathy's colleagues rallied to her needs.

"Get thee behind me." Lighting and its accompanying glare plague many visually-impaired people. Lighting, however, is one of the easiest problems to solve. Persons with glaucoma and other visual problems usually have mastered lighting requirements in their home environments. I find that facing a window destroys my visual acuity but as soon as I turn my back to the light source my vision is restored. I also find that if I choose a good lamp, preferably with a full spectrum bulb, I have no trouble reading—and I do a lot of that.

Just about every workplace is furnished with fluorescent overhead lighting. Jane, like me, has a serious glare problem. She switched her desk around with her back to the window taking advantage of ambient natural light and in doing so, reduced glare. She modified the harsh overhead lighting by removing one of the bulbs in the overhead fixture above her desk. Adele in accounting improved her ability to handle close work by adding a desk lamp equipped with a full spectrum bulb.

Most modifications of the workplace are low-cost and do not strain the company budget, but for some individuals such as George, a lawyer, computer adaptation became essential. Because of his poor sight, he needed voice-activated software. Computer usage compounds eye discomfort, work fatigue and stress. Since George had elected to confide his needs in his initial interview, he was able to work out his requirements for a state-of-the art computer with his company. Improvements in computer technology include flat screens, voice activation, a variety of background colors and font sizes. (See Chapter 14)

Extended time on the computer jeopardizes even the healthiest of eyes. If you spend a lot of time transferring hard copy to the computer, consider clipping your copy onto a stand. (Secretaries use them all the time). Upright print copy is easier to read than face-up copy on the desk. To relieve computer stress--palm. This is a simple exercise described elsewhere in Chapter 10. Rub your hands together. Close your eyes. Cup your hands over your eyes for a few moments. If you can spare five minutes--all the better. Your eyes will love it. Another very simple exercise is to raise your eyes and gaze at all four corners of the room in succession, a few minutes at a time. If you are near a window, gaze at a distant object. A few minutes are usually all you need to relieve feelings of stress. Close work requires a fixed eye accommodation that leads to strain. And for heaven's sake, if you've had a cataract operation make sure your correction is computer friendly.

Using multiple drops during the workday has been dramatically reduced for many glaucoma patients. With the range of medications now available no more than one or two instillations a day are usually needed. But if you are on maximum medical therapy and find it necessary to instill drops during the day and wish to do so unobtrusively take a bathroom break, find an unoccupied corner, or just walk into the hall on another floor. I never had a problem while on the job, for even if I were in a meeting, I took a few minutes out to instill a drop.

Instant face-recognition can be enhanced by studying the gestalt--gait, height, body contours, slope of shoulders, protrusion of abdomen, nervous tics and other mannerisms of individuals. It's amazing how slight a clue one needs to recognize a familiar individual.

Not to tell may not always be the wisest choice, especially if your condition is unstable. Side-effects of medications may cause digestive problems, eye tearing or blurring, dizziness, sleepiness, fogginess, and pain to name only a few problrms that may interfere with work performance. If you are on maximum medication, you may find that stepping down to a less-demanding position may better preserve both your work history and health. If you have kept your condition under wraps, your employer may be distressed to learn you need an expensive operation for a long-standing eye condition, both because of insurance issues and the need for another worker while you recoup.

We are all sensitive to any hint of being regarded as "other," or losing the respect of colleagues should we make frequent errors. When colleagues know, however, that with a few changes in routines and simple accommodations errors can be diminished, we become more comfortable, do a better job and the work atmosphere lightens up. Of course, past experiences in other jobs where your overtures were disregarded, pride, or fear of failure may color your decision. It's your choice, for only you are capable of assessing the stance you should take. But, if you realize after some time on the job and/or if your visual condition worsens that you cannot do without adaptive services, the law is behind you.

LEGAL PROTECTION

The 1990 passage of the *Americans with Disabilities Act (ADA)* cobbled together Titles I, II, III, IV and V covering employment, transportation, public accommodations, telecommunications, etc. entitling you to request these services from your employer. In 2008, the Senate approved a major civil rights bill to expand protection against workplace discrimination. A similar bill was passed by the House. Up front, should you reveal your needs and suspect that you do not get the position, or if you are already on the job, and your condition worsens, and if you feel you are being discriminated against, you are legally protected from bias. You are entitled to file a claim. The courts, however, are backed up with anti-discriminatory lawsuits and it may be months or years before your case is heard.

GETTING THERE

Generally, the fingers of the law have reached into public spaces, requiring access either in the form of ramps or elevators. Lighting, however, pardon the pun, is a gray area. Take the lighting in elevators for example. How often have you had to stoop and peer at the embossed metal buttons in the elevators? Auditory signals help somewhat if you're prepared to count the beeps; lighting in lobbies at times barely illuminates directories. While you may be able to read eye-level information, it becomes more difficult to read the higher tiers. As well, lettering is often too small to be read by the visually-handicapped. Signage is another daunting problem, especially in spaces such as railroad or subway stations. It becomes even more frustrating if you are in a hurry or happen to be in a station where an attendant is not available. Inability to read posted designations or directions can be stress- inducing. Street signs are a conundrum. They may be too high up for sidewalk reading or not easily located if on public transportation. Poor contrast can also create problems. If the bus driver or subway conductor does not announce the cross-streets or stations, you may find yourself late for work or for an appointment. Verbal directions can be confusing. How many times have you found verbal directions in error? Recently on my way to an appointment using the NYC transit I ended up in Brooklyn because the correct stop was named differently in one station than in the connecting station. Entering and alighting from subway cars or trains may be vexing if depth vision has been lost. For that matter, merely walking on the sidewalk can be hazardous. Glaucoma patients lose peripheral vision first and at times they find it difficult to concentrate both on what's ahead, what's on each side and what's happening at ground level. Reduced peripheral vision also affects balance. Furthermore, an impediment such an irregular sidewalk, a high curb, a metal surround protecting a street tree, an obtruding sign, chairs and tables for sidewalk dining, strollers, skaters, fast walkers—all can impact on getting there.

Can changes be made? Yes, slowly. Public awareness is the key. Some years ago, it would never have occurred to the drivers of buses to announce cross streets. In NYC, announcements are required much to the relief of both blind and visually-impaired riders. As with any change instituted with the handicapped in mind, announcements also benefit tourists and students. When sidewalks were adapted to meet the needs of wheelchair users, the general public greeted this accommodation with enthusiasm, for pushing baby buggies, shopping carts, and simply walking more safely at crosswalks became easier to negotiate. Change is usually stimulated through actions and/or demands on the part of consumer spurring government to make more accommodative changes.

Whatever your visual condition, if there is a job available where you feel you qualified, there is no reason that you cannot be considered a potential candidate along with other applicants. You have the tools to solve your work-related problems and the laws are there to back you up.

Chapter 14

Graceful Accommodation

○ ○

"It's them as take advantage that get advantage I' this world,"
George Elliot, Adam Bede (1859), 32.

Although the incidence of blindness resulting from glaucoma is dropping in developed countries, it is still at the near top of the list in poorer countries. Nevertheless, the dread of blindness or severely reduced vision haunts patients diagnosed with glaucoma, especially in the light of increased longevity. The first question a close colleague asked of a glaucoma specialist was, "When do I go blind." A stunned silence followed for she was asking the doctor to foretell the future. After deliberating, her doctor ventured she still had at least 15 years if she agreed to surgery to adequately lower her pressure. She was 55 at the time. With today's expanded life spans, a fifteen-year guarantee (if there can be such a thing) is cold comfort. Yet, in fifteen years, if the current impetus to unravel the intricacies of stem cell and gene rejuvenation takes root, the prospect of blindness from glaucoma may become history. At present, however, sight lost from glaucoma is irretrievable, a grim picture indeed despite the fact that loss of vision from glaucoma is minimal in most cases. Longevity, as mentioned above hovers like the sword of Damocles as people age into their 80's and 90'S. Needless to say, glaucoma patients impatiently await word that advances in medical treatment, stem cell research, regeneration of nerve cells and gene therapy will soon be available to at least conquer glaucoma's steady erosion.

Which brings us to the worrisome problem of living with reduced or lowered vision. While the majority of us do avoid total blackout, we cannot help but notice the diminishment of our vision especially when we're in the company of someone with normal vision who remarks on something that we've missed entirely. We are what Lorraine Marchi, Executive Director of the National Association of the Visually Handicapped, calls the "the-hard-of-seeing."

This problem may affect our quality of life. Findings from the *Collaborative Initial Glaucoma Treatment Study* cited that females, blacks and younger glaucoma patients, twenty-five-to-fifty-four, worried more about upcoming physical and psychosocial problems. Since this group was at the diagnostic stage, the authors suggested that this particular cohort be followed to determine quality of life as conditions changed.

Quality of life is indeed a serious issue. Fortunately, among the various resources, both non-profit and commercial, there is little need to suffer serious quality of life issues. Schepens Eye Research Institute devotes considerable time and resources to develop visual aids that promote an individual's ability to continue to work and live productively despite severe loss of vision. Some of the technologies they are exploring consist of an intraocular telescope implanted inside the eye, a bi-optic telescope on glasses for driving, telescopes built right into the lenses of eyeglasses that enhance vision up to twenty times, digital television technology to increase contrast and sharpness of the image, as well as expansion of visual field for patients with tunnel vision. Studies on improving quality of life through rehabilitative services using some of the techniques already developed for the blind have proven to be helpful for people who have lost considerable vision. There are centers available where you can learn to effectively use your remaining vision. When visiting a center, be sure to make a list of your goals.

Those of us, however, who have lost a percentage of vision acuity do manage quite well with surprisingly few aids. I've lost eighty percent of vision in one eye and although I measure 20/25 with my good eye in the doctor's office, I suspect that in the throb of city life I see no more than 20/40. My peripheral vision, however, has been affected in both eyes and I need to take special care in crossing streets. In our Group, several members also have lost most of the function of one eye, but this condition hasn't stopped them from continuing with most of their activities. Several with only one functioning eye regularly bicycle. The woman who helps puts our glaucoma newsletter regularly takes bicycle vacation trips in different European countries. Others like Betty, who has lost impressive function in both eyes, holds down a job, relying mainly on computer technology or magnification for all of her close work. Fortunately, abundant smart technology can reinforce remaining vision. Furthermore, a possible compensation to loss of sight may be improved memory and keener hearing. Researchers at Hebrew University, Jerusalem, found that people blind from birth did considerably better in recalling abstract words than seven people with normal vision. Generally, blind people do develop superior ability in their other senses, especially hearing and tactile, a faculty that continues throughout life.

Loss of vision, even when it's extreme, does not necessarily narrow your activities. An outsider (self-taught) artist, Tracy Carcione, draws. Picture making is apparently innate, a cognitive ability deeply imbedded in our brains. Famous artists also lose vision but soldier on with their work which often lacks detail but is compensated for in other dimensions. Claude Monet, with severe cataracts, painted from memory. Camille Pissaro had tear duct problems and couldn't go outside, so painted cityscapes from a window; Edgar Degas suffered *retinal* disease for nearly half his life and used peripheral vision to great effect in his painting. Photography also does not take a back seat. An article in *The New York Times* described blind individuals participating with a group called "Seeing with Photography Collection," sponsored by Visions (see Resources). Led by a seeing instructor, members of the group produced works expressing their inner anguish at loss of sight, but also did not neglect feelings of beauty. Cognitive scientists have found that many blind artists reproduce Renaissance tricks of perspective, probably hard-wired into the brain. Comfortingly, it appears that the brain is capable of making sense out of the world even with extreme loss of vision.

At times, diminishment of vision is equated with losing a part of self. If you despair, inventory your current abilities. You may still possess other faculties, may be in good health, may still be able to enjoy the arts with adaptive technologies and most important, still retain the love and respect of your family. There are changes you may need to make. Don decided that, when he could no longer read print, to sign up for Braille lessons. Emily entered a computer program especially designed for newly-diagnosed low-vision patients. Enid arranged to have a seeing-eye dog. Comeback stories abound. Richard Lane, who lost his sight due to a connective tissue disorder resulting in a detached *retina* that could not be repaired and which was followed by glaucoma, cataract and occluded cornea, lives a perfectly normal life. He is married and leads a competent social and professional existence made possible by use of a talking computer, a guide dog, his rolling cane, Braille material, and physical exercise. He is jarred only occasionally by dreaming in clear vision.

LOSS AS A PRESERVER OF VISION

Perfection most sought after but seldom attained might be applied to glaucoma treatment. Both the eye medications and surgical interventions, while preserving vision, are often accompanied by a loss of acuity. It is not uncommon to lose one or more lines on the Snellen chart (see Chapter 4)) after a surgical procedure. Likewise, the eye drops may cause some cloudiness, cataract formation, and myopia (near-sighted). In the third year of my using drops, I became severely near-sighted.

Somewhere along the line, you may be wondering whether low vision services can help you master your new needs. While your primary eye doctor is superbly equipped to handle all your medical glaucoma problems, he or she may have scant knowledge of low-vision services that may be available to you. Furthermore, the staff in your doctor's office may be so burdened with technical details that they are unable or unwilling to research these services. I often note how managing an active office—constantly vetting the phones, clients and doctors to arrange for optimum patient care, keeps the staff inordinately busy. Accepting this reality and depending upon the community you live in, you may need to search out low-vision care. In most cases, such services do exist, and many are supported by government resources. Agencies that serve the blind and visually impaired can be a good source. (See Resources)

VISUALLY CHALLENGED? DISABLED? LESS THAN HUMAN?

Throughout history, persons with handicapping conditions have been either treated as pariahs or extolled for their unique qualities, but for the average person with a disabling condition, human attitudes towards disease by the unenlightened have followed a sorry trail throughout history. In many societies (some still practicing today), disease and illness were or are believed to be caused by divine or supernatural causes and only the intervention of a priest, medicine man or someone equipped with exquisite powers has the ability to exorcise the demon causing the affliction. In Eastern religions there is still a strong belief that the afflicted one needs to work off the karma from a previous less than perfect life. But the most insidious observation is the notion, often unconscious, that the disabled are "less than human"; that is, they do not feel the same pains and discomforts as others. A severely handicapped man confined to a wheelchair confided that to his dismay people assisting him would wheel him into a corner facing the wall while they chatted with friends and colleagues. "Deposited like a bundle of rags," he complained.

There are changes of course. As to whether, in the long run, attitudes will change remains to be seen, for equal opportunity is an ongoing process. The first steps are now in place. The ADA (*Americans for Disability Act*) in its present form assures equal opportunity in the workplace and access to all public facilities. But to assure that those in need of services receive timely and adequate services requires constant vigilance. Budgetary restrictions may make inroads on the services that you should or are receiving. We suggest that you work with your state representative to assert your rights. Services are most often awarded to those who scream the loudest. Certainly, liaison services among low-vision centers, medical personnel, and government resources need strengthening. Perhaps, an unmet, but badly-needed service bedevils those who have lost vision but who are not yet labeled "legally blind." This is a gray area. You may still have better than 20/200 vision and not have tunnel vision, but nevertheless, have difficulty reading signs, literature, or just simply walking about. Currently, legal blindness is defined by 20/200 vision or lower in both eyes and/or a visual field of less than 20 degrees in both eyes.

When the prospect of blindness or decreased visual acuity appear to be inevitable, patients may go through a series of stages. Unless there is a major medical breakthrough where sight can be restored, or at the very least, progressive loss of vision halted, the inexorable decline in acuity is a grim scenario. Emotional distress may follow. At first, the patient is unaware of loss, but over time, a patient may begin to notice signs of diminished sight and visual capacity such as sensitivity to glare, contrast sensitivity loss, increased side effects of medication, and photophobia, to name some of the more common complaints. These disturbances may lead to falls and other injuries that add to the already disruptive and limited lifestyle imposed by faulty vision. Under current laws, resources to assist those with some of the above problems are scarce or non-existent. If the individual is working, particularly, and needs some assistance to continue on the job, help even at a minimal level may be non-existent.

When vision declines severely, patients may need time to adjust to this new situation. Psychologists involved with ophthalmological patients take a page from Dr. Elizabeth Kubler-Ross in her landmark book *On Death and Dying* (Simon & Schuster, 1970) to parrot similar stages that a glaucoma patient may pass through. At first there is denial and isolation leading to shock and disbelief followed by a refusal to admit to limitations. Patients still claim that they are still "whole". But this reaction can have a devastating effect on social contacts and set up resistance to seeking help from professionals and agencies equipped to help them.

With dawning realization during the second stage that blindness is permanent, denial gives way to anger that may lead to feelings of persecution. In this volatile situation, the individual may lash out at friends and family and even at the practitioners equipped to handle the case. Apparently gradual and inevitable loss of vision is harder to bear than a sudden blackout. Partially sighted children also do less well in adjusting than completely blind children. Perhaps when you can see a little bit, more is expected of you leading to frustration and anger.

By the third stage, bargaining or optional thinking replaces anger and desperation. Those with some vision make bargains with themselves, their God, their doctors or anybody else involved with their care, offering to do everything right—take the medication, eat the right foods and so on. They plead to keep whatever sight is left and begin to plan options for making the best out of a bad situation.

When bargaining and optional thinking no longer work, patients may enter a fourth stage of depression where it becomes difficult to stem feelings of fear, anger and sadness. The realization that family, friends, and services have not met their current needs (often because of limited resources), feelings of being overwhelmed may begin to swamp the individual. Yet there are those who accept their condition, seek out methods for retaining their position in society and continue to live a fruitful life. The bottom line—whatever your condition, fight back. Only with death does striving end.

GLARE

Glare and contrast sensitivity associated with the loss of nerve cells in the eyes plague many glaucoma patients, especially in the presence of bright light. Some glaucoma patients complain that glare from bright sunlight wipes out vision entirely, while others, myself included, experience an affinity with bright sunlight claiming to see better. Those who have severe glare problems and who drive should always have clean windshields, especially in the presence of a setting sun that strikes dirt particles on a windshield scattering light that then reduces clarity of vision. In all of these cases, a good pair of sunglasses (spotlessly clean) can help to restore acuity.

Sun-glasses are best purchased from a low-vision center for these establishments carry products affording protection from all dangerous ultra-violet rays. They are available in a variety of shades. Take time to test different colors in varying intensities of light to be certain that the glasses meet your need. Some people prefer grey (the color that is usually issued to you when you've had a cataract operation). Others prefer a sunnier shade such as amber or yellow. Whatever shade you choose, be sure that it meets the standards of UV/UVB protection. Standards are set by Prevent Blindness America, the American Optometric Association and The American Academy of Ophthalmology.

Corning produces sunglasses that adapt to different light intensities. Some people love these and others complain that the color changes are too slow especially upon entering a dimly-lit room or a hall such as a movie theater. Purchasing these glasses is risky if they are made up in your prescription, for they can't be returned. A better option may to try out a pair for a week or so with the provision that they can be returned if not suitable. Sunglasses developed for schussing down a slope may be another option. These glasses are tight-fitting, come in a variety of shades especially designed to temper bright light. To explore, visit the sports department of a store near you.

And don't forget to wear a brimmed hat. I'm never without my hat, for not only does it eliminate much of the glare, but the brim protects my facial skin as well from the sun's exposure. If you lower the brim to meet the bridge of your sunglasses, you'll find that you've eliminated at least seventy-five percent glare.

Low-Vision Services

The blind and visually-impaired have been served by agencies and governments perhaps longer than for most handicapping conditions. There is something about being blind that evokes a responsive chord in others. This may be one of the reasons that you can find a Commission for the Blind and Visually-Impaired or the equivalent in just about any state in the US and in other developed countries and large cities as well. Generally, these organizations provide services that encompass education, vocational rehabilitation, independent living, eye health, consumer advocacy, aids and appliances, consumer complaints, reduced-fare on public transportation, community-based programs and amenities including theater passes and other cultural events. If your doctor's staff does not know the address of your state office, consult directory assistance, or check *The Directory of Services for the Blind and Visually Impaired in the United States and Canada,* published by the American Foundation for the Blind (see the Resources section) for contact information and for other low-vision centers.

Specific services are available for those designated as blind and legally blind (in both eyes 20/200 and/or a visual field of 20 degrees or less). Those who are classified with legal blindness who have some usable vision are afforded the same services as the blind. Unless your condition falls into this narrow category, many low-vision services are unfortunately unavailable to you. Mark these distinctions, for they will be useful to help you differentiate between what you can receive from the government and what you need to seek out for yourself.

State laws do not always consider those with low vision who do not fall into the category of legal blindness as eligible for services. Here is an opportunity for you to advocate for services. Light a fuse by writing to your state legislators and congressional representatives, by sending letters to "Letters to the Editor" column of your local paper, and by enlisting others with similar problems or who are sympathetic to them to rally to the cause. Or start a blog and rally otj=hers in your condition to seek action. That's one part of it. The second part requires that you focus on achieving the best possible milieu to function independently, if possible. Realize there will be periods when you need help and it's best to have a sack of strategies to fill this gap.

In general, services are available to those who are legally blind and, to a lesser extent, those with low vision. When you enroll in a low-vision program, you may find a division of services--the Federal Government funds the required needs and possibly one or more social service agencies share responsibility for providing the services. Often a private organization will have developed comparable commitments to get you back on track. Most important, when your vision begins to fade, seek help immediately. It takes time for these agencies to grind out services and the sooner you register for help the better you'll be served.

SERVICES FOR THE LEGALLY BLIND

- Should your vision fall into the category of legal blindness described above, you are entitled to services for the legally blind.
- Step One--ask your doctor or someone on staff to complete the necessary paperwork for you to receive assistance from your state office of the blind and visually-handicapped. Many states have a mandatory form. Initiate the process, if not offered by your doctor or office staff, for you may find your doctor's staff is unaware of the services available. Once the state office receives the paperwork, the ball starts rolling. Within a short period of time, you should receive a registration number. This should be an indication that the state has forwarded your case to an agency equipped to provide support services and retrain you for the workplace, if that is an option. You may need to give your doctor, the state office and the referring agency gentle reminders to keep the process flowing. In other words, follow through and don't depend on a smooth ride. And, please seek out these services for they can help save your job, prevent accidents, and possibly save your life. And once you know that your case is in progress, be patient. Winding through the system may take several months.
- Should you lose sight precipitously, insist that you receive emergency services. Your doctor will need to initiate this procedure following the above protocols. Your case, however, should take priority.
- Ask a friend or family member to assist you in maintaining your doctor's visits. This may require nothing more than simply checking to see that you keep your appointments. If you need someone to

accompany you to your doctor(s), and should this help not be available, consider hiring a private escort. Lessened anxiety may be worth the price. Alternatively, depending upon your condition, social services in your community may provide an aide or be able to refer you to a voluntary service. In the US, transportation to doctors' visits must be fulfilled for the handicapped. A van will pick you up at your home and transport you to and from your appointment, but be prepared to wait between rides because these units serve a sizeable population.

- When undergoing a medical or surgical procedure, have someone accompany you. Anticipatory anxiety precedes any kind of invasive surgery and being accompanied and comforted by a loved one helps to relieve tension. Most likely you will need someone to drive you home following the procedure, especially if you have been given medication to relax you or put you to sleep or if your eyes have been dilated.
- Ambulette services may be available to you. Check it out with the hospital staff. There may be charges for this service but possibly, your private or government insurance may foot the bill.

HERE ARE SOME OF THE SERVICES YOU CAN EXPECT

- Computer skills training.
- Rehabilitative services.
- Ways to modify your workplace.
- Adapted vacations.
- Special transportation. The ADA Act requires that communities provide para-transit resource;
- Independent living skills training.
- Occupational therapy where needed.
- Mobility training   how to properly use a cane.
- Assigning the services of social workers and other specialists to help you sort through government forms for low-vision services in your area.

You may encounter refusals for procedures that you believed were covered by such governmental programs as Medicare and Medicaid. You have the right to appeal.

Finally, receiving aid is worth the struggle. Services include a variety of visual aids and mechanical devices that can help you remain independent and fully productive. Below are some of the aids on the market. Daily, however, more aids and technological tools are added to the mix. There is no end to it. Technicians are constantly developing new products at a dizzying speed with often beneficial results for your condition.

VISUAL AIDS

These products improve your ability to see. They range from inexpensive magnifying glasses to sophisticated telescopes that can be mounted on your eyeglasses. People with low vision often find these tools invaluable for maintaining their current life styles. They're easy to use, small enough to carry in your pocket or handbag, and can be transported from place to place. Furthermore, they are the least expensive visual aids.

MAGNIFIERS

Magnifiers are rated by power. In general the greater the power the smaller the magnifier lens. The power of a magnifier is labeled. For example, at 2X--material is magnified two times, 5X--five times. These measurements, however, are not standardized and differ among manufacturers of lenses. Some lenses are also labeled with diopter measurement. The unit diopter is the inverse of the distance that the lens is in focus. One diopter reads that the lens focuses at one meter, 20 diopters, at 0.05 meters or 5 cm. So, as the lens becomes more powerful it will provide more magnification but this means it must be closer to the material it is intended to magnify. People who wear glasses may be familiar with the diopter system. Near-sighted people have minus diopters in their eye-glasses. If you divide the dioptric label by four you have an estimate of magnification. (A 20 diopter lens is 5X.)

Magnifiers come in many sizes, shapes and devices—round, square, hand-held and/or stand, illuminated or non-illuminated. They range from 2X to 10X. The distance between the hand-held and reading material can be manipulated, the stand is in a fixed position. With a fixed magnifier you should use near glasses for best magnification; with the hand-held, distance glasses. Your corrective lenses need to be appropriate for the enhancement of magnification, for if not, you will be losing full benefit from your magnifier. Small powerful lenses function best when both the magnifier and the material are brought close to the eye. Reading-speed, however, may be lost as the field of vision narrows. Lower power magnifiers can provide a larger field of vision but magnification is reduced. Distortion at the edges is one of the drawbacks of manufacture. Even the best magnifiers may not eliminate the distortion of images and colors at the edges, but as you become accustomed to the device, this should bother you less. These magnifiers are portable and you can carry them around and use as needed.

Magnifiers like glasses may also be tinted, but it's better to use clear lenses, for the tints reduce light except in situations where bright light causes discomfort. Where maximum light is necessary, both hand-held and stand magnifiers are available with a built-in light source. Before purchasing a magnifier, "try it on." And do discuss your needs with a low-vision specialist. The best magnifier, like a glove or shoe, fits well--so spend the time to be sure you have the best, if not the perfect fit.

TELESCOPES

Depending upon the state of your vision and your desire to be completely independent, you may want to investigate the variety of telescopes that are on the market. Telescopes that can be mounted on your glasses may be especially appealing. One snappy model forms a bar or bridge across the top of your glasses. Telescopes are becoming less obtrusive and some versions do not advertise a visual handicap. One rather pricy option is to have a telescopic lens inserted into a pair of eyeglass frames. An intraocular telescope, the size of a pea, has been successfully transplanted into the eyes of people with severely damaged *retinals*. This option requires the same operation as that performed for cataract extraction. The FDA has approved the device, which is produced by VisionCare. A telescope can serve to obtain a limited-vision driver's license. For intermediate viewing, prescription or non-prescription telescopes can be attached to glasses. Magnification is 4X but field of vision is reduced. Hand-held telescopes give better magnification at 10X, but field of vision is also reduced. Electronic desk-mounted telescopes provide magnification up to 24X with a wide field of vision. The electronic head-worn telescopes provide magnification up to 30X, high contrast and wide field of vision.

ELECTRONIC READING ENHANCEMENT SYSTEMS CLOSED CIRCUIT TELEVISION (CCTV)

These systems provide magnification using either a television set or a monitor. They are easy to use and provide a large reading area that can be substantially magnified. A book, magazine or newspaper is placed on the equipment. Magnification can be adjusted to match your needs. Up to 72X magnification, wide field of view and high-contrast is possible. CCTVs are available in either black and white or color with options on monitor size--14, 17 or 20 inches. Designs vary. CCTVs can stand alone or be hooked up to your computer (PC or MAC). An additional feature includes a camera that can be used to display objects a distance away from the screen.

Portable Magnifiers

These small hand-held systems provide magnification up to 28X, a wide field of view, high contrast and are suitable for reading and writing. They're small enough to be carried in a purse or a backpack. The American Optometric Association's Low Vision Section provides a nationwide listing of optometrists who offer these services (see Resources)

Some companies will send a sales representative to your home to demonstrate the machine of your choice allowing you to test it out for thirty days. After trying out the instrument, should you decide against purchase for whatever reason, the company will refund your payment. When deciding to buy, be sure to include maintenance and a return policy in your contract.

Vision Enhancement Systems Regenerate Your Life and Improve Vision With Computers

If you haven't yet joined the ranks of computer users, what are you waiting for? The average computer is relatively inexpensive and, in most cases, because you can enlarge the size of fonts, it is adequate for most people with low vision. Enhancement always appears to be reaching higher levels. T.V. Raman, a Google employee, who lost his eyesight to glaucoma at the age of 14, works to make things easier for the blind and visually handicapped. Negotiating your computer, therefore, becomes easier. Should you be unable to read the highest magnification, there are computers that read to you or software can be added to your present computer. With the proliferation of newspaper, magazine articles and books available on the web, you can keep up with the times. Alternatively, if you enjoy writing you can write letters, documents or literary works on a computer and if you have difficulty with typing, speak into the computer and know that your words will be translated into text. Of course, computers need to be equipped with special software programs for these purposes and the latest versions include some of these in the package. When in the market to purchase or update your system, visit either a low-vision center or simply a store specializing in this equipment. Alternatively, you can call in a "techie" to help you through the process. For E-mail and internet access, you will need to sign up with an internet service provider (ISP). America on Line (AOL) is among the largest but there are hundreds of other companies offering service. Your best friend will probably tell you about a great ISP. You can get broadband packages which provide much faster speeds than dial-up internet connections. Cable service can be packaged with your TV cable service or DSL service can be packaged with your telephone service, or everything can be packaged under one vendor. Hooked up, you have access to online forums and mailing lists, libraries, electronic mail, shopping, news, weather, games, auctions, databases of all kinds, communication with other people, and so on, and if you're not careful, you can become a computer junkie. At times, those with disabilities feel like second-class citizens. The Disability Network http//:www.disabilitynetwork.com/ acts to level the playing field. By joining forces, you are adding your voice to the fifty-four or so million Americans with disabilities who want to eliminate the double standard that often applies to this group.

Both Windows and Macintosh offer built-in functions to assist the visually impaired to use the computer. Windows XP, Vista and later versions come with a program called Narrator that reads aloud dialog boxes, menu items, and text on the screen. A choice of voices and speed is available. You can also dictate your information if you can no longer see the keys or if typing is a chore. You can easily increase the font size, change the screen resolution, and enlarge the image on the screen to whatever is comfortable for you. The Accessibility Program is also available in earlier versions of Windows. For more information, go to www.microsoft.com/enable. To turn Narrator on, click on START, go to ALL ***PROGRAMS or the CONTROL PANEL, then to ACCESSORIES, then to ACCESSIBILITY***, then click on ***NARRATOR.***

Third party screen reader programs for Windows include: JAWS (Windows 95 or later) *www.freedomscientic.com/fsproducts/softwarejaws.asp.*

ReadPlease has several different versions ranging from free to under $100 that works with most versions of Windows. www.readplease.com.

IBM's **Home Page Reader** is designed specifically for E-mail and web pages and is compatible with Windows 2000 or Windows XP. *www.ibm.com/able/solution_offerings/hpr.html.*

There is a site on APPLE devoted to assistive technology. www.apple.com/accessibility. The updated version of Mac Os X (TIGER) will have a spoken word interface called VoiceOver built right into the system.

The Ability Hub *(www.abilityhub.com)* can be helpful in finding computer products to help the visually handicapped.

Magnification is practically a necessity for people who have lost vision. Most computers today come with a built-in screen magnifier. For Windows users, hit the start button located on the bottom left hand side of your screen;

then go to Programs, then Accessories, then Accessibility, then click on Magnifier. A screen will open up giving you a choice of magnification. Be sure to click on Apply.

To change your monitor's scheme select Properties, select Appearance tab. Select a scheme for High Contrast and hit *Apply*.

To change your monitor's screen area explore Options—some of which may make viewing better for you. Fewer pixels will make everything appear larger on your screen.

To change the browser system on your computer, open Internet Explorer and click on View at the top of the window; a drop-down menu will appear, then point to the TEXT or FONT SIZE; another menu will appear, click on Larger or Largest. You can also select Accessibility Options in Internet Explorer by going to Tools, then Internet Options and clicking on the "Accessibility" button. The text on some web pages won't adjust appropriately unless you select "ignore font sizes specified on web pages."

To use Netscape: open Netscape, click on EDIT at top of window, a drop down menu will appear, point and click on PREFERENCES, a new window will open up where you can select several options to improve viewing.

JBliss Imaging Systems has introduced a new internet browser PnC Net developed by the National Science Foundation enabling people with low vision to conduct productive internet sessions. You can learn more about this program at http:*www.jbliss.com/pncNet.htm.*

How to get training

If you have learned to type, you're one step up the ladder to computer training. The keyboard is the same as that of the typewriter. Mastery of the various features of both your PC (personal computer) and the Internet does require some training. First of all, the vocabulary is alien, and although computer lingo has become more familiar, you will still need to learn the meaning of certain expressions. The more dogged you are learning about your computer, the better you will feel about using this equipment. When I first ventured into computer world, I thought my level of frustration would erode any supposed benefits, and I yearned for the simplicity of the typewriter. But I realized I could no longer work effectively without the computer.

Training is relatively easy to come by. Check the libraries, senior citizen's centers, community centers, churches, colleges. Apple (runs a series of free lessons. The American Foundation for the Blind (see the Resources) provides a technological center that reviews all available computer technologies. Baruch College, part of the City University of New York, has a unique program for the blind and visually-handicapped, as does the Lighthouse.

Should you be in a position where you need retraining on the job and the computer is your best bet, your State Commission for the Blind and Visually Handicapped can help but if you want to learn the computer for personal purposes, this training will probably be denied.

For those using Braille, a program called *BRAILLE SYSTEMS* makes life easier: Braille NOTETAKERS transform Braille into speech, E-mail or word processing. There are a number of models on the market.

ONLINE ACCESS—THE ROYAL ROAD TO EVERYTHING

Computers today have built-in search engines. Google appears to be one of the most popular, but your service provider also has its own. Yahoo is another widely-used search engine. If you are doing a search, you may wish to use one or two search engines to make sure that you covered all bases.

Access to the internet can be appealing, revealing, frustrating and satisfying. At your fingertips, you are presented with a wide spectrum of information. Some of it rooted by scientific or double-blind studies providing references; others appear to be primarily opinions of the writers, or in some cases, clinical evidence with dubious credentials. That the Internet has become a favorite source of medical information is indisputable. In an article in one of the peer-reviewed journals, the authors reviewed the quality of medical information found on the net. Medical information on the Internet is neither monitored for accuracy nor standardized. It contains a mixture of opinions, controversies, and financial opportunities. Potential misinformation is mixed in with valuable medical information. The authors compared the information generated from a number of different search engines and found that commercial listings accounting for twenty-five percent of the listings were usually found at the top of the lists. Government/educational comprised another twenty-five percent and informational fifty percent. Sites you can trust with information about glaucoma include: The Glaucoma Research Foundation (*http://www.glaucoma.org*) and the Glaucoma Foundation (*http:// www.glaucoma-foundation.org /info*), Glaucoma Associates of New York, (http: //www.glaucoma.net/gany/index.html.) and Wills Eye Hospital Service Foundation to Prevent Blindness (http://www.willsglaucoma.org. Macular Degeneration sites include: Macular Degeneration Foundation, (http://www. eyesight.org/) AMDC: American Macular Degeneration Foundation, (*http:// www.macular.org/),* Macula Degeneration Help Center (*http://healthfinder.gov/ docs/doc04600.htm*). General eye information can be found on the National Institutes of Health, National Eye Institute website at (*http:///www.nei.nih.*

gov/. Health on the Net (HON) has created a Code of Conduct for websites that relay health information. It follows certain principles which can be found at (*http://www.hon.ch/HONcode/Guidelines/guidelines.html.*)

The above is heavy going for some people. You may decide that you want to use your computer for entertainment. You can access its multimedia capacity, listen to and download music (record to a disk or CD) and, should you have artistic inclinations, you can draw on the computer. You can create posters, flyers, announcements of parties, weddings and other celebrations on your computer and send this information to friends and family via your E-mail. Your computer is equipped with games including a number of card games and you can spend hours playing bridge, for example, if that's your passion.

Should you want to use a computer only occasionally, but do not care to purchase your own, check out your public library. Just about every library provides computers available for public use.

HELPFUL HINTS FOR GETTING THE MOST OUR OF YOUR COMPUTER

- Avoid staring at the screen. Raise your eyes to look around especially out of a window or at a far wall. Accommodative change is important to eye health. Get up every fifteen or twenty minutes—stretch, walk around, make a phone call. Hard to remember to do this? Click on (http://www.cutereminder.com/help/healthcare.php) or Workplace at (*http://www.workpace.com.*)
- Keep it clean. Weekly, use a soft cloth and wipe dust from the screen. You don't want anything to interfere with visual access.
- Blink, blink, blink. Working on a computer slows down your blink rate, a problem that may promote dry, tired eyes.
- Arrange your monitor in such a way that you gaze down at a 15-degree angle. This angle is better for eyes.
- Overhead lighting may produce glare. Try illuminating your screen with desktop lighting focused directly on your task.
- Avoid facing the window. Light streaming from outside creates glare and interferes with your view of the screen. This light also worsens contrast problems. Light from a window behind you may also cause glare. Before establishing a permanent position for your PC, check out the effect of light on the screen.
- Glare problems can be reduced with a good filter that fits over your screen.

- Distance yourself at least two feet from the monitor just to be safe from radiation exposure, although official data has not provided evidence that this exposure is harmful.
- Adjust your keyboard to be twenty-eight to thirty-one inches from the computer screen and your chair with an adjustable backrest to provide mid-back support.
- Stretch, walk around, rest your eyes, and ease your back to avoid aches and pains associated with sitting stiffly in one place.

LIGHT YOUR WAY

We all lose both visual acuity and a dimming of vision with age. Cataract formation accounts for the dimming, and loss of neurons for acuity. In normal eyes, this loss is incidental, but in glaucoma eyes, the loss can be dramatic. Under ordinary circumstances, visual reduction can be countered by stronger light and a stronger eyeglass prescription. Both are easy solutions. Your doctor can prescribe lenses to help you see better. But it's up to you to seek out the best lighting to make your life easier.

Those of us with glaucoma are keenly aware of the quality of lighting. Joel, who when younger, hardly ever turned on lights until darkness descended, now upon entering a room, immediately switches on the lights. He requires strong lighting for reading. Evelyn who has had cataract operations on both of her eyes, on the other hand, turns off all extraneous light that she now finds too bright. A flood of light makes her jittery.

The market, fortunately, has produced such a wide variety of lamps that Joel's and Evelyn's needs are easily met. If you are sensitive to conserving electricity (and we all should be), choose from a wide variety of fluorescent bulbs that are manufactured in various shapes and that will fit most lamps. Select full spectrum bulbs (equivalent to daylight). These are available as both fluorescent and incandescent bulbs, but be aware that with an incandescent bulb, heat builds up. Take care to use only the approved wattage registered for your lamp. Use of a higher wattage will burn connecting wires that may burn right through the socket causing difficulty in removing the burned out bulb. Natural spectrum lighting (like the Verilux lamps) are claimed to promote vitamin D production, reduce fatigue and help fight winter blues. Some glaucoma patients find fluorescent lights cause glare and consequently tire the eyes. While Community Services for the Blind and Partially Sighted recommends halogen lights, be cautious about using these lamps. They burn very hot and have been known to spontaneously ignite. Should special lamps be unavailable in your community, you can find a wide selection in mail order catalogues. National Association of the Visually Handicapped suggests contacting Robin Mumford at mumfynet@earthlink.net for expert lighting advice. They produce a desk lamp, The RobinSpring 32 light. Although it is a fluorescent, it is glare-free, and uses minimum electricity. (See Resources for more information.)

LOOK INTO LARGE-PRINT TEXT MATERIAS

Not too long ago as time is reckoned, large-print materials were available from only limited sources. But as the aging population has grown, publishers of materials have recognized that a substantial market for large-print materials exists. Large-print format is available in both hard and soft cover novels, history, romances, travel, reference and general non-fiction. And it's not necessary to purchase these materials. Both the public libraries and the National Association for the Visually Handicapped (NAVH) carry them. NAVH's library contains more than 8,000 titles for loan. (See Resources)

The *New York Times* publishes a large-print edition of its paper. Some cultural institutions offer programs in the large-print format. Some magazines geared to persons with visual problems automatically use large print. Unfortunately, you may find that some of your favorite magazines use not only a small font but do an artsy page layout using colored inks on colored paper. Some of these fonts are difficult to read even if you use a magnifying glass. Fancy lettering and colored backgrounds do attract attention, but for the visually- challenged, that print is frustrating to read. We don't know whether such magazines have the capacity to print up separate editions but it does no harm to write to the editor and make this suggestion. If the marketing division of the magazine in question receives a substantial number of requests, the editors may regard it as economically feasible to produce special editions or make it available on the web.

Similar problems may also exist with such innocuous items as your monthly statements from banks, utilities, medical institutions, and other services. Using larger print in these cases is a no-brainer. Yet, these institutions are slow to change their ways. Here again, some gentle consumer prodding may facilitate change to large print and/or bold copy providing contrast. Don't you hate to receive an official document printed in red or green ink in an 8pt font size?

The problem also exists in malls, department, grocery and other merchandising stores. Often the tiny print and particular form of lighting obscures labels, prices, clothing sizes and other information necessary to make an informed purchase. I find that I need to stoop, stand on tiptoe, twist my body at times, simply to read the price of a certain item, especially in grocery stores. And forget those items placed on high shelves. If I don't recognize the shape of the container, I've no idea what the can or package holds. One of my favorite health food markets has installed a type of fluorescent lighting that, for my eyes, blanks out written material. Here, the combination of poor lighting and small print often makes it impossible to read labels. If you find that sensitivity to the need for large print materials missing in your neighborhood stores, advocate for change. Many of us can see adequately with better lighting and enlarged print. If you regularly attend a cultural event, write to management and ask that they provide large-print materials. You might also request that your favorite restaurant produces a large-print edition of its menu. Have you ever tried to remember the items the waiter rattles off if you want to know the menu offerings? The brain simply cannot quickly absorb this spiel. I know of a glaucoma patient who will only order one thing when he goes out to eat because he's embarrassed to ask someone to read the menu to him.

E-Books

Want to read in bed, while taking a bath, having breakfast and at the same time have an entire library at your disposal? Then you're a candidate for an E-Book--a book-sized electronic device that can be carried wherever you go. Literally, this is a moveable world at your fingertips. This newest technology introduced by Amazon as the Kindle has spawned a number of versions—Sony Daily Reader, Coolreaders.com, the Nook byBarnes and Noble—and there are more to come. These readers may already be loaded with a library or provide for a 14-day lending library facility. Purchase of magazines, books, newspapers can be made through Barnes and Noble. Like the computer, E-Books are equipped with text enlargement and other features to make reading easier for visually handicapped.

Listen Up

Don't want to struggle with recreational reading? Then just tap into the wide selection of recorded books. These are provided by both the Library of Congress and general interest publishers. The Library of Congress provides a wide selection of recorded books and other materials along with the machines to play them on--all of which will be sent to you free of charge. As well, many local public libraries have books on tape for loan. Publishers, fortunately, have seized on this opportunity to expand their book sales and with best sellers, in particular, often provide books on tape. For access, see Resources.

An organization, *Recording for the Blind and Dyslexic*, a non-profit based in Princeton, New Jersey, has taped some 83,000 textbooks, many of which have not been available in Braille. But a typical book of four hundred pages requires six-to-eight cassette tapes. Now this organization has started recording these books on CD's that hold up to forty hours of recorded text that can be played on PC's or on special players (VisuAide or Plextor). (*www.rfbd.org.*)

A free service provided by National Federation of the Blind www.nfb. org, offers current events through your telephone. All you need is a touch-tone phone and you can listen to news coverage provided by your local paper. A variety of options include newspapers, a Local Information Channel and NEWSLINE news. You can scan for articles of interest simply by pressing a single key on your telephone pad. Call 410-659-9314 for an application.

Television and Movie Access is improving. The FCC (Federal Communications Commission) has issued guidelines to make television more accessible to persons with disabilities in hearing and vision. For the visually impaired, the user turns on a secondary audio programming channel where a narrator describes the action when speech is absent. Not all programs will be equipped but public access programs have this amenity in place. Descriptive action in the movie house is getting on the bandwagon. Rear Window ® Captioning and DVD Theatrical ® developed by Media Access Group at Boston public broadcaster WGBH has improved accessibility in theaters. DVD Theatrical provides concise narration of visual cues. This equipment is installed in theaters nationwide and Canada. For information on theaters carrying equipment and when a particular movie will be shown click on to *http://ncam.wgbh.org/mopix/nowshowing.html* or visit the MoPix website

General Access is Improving

Frustrated by navigating screen-activated ATM's? A lawsuit filed against Diebold, the parent organization of Rite-Aid, has resulted in installing ATM's that are voice activated.

Personal Organizers

The Magnifico Portable PDA Screen Magnifier (www.officeonthegogo.com) magnifies the tiny screen.

Cell phones and Ipods: who doesn't have one these days? But except for those with keen sight and nimble thumbs, who isn't challenged by the tiny instrument? Manufacturers are addressing this problem by producing software that speaks up. Cingular Wireless has a feature called *Talks* that is based on text-to-speech software made by ScanSoft, allowing users to navigate choices by listening and prompting. This option comes on a card that is inserted into the cell phone beneath the battery. The Nokia 6620 is equipped to handle the card. The package cost is pricey, but since it's one of the first on the market, prices may come down across the range of phones. Taking matters in her own hands, a senior research associate at the *Cornell Center for Policy Research in Washington*, Dr. Bonnie O'Day, who has low vision, filed a formal complaint with the Federal Communications Commission against her service provider, Verizon Wireless, and Audiovox. Results from this action transformed cell phones that talk such as Toshiba VM4050. The Telecommunications Act of 1996, Section 255, states that telephone makers and service providers must make their products and services accessible to those with disabilities. The *Cellular Telecommunications and Internet Association,* a trade group for mobile phone companies (website *www.accesswireless.org*), provides information about phones with features to help those with visual problems.

New products are constantly being developed. Systems are available to monitor your home and garage. People now install a global positioning device in their cars to map routes. It scans the area and tells you what's around you. (*senderogroup.com*)

MAKE YOUR LIFE EASIER IN THE HOME-- HELPFUL HOUSEHOLD PRODUCTS

I would often trot into my husband's study to proffer a jar I could not open. His large strong hands always served the purpose until I discovered the many jar openers available. I also found that a simple nut cracker was ideal in opening bottle screw on tops, especially those heavily sealed with plastic. Chopping up food is an arduous activity and when sight is diminished, a dangerous one. A food processor or a blender easily does the job. Or you may wish to use a slicing guide. This product possesses an adjustable frame that regulates slices of varying thickness for foods such as bread, fruit, vegetables, meat or cheese. It can be purchased with a knife but your own trusty knife is also adequate. Use a colander to strain and rinse the water from pasta and other foods. Find it hard to turn your gas flame to the correct heat? Try a simmer ring. Newer stoves have numbered settings.There are tools for the delicate job of separating yolk from the white of an egg and poaching eggs. Spaghetti-measures remove the guesswork from cooking up a pasta dish. And there's an inexpensive tool that pops open those carefully sealed jars of food and drink. What a relief to find this item.

Other useful helpers include dustpans that fold up into a funnel pouring spout making it easier to dump the refuse into a container, a pie starter consisting of an aluminum wedge that you bake into a pie providing easy access to remove the first slice. (I personally do not advocate using any aluminum cooking utensil because aluminum is a toxic metal.)

Talking items are proliferating. Clocks and watches have been on the market for some time. Now, just about every piece of equipment appears to have a voice box built into it. A talking prescription bottle tells you its contents, etc. Many of these items can be found in specialized catalogs, but department stores and even convenience stores carry some of them. It's rather a comfort to hear a voice or at least a beep on an electronic instrument telling you that you successfully completed an operation. Gift items, too, may be voice- activated. I recently received a plaster mold of Franklin D. Roosevelt equipped with a short speech. One of my fax machines gave me an approval message after I'd sent out a fax.. Also, voice-activated phones that automatically dial the number you request are available.

Sewing on a button can be a frustrating experience, especially when attempting to thread a needle. Don't despair. There are spread-eye needles and also a number of gadgets that do the threading for you. One that works nicely for me requires that you drop the needle into a funnel; lay the thread across the groove, press a button, and the needle is threaded. Self-threaders work for both hand-held and machine sewing. You can also use a sewing gauge to help space stitches for hems, scallops, or embroidery patterns, as well for general measurement. Hate to sew at all? You can glue down a hem or a patch. These items are easily accessed from catalogs or in a five-and-dime store if one still exists in your locality.

If you have the cash (about $900), a device called Color Talk can help you match shades in your wardrobe. This item has been developed in Japan.

Distinguishing between medical vials can be frustrating and potentially dangerous if your sight is diminished, especially if you are on multiple medications. Fortunately, the various eye medications come with color distinctive tops and in different size bottles, but prescriptions from your pharmacy most often come in uniform containers. Ask the pharmacist to use a magic marker to write the first letter of the medication on the container. Diabetics can take advantage of the click-count insulin syringes—each click on the syringe is equal to two units of insulin. Also available is a device, the "Mani-Build" Becton-Dickinson scale magnifier and needle guide that magnifies the entire length of the syringe scale. This instrument simplifies mixing insulin and helps to check for bubbles in your syringe. This sampling of available materials is merely an indication of the many items designed to keep you actively involved in your daily activates and medical management.

Simple activities such as signing checks can suddenly become a problem if you have trouble locating the proper lines for this purpose. Check-writing templates (plastic sheets with openings corresponding to standard line spacing) are available to ease this problem. Use a sharpie pen to provide better contrast.

The *National Federation of the Blind* has produced a "Low Vision Resource Kit," that contains playing cards, talking alarm clock key chain, dark marking pen, bold line writing pad, large print ruler, self-threading needles and needle threaders, check writing guide, small, medium and large clear dots for identification, and various catalogs. Cost is $30 plus $5.00 for shipping and handling.

Perhaps one of the most useful pieces of information you can access is "Sharing Solutions" produced by the Lighthouse. This publication contains hints from people who have lost some or all vision. The solutions are unique but easily replicated and they cover every aspect of everyday life, including continuing to work at a skilled job. Access this information either by signing up for cassette tapes, large print copy or use E-mail info@lighthouse.org. Phone: 800-829-0500.

Recreational activities need not take a back seat. Chess, backgammon, checkers, and tic-tac-toe, are just a few of the items available that are equipped with tactile features. Do-it-yourself items include specially-adapted measuring tools insuring that precision is not lost. Visiting another state or locality? Check out a tactile map of the United States or use the Internet where you can access information for your entire trip. Bird watching by song can be an exhilarating experience and there is an organization called the *Blind Birders* to prove it. Members study tapes and CD's of bird song and they compete in tournaments to sight the most birds. These events take place in Texas sponsored by the *Texas Parks and Wildlife Department* and by *Texas Health Department*. But there's no need to go to Texas, for all you need is recorded bird song to start you on your birding journey.

The above items and many similar ones discussed in this chapter are available through mail order. Check out the Resources for names and addresses of companies and organizations that provide a full line of items that make life easier. In these catalogs you'll also find items to help you cope with other health problems.

VISION REHABILITATION

There may come a time when your vision no longer serves you. This condition, however, should not deter you from getting about, for help is available either through training to use a seeing-eye dog or mobility training—using a cane to help guide you while walking. The importance of this training cannot be overstated, for it is the first step in maintaining your independence. Mastering such training is reassuring, for it helps to maintain your competence in performing your everyday affairs and it is one of the first services that organizations serving the blind and severely visually-handicapped offer. The training is deceptively simple. You learn to use a cane to "sweep" in front of you enabling you to detect potholes, crevices, depressions, or other obstacles in your path. Sidewalks bristle with obstructions that may include open-air restaurant services, venders, strollers and baby carriages, tree surrounds, the unloading of vans, utility dig-ups and countless other improbable objects. A cane helps you to navigate a secure pathway. Even those of us who have decent vision may find ourselves tripping over a small extension or a larger object that our faulty peripheral vision did not detect.

Several types of canes are available. The touch technique cane is equipped with a pencil tip allowing the user to tap the area just in front of the trailing foot to detect objects in the pathway.

The rolling tip cane has an embedded ball-bearing at its tip. It is in contact with the ground at all times, and may provide greater stability and avoid a potential problem with the tapping cane. If the tip of the tapping cane gets stuck in a crack, the user may be jabbed in the stomach and possibly destabilized. Falls have occurred with this cane.

Some aspects of vision rehabilitation require different strokes for different folks. People with macular degeneration are taught Eccentric Viewing— learning to use the intact peripheral vision. To test how it works, look at a well-lighted doorknob which, depending on the condition of your eyes, you may not be able to see. Now look two feet to the right of the knob and it will float into view.

Have trouble reading the traffic light signal? You're not alone. Various companies are investigating products that provide an auditory signal that will be loud enough to be heard over the drum of traffic but not so loud that the sound is annoying to others. This is an area where advocacy can move the technology into daily use.

Ever expect the tongue to be a transmitter of information other than the taste of food? Researchers at the University of Wisconsin have developed a grid of gold-plated electrodes that when placed on the tongue can transmit visual cues to the brain.

And there is now evidence that your ears can help you see. A research scientist in the Netherlands has developed a technology called vOICe that translates sounds into sight. The device consists of a tiny camera, a laptop and headphones. The camera is mounted on the head of the patient and sends video input to the laptop where the information is converted to a soundscape. This device has been used by both blind people from birth and those who have gone blind, and Harvard researchers conducting brain scans, found in both cases, many responses equal that of a sighted person. The device, fortunately, has undergone modification and a simplified version connecting the camera to a cell phone is now being studied. *(www.seeingwithsound.com/voicefrl.htm)*

There is no end to the stretch of technology. Glasses and contact lens may soon be enhanced to not only make things clearer but to provide electronic images, virtual information such as maps, etc. The new world is coming in fast.

You may even be blessed with unusual taste buds. Yes, there is something called *synesthesia,* a sensory phenomena in which a sound evokes an experience of color. Some people can taste a word and in a rarer occasion taste tone intervals. The body's capacity for adaptation appears to be endless. We know of a blind individual who can identify color.

Aside from technology, at times the brain fills in the missing information. There is the case of a doctor left blind from two successive strokes. Researchers asked him to navigate an obstacle course. At first he declined, but then agreed to try and navigated the course successfully. Researchers called this phenomenon blindsight, the primitive part of the brain using the brain's subsconscious to see. For more information, click on: *www.beatricedegelder.com.*

Medical coverage for certain treatments among the insured can raise thorny problems, especially when the treatment is considered unproven. Congress has recognized the need for Medicare beneficiaries to challenge policies that affect them. When you are affected by a Medicare denial of coverage, you can join with any number of senior organizations to pressure the Department of Health and Human Services (HHS) to take action redressing this need.

Helpful resources can be found locally in many communities. Check with your social services agency or better yet, form a support group and become an activist. (see below)

THERE'S NO GROUP LIKE A SUPPORT GROUP

A support group can serve many functions. It helps to unite a group of people with similar problems, especially those with a chronic disease such as glaucoma. A support group, whether it is virtual (web-based) or one where people meet together weekly, monthly, or even occasionally in a designated place, is an invaluable method for airing problems, learning more about glaucoma, and sharing concerns. It also offers an ideal venue for mutual assistance, lending an empathetic ear to those distressed by their conditions, as well as providing assistance in handling technical problems. It promotes the sharing of medical and general information useful for making important decisions in self-care. When a member experiences visual impairment, other members of the group can be of assistance by sharing similar experiences and offering advice to help cope with the situation. This support can help guide the individual to find a satisfactory lifestyle when vision is diminished. The support group is especially important if glaucoma strikes during one's most productive years and if severe vision loss occurs. Members who likewise have been affected offer valuable assistance in helping to select proper adaptive materials.

A vital support group is not limited to adults. Parents of children with glaucoma find solace in sharing information to help manage their children's medical and surgical needs.

A Support Group can help to

- Interact with other patients.
- Share information with others.
- Gain emotional support.
- Establish a phone network that will be available in case of emergency.
- Strengthen doctor-patient relationships.
- Provide information enabling better understanding of glaucoma.
- Share similar problems and coping solutions to its members.
- Educate by inviting speakers from different branches of the medical profession and health field including complementary therapies such as herbal and vitamin supplementation, yoga, acupuncture, and other specialties. Be cautious when inviting complementary therapists. Check qualifications for information buttressed by research.
- Learn early about new applications based on the latest research.
- Set up separate small counseling sessions headed by a psychologist.
- Establish an advocacy committee to promote awareness in the business community and the public at large of the need to modify transportation, written materials and practices. Some examples include: modifying lighting in restaurants, restrooms, and grocery stores; adapting various forms of recreation; providing street announcements by transportation operators; equipping public facilities with voice-activated speech, such as in elevators and directories in buildings supplying yellow strips on bottom stairs and large letter street signs; developing good contrast written materials and large print on documents including bills, medical forms, insurance forms, restaurant menus, entertainment programs and such, and improving visibility on display menus on technological equipment. The list is endless. The support group chooses a target to improve access.

- Empower self and other members to take a voice in glaucoma treatment, manner of research, life style issues, and to some extent exert influence over the manufacture of supplements and materials that may be of benefit.

READY TO BEGIN

Congratulations! You are about to start a new phase as an empowered glaucoma patient. By taking charge of your own health, by learning more about glaucoma, by sharing your concerns with others, and by creating a venue where all the above can be aired, you will be broadening your horizons, and strengthening your ability to cope with glaucoma.

Sponsorship

It may be possible for a local health organization or a hospital to sponsor your group. This can be an advantage, since such an organization may elect to provide space for your meetings. Depending upon the resources of the organization, you may also be able to use mailroom facilities.

Advertising the Group

Telephone trees are serviceable in the beginning, but most people like to have a flyer in hand for referral. Also, producing flyers announcing your next meeting is a good way to advertise your group, since the flyer can be posted in doctors' offices, hospital waiting rooms and senior citizen centers. Flyers provide an excellent method for recruiting new members. Ask members of the group to post flyers in libraries, drug stores and in their personal doctors' offices. (See sample flyer)

Financing

At the very least, you will need some money to send out notices, especially as your membership list begins to grow. You may want to charge minimum yearly dues just to cover expenses, or seek a small grant from one of your local institutions such as a bank. If you do have a sponsor, you may be able to arrange to have the flyers printed and mailed under its auspices. Once your group is established, note that in the US, it is possible to send out flyers free as long as you stamp "free matter for the visually handicapped" in the right hand corner where the stamp would ordinarily go. Keep in mind that the mission of a support group is to bring together people with similar problems. If the support group is engaged in large projects requiring substantial funding, the original purpose of the group may be set aside

Essential Requirements for a Support Group

1. A permanent meeting place.
2. A register of members
3   Method of member communication.
4. Funding, however minimal, to cover expenses.
5. Commitment of the coordinator to oversee all the necessary functions.
    a. solicit speakers if that is one of the missions.
    b. run the meetings.
    c. publicity to: doctors, local newspapers, health organizations, senior citizen centers, etc.
6. Not absolutely essential, but a newsletter summarizing your meetings helps to bind the group together. This newsletter can be an E-mail attachment thus saving on postage.

How to begin

One of the most obvious venues for starting a support is to approach your eye doctor or the clinic you visit. You may find that although your doctor or the clinic director is in favor of a group, he or she doesn't have the time to devote to its formation. Try to obtain permission, therefore, to discuss plans with fellow patients. The waiting rooms of eye clinics or eye doctors' offices are ideal settings for interaction with patients who have glaucoma and who may welcome the possibility of forming a support group. These patients may well become the nucleus of a group. Our group, initiated by a doctor who teamed with Prevent Blindness America, was instrumental in drawing together three or four patients. The Group has grown to well over 300 members.

If you visit a doctor in a teaching hospital, you may find a receptive audience with the Glaucoma Fellows who are generally interested in learning more about patients' responses. They may be helpful in recruiting members, providing space and serving in a general advisory capacity.

Should the medical community be unresponsive or too busy to accommodate a support group, you might turn to your local church, mosque, synagogue, YMCA or WMHA, public library, local school, community center or any other public or religious facility to assist you in both forming a group and providing space. While there may be a charge for space, it is generally minimal.

Essentially you will want to

1. Develop a nucleus of people dedicated to help and support themselves and other patients. As few as three or four individuals can provide the core.
2. Enlist your doctor's cooperation to inform patients of the support group's existence. Ask his/her help to request other doctors to do the same.
3. Contact local pharmacists who may be helpful in recruiting both members and sponsors/speakers.
4. Tap the glaucoma services in local hospitals for potential members and doctors who can support your group.
5. If hospitals have newsletters for patients, ask to have an item about your support group inserted.
6. Send out news releases to local papers and health newsletters.
7. Announce the formation of the group on the Internet, especially on local health newsgroups.
8. Inform Scott Christensen, CEO, The Glaucoma Foundation, 80 Maiden Lane, New York, NY. 10038, Director of the World Glaucoma Patient Association (WGPA) once the group has formed.

Define your goals at your first meeting

Below are just a few of the questions that will form your group. As your group develops, you will probably find that your members' desires will crystallize. In the beginning, therefore, maintain a flexible agenda until the group's direction emerges.

Please keep in mind that a support group should be fashioned by the perceptions of its members. It can be entirely patient-focused as is The New York Glaucoma and Support Group that is run by a Steering Committee. Primarily, this Group invites speakers to each of its meetings, setting aside time for patient interaction and support at the beginning of the program. In addition, it publishes a newsletter. Three-quarters of its members are homebound, but are still actively involved, drawn to retain membership because they wish to receive the newsletter. It is one of the chapters of the The Glaucoma Foundation that provides technical support.

Possibly, support group services can be formalized similar to Glaucoma Australia, Inc. This group was formed to increase community awareness, to provide information and support for glaucoma patients and their families, and to develop financial resources to fund research. A Steering Committee was formed by a group of ophthalmologists and patients. This group grew into a national organization that distributes, at no charge, pamphlets and information sheets on glaucoma, and produces a newsletter, *Glaucoma News* that reaches over 6,000 people. It has spawned support group meetings in Perth, Hobart, Melbourne, Adelaide, Canberra, Sydney, Armidale and Newcastle. It has also produced a handbook that has been translated into a number of languages. The national organization conducts an annual fund-raising appeal that has enabled it to provide funds to various research projects. Because of its large volunteer base, it needs only two full-time and one part-time staff members.

Some questions to ask as you set up your group

- Should your meetings focus solely on mutual support?
- Should you have a speaker in the health field at each meeting?
- Should there be a mix of both?
- Should your group develop a charter, by-laws, etc., where you elect officers each year?
- Should you establish an informal structure led by a Steering Committee?
- Should you publish a newsletter? If so, will the newsletter be a chatty account of members' concerns or a more formalized structure summarizing your lecturer's talks?
- Will this be a dues-paying organization?
- Will you make fund-raising for glaucoma research a part of your program?
- Will your focus be on patient advocacy?

Your first meeting

1. Ask for volunteers to carry out various functions e.g. coordinator, secretary, treasurer, newsletter editor, production manager, newsletter distribution, speaker contact, and telephone and email support.
2. Pass around a sheet of paper with suggested topics. Ask members for additional suggestions.
3. Serve refreshments if possible. Be sure to include snacks suitable for diabetics.
4. If you do not have a speaker, don't attempt to answer medical questions, but focus on ways to cope with glaucoma and visual impairments. When you have a speaker, please leave enough time for patients to ask questions.

5. Announce the formation of the group on the Internet, especially on local health newsgroups, and/or *glaucoma@yahoogroups.com*. This site allows posts of meeting notices for local groups.

Topics That May Be Of Interest To A Support Group

Medical:
1. Medications
2. Laser treatment, (trabeculoplasty and other laser procedures)
3. Filtration (trabeculectomy)
4. Cataract surgery

Types of glaucoma
1. POAG (Primary open angle glaucoma)
2. Normal-Tension glaucoma
3. Pigmentary Dispersion Syndrome
4. Exfoliation Glaucoma
5. Ocular Hypertension--high tension but no sign of glaucoma damage yet
6. Narrow/Acute Angle Closure Glaucoma
7. Glaucoma and macular degeneration
8. Glaucoma in children and juveniles
9. Glaucoma associated with diabetes mellitus
10. Rarer forms of secondary glaucomas.
11. Low Vision and visual aids

Diagnosis
1. Examination
2. Gonioscopy
3. Central Corneal Thickness
4. Intraocular pressure
5. Optic nerve evaluation
6. Visual field test
7. Nerve Fiber Analyzers (GDx.OCT, etc.)

Related Health Issues
1. Services for legally blind
2. Living with a chronic condition—quality-of-life issues
3. Nutrition
4. Supplements including herbal treatments.
5. Eastern forms of relaxation (meditation, yoga, etc)
6. Exercise

SPEAKERS

Since you will probably not have a budget to pay an honorarium to a speaker, you will need to find speakers who will address your group free of charge or pro bono. This is usually not difficult to do because most healthcare professionals consider it a public health service to speak to a group. If you are able to enlist your ophthalmologist in supporting the group, he or she will be able to recommend speakers. In many cases, those who have had glaucoma for a number of years will occasionally need to be evaluated by ophthalmologists specializing in the *retina*, cornea or other parts of the eye. Tap these specialists also as speakers.

When you have arranged for a speaker, be sure to offer the speaker choice of a particular topic and include in your confirming letter (see sample below) time, place, address, Room #, etc. Be sure to include all pertinent information. Also ask the speaker if he or she plans to do a power-point presentation. If you are holding your meetings in a hospital, chances are that audiovisual equipment will be available. Otherwise, the speaker may need to provide the equipment. You will probably arrange for a speaker over the phone, or personally if the speaker is your own physician. After setting a date, it is wise to confirm the event either through E-mail or snail mail even if it is just a short note, thanking the speaker for agreeing to address the meeting. (See sample letter)

It is wise to contact the speaker a few days before the meeting date as a reminder.

Following the presentation, you will want to thank the speaker either via E-mail or letter. (See sample) This is an important step since speakers are interested in feedback from the Group and a heartfelt thank-you may encourage the speaker to return on another occasion.

Of course, a support group can exist without speakers, but don't be disappointed if the group membership dwindles after a number of meetings. Participants of a group often find that when their primary emotional needs are met, they no longer have the urgency to share experiences. It is, therefore, important that recruitment be an ongoing activity.

Some patients tend to just want to keep talking about their experiences, especially if they have a particular problem. This situation usually causes the group to become restless. <u>Allow sufficient time</u> for the individual to air the problem, and then gently move onto another participant.

SAMPLE LETTERS TO HELP FORM A SUPPORT GROUP

Sample Application Form

(Insert name, address, phone number and E-mail of your Group)

Welcome! You are about to join a large group of patients who are interested in self-empowerment to help cope with glaucoma. Membership in the Group entitles you to monthly free lectures by physicians and other health professionals. Meetings are held on (insert schedule of meetings) at the (insert location, room, time, etc.). Along with monthly flyers announcing the next meeting, you will receive a quarterly newsletter that recaps the lecture material. To keep this organization viable, we request, if possible, a donation of $25. Should you choose to increase your donation, this additional funding will be directed to a glaucoma foundation for research purposes (or to the organization with which you are affiliated.)

Send this half to (Insert Name of Your group):

PLEASE PRINT:

NAME_____ADDRESS_____

CITY_____STATE_____

ZIP_____

PHONE:_____HOME_____

BUSINESS_____

E-MAIL_____

Can you participate in helping out with writing articles, administrative matters, working on the newsletter, the mailings and attending two planning sessions a year?

Yes ☐ No ☐ I cannot help now, but keep me in mind if you really need me. ☐

Signature: _____Date_____

Donation_____

Confirmation letter to speaker

Date:

Address of Speaker

Dear,

Thank you for agreeing to participate in our lecture series.

Your lecture is scheduled for (DATE) at (TIME) in the (PLACE, ADDRESS, ROOM #). If you plan to use audiovisual or power-point, please advise us immediately so that we can arrange to have the equipment available.

As we discussed over the phone, our group is particularly interested in learning more about the various surgical techniques that are used to control the progression of glaucoma. Some of our members are in the process of grappling with the question of whether to have glaucoma surgery and are eager to know all implications of such surgery. We are, therefore, most interested in a lecture updating us on the current practices of filtration surgery. This is a sensitive topic for glaucoma patients, so there will probably be a lot of questions.

We will be sending out a flyer to members and for this, we will need your CV, both in order to introduce you and for information to be placed on the flyer. Below is a suggested title. You are, of course, free to change it to one you consider more suitable.

WHEN IS THE RIGHT TIME FOR FILTRATION SURGERY?

You can fax this information to me at (FAX number) or mail it to (MAILING ADDRSS), or E-mail: (E-MAIL ADDRESS)

(Optional) We publish a summary of your lecture in our newsletter that is sent to our members as well as to a group of doctors. Thank you again and we are looking forward to your being with us.

Sincerely,

Thank you letter
DATE
SPEAKER'S ADDRESS

Dear

On behalf of (NAME OF GROUP), we want to thank you for your amazing lecture on (DATE). We are deeply grateful that you took the time out of your busy schedule to meet with us. Any information we can bring to the Group that will enlighten them about health and its influence on the eyes is greatly appreciated and we feel that your lecture did just that. Members attending voiced their deepest appreciation for the information you imparted to us.

(Optional) As you may recall we reprise your lecture and plan to include in one of our quarterly newsletters. Enclosed is the article (or) I've emailed you the article. Please feel free to make changes that will representative your point of view. Your lecture contained a wealth of information and we could not include all of it.

Is it possible for you to email or mail your corrected copy of the attached material by (DATE)?

Again thank you for presenting this very important workshop.

With best wishes,

INTRODUCTORY FLYER OR LETTER FOR DOCTORS' OFFICES, HOSPITALS, ETC.

PLEASE POST

THE GLAUCOMA SUPPORT AND EDUCATION GROUP

A chapter of
THE GLAUCOMA FOUNDATION
Presents

FREE Saturday Lecture Series

MAY 21, 2009
10:30 AM

New York Eye and Ear Infirmary
310 East 14th Street at Second Avenue
3rd Floor Conference Room

UNDERSTANDING GLAUCOMA

AS THE RESULTS ON STUDIES BEGIN TO EMERGE, THE FUNDAMENTAL CONCEPTS ABOUT GLAUCOMA BECOME CLEARER. HERE'S AN OPPORTUNITY TO LEARN MORE.

Speaker: (Give name and affiliation)

Selected Bibliograhy

PART I

DIAGNOSIS

Albekioni, Zurab, et al, "Correlation Central Corneal Thickness and *Scleral* Thickness", *Rounds, New York Eye and Ear Infirmary, New York University, Manhattan Eye, Ear and Throat Hospital, New York Medical College, Rounds, 2004.*

Boas, Gary, "OCT Images Blood Flow with Complex Geometries", *Biophotonics International, April,2004:12*

Brownlee, Michael, MD, "Benfotiamine study*, http:ww.benfotiamine.org/ Brnlee. Htm, 2/162003*

Cunningham, Emmett T., Jr., MD, PhD, MPH, "Diagnosing Uveitis," *Review of Ophhalmology, Jan. 1999:46-55*

Drance, Stephen, OC, MD, et al, "Risk Factors for Progression of Visual Field Abnormalities in Normal –Tension Glaucoma," *American Journal of Ophthalmology, 131:6:699-707*

EyeMDLink, "Optic Nerve Imaging," *http://www.eyemdlink.com/Test. asp?ID=24*

IBID, "Ultrasound Examination," *http://www.eyemdlink.com. Test.asp?ID-31*

IBID, "Pachymetry," *htpp://www.eyemdlink.com. Test.asp?ID=24*

IBID, "Corneal Cell Count," *http://www.eyemdlink.com. Test.asp?ID=6*

Fisher, Anne L, "Telemedicine is changing the way we maintain health by diagnosing and treating illness remotely," *Biophotonics International, Oct. 2004:42-45.*

Fishman, G.R, et al, "Central Corneal Thickness Measurement by Optical Coherence Tomography", *Rounds Conference, New York Eye and Ear Infirmary*

Foroozan.Rod, MD & Savino, Peter J.MD, "How to Uncover the Case of the Swollen Optic Nerve," *Review of Ophthalmology:June 2001:99*

Furchgott, Roy, "For an Ailing *Retina*, Instant Diagnosis From Afar." *The New York Times, 7/3/2003*

Goldberg, I, et al, "Multifocal object perimetry in the detection of glaucomatous field loss," *Am Ophthalmol, 2002:133:29-39*

Greenfield, David S., "Clinical Assessment of Optic Nerve and Nerve Fiber Layer in Daily Practice", *Comprehensive Ophthalmology Update:1:2; Mar/ Apr 2000.87-96*

Hepson, Ibrahim F. Everekliouglu, "Defective visual field tests in chronic heavy smokers," *Acta Opthalmologica Scandinavia, 2001:79: 53-56*

Higginbothem, Eve J. MD "Advances in Glaucoma Diagnosis," *Ocular Surgery News: 9/1/200*

Hogan, Hank, "High Sensitivity," *Biophotonics, Jan., 2004:64*

IBID, "The image that came in from the cold," *Biophotonics, Jan/Feb. 2003:57*

IBID, "Raman spectroscopy measures eye pigment, *Biophotonics, Sept. 2003:22*

IBID, "Scanning eyes to track blood flow," *Biophotonics International, Dec.2002:17*

IBID: "Imaging neurons as they two-step," Biophotonics International, December 2004:32-=3

Hood, Donald C., et al, "Detecting Early to Mild Glaucomatous Damage: A Comparison of the Multifocal CEP and Automated Perimetry", *Investigative Ophthalmology & Visual Science, Feb, 2004.5:2:492-498*

IBID, "An Intraocular Comparison of the Multifocal VEP; A Possible Technique for Detecting Damage to the Optic Nerve, *Investigative Ophthalmology and Visual Science, May, 2000:41;6:1580-7*

Hsiung, Pei-Lin, Et al, "Laser Advances Benefit Optical Coherence Tomography", *Biophotonics International, Nov. 2003: 36-40*

Hyvarinen, Lea, Quantitative Color Vision Test P-16 Manual, *Precision Vision, 944 First Street, La Salle, IL 61201, USA*

Ishikawa, Hiroshi, "Can the Newer Sophisticated Instruments Tease out Vision Loss?" *Lecture to New York Glaucoma Support and Education Group, published in newsletter, Living With Glaucoma: Aug/Sept. 2000*

Ishida, Kyoka, Et al, "Disk Hemorrhae Is a Significantly Negative Prognostic Factor in Normal-Tension Glaucoma", *American Journal of Ophthalmology, June 2000, 707-714*

Johnston, Cameron,,"Sleep Position Linked to Glaucoma Symptoms," *DG News, Dallas, TX 11/1/2000 Report on AAO Conf.*

Jones, L.A., et al, Low Vision Intervention Clinical Trial Pilot Study Results, *Association for Research in Vision and Ophthalmology, March 15, 2001*

Kahana, MD Ph D, Gottlieb, Justin, L, Ophthalmology on the Internet, *Arch Ophthalmol:122: Mar 2004: 180-3*Hogan, Hank, "High Sensitivity," Biophotonics International, Jan. 2004: 65

Kent, Christopher, *Review of Ophthalmology,* June, 2009, "New Prospectives on Glaucoma Progression.

Kommshi, Ernest W., MD & Latina, Mark A., MD, "Will LASIK, PRK delay diagnosis of glaucoma?" Ophthalmology Times, Oct. 15, 2004:

Mutlukan, Erkan, MD, PhD, and Katz, Jay, MD, "What You Need to Know About Faster Visual Field Tests, *Review of Ophthalmology, June 1991:1-4*

Noirk, T, Michael, MD, et al,"Swelling and Loss of Photoreceptors in Chronic Human and Experimental Glaucoma", *Arch Ophthalmol: 118: Feb 2000:133-43*

Quinn, Christopher J., OD, & Chaglasian, Michael, OD, "HRT vs. GDx," *Review of Optometry, 7/15/200,:62`-64*

IBID, "Glaucoma: Is it H. Pylori Related?" *Review of Optometr: 139:07:7/15/02*

Patel, Avimash, S., King, MD John S., Netland, Peter A.MD,"How To Choose the Right Automated Perimetry Unit," *Review of Ophthalmology: June, 2001:105-10*

Photonic crystal may allow glucose test based on eye color," Biophotonic's International, May, 2003

Podolsky, Morris, MD, "Primary Care Physicians are Instrumental in Early Detection," *Postgraduate Medicine: Glaucoma: 103: May 1998:131-48*

Reichert Ophthalmic Instruments, "Applanation tonometry and corneal viscoelasticity,: *http://www.reichert.com/org*

Reiss, Susan M, "Confocal method reveals neurodegenerative process," Biophotonics International: October 2004:28

Ritch, Robert, Pigment Dispersion Syndrome—Update, 2003, *Glaucoma, Ritch 20.02.2004:177-191*

IBID, "New imaging tools promise accuracy in diagnosis and in following the progression of glaucoma damage," *EyetoEye, newsletter, The Glaucoma Foundation, spring/summer, 2003*

Sample, Pamela AZ, "Glaucoma is present prior to its detection with standard automated perimetry: is it time to change our concepts?" *Graef's Arch Clin Exp Ophthalmologyl: 2003: 242: 168-9*

Schlotzer-Schrehardt, U, et al, "Increased extracellular depositions of fibrillin-containing fibrils in pseudoexfoliation syndrome," *Investigative Ophthalmology and Visual Science: 38:870984*

Scerra, Chet, "OCT offers early insights into risk of visual-field deterioration," *Ophthamoogy News, 8/1/2003: 10*

Sherman, Jerome, OD, FAAO, "New Insights in Glaucoma Detection and Monitoring," *Eyetech Update May June, 2000:*

"Two Photon Images Capture Blood Flow," *Biophotonics International: Nov.2003:13*

Zangwill, Linda H, PhD, et al, "Racial Differences in Optic Disc Topography", Arch Oohthal:122, Jan, 2004: 22-28 *http://www.retinalspec.com/erm.htm* "Epiretinal Membrane

GLAUCOMA/GENERAL INFORMATION

Ackerman, Diane, "I Sing the Body's Pattern Recognition Machine,:" *The New York Times, June 15. 2004*

Alshari, Natalie A., MD, "What's New in Cornea and External Disease," *Review of Ophthalmology, April, 2004: 71-5*

Anderson, Lynn, PhD, "A Good Lens Tech May Make the Right Fit," *Review of Ophthalmology, April, 2004:17-18*

Angle Recession Glaucoma, July 8, 2004: *http://www.emedicinehealth.com/articles.41766-1.asp,*

Aret, Ahmad A., BS and Schmitt, Breian P. MD, MPH, FACP, "Open-angle glaucoma: Tips for earlier detection and treatment selection," The Journal of Family Practice, February, 2005:54:2:117-24

Blakeslee, Sandra, "When the Brain Says, 'Don't Get Too Close'", *The New York Times, July 15, 2004*

IBID "Eye Cells May Help Regulate Body's Clock," *The New York Times, , February 8, 2002*

IBID "How the Brain Works: A New Theory of Consciousness," *The New York*

Times, March 25, 1995

Central *Retinal* Vein Occlusion, *University/Iowa, Department of Ophthalmology and Visual Sciences, http://webeye.ophth.uiowa.edu.dept.crvo.01.HTM*

Bowling.Earnest L. OD, MS,, FAAO, & Mann, Daryl F. OD*: Anterior Uveitis: "A Review for the Practicing Optometrist" Contemporary Optometry. Vol. 9, #2, February 2005. PP 1-7.*

Coleman, Anne L, "Glaucoma," *The Lancet, 354:11/30 ,1999:1803-9*

Central *Retinal* Vein Occlusion, *http://www,emedicine.com/oph/byname/central-retinal-artery oc...*

Charters, Linda (reviewed by George Spaeth, MD, "Individualized treatment essential with ocular hypertension," *Ophthalmology Times, April 1, 2004*

Dell'Osso, Louis F., PhD, "Novel Surgery for Nystagmus: Initial Trial Results," *Research to Prevent Blindness, Seminar*

Dreyer, Evan Benjamin, MD, PhD, & Lipton, Stuart A., "New Perspectives in Glaucoma," *JAMA Jan 17 1999:281:4:306-8*

"Eye on Inflammation" The H*ealth Resource Newsletter, : 19:1:2003*

Foster, C. Stephen, "Characteristic of Uveitis Presenting for the First Time in the Elderly," *http://wwwmeei.harvard.edu/*

IBID "Ocular Inflammatory Disease Review of System Questionnaire," *IBID*

IBID "Secondary Glaucomas" IBID

IBID "Limbal Stem Cell Transplantation" *IBID*

Fuchsjager-Mayrl G, et al, "Ocular blood and systemic blood pressure in patients with primary open- angle glaucoma and ocular hypertension," *Invest Ophthalmol Sci, 2004:45:835-39*

Geddes, Chris D., MD, et al "Contact lenses May Provide Window to Blood Glucose," *Biophotonics International, Feb. 2004"50-3*

"Glaucoma and Pregnancy," *The Newsletter of the Glaucoma Foundation, Winter, 2003*

"Glaucoma," *The Johns Hopkins White Papers, Johns Hopkins Medical Institutions, Baltimore, MD, May 1999:25-37*

Gordon, Mae O., PhD, et al "The Ocular Hypertension Treatment Study" *Arch Ophthalmology: 120: June 2002: 714-19*

Harris, Alon, PhD, et al, "Reduced Cerebrovascular Blood Flow Velocities and Vasoreactivity in Open- angle Glaucoma," *American Journal of Ophthalmology, Feb., 2003: 135:2 144-7*

Hitchings, Roger A, MD FRCS, "Glaucoma in the New Millennium," *From the Moorfields Eye Hospital and Institute of Ophthalmology, London, England, 12:1:Dec. 1999: 51-31*

Hosking, S. I., et al, "Ocular haemodynamic responses to induced hypercapnia and hyperoxia in glaucoma," *British Journal of Ophthalmol 2004:88:406-11*

Johnson, Douglas H., MD & Bruvaker, Richard F., MD, "Glaucoma: An Overview," *Mayo Clinic Proceedings 61:59-67, 1986*

Kellogg, Sarah. "Doctors Predict Uptick in Vision Problems," *Aug. 23, 2004 http://newhousenews.com/archive/kellogg082304.html*

Kent, Christopher, Senior Editor, *"Glaucoma Risk: The Nutrition Connection," Review of Ophthalmology,* Nov. 2008, PP 118-122

Kolata, Gina, "Studies Find Brain Grows New Cells," *The New York Times, March 18, 1998*

Krichevs, Anna & Kosik, Kenneth, "RNA nuggets at Synapse May Fuel Memory, Learning, *Focus, News From Harvard Medical School: A special Edition Featuring News on Neurobiology*

"Los Angeles Latino Eye Study Issues: Principal Investigator Speaks at Capitol Hill Briefing on Vision Health Disparities Research:" *ARVO NEWS, Winter Newsletter, 2004*

Moshfeghi, Darius M. MD, et al, "Ocular Hypertension and Early Primary Open-Angle Glaucoma," *Comprehensive Ophthalmology Update, 1:3: May/June 2000:136-44*

Lee, David A., MD & Netland, Peter A, MD, Ph.D, *"What's New in Glaucoma Research," Review of Ophthalmology, May 1998: 86-95*

Lee, Seung-Iae & Montell, Craig, "Unexpected mechanism causes light-induced blindness;" *reported in Biophotonic's International: February 2005: source, Curremt Biology,. Dec. 14:2004: 2076*

"Multiple neurotransmitter vesicles released at synapses?" *Biophotonics Intrernational, September 2002:40*

Murphy, Bob, "New Approaches to Diabetic Retinopathy," *Review of Ophthalmology, August, 2002:47-51*

Neri, P et al, "Incidence of glaucoma in patients with uveitis," *J. Glaucoma: 2004:13:6:461-65*

Netland, Peter A., MD, PhD, & Lee, David A., MD "What's New in Glaucoma Research," *Review of Ophthalmology, May 1999: 102-110*

Netland, Peter A., "What's New in Glaucoma at ARVO," *Review of Ophthalmology, May 2001: 67-75*

Netland , Peter A. MD, PhD, "What's New in Glaucoma?" *Review of Opthalmology, May, 2003: 82-85*

IBID "What's New in Glaucoma," *Review of Ophthalmology, April, 2004: 93-98*

Pilcher, Helen R., "Un-blinded by the light," *http://www.nature,com. nsul.030303/030303-1.html*

Piltz-Seymour, Jody R, MD, "Does Your Patient Have Glaucoma", *Review of Ophthalmology, June 1999:86-99*

Pinnolis, Michael, MD, "Central *Retinall* Vein Occlusion": *www. harvardvanguard.org/visualservices/vscrvo.html*

Pollock, Andres, "RNA Trades Bit Part for Starring Role in the Cell," *The New York Times, Jan. 21, 2003*

Porter, John D., PhD, "Muscles of a Different Order: Using the Eye as a Window into Neuromuscular Disease," *University Hospital of Cleveland and Case Western Reserve University*

Prather, W. C., et al, "Spectroscopic Methods for Quantifying Surface Protein Accumulation on Human-Worn Contact Lenses and Subsequent Protein Removal in Simulated In-Eye Use of Lens Rewetter Products, *Allergen*

Ritch, Robert, MD, :"Glaucoma Pigmentary," *http://www.emedicine.com/oph/topic136.htm*

Scerra, Chet, "Ocular circulation: New significance in glaucoma," *Ophthalmology Times,2/15/98:36-7*

Schlotzer Schrehardt, U., et al, "Mechanisms of glaucoma development in pseudoexfoliation syndrome," *Department of Ophthalmology, University Exlangen-Nurnbverg, Erlangen, Germany*

IBID, "Trabecular Meshwork in Pseudoexfoliation Syndrome with and without Open-Angle Glaucoma," *Investigative Ophthalmology & Visual Science, Aug, 1995:36:9:1750-64*

"See Change—New Views on Vision, "*Bostonia, Fall 2003*

Sommer, Alfred, "Doyne Lecture, Glaucoma Facts and Fancies," *Eye (1996):10+295-301 Royal Collee of Ophthalmologists*

Spears, Carl, OD, :"Controversies in Glaucoma Care," *Review of Ophthalmology, July 15, 199: 89-99*

Sullivan, Brian, R., MD, "Glaucoma, Angle Recession," *updated, 12/7/2003, Department of Ophthalmology, University of Texas, Southwestern Medical Cente*

Uveitis/Inflammatory Disease Research, *index.aspindex.asp*

Yang-Williams, Kathy, OD, "Insights into risk factors, diagnosis and treatment,"

Review of Optometry, http://www.revoptom.com/index.asp?page=2-539.htm

LASER

Butterworth-Heinemann, "Summary of ophthalmic lasers: their primary characteristics and applications," *Wormington CM, 2003*

Choplin, Neil T., MD, "New Tack in Scanning Laser Polarimetry," *Review of Ophthalmology, June 2003: 92-5*

Cioth, George A., et al, "Argon versus Selective Laser Trabeculoplasty," *Glaucoma: 13:2: April 2004: 174-7*

Higginbotham, Eve J, MD, "Reaffirming the Role of Laser in Glaucoma Management," *Arch Ophthalmol: 117: Aug 1999:1073-6*

Mizota, Atsushi, et al, "Experimental Science: Internal Sclerostomy With the Er:YAG Laser Using a Gradient-Index (GRIN) Endoscope," *Accepted for publication, July 28, 2001, http://www.osli.com/showAbst.asp?thing=2330*

Nataloni, Rochelle,,"Laser options are on the rise for glaucoma treatment," *Ocular Surgery News Europe/Asia-Pacific Edition June 2000. http:www. osnsupersite.com/view.asp?ID=495*

Park, Carl H, MD, et al, Developments in Laser Trabeculoplasty," *Laser Surgical Review, April/May 2000:315-22*

"Professional society releases lasik guidelines," *Biophotonic's International July/ Aug 2002:15*

Reiss, Susan M., "Ophthalmology Techniques Get a Boost," *Biophotonic's International, March 2003: 52-5*

Scerra, Chet, "Glaucoma specialists explore effectiveness of laser therapy," *Ophthalmology Times, March 15, 1999: 8,57*

Steinert, R.F., et al, "Cystoid macular edema, *retinal* detachment and glaucoma after Nd:YAG Laser posterior capsulotomy,": *Am J Ophthalmology: 1991: 112-4:373-80*

"Ultrafast laser ablation facilitates microfabrication of scaffolds," *Biophotonic International, May 2005:54-5*

Weinreb, Robert N., MD, "Laser Therapy,:" Focus on Glaucoma, newsletter, XVII:1:2000:4-6

MEDICATION

Abelson, Mark B. MD, "The 3 Myths of Topical Adrenergic Agents," *Review of Ophthalmology; May,1997, 114-15*

Sang, A, et al, "Long term use of latanoprost on *intraocular pressure* in normal tension glaucoma, *Br J Ophthalmology, 2004:88:63034*

Anwaruddin, Raana, MD et al, "Effect of Preservative on the Ocular Surface in Chronic Glaucoma Therapy," *Study, University of Arizona, Department of Ophthalmology, Tucson, AZ*

"Breathing Problems in Older Adults Using Beta-Blocking Eye Drops for Glaucoma:" *Worst Pills Best Pilla:9:2 :Feb. 2003:15*

"Cancer Drug May Save Sight of People With Macular Degeneration" *news release, 32, 2005 "Avastin Blocks Protein That Causes Abnormal Blood Vessels,"*

Diggory, Paul, & Franks, Wendy, "Medical Treatment of Glaucoma—A reappraisal of the risks," Department of Elderly Medicine & The Glaucoma *Unit,* Mayday & Moorfields Eye Hospital, London

Fackelmann, Kathleen, "Blocking nitric oxide protects eyes from glaucoma", *USA Today, 8/17/1999*

"Glaucoma Medications," *Review of Ophthalmology, May, 1997:41-2*

'Glaucoma Medications," *Supplement to Review of Ophthalmology, May 15, 2002;1-14*

Groves, Nancy, "Transscleral drug delivery system under development," *Ophthalmology Times, 8/12003:24*

Grunwald, Juan E., MD, et al, "Acute Effects of Sildenafil Citrate (Viagra) on *Intraocular pressure* in Open-angle Glaucoma," *American Journal of Ophthalmology,:132:8:872-4*

IBID, "Effect of Sildenafil Citrate (Viagra) on the Ocular Circulation," *American Journal of Ophthalmology, 131:6:751-5*

IBID, "Effect of isosorbide mononitrate on the human optic nerve and choroidal circulation," *British Journal of Ophthalmology, 1999:93:162-67*

Howlett, Allyn, PhD & Johnson, Jeff, PhD, "Cannabinoids Receptor and Ligands," *Cayman Currents, Winter, 2003:13*

Jou, Diana, et al, "Glaucoma Medications, First, Do No Harm", *Review of Ophthalmology,:June,1998:84-90*

Kountouras A, Jannis, MD et al, "Eradication of Helicobacter pylori May be Beneficial in the Management of Chronic Open-Angle Glaucoma," *Arch Intern Med:162: June 10,2001:1237-1242*

Kurtz, S. and Shemesh, G., "The efficacy and safety of once-daily versus once-weekly latanoprost treat for increased *intraocular pressure,* "*J Occl Parmacol Ther, 2004:20:4:321-27*

Lauerman, John F., "Marijuana? A maligned drug edges toward the mainstream," *Harvard Magazine,Mar/Apr 2001:26-7*

Lee, A.G., et al, "Presumed 'sulfur allergy' in patients with intracranial hypertension treated with Acetazolamide or furosemide: cross-reactivity, myth or reality," *Am J Ophthalmology, 2004:138:114- 18*

Lee, David A., MD "A Sound Option for Replacement Therapy," *Eyenet Magazine, Feb.,200026-*

Ophthalmology: May, 2001:117:21

Lewis, Thomas L, OD, PhD, "Glaucoma: New methods of drug delivery and new ways to monitor IOP, may be available to your patients one day soon," *Review of Optometry, ARVO Meeting Report, 2003*

Liang, C., et al, "Toxicity of intraocular lidocaine and bupivacaine," *American Journal of Ophthalmology,:125:2: 191-6*

Maxey, Kirk, MD && Johnson, Jeff, PhD, 'no; Recent Developments", *Cayman Currents, #11, Winter 2002*

McGwin, Gerald, Jr., MS, PhD, et al, "Statins and Other Cholesterol-Lowering Medications and the Presence of Glaucoma," *Arch Ophthalmol:122:Junw, 2004*

Memantine for Alzheimer's Disease," *The Medical Letter, #45:11651: 9/15/2003:7304*

Mermer, Cory, "Just say NO! (Nitric Oxide that is), "*The Townsend Letter for Doctors and Patients, December,2000:72-4*

Netland, Peter A., MD, Ph.d, "What's New in Glaucoma—Drugs-Miscellaneous," *Review of Ophthalmology, April, 2004 95*

Novack, Gary D., PhD, et al, "New Glaucoma Medications in the Geriatric Population: Efficacy and Safety, *JAGS, 50:956-962, 2001*

"Ophthalmic Preservatives: Consideration for Long-term Use in Patients with Dry Eye or Glaucoma," *Continuing Medical Education, Review of Ophthalmology, June, 2001: 73-8*

Pollock, Andrew, "In Trial, Drug Aids Vision of Elderly," *The New York Times, May 24, 2005*

"Punctal Occlusion in Normal Eyes Charted," *Amer Journal Ophthalmol 2001:131:339-344 (reported in Review of Ophthalmology, June 2001)*

Reiss, Susan M, "Working to Make a Good Technology Better,:" *Biophotonics International, June 2002: 41-6*

Than P, MS, OD, "New Perspective on Managing Glaucoma," *Optometry Today: April, 1998: 44-7*

Schachat, Andrew P MD, Section Editor: Higginbotham, Eva J. MD, "Initial Treatment for Open-Angle Glaucoma—Medical, Laser, or Surgical? Medication is Treatment of Choice for Chronic Open-Angle Glaucoma: Jampel, Henry J., "Laser Trabeculoplasty if the Treatment of Choice for chronic Open- Angle Glaucoma," *Arch Ophthalmol 116: Feb., 1998: 239-40*

Smit, Barbara A., MD. PhD, "Effects of Viscoelastic Injection into Schlemm's Canal in Primate and Human Eyes," *Ophthalmology 109:4: April, 2002:786-82*

NEUROPROTECTION

Abmad, Iqbal, "Stem Cells: New Opportunities to Treat Eye Diseases," *IOVS Nov. 2001:42:12:2743- 7:*

Brooke, James, "Without Apology, Leaping Ahead in Cloning," *The New York Times, 5/31/2005*

Celia, Frank, "Understanding Apoptosis: The key to Neuroprotection in Glaucoma," *Review of Optometry, Jan. 15, 2005*

Friedlander, Martin, MD, PhD, et al, "Stem Cell Procedure Protects Mice from Degenerative *Retinal* Diseases: May be Promising for People with Similar *Retinal* Diseases, *Journal of Clinical Investigation, Sept .15, 2004*

Gidday, Jeffrey M, PhD, "Protection of *Retinal* Ganglion Cells by Hypotoxic Preconditioning," *Eye to Eye, Newsletter, The Glaucoma Foundation, Spring/Summer,2004.*

Hogan, Hank, 'Saving Sight with Stem Cells," *Biophotonics International, Jan. 2005:22*

IBID "Drug May Block Gene Damage," Biophotonics *International, Inc., Dec. 2004:65*

IBID Dual-color fluorescence labeling of embryonic stem cells," *Biophotonic's International, Aug. 2004:37*

IBID "Tracking gene delivery optically as never before," *Biophotonic's International, 2005:56*

Disorders," *Arch Ophthalmol: 122: April 2004*

IBID "Stem Cell Therapy for Ocular Disorders," *The Glaucoma Foundation's Ninth Scientific Think Tank,: Stem Cells and Glaucoma. 9/2/2004*

Kausik, S, et al, "Neuroprotection in Glaucoma," *J Postgrad Med 2003:49:90-55*

Kessler, Bakalash S., et al, "Antigenic specificity of immunoprotective therapeutic vaccination for glaucoma," *Invest Ophthalmol Vis Sci. 2003 Aug .44:8:3374-81*

Lanza, Robert and Rosenthal, Nadia, "The Stem Cell Challenge," *Scientific American, June 2004: 93-9*

Litinsky, Steven, MD, "The Importance of the Optic Nerve in Glaucoma Management," *Gleams, Newsletter, The Glaucoma Research Foundation:22:1: Sept. 2004*

Lottery, A. J., "Glutamate excitotoxicity in glaucoma: truth or fiction?" *Eye: 2005:19:369-70*

Miller, Neil R., MD, "Optic Nerve Protection, Regeneration,. And Repair in the 21st Century: LVIII Edward Jackson Memorial Lecture," *American Journal of Ophthalmology December 2001:812-17*

Pollock, Andrew, "Method to Turn Off bad Genes Is Set for tests on Human Eyes," *The New York Times, Sept. 14, 2004.*

Prasanna, Ganesh, PhD, "Endotheliopathy, Gliosis, and Glaucoma," *Eye to Eye, Newsletter, The Glaucoma Foundation, Spring/Summer, 2004*

"Presentation Abstracts," *8th Annual Think Tank, July 2021, 2001, The Glaucoma Foundation*

"Regenerating the Optic Nerve," Biophotonic's International, March 2005:10

Scerra, Chet, "Update presented on glaucoma neuroprotection research," *Ophthalmology Times, April 1, 1999:51-4 (Reviewed by Joseph Caprioli, Md, Yvonne M. Buys, MD and Evan Dreyer, MD, PhD.*

Schepens Scientists Regenerate Optic Nerve for the First Time, Boston MA, 2005, news release

Schwartz, M, "Neurodegeneration and neuroprotection in glaucoma: development of a therapeutic neuroprotective vaccine: the Friedenwald lecture, *Invest Ophthalmol Vis Sci: 2003:44:1407-11*

Shaberman, Ben, "Genetics in RP and *Retinal* Degenerative Diseases: Discoveries, Breakthroughs, and Challenges," The Foundation Fighting Blindness, Science and Research: Review articles2004

Shaw, Jonathan, "Stem Cell Science," *Harvard Magazine, July/Aug, 2003:*

Tsai, James C, MD, "A New Era for Glaucoma Neuroprotection?" *Review of Ophthalmology, October 2004:105-9*

Weinreb, Robert N, MD, "Neuroprotection in Glaucoma," Ophthalmology *Times, vol. 32, #9.May 2007*

Young, Patrick, "Glaucoma and Neurodegeneration," *Research to Prevent Blindness, report*

PEDIATRIC GLAUCOMA

Altman, Lawrence, MD, "Staving Off Blindness in the tiniest of Infants," *The New York Times, March 2, 1999*

"Handheld scanning laser ophthalmoscope assessed in children," Biophotonic's International, May 2001: 61

Henriques, M. J., et al, :"Corneal thickness in congenital glaucoma, *Glaucoma: 2004:13:185-88*

Landers, Aaryn, "Young and Under Pressure," *The Newsletter of the Glaucoma Foundation, 12:1, Spring, 2001*

McCormick, MD, "The Phakomatoses," *(Outline presented here relies heavily on Section 6 of the Academy's Basic and Clinical Science Course).*

Walton, David, MD, "Juvenile Glaucoma," 2-10 *http://www.emedicine.com/oph/toppic333.htm*

RETINAL THERAPIES

"A Second AMD Gene Discovered by FFB-Supported Team," *reported in July 22, 2004 New England Journal of Medicine; emailed by Foundation Fighting Blindness, 7/23/2004*

Abelson, Mark B., MD, et al, "AMD: New Therapies, New Mechanisms," *Review of Ophthalmology, June 2004:76-8*

Boas, Gary, "Artificial synapse chip could act as a *retinal* prosthesis," *Biophotonic's International, Sept 2004:23-7*

Hoagland, Tom, Foundation Sponsored Meeting Provides Glimpse of Gene Therapy's Future, *Fighting Blindness News, Newsletter, The Foundation Fighting Blindness, Fall 2002.*

Hogan, Hank, "Laser system helps quantify PDT drug concentrations," *Biophotonics, International, Sept 2004:16*

Klancnik, MD, "New Directions for Treatment of Macular Degeneration," *Living With Glaucoma, Newsletter, The Glaucoma Support and Education Group, 17:1, Nov 2003*

Patterson, Sally B, "Microchip implant tested on retinitis pigmentosa patients," *reported in Archives of Ophthalmology: April, 2004:46069, Biophotonic's International, May, 2004: 23-4*

Paul, Edward L Jr., OD, PhD, "The Treatment of *Retinal* Diseases With Micro Current Stimulation and Nutritional Supplementation," *presented to the International Society for Low-vision Research and Rehabilitation (ISLRR) Goteburg University, Sweden*

Reiss, Susan M., "PDT Is Key to New Eye Treatments," *Biophotonic's International, Sept 2004:38-41*

Regillo, Carl, MD, "What's New in *Retina*," *Review of Ophthalmology, April, 2004: 54-60*

Richman, Elaine A., PhD, "Neurotech Clinical Trial Moves Closer to RP Therapy," *In Focus, Newsletter, The Foundation Fighting Blindness, Spring, 2004*

Weiner, Jon, "USC Ophthalmologists Review Progress of Permanent *Retinal* Implant Study, *News Release, Dec. 2002*

SURGERY

Baerveldt, G. S., "Surgical outcomes utilizing the TRABECTOME in adult open-angle glaucoma— novel surgical device," *presented at American Glaucoma Society Annual Meeting: March 6, 2004 (abstract 19)*

Blecher, Mark H. MD "What's New in Cataract," *Review of Ophthalmology, April, 2004:44-9*

Brown, R.H., et al, "New Glaucoma Drainage Implant Progresses to Phase III," Glaucoma device under a scleral flap in high-risk cases, *paper, American Academy of Ophthalmology Annual Meeting, April 36, 2004: #1057*

"Cataract Development Linked to Lead Exposure at Levels Commonly Experienced by U.S. Men," *Vitamin Research News: 191, Feb. 2005*

Charters, Linda, "Therapeutic statins not associated with cataract formation," *Ophthalmology Times," May 1, 2002:27:9:1-2*

Faulkner, Wade, MD, "Should Viscoanalostomy Be the New Standard of Care?" *Review of Ophthalmology, June, 1999 (Discussion)*

Fischer, Anne I, "Eye surgery outcome affected by environment," *Biophotonics International, June 2004 (reported in the Journal of Cataract and Refractive Surgery, April, 2004, 794-803.)*

"Glaucoma Valve Implants," *GLEAMS, newsletter, The Glaucoma the Research Foundaiton, #18:3:Jan. 2001*

Guttman, Cheryl, "IOL Design mimics optic shape change of natural lens," *Ophthalmology Times, Aug 1, 2003 (Reviewed by John D. Hunkeler, MD & Randall L. Woods, OD*

Johnstibem M.A., "The aqueous outflow system as a mechanical pump: evidence from examination of tissue and aqueous movement in human and non-human primates, *J Glaucoma, :2004:13:421-38*

Khow, P.T, et al, "Surgery for glaucoma in the 21st century," *British Journal of Ophthalmology, 86:710-11, 2002*

Mackool, Richard J., MD, "New Technology Decreases Risks in Cataract Operations," *Living With Glaucoma, Newsletter, The New York Glaucoma Support and Education Group, 17:4, Summer, 2004*

Maloof, Anthony, et al, "Selective and specific targeting of lens epithelial cells during cataract surgery using sealed-capsule irrigation, *"Journal Cataract Refract Surg:29:Aug 29, 2003:8:11566-8*

Noccker, Robert, MD, "No, It Lacks Trabeculectomy's Proven Track Record,"

Review of Ophthalmology, June, 1999 (Discussion

O'Bart, D.P, et al, "A randomized prospective study comparing trabeculectomy with viscocanalostomy w adjunctive antimetabolite usage for management of open-angle glaucoma uncontrolled by medical therapy, *BR J Ophthalmology, 2004: 88:1012-17*

Pablo, L.E., et al, "Contact-topical intracameral Lidocaine versus peribulbar anesthesia in corneal surgery," *J Glaucoma, 2004:13:6:510-15*

Rodriguez-Prats, J.L, et al, "Milling trabeculoplasty for nonpenetrating glaucoma surgery," *PubMed: www.ncbi.nlm.nih.gov/entrez/query.fcgi?cmd=Retrieve&d.*

AquaFlow Holds for Glaucoma Patients," *Review of Ophthalmology," June, 2002:65-71*

IBID, "What Role for Non-=penetrating Filtration Surgery? *Review of Ophthalmology, June, 2001, 47- 50*

Sidoti, Paul, MD, "It's Operation Time," *Living With Glaucoma," Newsletter, The New York Glaucoma Support and Education Group, 18:4: Fall, 2004*

Singh, Kuldev, MD & Greenfield, David S., MD, Program Directors. "Glaucoma 2003, Trials and Tribulations, *presented by The American Academy of Ophthalmology in conjunction with The American Glaucoma Society, Anaheim, Ca.11.15/2003*

Szymanski, A., "*Scleral* free auto-implant plug with mitomycin as limitation of trepanosclerectomy flow in glaucoma filtering surgery," *International Ophthalmology 20:1-3:89-94, 1996-7* Wang, Xiaofei, et al, Oxidative Damage to Human Lens Epithelial Cells in Culture: Estrogen Protection of Mitochondrial potential, ATP, and Cell Viability,
"*Investigative Ophthalmology & Visual Science, May 2003; 44:5:2067-2075*

PART II

LIFE STYLE AND SELF HELP

Abelson, Reed & Brown, Patricia Leigh, "Alternative Medicine is Finding Its Niche in Nation's Hospitals," *The New York Times, April 13, 2002.*

Bakalar, Nicholas, "Sweet and Sour Tones for The Record Books," *The New York Times, March 8, 2005*

Barry, Patricia, "The Real Value of Drugs," *AARP Bulletin, March, 2005:14-15*

Berger, Leslie, A Therapy Gains Ground: Meditation, *The New York Times, Nov. 23, 1999*

Berk, L.S., et al, "Modulation of Neuroimmune Parameters During the Eustress of Humor Associated Mirthful Laughter," *Alter Therapy Health Med, 2001, Mar: 7:2:62-72, 74.6.*

Blumenthal, Ralph, "For Blind Birders, a Contest Becomes 'Name that Tune,'" *The New York Times, April 13, 2004*

Brody, Jane, "A Second Opinion on Sunshine: It can be Good Medicine After All", *The New York Time, June 17, 2003*

Casura, Lilu Giambarba, ʹ "RX for Winter Health: Breathe Green Air "Clean Air Plants and Winter Indoor Air Quality," *The Townsend Letter for Doctors and Patients, 1997:68-74*

Castleman, Michael, "Natural Stress Relief," *Herbs for Health, March/April 2000. 56-61*

Chan, Erin, "Photographers Make Art as AnotherWay of Seeing," *The New York Times, September 29, 2003*

Corsello, Serafina, "Stay Uplifted & Connected" *The Townsend Letter for Doctors and Patients, January, 2000: 98-103*

Davis, Robert J., "Persistence Co-pays," *WebMD the Magazine: April/May 2005* Dean, Ward, "Mitochondria Dysfunction, Nutrition and Aging," *Vitamin Research News, 16:10: 1-8*

Doobinan, Peter, "Get in Touch With Your Inner Strength Through Meditation," *Living With Glaucoma, 17:2:7-9*

Duenwald, Mary, "How Patients Can Use the New Access to Their Medical Records," *The New York Times, May 11, 2004*

Elliot, J.L., et al, "Self-Reported Mobility Performance Among Older Veterans Completing a Blind Rehabilitation Program," *Poster, Association for Research in Vision and Ophthalmology, Poster, Mar 15, 2001*

Epstein, Randi Hutter, "Sifting Through the Online Medical Jumble," *The New York Times, January 28, 2003,*

Fitzgerald, Thomas J., "Step by Step Prompts Puts the Blind on Track", *The New York Times, October 17, 2002*

Friedman, Richard M., MD, "Should a Doctor Fire a Patient?" *The New York Times, Sept. 27, 2005*

Galland, Leo, MD "Drug-Supplement Interactions: A Counter-Offensive", *The Townsend Letter for Doctors and Patients, April, 2005: 50-2*

Goldberg, Ivan, "Thyroid Disease and Glaucoma", *Article written for the Glaucoma Service, Department of Ophthalmology , Sydney Eye Hospital and University of Sydney*

Goode, Erica,"Can an Essay a Day Keep Asthma or Arthritis at Bay?" *The New York Times, April 14, 1999*

Greenman, Catherine, "Books for the Blind Go Digital" *The New York Times, July 12, 2001*

Groopman, Jerome, MD, "The Anatomy of Illness", *Random House Publishing, New York, 2004*

Grossman, Marc & Swartwout, Glen, "Natural Eye Care,"*Keats Publishing, 1999.*

Guthrie, Jane, "Magnets—Not Just for Your Refrigerator Anymore", *The Health Resource, 20:2:1*

Hall, Stephen S., "s Buddhism Good for Your Health?" *The New York Times Magazine, September 14, 2003:46-47,49*

Hattersley, Joseph G. & Treacy, Kevin J., "Overbreathing: Its Effects and What you Can Do About It," *The Townsend Letter for Doctors and Patients, January, 1998,:92-95*

Karmel, Miriam, "Southern Exposure: Buying Drugs in Mexico is Cheap, Hassel-free…and Risky," *AARP, July/August, 2003*

Kitchen, Judy, "Hypochlorhydria: A Review—Part I," *The Townsend Letter for Doctors and Patients, October, 2001:96-60*

Kolatch, Jonathan, "When Shadows Float Before Your Eyes" *The New York Times, January 25, 2005*

Kozak, Sandra Summerfield, *"BreathSounds" Lotus Press, www.lotuspress.com*

Hu, Winnie, "Violent Sounds of Escape from the 71st Floor," *The New York Times, October 7, 2001*

Kruglinski, Susan, "When Vision Goes, the Hallucinations Begin," *The New York Times, September 14, 2004*

Lawrence, Ronald, "Brain-Boosting Nutrients can Help Enhance Visual Health,"*Journal of Longevity, 7:10:39-40*

Levine, Meredith, "Tell the Doctor All Your Problems but Keep it Less Than a Minute," *The New York Times, June 1, 2004*

Lipschitz, I, et al, "Intraocular Telescopic Lens for Patients With Macular Degeneration," *Association for Research in Vision and Ophthalmology, Poster, March 15, 1999*

Martin, Nina, "Multitasking Makes You Sick," *Organic Style, Nov/Dec. 2003: 55-60*

McCullough, Lynda, "Integrative Medicine Goes Mainstream," *Herbs for Health, December 2004, 52:4*

McEwen, Bruce, "The End of Stress-AS We Know It", *Joseph Henry Press, Washington, DC, 2002*

McGwin, G. et al, "Statins and Other Cholesterol Lowering Medications and the Presence of Glaucoma," *Arch Ophtholmol, 2004:122:622-6*

McWilliams, Charles, DAc, Dhom, "A Rational View of Chinese Acupuncture, Massage, and Medical Gymnastics—Part 2," *The Townsend Letter for Doctors and Patients, November, 1997: 69-71*

IBID "A Brief Overview of Immunity," *IBID, May 2001, 102-4*

Ogilby, Peter R., "Digital Infrared Microscopy Reveals Singlet Oxygen," *Biophotonics International: May 2004:20*

O'Neal, John, "Lead's Link to Clouded Vision", *The New York Times, December 14, 2004*

Pollock, Barbara, "The Art of Healing", *Columbia, Fall, 2003*

Raash, T. W., et al, "Low Vision Intervention" Clinical Trial Pilot Study Program, *Poster, Association for Research in Vision and Ophthalmology, March 15, 2001*

Rehm, Donald, "The Truth About Nearsightedness," *The Townsend Letter for Doctors and Patients, Feb/Mar 1999, 112-14*

Rimer, Sara, "Turning to Autobiography for Emotional Growth in Old Age," *The New York Times, Feb. 9, 2000*

Roberts, Josh P., "Red Light Treatment May Prevent Blindness," *Biophotonics International, May, 2003, 115*

Rosenbaum, Michael, MD, "Natural Immune Modulation Therapies for Chronic Fatigue Syndrome," *The Townsend Letter for Doctors and Patients, Aug/Sept. 2003:115-16*

Rubin, Jordan, NMD, CNC, "Attacking the Seven Causes of Inflammation," *The Townsend Letter for Doctors and Patients, Feb/Mar 2003:111-14*

Rubin, G. S., et al, "The Interaction of Vision and Hearing Impairment and Their Impact on Physical Disability in an Older American Population," *Association for Research in Vision and Ophthalmology, Paper, March 15, 2000*

Schaumberg, D.A., et al, "Waist-Hip Ratio (WHR), Body Mass Index and Cataract in Men," *Paper, Association for Research in Vision and Ophthalmology, March 15, 1999*

Schwartz, Jeffrey M. MD, and Begley, Sharon, "The Mind & The Brain", *Regan Books, 2003*

"Sightings", *Spring, 2004, Schepens Eye Research Institute,* general information

Stolberg, Sheryl Gay,"Alternative Care Gains a Foothold," *The New York Times, Jan. 31, 2000*

"Interview with Dr. Bernie Siegel," *Townsend Letter for Doctors and Patients,* Jan. 2006,

Wingfield, Benjamin R., B App Sc (Chiro) and Gorman R. Frank MBVS, DO, FRACO, "Treatment of Severe Glaucomatous Visual Field Deficit by Chiropractic Spinal Manipulative Therapy," *JMPT, :23:6: July/Aug, 2000*

Wren, P.A., et al, "Baseline Quality of life Findings From the Collaborative Initial Glaucoma Treatment Study" (CIGTS) Poster, *Association for Research in Vision and Ophthalmology, March 15, 1998*

Yarkovsky, S., MD, "The Thyroid Gland:, Cures, Fallacies and Fixes," *The Townsend Letter for Doctors and Patients, May, 2001, :84-9*

Zabloski, Elaine, "Medical Students Learn Mind-Body Methods," *The Townsend Letter for Doctors and Patients, Nov. 2004: 83-5*

NUTRITION

Atti, Maria Roberta, "Nutrition, Immunity, and Spiritual Growth", *Roberta Marie Atti, PO Box1258, Maplewood, NJ 07040*

Bradley, Ronald, "Living Foods," *Townsend Letter for Doctors and Patients, October, 2001, pp 68-69* Bradshaw-Black, V. "Unrefined Salt vs. Industrial Grade Sodium Chloride" *Ibid, February/March, 2004, pp 134-137*

Fallon, Sally & Enig, Mary G., "Tragedy and Hope," *The Third International Soy Symposium, Part I,* IBID, *July, 2000, pp 66-81.*

Hattersley, Joseph G., "The Nearest Thing to a Perfect Food," *Ibid, Part I May, 2002, pp 70-73, Part II June, 2002, 86-90.*

Heltman, Robert (Bob) F., "Organic Food Is More Nutritious," *Ibid, November, 1997, pp 12-13*

Johnson, Terri, ND & John Keoni Teta, ND, *"The Healthy Side of Saturated Fats," Ibid, Feb/Mar, 2003, pp 68-70*

Misner, Bill, PhD CSMT, "Does The Growth of Aerobic Bacterial Cells in Organic Plant Foods Reflect the Health Potential of That Food in Human Cells? *Ibid, Aug/Sept, 2004, pp 78-80*

IBID. "Food May Not Provide Sufficient Micronutrients to Avoid Deficiency," *April, 2005, pp 49-51.*

Nick, Gina L, PhD, ND, "Whole Food Protection from Age-Related Cognitive and Neurodegenerative Disorders*", Ibid, July, 2002 144-147*

IBID, "Impact of Glutamine-Rich Food on Immune Function," *April, 2002, pp 148-149*

IBID. "Medicinal Properties of Whole Foods," *April, 2004, pp 131-132*

Sardi, Bill, "They're Taking the Joy Out of Soy," *Ibid, October, 2000, pp 105-108*

Williams, Rose Marie, "Wild Salmon Don't Do Drugs and Other Fish Stories*," Ibid, Feb/Mar, 2003n, 46-48*

Gittleman, Ann Louise, PhD, CNS, "Understanding Salt and Sodium," *Herbs for Health, Mar/Apr, 2003, p 12,*

Giuffreda, L., et al, "Polyunsaturated Fatty Acids Dietary Supplement in Retinitis Pigmentosa Analysis via Visual Evoked Potentials," *Poster Presentation, Association for Vision and Research in Ophthalmology, 3/15 2001*

Hunter, Beatrice Trum, "The Healing Miracles of Coconut Oil*" Health Wise Publications, PO, Box, 25203, Colorado Springs, CO, 80936, USA*

Kang, Jae. H, et al, "Dietary Fat Consumption and Primary Open Angle Glaucoma," *American Journal of Clinical Nutrition, 2004, 79:755-64*

Leigh, Evelyn, "Boost Your Immunity With Tea," *Herbs for Health, June, 2004, pp 14*

Mitchell, P, et al. "Diet and Cataract," *The Blue Mountain Eye Study, Association for Vision and Research in Ophthalmology, Paper Presentation, March 15, 1999.*

SUPPLEMENTS

Batchelder, Tim, "Cannabis Sativa and the Anthropology of Pain," *The Townsend Letter for Doctors and Patients, March, 2004, pp 156-63*

Ibid, "Cannabis and Culture," Ibid, *January, 2000, 50-51*

Bioflavonoids/flavonoids: Health Benefits of Hesperidin*", Acu-Cell Nutrition, http://www.acu- cell/bio.html*

Bone, Kerry, "Ginkgo: Clinical Studies of Novel Applications*", Ibid, October, 2000, p 122*

Bone, Kerry and Morgan, Michele," Herbs and Heavy Metal Detoxification," *The Townsend Letter for Doctors and Patients, January, 2006, pp 51-8*

Chang, Kenneth," Supplements Work to Treat Vision Loss in Elderly," *The New York Times, Oct, 12, 2001*

Chung, Hak Sung, et al, "Ginkgo Biloba Extract Increases Blood Flow Velocity," *Journal of Ocular Pharmacology and Therapeutics, 15:3, 223-39*

Crayhon, Robert, MS, Warned of Pitfalls with Some Multivitamins and Vitamin Wafers,' *The Townsend Letter for Doctors, , October, 2004, p 16*

Ibid,"The Clinical Benefits of Acetyl-L-Carnitine," *The Townsend Letter for Doctors and Patient, Aug/Sept. 2002, p125-6*

Dash, S. K, PhD, "Selection Criteria Probiotic Supplements," *Ibid, Feb/Mar, 2003, 99-201*

Dean, Ward, "Mitochondrial Dysfunction, Nutrition and Aging: The Most Effective Nutrients For Defending Against Age-Related Mitochondrial Decline,"

Ibid, *16:3, 2003, 103-, Vitamin Research News, March, 2002, pp 6-7*

IBID, *"Melatonin: Unique, Potent, Life-Extending Nutrient," Ibid, 18-7, pp1-7*Ibid, "Carnosine: Multipurpose Anti-Aging Nutrient," *Ibid, 18:9, 1-7*

IBID, *Glutathione: Life-Extending "Master Antioxidant"*,

IBID, 18:2 pp1-6

Fox, A, et al, Calcium and Lead Induct Rod Cell Apoptosis By Switching the Mitochondrial Permeability Transition to a High-Conductance State," *Paper Presentation, Association for Research in Vision and Ophthalmology, 3/15/99.*

Gaby, Alan R, MD, "Ginkgo Biloba Extract for Normal Tension Glaucoma," *The Townsend Letter for Doctors and Patients, Aug/Sept. 2003, p 45-6*

IBID, "Quercetin: A Potentially Harmful Flavonoid," *Ibid, May, 1998, pp 102-3*

IBID, "Vitamin A for Dry Eyes," *Ibid, Oct. 1998, p36*

Gissen, Adam & Morgenthaler, Adam, "Riboflavin The Dose That Makes The Poison," *Ibid, June, 2003, p135*

Head, Kathleen, "Natural Therapies for Ocular Disorders Part II: Cataracts and Glaucoma", *http://www.thorne.com/altmedrev/.fulltext/6/2/141.html*

Holick, Michael F., MD, "Vitamin D Deficiency, The Silent Epidemic," Interview," *Nutrition Action Newsletter, October, 1997, pp 3-6*

"How Does Chocolate Measure Up?" *Prevention, Feb., 2003, pp130-33*

Hurley, Dan, "Medical Marijuana on Trial", *New York Times, 3/29/2005*

Harris, A, , et al, "Estrogen Replacement Therapy Improves Oxygen Hemodynamics in Women," *Poster Presentation, Association for Research in Vision and Ophthalmology, 3/15/2001*

IBIS, "The Integrative Body Mind Information System," http "Integrative Medical Arts Introduces Guide to Drug-Herb and Drug-Nutrient Interactions," *IBICmedical.com, The Townsend Letter for Doctors and Patients*

Jampel; Lee M., MD, 'Antioxidants, Zinc and Age-Related Macular Degeneration :Results and Recommendations,' *Research to Prevent Blindness, 2004 (on web), pp 4.*

Khalsa, Karta Purkh Singh, "The Eyes Have It, Herbs for Health," *Aug 2001, 38-42*

Leuing, I.V.F. et at; "Absorption of Zeaxanthin in Human Subjects After Ingestion of Fructus" *Lych, Association for Research in Vision and Ophthalmology, Poster, March 15, 2001*

Liebman, Bonnie, "Antioxidants: No Magic Bullet," *Nutrition Action Newsletter, April, 2002, pp 4-8* "Life Extension, Phosphatidylserine, The Essential Brain Nutrient," *Life Extension, September 2002, 41-44*

Maris,-Perlman, et al, "Relationship of Zinc from Food and Supplements to Age-Related Maculopathy" *Third National Health and Nutrition Examination Survey, (NHANES III), Association for Research in Vision and Ophthalmology, Paper Presentation, 3/15/2000*

Minami, M., et. Al, "Green Tea Inhibited Oxygen-Induced *Retinall* Neovascularization in the Neonatal Rat", *poster presentation, Ibid*

Moss, Jeffrey, DDS, CNS, CN, "A Perspective on Quality Control of Supplement Manufacture, Part I," *The Townsend Letter for Doctors and Patients, Feb/Mar, 1999, pp127-30*

Murray, Michael T, A , "New Breed" of Antioxidant: Alpha-Lipoic Acid," *Healthy Talk, October, 1991* Nick, Gina L, PhD, ND,"The Anti-Infective and Anti-Inflammatory Effects of Glutamine,"*The Townsend Letter for Doctors and Patients, May, 2005, pp 106-11*

Orgianisciak, D.T. et al, "Antioxidants Alter Apoptosis Cell Death in *Retinall* Light Damage," *Poster Presentation, Association for Research in Vision and Ophthalmology, Aug, 3/15, 2001*

Palmberg, Paul, MD, "Chat Highlights, Alternative Glaucoma Treatments" http://www.wills- glaucoma.org/digichat/altchat2_23_00.html.

Rhee, Douglas, J., MD, et al, "Complimentary and Alternative Medicine for Glaucoma," *Survey of Ophthalmology, Vol. 46:1, July/Aug, 2001*

Riddle, Judith Springer, "Can Nutrient Supplements Benefit Ocular Health?" *Review of Ophthalmology, Feb., 2004, pp 57-6*

Ritch, Robert, MD, *Potential Role for Ginkgo Biloba Extract in the Treatment of Glaucoma, Medical Hypotheses, 2000, 54:2, 221-35*

Rubin, Jordan, PhD, NMD, "The Case for Whole Food Nutritional Supplements," *The Townsend Letter for Doctors and Patients, Feb/Mar, 2004, pp 93-6*

Schardt, David, "Are Supplements Safe?" *Nutrition Action Health Letter, Nov., 2003, pp 106\ Schaumberg, Debra, ScD, OD, MPH, "Hormone Replacement Therapy and Dry Eye Syndrome," JAMA, Nov.7, 2001, 286,2114-9*

Snodderly, D. Max, PhD, et al, "Improved Nutrition Could Prevent Vision Loss" *Investigative Ophthalmology & Visual Science, Feb. 1998, Vol. 39:2*

Stough, Con, Ph.D,, "An Examination of the Effects of the Antioxidant Pycnogenol on Cognitive Performance, Ser um Lipid Profile, Endocrinilogical and Oxidative Stress Biomarkers," *Psychopharmacol ,Dec.2008;22(5)553-62*

Taylor, Hugh R, MD, "Supplement Vitamin A and Risk of Cataract and AMD: Results from the ECAT Study," *Association for Research in Vision and Ophthalmology, Minisymposium, March 15, 2001*

Wright, Jonathan V., MD, "Lithium, Part I, Protect and Renew Your Brain," *The Townsend Letter for Doctors and Patients, Feb., 2004, 78-81*

POLLUTANTS AND TOXINS

Berenson, Alex, & Bayot, Jennifer, "Vision Loss is Reported in a few Users of Viagra," *The New York Times, May 28, 2005*

Brudnick, Mark A., PhD,"Acrylamide in Food Supplies: Danger or Just Dander?" *The Townsend Letter for Doctors and Patients, Aug/Sept, 2003, pp 17*

Burros, Marian, "Acrylamide in Food, How Big the Risk?" *The New York Times, July 31, 2002.*Casura,

Lily G.., " Strange Brew; What's Really in Our Water, Bottled and Otherwise," *The Townsend Letter for Doctors and Patients, Aug/Sept, 2002, 170-3*

Bannin, E., et al, "Ocular Toxicity of high-dose Tamoxifen," *Association for Research in Vision and Ophthalmology, Poster, March 15, 1999*

Clapp, Richard, "Dioxin for Dinner" *Nutrition Action Health Newsletter, Oct.,2000, pp 4-7*

Crinnon, Walter J., "Environmental Medicine: Excerpts from Articles on Current Toxicity, Solvents, Pesticides and Heavy Metals," *The Townsend Letter for Doctors and Patients, Jan, 2001, pp 64-72*

Droy-Lefraix, M., "Role of Oxygenated Free Radicals of Light-Induced Apoptosis," *Association for Research arch in Vision and Ophthalmology, Paper, March 15, 1999*

Elliott, W.R., et al, "Oxidative Stress in *Retinal* Photoreceptors after Acute Laser Lesion:2.7 Dichlorodhdrofluoresciendiacetate In The Small Eye," *Association for Research in Vision and Ophthalmology, Poster, March 15, 1999*

Hepsen, Ibrahim F. et al "Defective Visual Field Tests in Chronic Heavy Smokers,"*Acta Ophthamologica, Scandanavia, 2001*

Krishnaiah. S, et al, "Smoking and its Association with Cataract: Results of the Andhrapradesh Eye Disease Study From India,:"*Investigative Ophthalmol Vis Sci., 2005 Jan: 46:1:58-65*

Liebman, Bonnie, "MSG: Safe or Sinister?" *Nutrition Action Newsletter, Dec. 1991, pp4-5*

Marquis, Christopher,"U.S. Seeks 54 Exemptions on Pesticide Ban," *The New York Times, Jan,7, 2003*

Gaby, Alan R., MD, "Is Aspartame Safe?" *The Townsend Letter for Doctors and Patients, May, 200589-90*

Matossian, Mary Kilbourne, "Poisons of the Past: Molds, Epidemics and History," *Yale University Press, 1989*

Mirtchell, Paul, MD, PhD, et al, "Smoking and the 5-Year Incidence of Age-Relat*ed* Maculopathy," *Arch Ophthalmology, : 2002120:1357-1363*

Null, Gary, PhD, "Stop Fluoridation Now. New Research on Fluoride's Brain and Thyroid Toxicity," *The Townsend Letter for Doctors and Patients, April, 2005, 56-60*

PP 10-11

"Pesticides*" EPA's Efforts to Collect and Take Action on Exposure Incidence Data, GAO/RCED-95-163, U.S.General Accounting Office, PO Box 6015, Gaithersburg, MD 20884-6015*

Revkin, Andrew C., "Broad Study Finds Lower Levels of Old Chemicals, but New Trends are Found Worryin*g*," *The New York Times, Feb. 1, 2003*

Roberts, H. J. MD, FACP. "Pseudotumor Cerebri Due to Aspartame Disease,"*The Townsend Letter for Doctors and Patients, June, 2002, p 65-8*

IBID, "Aspartame-Induced Dyspnea and Pulmonary Hypertension," *IBID, Jan. 2003, pp 64-5*

IBID, "Aspartame-Induced Arrhythmias and Sudden Death," *IBID, May, 2004. 121*

"Scorecard," *Chemical Profiles, http://www.scorecsrd.org/chemical-profiles. tcl?html*

Williams, Rose Marie, MA, "Health Risks and Environmental Issues," *The Townsend Letter for Doctors and Patients, Jan. 2001, pp 28-9*

IBID, Dioxin: A Universal Toxin, Part I" ibid, *April, 2001, 158-60* IBID "Pesticide Neurotoxicity", IBID*, July 2002, pp 30-2*

IBID, "Cosmetic Chemical and Safer Alternatives," *ibid, Feb/Mar, 2004, pp 32-4*

IBID, "More on "Inerts"," *ibid, July, 2004, 150-2*

Yanick, Paul Jr., PhD, "Mycotoxicosis: A New Emerging CoFactor in Alzheimer's Environment, and Treatment-resistant Syndromes," *The Townsend Letter for Doctors and Patients, July, 2002, 154-6*

Wertheim, Alfred H., "The Ubiquitous Toxic Flavor-Enhancer Monosodium Glutamate (MSG)," *The Townsend Letter for Doctors and Patients, Aug/Sept 2000 pp 97*

Winkle, R. K., et al, "Weight Lifting With and Without Valsalva and *Intraocular pressure," Association for Research in Vision and Ophthalmology, Poster, March 15, 1997*

Glossary

Accommodation: adjustment of the eye to focus on objects at varying distances

Acetylcholine: neurotransmitter

Acetylcholine: medications that constrict the pupil

Acetylcholinesterase: an enzyme that breaks down acetylcholine to form acetic acid and choline.

Acuity: visual acuity is determined by the smallest object that you are able to see at a specific distance. The Snellen chart is used to measure visual acuity determining what you can see as compared with normal vision at a distance of 20 feet

Acupuncture; a traditional Chinese therapeutic technique using fine needles inserted under the skin at specific sites to stimulate different organs and systems

Adenosine Triphosphate: an energy source in all metaolic reactions

Adinonectin: fat cells.

Adrenergic drug: one of a class of drugs used to control glaucoma by increasing aqueous outflow and decreasing aqueous production

Agonist: In ophthalmology, a term used to describe the action of certain medications.

Aldehyde: Any of a class of highly reactive organic chemical compounds obtained by oxidation of primary alcohols

Amblyopia: "Lazy eye." If not attended to early on will develop into blindness in that eye

Angiogenesis: blood vessel development

Aniridia: congenital absence of all or part of the iris.

Angiogram: A photographic image of blood vessels

Angle: The area in the anterior (front) part of the eye where the *iris* and cornea meet

Anterior chamber: The front portion of the eye that contains the aqueous humor bounded in front by the cornea, behind by the iris and lens

Antigen: a protein marker on the surface of a cell identifying it as self or non-self

Antioxidant: A chemical compound or substance that neutralizes the oxidant substance that causes damage to the tissue

Aphakia: Absence of the eye's natural lens

Applanation: Flattening of the cornea to assess the level of pressure in the eye

Apoptosis: Disintegration of cells; programmed cell death

Aqueous humor: A nutritional fluid produced by the ciliary body that fills the anterior chamber of the eye; also called the aqueous fluid

Argon laser: a type of laser used to treat glaucoma by placing minute burns on the trabecular meshwork, *iris*, *retinal*, and/or abnormal blood vessels in the eye

Benzalkonium (BAK): a detergent preservative

Behcet's syndrome: a disease causing blindness and other physical disorders

Benzododecinium: detergent preservative

Beta-adrenergic blocker: any of a class of drugs that block the stimulating effect of epinephrine. Used to treat glaucoma, these drugs inhibit the secretion of aqueous humor by the ciliary body; also called beta-blockers.

Biochemical marker: any biochemical compound sufficiently altered in a disease to serve as an aid in diagnosis

Bioflavonoid: any of a group of aromatic biological pigments or compounds, widely distributed in higher plants that account for yellow, red, and/or blue pigmentation. Many have antioxidant properties

Bipolar cells: type of neuron--in the eye-retinal cells that connect the rods and cones with the ganglion cells

Blastocyst: a ball of undifferentiated cells formed in first few days of fertilization

Bleb: a reservoir created in a glaucoma filtering operation to aid in the drainage of fluid from the eye **Blepharitis:** inflammation of eyelids involving hair follicles and glands; may be ulcerative or non-ulcerative

Blind spot: the area where the retina, non-sensitive to light, joins with the optic nerve, forming a funnel, and from which the nerve extends to the brain.

Brucellosis: wide spread infectious disease, mostly in cattle, swine and goats, but can affect humans

Calcium-channel blocker: a type of drug used to treat high blood pressure by decreasing total peripheral resistance

Campimetry: a method of detecting defects in the central portion of the visual field

Canal of Schlemm: a ring-shaped network of passages through which aqueous humor drains into the bloodstream

Capsule: the transparent sac attached to the ciliary body that contains the lens

Capsulotomy: an Nd:YAG laser procedure performed to correct capsular clouding after implantation of an intraocular lens a surgical procedure performed

Carbonic anhydrase inhibitor: a chemical compound that suppresses the formation of the enzyme carbonic anhydrase in the eyes, decreasing the formation of aqueous humor

Cataract extraction: removal of deceased intraocular lens

Carotid artery: either of two major arteries in the neck that carry blood to the head

Catabolize: to break down a complex substance into simpler substances

Cataract: opacity of the crystalline lens

Catecholamine: any of a group of natural substances in the body that stimulate the sympathetic nervous system. Among them are epinephrine, norepinephrine, dopamine, and nomethylepinephrine

Chlamydia pneumoneumon: parasitic disease found in animals and humans commonly transmitted sexually

Cholinergic: activated by or capable of liberating acetylcholine

Choroid: the highly vascular tissue layer beneath the *retinal*; provides the blood needed to nourish the retina

Ciliary body: a ring-shaped structure that joins the iris and choroid and which produces aqueous humor

Ciliary body glaucoma: Malignant glaucoma following surgery caused by aqueous humor becoming trapped behind the vitreous

Ciliary muscles: finger-shaped extensions of the ciliary body to which the zonules are attached

Ciliary processes: layers of cells arranged in folds to make up the ciliary body. They are responsible for the production of aqueous fluid

Circadian rhythm: the biological clock

Coccidloldomycosis: an infectious fungal respiratory disease

Collagen: a fibrous protein found in the connective tissue, including skin, bone, **Cartilage** and ligaments There are four types of collagen in the eye.

Cone cells: light-sensitive cells concentrated in the macula

Conjunctiva: the mucous membrane lining the insides of the eyelids and covering the exterior part of the eye

Confocal laser scanning ophthalmoscope: a diagnostic instrument

convergence: The eyes' effort to maintain binocular vision; seeing objects with both eyes simultaneously.

Cornea: clear tissue that makes up the forward central part of the eye, responsible for the majority of the eye's focusing power

Corneadygenisis: abnormal cornea

Corneal edema: a condition in which the cornea swells with water and becomes cloudy

Corneal decompensation: failure of cornea to maintain structure

Corneal endothelium: the innermost layer of the cornea. Only one cell thick, it regenerates rapidly if damaged

Corticosteroid:. a steroid produced by the adrenal cortex; cortisone derivative

Count fingers test: A test of low visual acuity, determined by a person's ability to count fingers presented over two feet away

Cow's eye: a bulbous eye where trapped fluid expands the flexible tissue of an infant's eye

Cup: in ophthalmology, a concave area in the optic disk that represents nonfunctioning retinal cells

Cupping: a term used to describe the appearance of a damaged optic nerve. A measure for evaluating the progression of glaucoma

Cyclocryotherapy: therapeutic destruction of tissue by freezing

Cyclophotocoagulation: the use of laser to therapeutically coagulate part of the ciliary body

Cyclodestruction: a general term for the use of either extreme cold or laser energy to destroy part of the ciliary body

Cystoid macular edema: retinal swelling and cyst formation in the macular area

Cystercicosis: parasitic infection

Descemet's membrane: basement membrane lying between the stroma and the endothelial layer of the cornea

Deoxyribonucleic acid (DNA): a complex nucleic acid that contains the genetic "code" within each living cell.

Diabetic retinopathy: condition associated with diabetes mellitus in which blood vessels proliferate over the retina damaging it..

Digital tenometry: judgment of intraocular pressure by pressing a finger against the eyeball to test its resistance.

Diurnal: happening in the daytime

DNA: deoxyribonucleic acid

Drusen: small pathological growths formed in the retina; may be a sign of macular degeneration.

Dry eye: uncomfortable condition resulting from either by a defect in the composition of the tears or incomplete closure of the eyelids

Edema: body tissues containing an excessive amount of fluid

Elastin fibers: thick yellow connective-tissue fibers

Electrochemical: eonversion of chemicals in the cell into electrical energy

Electroretinography (ERG): a technique for measuring the retina response to light

Electroretinogram: a record of an ERG test

Endogenous: arising from within a cell or organism

Endocapsular: occurring or appearing within the lens capsule

Endogenous endophthalmitis: parasitic infection in the eye; serious

Endothelium: the innermost tissue lining of many structures, including blood vessels and the cornea

Episcleral: overlying the sclera of the eye

Epithelium cells: membranous tissue, usually a single layer of closely placed cells that cover most internal and external surfaces and organs and outer surfaces of the body

ERG: electroretinography

Eukaryote: one of the first organisms to appear on earth; cells contain a distinct membrane-bound nucleus

Exfoliation: a general term for processes whereby flakes of tissue are shed in the eye and in other organs in the body

Extracapsular: occurring or appearing outside the lens capsule

Extracapsular cataract extraction: surgical cataract extraction procedure in which the anterior lens capsule is partially or completely removed

Extracellular: outside the cell

Extraocular muscles: the muscles attached to the outsides of the eyeballs and the insides of the eye socket responsible for moving the eyeball

Eye muscles: muscles are responsible for movement of the eyeball: lateral rectus, superior oblique, superior rectus, inferior oblique, inferior rectus,

FDT: frequency doubling technology for visual field test

Fibrin: fine filaments involved in clot formation

Fibroblast: a connective tissue cell. Fibroblasts form the fibrous tissues of the body, and also proliferate at sites of chronic inflammation

Fibrocytes: a mature fiber forming cell

Filtering operation: a surgical procedure to open a channel through which the aqueous fluid may pass

Fixation: focusing on a target

5-Fu: fluorouracil, an antimetabolite used to stop formation of scar tissue

Floaters: dark specks or lines that appear to float before your eyes, caused by cells or other nontransparent material floating in the vitreous fluid and casting shadows on the retina

Fluorescein angiography: an imaging technique in which the dye fluorescein is injected into a vein and its circulation tracked by x-ray. it can be used to assess circulation in the retina and choroid

Fovea: the area in the center of the macula that provides clear and long-distance vision

Free radical: an atom or group of atoms having at least one unpaired electron, making it highly chemically reactive

Fuch's syndrome: progressive corneal disorder that can lead to blindness

Fundus: the interior of a hollow organ such as the eye

Ganglion: a mass of nerve tissue containing nerve cells that comprise the optic nerve and which are also found in the spinal cord

Gene: the basic unit of heredity

Glutathione peroxidase: a compound synthesized from the amino acids glutamate, cysteine, and glycine, widely distributed in animal and plant tissue. It destroys peroxides and free radicals; is a cofactor of enzymes; and detoxifies harmful compounds

Glutathione Transferase: enzyme transferring from one chemical to another

Glycogen: a carbohydrate, the form of which glucose is stored in the liver

Goldmann visual field: an instrument that uses a kinetic approach to measure the field of vision. **Goniolens:** an optical device used for examining the anterior (front) section of the eye

Gonioscopy: examination of the anterior chamber using a goniolens

Goniotomy: surgical procedure to remove obstructions to allow free flow of aqueous fluid

Granulomatous uveitis: chronic inflammation of the uvea

Haptic: a hook on an intraocular lens implant to hold the implant in place

Histoplasmosis: fungal infection

Humphrey or Octopus visual field: a computerized visual field testing instrument that uses a static approach to measure the field of vision

Hyaloid face: the thin membrane that surrounds the vitreous and interfaces the anterior and posterior sections of the eye; also called the hyaloid membrane

Hyaluronic acid: a component of the vitreous and aqueous fluids

Hyperopia: Refractive error where light falls in front of the retina rather than behind the retina. .

Hydrocephalus: fluid on the brain

Hyperplasia: a non-tumorous increase in the number of cells in an organ or tissue

Hyphema: Collection of red blood cells in the anterior chamber of the eye.

Hypothalamus dysfunction: precocious puberty.

H-pylori (thaliocobactereria pyloria): an infection in the stomach believed by some to affect glaucoma adversely

Hypotony: abnormally low intraocular pressure

Iatrogenic disorder: an adverse mental or physical condition induced by medical treatment

Intracapsular cataract extraction (ICCE): surgical cataract extraction procedure in which the lens is removed

Intraocular lens (IOL): an artificial lens implanted in the eye after surgical removal of a cataractous natural lens to correct refractive error

Intraocular pressure (IOP): in glaucoma, a high intraocular pressure is one in which the patient continues to lose field of vision

In Vivo: within a living organism

In Vitro: outside of living organism.

iridiodygenisis: destruction of the iris

Iridectomy: surgical removal of part of the iris, performed to control intraocular pressure

Iridotomy: creation of a small puncture in the iris; a laser is often used for this **procedure**

Iris: The pigmented vascular ring-shaped structure in the front of the eye that controls the amount of light passing from the pupil to the retina. It is attached at the outer edge to the ciliary body.

Iris root: the portion of the iris that is attached to the ciliary body.

Ischemic optic neuropathy: obstruction of blood flow to the optic nerve

Juxtacanalicular: connective tissue of trabecular meshwork and the inner wall of the Schlemm's Canal

Keratic: pertaining to the cornea.

Kerotocyte: a corneal cell

Krukenberg's Spindle: symptom associated with Pigmentary Dispersion Syndrome.

Lacrimal apparatus: the system that produces tears and allows them to drain from the eye. It includes the lacrimal glands, the puncta (the opening inside each upper and lower lid), the lacrimal sac, and the tubes and ducts that drain tears into the nasal passages.

Laser: a device that uses a concentrated beam of light to cut or burn objects, including tissue. Lasers are used for a number of procedures to treat glaucomatous conditions. The word is an acronym for light amplification by stimulated emission of radiation.

LASIK: a corneal operation to correct refraction for either the near-or-far-sighted

Lateral Geniculate Nucleus (Body): Upper end of the brain stem where optic track fibers connect.

Lenticular: like a lens; usually refers to the crystalline lens of the eye

Leptin: fat cell

Lupus erythematosus: chronic rashes

Leukotrienes: a group of arachidonic acid metabolites that function as mediators of inflammation

Lyme disease: an infection transmitted by a tick that causes arthritis and other physical problems

Lysozyme: an enzyme that occurs naturally in tears and is capable of destroying some bacteria, thereby acting as a mild antiseptic

Macrophage: a type of white blood cell that removes debris, dead tissue, and foreign substances from tissue

Macrocephaly: abnormal enlargement of the head

Macular: a small yellowish area of the retina where rods and cones are most densely packed. The macula is responsible for fixation.

Magnetic resonance imaging (MRI): computerized scanning using a strong magnetic field; often used in diagnosis of nerve fiber disorders

Magno cells: specialized cells in the retina defining objects

Malignant glaucoma: a condition in which the ciliary body rotates and blocks off the flow of aqueous fluid most likely to occur as a complication of filtration or cataract-removal surgery.

Melatonin: hormone produced by the pineal gland involved in the sleep cycle

Meninges: Membranes surrounding the brain.

Metabolic: physical or chemical change; breaking down

Micropolysaccarides: lots of tiny sugar molecules.

Microcephaly: abnormally small head and brain

Miosis: constriction of a pupil

Mitomycin C: an antimetabolite used to prevent scarring of tissue

MRI: see Magnetic resonance imaging

Mutlifactorial: more than one factor involved

Mydriasis: dilation of the pupil

Myopia: refractive error causing nearsightedness

Myelin: protective sheathe on nerves

N-acytl-cysteine: an amino acid supplement

Nanophthalmos: abnormally small eyeballs

Nanotechnology: science and technology of building electronic circuits and devices from single atoms and molecules.

Narrow-angle glaucoma: glaucoma characterized by a buildup of aqueous fluid in the anterior chamber resulting from closure of the angle. It can be a result of the structure of the eye (shallow angle) and/or other ocular bodies inserting into the angle.

Neovascular glaucoma, neovascularization: glaucoma associated with the abnormal formation of new blood vessels

Nephritis: inflammation of kidney

Nerve fiber layer: the layer of tissue in which retina nerve cells converge to form the optic nerve

Neurotransmitter: a substance used to transmit signals from one nerve cell to another.

Nocturnal: occurring in the nighttime

Occipital lobe. the rear part of the brain; responsible for visual perception

Octopus visual field. see Humphrey or Octopus visual field

Open-angle glaucoma. glaucoma in which the angle is open, but the outflow of fluid is otherwise impaired resulting in a buildup of aqueous fluid in the anterior chamber

Ophthalmologist: a medical doctor who specializes in the treatment of eye diseases

Ophthalmoscope::an instrument to examine the back of the eye

Optic nerve:. a bundle of nerve fibers connecting the retina to the visual cortex of the brain.

Optic neuropathy: degeneration of the optic nerve

Opsin: protein portion of the rhodopsin molecule

Optical coherence tomography: a class of instruments used in diagnosis.

Oxidation: a chemical reaction in which an oxygen molecule encounters another substance and snaps up or sheds one of its electrons to combine with that substance

Pachymetry: measurement of corneal thickness

Pallor: unnatural paleness; in ophthalmology, it is a term used to refer to paleness of the optic nerve head, which may indicate lack of blood flow

PAM: see potential acuity meter

Parasympathetic nervous system: part of the autonomic (involuntary) nervous system controlled by the neurotransmitter acetylcholine

Parvo cells: a specialized group of cells that discriminate features of the object and which are found in the retina.

PEDF: pigment epithelial derived factor

Periocular injection: injection into the eyeball

Phakomatoses diseases: group of congenital diseases probably of hereditary origin

Phacoemulsification: part of a cataract removal procedure in which ultrasound vibrations are used to liquefy the diseased lens, which is then extracted through a tiny incision

Phagocyte: a scavenger cell that engulfs and absorbs waste matter and invading microorganisms in the body

Photocoagulation: condensation of protein material by laser beam; in ophthalmology, it is used primarily to treat retinal detachment, destroy abnormal retinal blood vessels, and destroy part of the ciliary body.

Photodynamic therapy: used primarily as a therapy for macular degeneration involving the combined use of a drug and light stimulation

Photon: the smallest unit of light energy; sometimes described as a particle or quantum

Phthisis bulbi: shrinkage of a damaged or diseased eyeball

Pigment: organic coloring matter

Pigmentary-dispersion glaucoma: glaucoma associated with the flaking off of pigment from the iris; the pigment disperses into the anterior chamber and causes blockage of aqueous flow

Plateau iris: a configuration of the iris that may result in blockage of the trabecular meshwork

Pneumotonometer: a tonometer that uses a puff of air to measure intraocular pressure.

POAG: see Primary open-angle glaucoma.

Polygenic: more than one gene

Posterior chamber: the portion of the eye behind the iris containing the crystalline lens and vitreous humor

Potential acuity meter (PAM): a device used to measure potential visual acuity in eyes with cataracts

Prelaminar layer: the layer of tissue where the nerve fibers converge to take a 90-degree turn to form the optic nerve

Primary open-angle glaucoma: the angle where the cornea and iris meet is open, but other factors are responsible for the glaucoma condition.

Prostaglandin: any of a group of body chemicals synthesized from fatty acids and serving as mediators of many physiologic processes

Pseudoexfoliation syndrome: a condition in which white flakes appear on the tissues and structures of the eye and clog the outflow passages

Ptosis: drooping of the upper eyelid

Pupillary block: blockage of normal aqueous flow through the pupil from the back to the front of the eye

Raynaud's disease: a peripheral vascular disorder

Resisten: fat cells

Retina. the innermost layer of the eye comprised of light-sensitive tissue

Retinal detachment: Complete or partial separation of the retina from the choroid.

Retinol: the form of vitamin A used by the body and which is stored in the liver--needed by the rod and cone cells

Rheumatoid arthritis: a connective tissue disease producing pain and inflammation of the joints; it is also associated with thinning of the sclera, red and dry eyes, and juvenile glaucoma

Riboflavin: vitamin B2

Rods: light-sensitive cells that primarily serve for night vision

Scanning laser polarimetry: a diagnostic instrument

Sclera: the tough, fibrous, white tissue that forms the outer layer of the eye

Scleral spur: the band of scleral fibers located between Schlemm's canal and the ciliary muscle, which serve in part as anchor for the ciliary muscle

Sclerostomy: surgical creation of a hole in the sclera for the purpose of producing another channel for fluid drainage

Scotoma: an area in the visual field where vision is impaired or absent

Shiatsu: a form of massage based on the principles of acupuncture; instead of needles, pressure of the thumbs and forefingers is used to stimulate specific points on the body

SITA: Swedish interacting threshold algorithm to measure visual field defects

Sjogren's syndrome: thought to be an immune disorder occurring in postmenopausal women causing dry eyes and including arthritis

Slit lamp. an instrument that projects an elongated beam of light on the structures of the anterior segment of the eye, allowing a doctor to view the eye's interior

Snellen chart: the standard chart used to measure visual acuity

Sphincter: A general anatomic term for a circular (ring-shaped) muscle, such as the pupillary sphincter.

Stabilized oxychlora: (complex SOC) oxidative preservative

Stem cell: a cell that has the potential of becoming any type of organ or tissue

Stroma: foundation supporting tissue of an organ.

Superior oblique muscle: the muscle that moves the eyeball outward.

Superior rectus muscle: the muscle that moves the eyeball upward

Superoxide dismutase: an enzyme that produces peroxide that is a free radical which can kill bacteria or damage tissue in some cases

Suture: stitching; the thread used to close an incision following surgery

SWAP: short wave length automated perimetry

Tendon: a strong fibrous band of tissue that attaches muscle to bone

Thromboxane: a vasoconstrictor

Tonometer: an instrument that measures intraocular pressure by assessing the eyeball's resistance to flattening (applanation)

Toxocanasis: parasitic infection

Toxoplasmosis: parasitic infection

Toxoplasmic retinochoroiditis: inflammation of the retina

Trabecular meshwork: the porous structure through which aqueous humor drains, located in the anterior chamber angle where the cornea and iris meet

Trabeculectomy: a surgical procedure in which tissue is removed from the trabecular meshwork to create a new channel for the outflow of aqueous fluid; also known as filtration surgery

Trabectome: minimally invasive glaucoma procedure to improve drainage; may replace **trabeculectomy in some cases**

Trabeculoplasty: a laser procedure creating burns on the trabecular that increases fluid outflow

Ultrasound: the use of high-frequency sound waves for diagnosis and/or treatment.

Uvea: pigmented tissue of the eye that contains the majority of blood vessels. Composed of the choroid, ciliary body, and iris, it is considered a whole system

Uveoscleral pathway: second pathway for discharge of aqueous fluid.

Vascular: the blood vessel system

Vasoconstrictive: tending to constrict blood vessels

VEGF: vascular endothelial growth factor

Visual cortex: the area of the brain responsible for interpreting visual information located on the occipital lobe, in the back of the brain

Visual evoked potential: analysis of what is seen and interpreted by the brain

Visual field: the entire field of vision; most often referred to as a test of the visual field to determine extent of glaucoma damage

Vitreous body: located in the back of eye, this gel filled body is partly responsible for the eye's rigidity

Vitreous humor: the transparent gelatinous mass that fills back of the eye

Whipple's disease: rare disease characterized among other symptoms of inability to absorb nutrients

Zonular fibers. tiny ligaments that attach the edge of the lens capsule to the ciliary body.

Zonule: a zonular fiber.

Glaucoma Patient Support Groups

The following organizations are all affiliated with World Glaucoma Patient Association (WGPA). This is an international group of patients and professionals dedicated to promote patient awareness, empowerment, research and support.

ANTIGUA/WEST INDIES
Support Glaucoma-Antigua/
Milburn House, Old Parham Rd,
St. John's , Antigua & Barbuda
Tel: (268) 462-1513,
Fax (268) 462-5622
E;mail:jilliab@gmail.com
Dr. Jillia Bird, Optometrist
Meets once a month

AUSTRALIA
Contact: Beverly Lindsell
Supporting Physician: Dr. Ivan Goldberg
Glaucoma Australia National Association foundation
PO Box 429, Crows Nest, New South Wales 1585, Australia
Tel: 02-9906-6640/toll free 1-800-500-880
Fax: 02-9439-8736
E:Mail: glauacom@glacoa.org.au
www.glaucoma.org.au
Newsletter Dues

BRAZIL
Brazilian Patient Association
Contact: Elisabete Fruchi
Rua Botucatu, 822,
Vila Clementino, Sao Paulo, SP, Brazil
Tel: 55-11-5575-2302
E:mail: mailto:abrag@abrag.com.br
http://www.abrag.com.br
Quarterly newsletter

CANADA
Pediatric Glaucoma and Cataract
Family Association
Contact: Michael Atwell
Address: 939 Lawrence Ave E, Suite 667, Don Mills, Ontario M3C 3S7, Canada
Phone: 416-444-4536
E:mail: webmaster@pgcfa.org
http://www.pgcfa.org
Parents and professionals dealing with daily challenges of pediatric glaucoma and cataract. PGCFA--registered charitable organization.

CHINA
Glaucoma Patient Club in PUEC
Contact: Chun Zhang, MD,
PhD Peking University Eye
Center, Third Hospital of Peking
University Beijing, 100083, China
E;mail: zha ngcl@yahoo.com

DENMARK
Dansk Glaucom Forenin
Contact: Anders Christensen
Supporting Physician:
Dr. John Thygesen
Skovbakken 70, DK
3520 Farum, Denmark
Tel. DK 70200393
E-mail:post@glaucoma.dk
4-5 meetings per year
Dues: DKr 150 = USD 25
Newsletter: in Danish

FRANCE
Association France Glaucome
(AFG)
Contact: Didier Lambert, President
Supporting Physician: Dr. Yves
Lachkar
Foundation hospital St. Joseph,
185 rue Raymond Losserand,
75674 Paris cedex 14, France
Tel: 0800 505 501
E-mail: afglaucoma@wanadoo.fr
www.franceglaucome.fr.st
Meets once a month.
Speakers and Group discussions.
Dues: 30 Euros, Newsletter

GERMANY
Initiativkreis zur
Glaukomfrüherkennung
Contact: Dr. R. Gerste,
Generalsekretar
Supporting Physician: Dr.R.Gerste
1718, 82102, Germering (Germany)
E;mail: rdgerste@aol.com
In existence 13-14 years;
very active. Main goal to raise
awareness of glaucoma in
Germany, Switzerland and Austria.

GHANA
Glaucoma Association of Ghana
(GAG)
Contact: Harrison Kofi Abutiate
PO Box CT 2584,
Cantonments, Accra, Ghana
Tel: 0223 21 761502
E:mail: Harrison@africaonline.
com.gh
Voluntary association open to
anybody with or without glaucoma.

ISRAEL
Israel Glaucoma Patient
Support Group (IGPSG)
Contact: Dan D. Gaton, MD
Chairman, The Israel Glaucoma
Society
Self-Help monthly Meeting
19 Sokolov St. Tel Aviv 02485
Tel: 972 3 6850143 Fax: 972 3
6050143
E-mail: gaton@post.tau.ac.il

HONG KONG
Hong Kong Glaucoma Patients' Association Contact: Mr. Liu Kaishing
Supporting Physician: Dr. Hui Siuping
HK Kornhill Centre, G/F., Block 6, Kornhill Garden, 1120 King's Road, Quarry Bay, Hong Kong
Tel: 00 852-2573 7788
Fax: 00 852-35733535
E;mail: hkgpa@sinatown.com
Dues: quarterly Newsletter:

JAPAN
Glaucoma Friend Netwo
Contact: Mr. Yasuhide Noda
Supporting Physician:
Dr.Yoshiaki Kitazawa
Claire Ropongi 1101
Roppongi 2-2-7, Minato-Ku, Tokyo 1-6-0032 Japan
Tel: 81 3-3585-3433
Fax: 81 3 3568 2230
E-mail: info@gfnet.gr.jp
Newsletter

LITHUANIA
Lithuania Support Glaucoma Foundation
Contact: Saulius Galgaukas
Vilnius Zemynos 19-14 Lithuania
Tel: 370 85 2471637
Fax: 370 85 2490644
E:mail: saulius.galgaukas@santa.it

NEPAL
Glaucoma Support Group Nepal (GSGN
Contact: Dr. Suman S. Thapa, MD or Ms Yogi Gurung

Supporting Physician:
Dr. Suman S. Thapa
Tilganga Eye Center, P.O. Box 561 Kathmandu 561, Nepal
Tel: 977-1-5524927 Fax: 977-01-`4474937
E-mail: yogigurung_@yahoo.com
www.tilganga.org Newsletter:

NETHERLANDS
Glaucoom Vereniging
Address: Rijnsburgerweg 159 2334 BP Leiden, The Netherlands
Phone: +31 71 5174242
Fax:**+31 71 5175835**
Email:informatie@ glaucoomvereniging.nl
Webpage: http:www. glaucomeniging.nl
Quarterly Newsletter:
"Oogappel" – apple of the eye.

NEW ZEALAND
Glaucoma New Zealand
Contact: Heather Highland Dept of Ophthalmology,University of Auckland PB 92019, Auckland, NZ
Tel: 09 373 8779 Fax: 09 373 7947
E;mail: admin@glaucoma.org.nz
www.glaucoma.org.nz
quarterly newsletterlocal public meetings around the country.

NIGERIA
Contact: Austen Uwosomah (Secretary)
Glaucoma Care Foundation:

Multipurpose Cooperative Society (GCFMCS)Federal Housing Estate Street 8, Flat 15, Ikpoba Hill, Benin City, 300221 Edo State. Nigeria Tel: 234083052311 E;mail glaucomacare_foundation@yahoo.com glaucoma-cooperative.ng@hotmail.com Area of operation covers towns and local government areas in Edo State region and such other areas, Meets once a month

NORWAY
Norsk Glaukomforening
Contact Per Kaland
Supporting physician: Jan Erik Jakobsen, MD, Ophthalmologist Vestbyv. 23h, Oslo, 976, Norway Tel:(47) 22 25 48 46
E:mail: pergru@aolonline.no
www.glaucom.org
Newsletter

SINGAPORE
Glaucoma Society Singapore
Contact: John S.Y. Tan ,
Annie Leow (annyleow@yahoo.com Supporting Physician: A/Prof Paul Chew,
Dr. Jovina See 150 Orchard Rd #07-14, Orchard Plaza, Singapore 238841, Tel:065 6733 2922
Internet mailing list
Fax: 065 62353 3530
E:mail: cipremie@signet.com.sg
www.glaucoma-singapore.org
Dues   Newsletter

UNITED KINGDOM
International Glaucoma Association
Contact: David Wright
Woodcote House
15 Highpoint Business Village,Hempstead
Ashford Kent TN24 8DH
United Kingdom Tel:01233 648170
Fax:01233 648178
E-mail: dwright@iga.org.uk
www.glaucoma-association.com

USA

CALIFORNIA
Jules Stein Eye Institute
Glaucoma support
group Contact Yvonne
Goto,Supporting Physician: Joseph Caprioli, MD 100 Stein Plaza, UCLA, Los Angeles, CA 90095, USA Tel: 310-206-3063   E:mail: goto@jsei.ucla.edu

Marin County Glaucoma Support Group Contact: Jennifer Rulon, Glaucoma Research Foundation Redwoods Retirement Center, 40 Camino Alta, Mill Valley, CA 94941, USA
Tel:800-826-6693 or 415-986-3162
E;mail: info@glaucoma.org
Camino Medical Group Contact: Chris Saleh, Moderator/President or Sally Twestens,Health Education Department, Supporting Physician: Dr. Elizabeth Snedden Camino Medical Group, Urgent Care Ctr. Conf.Rm 2,,201 Old San Francisco Road, Sunnyvale, CA 94086 USA Tel:408-8479/408-523-3221E-mail:

Chris Saleh chris.saleh@sun.
com or Sally Twestens twestens@
caminomedical.org
www.caminomedical.org   Meets
the 4th Wed of every month except
November.

ILLINOIS
Contact: Dawn Bach
ILLINOIS EYE CENTER 5401
N. Knoxville, Basement classroom,
Peoria, IL 61614, USA
Tel: 309-682-9641 x 402
E;mail: dbach@illinoiseyecenter.
com
:www.illinoiseyecenter.com

NEW YORK
`THE GLAUCOMA
FOUNDATION
80 Maiden Lane
New York, NY. 10038, USA
212-285-0080
www.glaucomafoundation.org

SUPPORT GROUP CHAPTERS
New York Chapter
New York Eye and Ear Infirmary
310 East 14 St.
New York, NY 10003
Contact: Edith S. Marks
`& Janice Ewenstein
E-mail:edithmarks@nyc.rr.com
Supporting Physician:
Robert Ritch, MD
Dues Quarterly Newsletter

Chicago Chapter
Contact: Lianne Seyk
Tel: 815-341-1989

E:mail: Chicago@
glaucomafoundation.org

Long Island Chapter
Nassau/Suffolk Counties
Contact: Diana Falk
E-Mail: dfalk@optonline.net

New England Chapter
Serving Vermont, New Hampshire,
Maine, Massachusetts,
Rhode Island, Connecticut
Adult and Pediatric Groups
Contact: Catherine Duffek
Box 162 Boston, MA 02133
Tel: 617-797-6976
E-mail: cduffek@
glaucomafoundation.org

UVEITIS SUPPORT GROUP
New York Eye and Ear Infirmary
310 E. 14 St.
New York, NY 10003
212-979-4390

**Macular Degeneration Support
Group**
New York Eye and Ear Infirmary
310 E. 14 St.
New York, NY l000w
212-979-4390

MASSACHUSETTS
Uveitis/OID Support Group
Physical meeting place
Massachusetts Eye and Ear
Infirmary
243 Charles Street, Boston, MA
www.uveitis.org/patient/support/
newsletters/default.html
Maintains 3 web-based resources;

meetings on site 6x year
Supporting Physician: C. Stephen
Foster, MD

OREGON
Devers Low Vision Support Group
1040 NW 22nd Ave. #168,
Portland, OR 97229, USA
Contact: Linda Grana, Low Vision
Outreach Coordinator
Tel:: 503-413-8499
E:mail: lgrana@ihs.org

INTERNET GROUPS
Glaucoma and Ocular Hypertension Patient Advocacy Center (GLOHPAC)
Web based message board
Contact: Hank
Address: USA
Email: GLOHPAC@aol.com
www.glohpac.proboards?com

YOUNG PATIENTS UNDER PRESSURE
Internet mailing list
Contact: Aaryn Landers Lamb
or Scott Christensen
The Glaucoma Foundation
80 Maiden Lane, New York, NY
10038
E ;mail: yup@aarynandty.co
http://health.groups.yahoo.com/ group/
www.glaucomafoundation.org/info.
php?i-40

ADULT PATIENTS UNDER PRESSURE
www.health.groups.yahoo.com/
group/apup

HOSPITAL GLAUCOMA SERVICES
Virtual Patient Support Group
of the **Glaucoma Service Foundation**
Wills Eye Hospital
Supporting Physician:
Richard Wilson, MD
Provides support, information
on diagnostic testing, treatments,
medications, and research;
its support group component
includes a live online chat room
on Summarized as "chat highlights"
available to site visitors.
www.wills-glaucoma.org
Link to the Bionic Eye, (see below)

BIONIC EYE
Web based Internet chat and a
message board **Contact: Vivian Werner, Webmaster/Chat master Wills Eye Hospital, 840 Walnut St., #1130, Philadelphia, PA 19107-5598**
Mon – Fri 9-5 pm) Tel: 215-928-
3190
Fax: 215-928-3194
E ;mail: VW@scanmaster.org
www.willsglaucoma.org

GLAUCOMA MAILING LIST
Internet mailing list
Contact: Sherry Holthe
Supporting Physician: Dr. Robert
Ritch, MD **E-mail:** glaucoma-
owner@yahoogroups.com
http://groups.yahoo.com/group/
glaucoma/
A moderated internet mailing
list for Glaucoma patients and
medical professionals to support
patients.

DIABETES
Internet mailing list
Contact: Bernie Holt
E;mail: bigdogbernie@yahoo.com
http://health.groups.yahoo.
com/group/Glaucoma
**Diabetessupport@yahoogroups.
com**

GLAUCOMA SOCIETIES
The following are some of the
professional glaucoma societies.
Contact them for further
information about glaucoma
services they can recommend

THE INTERNATIONAL
GLAUCOMA ASSOCIATION
(IGA) *WWW.IGA.ORG.UK* A
registered charity offering advice
and support; campaigns for
improved glaucoma services; aims
to increase public awareness; funds
considerable clinical research.
Discussion board available. Website
provides accessible, high-quality
information on support services
to glaucoma patients, the general

public and professionals working
in ophthalmic and ophthalmologic
fields.

WORLD GLAUCOMA
PATIENT ORGANIZATION
(WGPO)
MISSION STATEMENT AND
GOALS: A liaison group facilitating
a flow of information from patient to
professional organizationsincluding
AGIS, Association of International
Glaucoma Societies, an international,
independent, impartial, ethical, global
organization for glaucoma science
and care. **WGPA** promotes patient
support--information, guidance,
education, and empowerment. Also
identifies glaucoma specialists for
patients who reside in outlying areas.
Disseminates information through:
--Chat rooms, interactive glaucoma
groups and the WGPA website
http://wgpa.org.--Support Group
meetings in hospitals, churches,
clubs or other physical spaces--Print
Media: Informative brochures, and
recommends written material **WGPA**
also assists in formation of support
groups to form and promote patient
advocacy, including disability rights
as defined by the Americans with
Disabilities Act (ADA) and the
British Disability Act and fine tune
these methods to meet the needs of
glaucoma patients, especially those
with low vision problems.--Patient
Advocacy also involves funding for
affordable medications, medical
research, neuroprotection options,
quality of life issues, and research

into whether conditions such as systemic high blood pressure, diabetes mellitus, thyroid disease, cancer, and other medical and environmental issues affect glaucoma. **WGPO** also identifies and helps groups promote services for those patients who have lost considerable sight or become blind because of glaucoma.

American Glaucoma Society
North American Glaucoma Society'
PO Box 45161
415-561-8587
Fax: 415-561-8531
E-mail ags@aao.org

Asian-Oceanic Glaucoma Society
National Taiwan University
Hospital
7 Chung-Shan South Road
Tapei100, Taiwan
886-2-2312-3455 x5186
Fax:886-2-2341-2634
Email:portying@ntu.edu.tw

Australia-New Zealand Glaucoma Interest Group
394 Albert St.,.East Melbourne,
Victoria 3004
Australia 613-9 662 1441
Fax: 613 9662-2340
E-mail amybrooks@bigpond.com

Canadian Glaucoma Society
Totonto Western Hospital
399 Balhurst St. ECW 7-042
Toronto, ON MST 258
E-mail:y.buys@utoronto.ca

Chinese Glaucoma Society
Zhongsham Ophthalmic Center
of Sun Yat-sen University
Guangzhou 510060
E-mail max-yu@tom.com

European Glaucoma Society
Western Eye Hospital
Marylebone Rd., London NW1
5YE
44-171-866 3258 Fax: 44-171-886 3259
E:mail: Cmigdal@compuserve.com
www.eugs.org

Glaucoma Society of India
91-048-2825 8267/2360 8262
Fax: 044-2825 4180
E:mail:drbs@snmail,org

Glaucoma Research Society
Bascom Palmer Eye Institute
900 NW 17 St.
Miami, FL 33136
305-326-6389
Fax: 305-326-6478
E:mail: rparris@med.miami.edu

International Society for Glaucoma Surgery
Jules Gonin Eye Hospital
Av. De France 15 Lausanne, 1004
Bron, Switzerland
41-21 626 8224 Fax; 41-21 626 6240
E:mail shaarwy@glaucoma-surgery.com
www.glaucoma-surgery.oom

Japanese Glaucoma Society
501 Asai Bldg 7-2-4 Honjo
Bunkyo-kuTokyo 113-0033
81-3-3811-0309
Fax:81-3-3811-0670 E:mail
kondo@g-jimukyoko.jp

Latin American Glaucoma Society
Av S Gaulter
91 Pinheiros Code 45455-000
Sao Paulo, Brazil
55-11-3022-5172
Fax: 55-11-3022-4300
E-mail: wilmalb@uol.co.br

Optometric Glaucoma Society
51 Hacienda Drive
Dublin, CA 94568 USA
1-925-587-4180
Fax: 925-557-4182
E:mail m.patella@mediloc.zeiss.com
www.optometricglaucomasociety.
org

Pan American Glaucoma Society
Av Sante Blanco 2073 Lo
Santiago, Chile
22-15-3537 Fax: 22-17-1522
E:mail:eumadecu@ctemundo.net
www.panglaucoma.net

**Pan Arab African Glaucoma
Society**
3A El Gamat Dowal Al Arabia
SphiniXSq
Cairo 11553, Egypt
+20 (2) 34777400-3477800-
2623990F
Fax: 20 (2) 3472090=2623995
E;mail:magdihelal@hotmail.com

South African Glaucoma Society
P. Gous
PO Box 56184 Arcadia,
0007 Pretoria, South Africa
Arcadia, 0007 Pretoria,
South Africa
+27-12-343 8035 Fax: +27-12-343
8038
E;mail: pgous@global.co.za
http:www.eyenet.co.za/glaucoma

**South East Asian Glaucoma
Interest Group**
Seng Kheong Fang
The Tun Hussein Onn National Eye
Hospital
Lorong Utara B46200
Petaling Jaya, Selangor Malaysia
603-79561511 Fax:603-79576128
Email: skfang@streamyx.com
www.seagig.org

Resources

ORGANIZATIONS—INVOLVED WITH VISION SERVICES

Unless otherwise specified, these agencies provide a variety of services ranging from information and support to rehabilitation services such as training in independent living skills, vocational training, and counseling and support services. Each community provides some services. Check social services to determine availability.

This is a sampling-more can be found on the WEB

American Academy of Ophthalmology
655 Beech Street
P.O. Box 7424
San Francisco, CA 94120
415–561–8500
http://www.aao.org
Provides information materials on glaucoma and co-sponsors the National Eye Care Project for persons over sixty-five who are medically underserved (800–222–EYES
Eye Care America

The American Academy of Optometry
6110 Executive Blvd.

Suite 506
St. Louis, MO 63141
800–365–2219
314–991–4100
Fax: 314–991–4101
www.aoa.org
;provides literature and doctor referral.

American Foundation for the Blind
Suite 300
11 Penn Plaza
New York, NY 10021
212-502-7600
Fax: 212-502-7777
Email: afbinfo@afb.net
Comprehensive coverage of many

issues and services; publishes the *Directory of Services for the Blind and Visually Impaired in the United States and Canada.*

American Macular Degeneration Foundation, P.O. Box 515
Northampton, MA 01061-0515
413-268-766- 888-622-8527
Fax: 413-505-2788
E-mail:amdf@macular.org
Works for prevention, treatment and cure,
provides information and help with macular degeneration

Blinded Veterans Association
477 H Street, NW
Washington, DC 20001-2694
1-800-669-7079 Fax: 202-371-8258
E:mail: bva@bva.org www.bva.org
Chartered by Congress to represent blinded veterans, generally
advocates for rights and rehabilitation

College of Optometrists in Vision Development
215 W. Garfield Rd,.
Suite 210
Aurora, OH 44202
330-995-0718
Fax; 330-995-0710
Non-profit--behavior and developmental vision therapy and vision rehabilitation;
recommends practitioners; provides tnformational literature

Contact Lens Association of Ophthalmologists
2025 Woodlane Drive
St. Paul, MN 55125-2918
8777-501-3937
Fax: 651-731-0410
http://www.eyes.clao.org
Information on contact lenses and list of doctors

Council of Citizens with Low Vision International
1155 15th St. NW Suite 1004
Washington. DC 20005
1-800-733-2258
Regional chapters; offers scholarships to students with low vision; advocates access, educate general public about needs for people with low vision.
Affiliate, American Council of the Blind Information on affiliates at www.cclvi.org.

EARS: Enrichment Audio Resource Services
1202 Lexington Ave.
Ste. 316
New York, NY 10028
212-717-2377
Free audio cassette training for those with low-vision
enhancing indoor mobility

Foundation Fighting Blindness
11425 Cronhill Dr.
Owings Mills, MD 21112
800-683-5555 410-568-0650
E-mail: info@ foundationfightingblindness.org
Information on retinitis pigmentosa, macular degeneration and other retinal diseases, regional offices

The Glaucoma Foundation
80 Maiden Lane, Suite 1208
New York, NY 10038
800-GLAUCOMA (toll-free
worldwide)
212-285-0080
Fax: 651-1888
http://www.glaucomafoundation.
org
Funds research to find a cure for
glaucoma. Publishes a quarterly
newsletter
Eye to Eye; a booklet, *Doctor, I Have
a Question;* and a patient's guide.
Will respond to written or telephone
queries. Sponsors Glaucoma
Support
Groups (see above)

Glaucoma Research Foundation
251 Post Street, Suite 1042
San Francisco, CA 94108
800–826–6693
415–986–316
http://www.glaucoma.org
National, non-profit dedicated to
preserve the sight and independence
of individuals with glaucoma
through research and education, with
the ultimate goal to find a cure. For
over 25 years, GRF has funded cutting
-edge research, provided the latest in
glaucoma education, and organized
support programs and services for
patients living with glaucoma. Free
educational resources to encourage
early detection of glaucoma and the
continuing education of glaucoma
patients.

**National Association for Parents
of the Visually Impaired
(NAPVI)**
PO Box 317 Watertown, MA 02471
800-562-6269 617-972-7441
Fax; 617-972-7441
E:mail: napvi@perkins.org
www.napvi.org
National organization providing
leadership,information, resources and
support for parents to help children
reach their potential. Partnership with
The American Foundation for the
Blind-chapters in states throughout
the US and worldwide.

Guilds for the Blind
www.guildfortheblind.org
Check with your local Catholic
Charities and Jewish Guilds for more
information.

Guide Dogs for the Blind, Inc
350 Los Ranchitos Rd.
San Rafael, CA 94903
415–499–4000
Oregon Site: 32901 SE Kelso Rd.
Boring, OR 97009
503-668-2100'Fax: 503-668-3141
Nonprofit: provides training in the
use, handling, and care of guide dogs,
plus follow-up services, at no charge
to the blind or legally blind.

Guide Dog
The Seeing Eye
10 Washington Valley Rd.
Morristown, NJ 07960-3412
973-539-1425
Fax: 973-539-0922
www.seeingeye.org

International Eye Foundation
10801 Connecticut Avenue
Kensington, MD 20895
240-290-0263
Fax: 240-290-0269
E:mail: ief@iefusa.org
www.iefusa.org
Regional Associations in:Africa,
Bulgaria, Egypt, Guatemala,
Honduras, India, Latin America,
Tanzania

**Helen Keller National Center
for Deaf-Blind Youth and Adults**
141 Middle Neck Road
Sands Point, NY 11050
516-944-8900 Fax: 516-944-7302
E-mail: hkncinfo@hknc.org
www.hknc.org
National organization with
regional centers to meet needs
for social, rehab and ind.living

National Federation of the Blind
1800 Johnson Street
Baltimore, MD 21230
410–659–9314
www.nfb.org
NFB-NEWSLINE 866-504-7300
Strong advocacy group; provides
information services and sells
products for visually handicapped.

Prevent Blindness America
211 West Wacker Drive
Suite 1700 Chicago, IL 60606
800–331–2020
E:mail: info@preventblindness.org
http://www.preventblindness.org
Maintains free center for
information

on a broad range of eye health and
safety topics; funds various research
projects; headquartered in Illinois
with affiliates throughout the
country.

Research to Prevent Blindness
645 Madison Ave.
New York, NY 10022-1010
1-800-621-0026
212-752-4333
Fax: 212-688-6231
E:mail-inforequest@rpbusa.org
Mobilizes financial resources in
support of eye research.

Other

**American Association of
Retired Persons (AARP)**
601 E Street, NW
Washington, DC 20049
800-687-2277
Spanish: 800-627-3350
TTY 202–434–6554
Intnl: 202-434-3525 http://www.
aarp.org
Disability literature on written
request; resource guide, Americans
With Disabilities Act (ADA)
guidelines, Pharmacy Service,
retirement planning, travel guide,
drug safety, effectiveness and costs
www,aarp.org/health/compared
drugs.The *AARP Guide to Pills*:
Membership fee.

**National Institute on Aging
Information Center**
Office of Communications
and Public Liaison

Bldg 31 Rm 5C27
31 Center Drive, Msc 2292
Bethesda, MD 20892
800-222-2225 TTY 980–222–4225
Fax 301–589–3014
E:mail: info@niapublications.org
www.nia.nih.gov/healthinformation/
pulications
Resources for all manner of aging.

Products and Technology

ABLEDATA
8630 Second St.
Silver Spring, MD 20910-3319
800-227-0216 Fax: 301-608-8958
E:mail: abledata.com www.abledata.
com or www.abledata@orcmazcro
National data base on assistive
technology products; databases
for rehab, research,programs
& newsletters; sponsored by
National Institute on Disability and
Rehabilitation Research, Office of
Special Education Services,USA

Alliance for Technology
1304 Southpoint Blvd.
Suite 240 Pettaluma, CA 94954
800=390-2696 800-910-0706
Fax:707-265-2080
www/atnet.org
Email: ATAinfo@ATAaccess.org
California (govt) based organization
to people with disabilities

American Foundation
for the Blind
National Technology Center
11 Penn Plaza New York, NY
10001 800–232–5463 or 212–502–
7600

http://www.afb.org/afb
Adapts, evaluates, manufactures,
& sells special aid devices and
products.

Freedom Scientific
11800 31sst Court North
St. Petersburg, FL 33716,
800–444–4443
Email:info@FreedomScientific.com
http://www.FreedomScientific.com
Sells screen reading software,
developed JAWS.

C-Tech
2 North Williams Street
Pearl River, NY 10965-9998
800–228–7798
Distributor of variety of reading
Machines and systems.
www.lowvisionproducts.com

Independent Living Aids, Inc.
200 Robbins Lane
Jericho, NY 11753
800–537–2118
fax 516–937-3906
E-mail: can-do@
independentlivingaids.com
http/www.independentliving.com
Sells various products; free catalog..

Kurzweil Educational Systems
100 Crosby Drive
Bedford, MA 01750-1402
800–544-8747 USA & Canada
303-631-2829 – all other
www.kurzweilledu.com
Sells reading machines and systems.

L.S&S. Group
145 River Rock Road
Buffalo, NY 14207
1-800-468-4789 Fax: 847-498-1482
716=346-3500
Email: info@lssproducts.com
http://www.products.com
low vision products, catalog.

Lighthouse International
111 East 59th Street
New York, NY 10022
212–821–9200 800–829–0500
Email: jjenkins@lighthouse.org
http:///www.lighthouse.org
Careers Network (online service
for blind) Publishes Self Help Mutual
Aid and Support Groups Guide for
Visually. Impaired
Older People:visions services and
products available in New York City
On-line and free print catalog...

Maddak, Inc.
6 Industrial Road
Pequannock, NJ 07440-1977
800–443–4926
973-628-7600
Fax: 973-305-0841
Email: customerservice@maddax.
com
http://www.maddak.com
Sells various products, free catalog.

Macular Degeneration Support
www.mdsupport.org/resources.html
search engine for eye problems.

Maxi Aids
42 Executive Boulevard
P.O. Box 3209

Farmingdale, NY 11735
800–522–6294 or
631–752–0521
Fax: 631-752-0689
www.maxiaids.com
Sells various products; free catalog

National Federation of the Blind
1800 Johnson Street
Baltimore, MD 21230
410–659–9314
Fax; 410-685-5653
www.nfb.org
International org, 50,000
membership, sells large assortment
of visual aids and appliances.

Optelec-
303 Enterprise Court
Suite D
Vista, CA 92081
800–826-4200
Shoplowvision.com
Reading machines/systems and
low vision aides. NA distributor of
Optelec

TeleSensory
4545 Stockdale Highway
Bakersfield, CA 93309
800–804–8004 (for products for
the visually impaired http://www.
telesensory.com
Mfg plant: Plo 160, Jalan Cyber 2
Senai Industrial Estate
81402 Senai, Johor, Malaysia
(60) 7 598-0985 (60) 7 598-9290
Sells both black-and-white and
color closed-circuit television
systems.

Visuaide
841 Jean-Paul-Vincent Boulevard
Longueuil, Quebec J46 1R3
Canada. 450-463-0120
Sells reading machines/systems,
devices to enhance daily living,
and technology
info@visuaide.com

**U.S.Consumer Product Safety
Commission**
Washington, DC 20207
800–638–2772 (hot line)
Provides information on product
safety.

RECREATION

Art Education for the Blind
160 Mercer Street
New York, NY 10012
212–334–3700
fax 212–334–8714
Through use of tactile information
teaches the visually handicapped to
"see" paintings. Conducts
workshops
and consults with museums,
working
on a twenty-volume art history
textbook for the visually impaired,
Art History Through Touch and
Sound
The Arts, Books, etc.

Hospital Audiences, Inc. (HAI)
548 Broadway
New York, NY 10012
212-575-7663
Fax: 575-7669
Email: hai@hospaud.org

www.hospaud.org
provides access to art
Publishes "Access for All:
A Guide for People With
Disabilities to New York
City Cultural Institutions."
Also has a program for the legally
blind in which a sighted individual
accompanies the person to theatrical
performances and describes the
action to him or her. This is an
expanding program world-wide and
access may be available in your
community.

Media Access Groups

WGBH 125 Western Ave.
Boston, MA 02134
1-800-333-1203
http://www.wgbh.org/dvs
Provides narrated descriptions of
televisionbroadcasts and current
films; concise narration. theater
accessibility in participating theaters.
Click on MOPIX for a theater near
you

The Laboratory of Ornithology
159 Sapsucker Woods Road
Ithaca, NY 13440
607–254–2400
Produces a bird song tutor on
tape that may be purchased
from the Laboratory or borrowed
from National Library Services

**North American Riding
for the Handicapped
Association**
P.O. Box 33150

7475 Dakin St Denver, CO 80233
303–452–1212 www.narha.org
Teaches horseback riding to
the blind and visually handicapped.
Has 460 centers throughout the
U.S. and Canada; will send a list of
centers in your state upon request.

AUDIO BOOKS. TAPES. AND LARGE PRINT

Aurora Ministries/Bible Alliance, Inc.
PO Box 621
Brandentown, FL 34206
941-748-3031
Fax 941-748-2625
E-mail: tapes@aurora.org
www.visionaware/aurora_ministries
Bible Cassette in 46 languages free

Basic Health Publications, Inc.
8200 Boulevard East
North Bergen, NJ 07047
Publishers "user's guides" on many
subjects

Blackstone Audio Books
P0 Box 969
Ashland, OR 97520
www.learnoutloud.com/resources/
publisher
by Blackstoneaudiobooks
Rent or purchase—over 2,000 titles
1-800-729-2665 (USA)

Bookshare
A searchable on-line book
library offering more than
50,000 digitalized books in
partnership with major publishers.

Membership available to those
with a visual disability/physical
or learning disability
www.bookshare.or

Choice Magazine Listening
85 Channels Drive
Port Washington, NY 11050
516–883–8280
Fax; 516-948-6849
E-mail: choicemag@aol.com
www.choicemagazinelistening.org

Blindskills, Inc.
PO Box 5181 Salem, OR 97304-
0181
1-800-860-4224 503-581-0178
Fax: 503-581-0178
Email: blindskl@teleport.com
Non-profit corporation publishing
magazine intended to enhance
quality of life. It covers a wide
range of subject matter on
all aspects of life. Offers free
service for persons unable to read
regular print. Every other month,
subscribers receive 4-track cassettes
containing eight hours of articles,
fiction, and poetry.
Cassettes are playable on Library of
Congress talking book & cassette
player, free of charge. Readings
cover well-known print magazines.

In Touch Networks, Inc.
15 W 65 St.
New York, NY 10022-1202
1-800-284-4422
212-769-6270
E-mail: inmtouchinfo@jgb.org
www.jgb.org/intouch

National Volunteer service allowing visually-impaired to listen to readings of articles from more than 100 news papers & magazines, 24 hours a day.

Library of Congress
National Library Services for the Blind
1291 Taylor Street, NW
Washington, DC 20011
1-800-424-8567
Fax 202-707--0712
http://www.loc.gov/nls
Provides braille and recorded books and magazines for the blind and physically handicapped; talking books, plays, catalogs and bibliography, music scores, and music nstructional materials.
Materials may be accessed directly from the library.
ALSO: **Library of Congress at**
101 Independence Ave.
Washington, D 20540
202-707-5000
General information

Lutheran Braille Workers, Inc.
PO Box 5000
Yucaipa, CA 92399
909-795-8977
Fax 909-795-8970
Provides Christian related large print and Braille books free of charge all over the world in 40 different languages

Matilda Ziegler Magazine
80 Eighth Avenue, Room 1304
New York, NY 10011

212–242–0263
Publishes Ziegler Magazine in Braille, monthly' provides tapes free.

National Braille Press
88 St. Stephen's Street
Boston, MA 92115
Braille publications; free catalog available. Also provides transcription services.
800–548–7323 or 617–266–6160
www.nbp.org
541-482-9239 (outside USA)

The New York Times
Large Type Weekly
Mail Subscription
Magazine City
650 Jefferson Parkway
Charlottesville, VA 22911
1-800-787-1414
www.magazinecity.com;nylp-52.html
Offers a weekly large-print newspaper
.

Reader's Digest
Large-Type Publication
P.O. Box 525
Pleasantville, NY 10570
800–877–5293
www.rd.pfs.org
Sells a large-type version of the monthly magazine

Soundelux Audio Publishing
7080 Hollywood Boulevard
Ste 1100
Hollywood, CA 90028
323-603-3200

Sells books on tape; free catalog

Thorndike: G.K. Hall Large Print Books
Amazon.com
Large selection new and used books on Amazon.com

UlversCroft Large Print Books
950 A Union Rd.
Suite 427
W. Seneca, NY 1422
800–955–9659
Main Office:The Green
Bradgate Rd.
LE 77FU
Sells soft-cover large-print books

OTHER

Lighting
Customized lighting can be accessed by contacting Robert Mumford
@ mumfynet@earthlink.net

Visions
500 Greenwich St.
New York, NY 10022
212–625-1618
Fax: 212-219-4070
Provides rehabilitation services for children and adults; serves NY, limited NJ & CT.

Eye Care America
Glaucoma help: 800-391-3937
Provides services to U.S. citizens or legal residents sixty-five or older who do not have access to an ophthalmologist. Medicare assignment accepted as full payment.

Eye Bank Association of America
1015 18th St. NW, Suite 1010
Washington, DC 20036-5504
202-775-4999
Fax" 202-429-6036
www.restoresight.org

Blindness Resource Center
New York Institute for Special Education
A comprehensive site on glaucoma and other eye diseases
www.nyise.org/eye.htm

**Glaucoma Screening
Congressional Glaucoma Caucus**
1083 Marcus Street
Lake Success, NY 11042
877-611-4232
www.glaucomacongress.org
does mass screening, supported by members
of congress

**Nutrition Action Healthletter
Center for Science in the Public Interest**
PO Box 96611
Washington, DC 20000-6011
Website: www.Nutrition Actiion Healthletter

National Disease Research Interchange
1880 John F. Kennedy Blvd. 6th Floor
Philadelphia, PA, 19103

800 222-NDRI (6374)
Ndnresearch.org

Phillips Life Line Systems
111 Lawrence St.
Framingham, MA 01702-8156
1-800-380-3111
Purveyor of products for independent living,medical alert systems, help, etc.

Medic Alert
2323 Colorado Avenue
Turlock, CA 95381-9015
800–863–3420
For an initial registration fee and an annual renewal fee, provides an emblem engraved with an ID number and a twenty-four-hour hot line number to supply vital medical information about the registered individual o
www.medicalert.org

Xal-Ease
Free eye dropper to help instill drops
1-866-846-9006

HELPFUL WEBSITES

Pub Med
http://www.pubmed.org
National Library of Medicine data base.
Hint: to access an item, for example, enter glaucoma—you'll get abstracts on latest research.

Med Watch
Food and Drug Administration (FDA)
 website disseminating drug safety information
www.fda.gov/cder/drug/DrugSafety/DrugIndex.htm
Have a problem with a drug?
Call 1-800-322-1088
Review of the scientific evidence on drugs
and their prices, Consumers Union (Spanish and English)

Consumer Reports.org—free reports on drugs
ww.crbestbuydrugs.org

National Library of Medicine: government site covering information about marketed drugs, supplements and other medical matters, Dailymed.nlm.nih.gov

News
http://www.google.com
http.//www.ivu.org/news/veg-news/
http:www.nytimes.com/mem/tnt.html.

MEDICAL AND FINANCIAL ASSISTANCE

Eye Care America
Low Vision Services
Patient assistive program
303 Enterprise Court
Suite D
Vista, CA 92801
800-826-4200

Fax: 800-368-4111
Eyecareamerica.org

Alcon Labs Humanitarian Service
(Azopt, Betoptic S, Timolol,
Travatan)
800-222-8103
www.alconlabs.com

Allergan Patient Assistance Program
(Alphagan, Betagan, Lumigan,
Propine)
www.patientassistance.com/profile
800-553-6783

Helping Patients.org
888=331-1102
Information in Spanish & English—
can view all companies participating
in available drugs; can also view and
print application forms
Free or low-cost prescriptions
Pparx.org
A comprehensive listing of
pharmaceutical organizations
offering service

FIND A DOCTOR IN YOUR VICINITY

American Association of Ophthalmology
PO Box 7424
San Franncisco, CA 95120
415-561-8500
E-mail: aaoeåao.org
http://www.aao.org

Vision USA
American Optometric Association
243 N. Lindbergh Blvd.
St Louis, MO 63141
800-365-2219
www.aoa.net.org/visioinusa/index.as
helps uninsured and low-income get
eye help

Merck Patient Assistance Program
800 727-5400

Pfizer
Xalatan
PO Box 515
Doniphen, MO 63735-0515
888-812-5152

Knights Templar Foundation, Inc.
6022 Knights Ridge Way
Alexandria, VA 22610-1635
703-071-3220
Fax 703-993-0655
www.knightstemplar.org

The Medicine Program
PO Box 515
Doniphan, MO 63935-0515
573-996-3333
Email: help@themedicineprogram.com
www. themedicineprogram.com

Seniors Eyecare Program
Eye Care America
800 222-EYES (3937)
For more information on agencies
in your area that offer services to
the blind and visually impaired,
check the publication or the web

address of the American Foundation for the Blind. In addition, your state Department of Rehabilitation may provide such services as instruction in Braille, daily living skills, independent travel, job preparation and placement, and medication consultation. If you are a veteran, you may qualify for rehabilitation services provided by the U.S. Veterans' Administration. The Veterans' Administration also produces audiotapes on subjects from medical care, housing, and living arrangements to consumer issues, financial matters, health and nutrition, and long-term care. You can also check with your local telephone and electric companies to determine if large-print statements are provided. Consult with state and local commissions and other public agencies for access to job counseling, rehabilitation, and placement services. Lastly, use the internet to find services in your area. Just about all organizations provide a website describing its services.

Travel and transport

Greyhound offers a free travel ticket for a sighted person accompanying a low-vision or blind person (pay for one ticket, get one free.)

Parking: Handicapped parking permits/placards are available from your state's Department of Motor Vehicles at no charge.

Para-Transit Service: It's the law
If the public transportation system serving your area cannot accommodate you, your community must provide para-transit by van, taxi, or some other vehicle.

Eye Bank Donations
When you donate your eyes upon death for research purposes, you are helping scientists in their quest for a cure of eye diseases. You can register at **The Eye-Bank for Sight Restoration** 120 Wall Street New York, NY 10005-3902 (212) 742-9000
E-mail: info@ebsr.org

Index

A

Acesulfame-K 364
Acetaminophen 187, 324
Acetazolamide 132, 157, 194, 315, 463
Acetone 360, 361
Acetylcholine 134, 272, 280, 326, 327, 336, 479, 481, 487
Acidosis 132, 133, 315
Acupressure 246, 262, 264, 270
Acupuncture 239, 242, 246, 262, 263, 444, 471, 479, 489
Adenosine triphosphate (ATP) 323, 479
Adrenal gland 61, 131, 243, 288
Adrenaline 123, 131, 243
Advanced glaucoma intervention study (AGIS) 91, 120
Advocacy 269, 425, 442, 444, 448, 496, 497, 504
Age-related 13, 64, 198, 289, 296, 322, 323, 325, 356
Age-Related Macular Degeneration 62, 64, 289, 322, 325, 356, 475
Agonists 129, 130, 131, 138, 143
Ahmed shunt 184
AIDS 44, 219, 220, 326
Alachlior 359

Alcohol 67, 137, 310, 333, 334, 341, 347, 353, 357, 365, 371
Alpha-chymotrypsin 390
Alphagan. *See* Brimonidine (Alphagan)
Alpha linolenic acid 346
Alpha lipoic acid 221, 312, 313, 326
Amblyopia 69, 73, 80, 365, 479
Amino Acids 168, 202, 217, 219, 290, 295, 296, 305, 324, 327, 334, 344, 365, 370, 484
Amitriptyline (Elavil) 391
Analgesics 390
Anemone pulsatilla (Pasque flower) 278
Anesthetics 37, 174, 175
Angle xi, 8, 11, 12, 13, 20, 23, 24, 25, 26, 30, 32, 35, 36, 37, 38, 39, 41, 44, 45, 51, 53, 54, 56, 57, 58, 59, 61, 73, 75, 81, 82, 83, 84, 86, 89, 95, 101, 118, 132, 135, 136, 137, 143, 145, 150, 152, 156, 158, 159, 160, 161, 163, 167, 168, 174, 182, 185, 186, 192, 212, 222, 225, 285, 304, 326, 331, 338, 342, 357, 375, 382, 389, 390, 391, 392, 393,

410, 434, 449, 458, 459,
460, 461, 463, 464, 467,
468, 473, 479, 487, 488, 490
Angle-closure glaucoma xi, 8, 36,
38, 45, 53, 56, 58, 59, 61,
95, 135, 160, 167, 225, 389,
391
Aniridia 68, 73, 83, 174, 226, 479
Ankylosing spondylitis 44, 257
Antagonists 331
Anthocyanidins 277, 290, 294, 317
Anti-arthritis drugs 390
Antibiotics 179, 184, 191, 210,
242, 297, 300, 304, 306,
331, 336, 367, 371, 392, 394
Antibodies 30, 177, 219, 242, 287,
298, 333, 334, 336, 367
Anticholinergic agents 391
Antidepressants 37, 65, 300, 371,
385, 390, 391
Antigens 223, 230, 287, 298
Antihistamines 390
Antimetabolites 120, 176, 177,
191, 209
Antinausea drugs 391
Antioxidants 65, 221, 291, 298,
307, 312, 313, 315, 316,
317, 320, 321, 325, 326,
327, 328, 338, 340, 341,
349, 475
Anti-Parkinson agents 390
Antispasmodics 37, 390
Anxiety 37, 110, 112, 126, 129,
131, 188, 243, 248, 250,
280, 281, 340, 376, 381,
384, 411, 427
Applanation tonometry 6, 457
Apraclonidine (Iopidine) 129, 130,
157, 159, 167
Apresoline 391. *See* Hydralazine

Aqueous humor 5, 10, 11, 12, 25,
46, 56, 123, 125, 129, 131,
132, 161, 163, 167, 174,
177, 181, 206, 314, 315,
479, 480, 481, 490
Arachidonic acid 46, 221, 282,
285, 347, 486
Aralen 390. *See* Chloroquine
Argon laser 28, 152, 153, 161, 166,
480
Argon laser sphincterotomy 166
Arsenide 153, 154
Artane 391. *See* trihexyphenidyl
Arthritis 24, 44, 47, 61, 85, 129,
216, 221, 266, 275, 290,
295, 298, 301, 322, 329,
335, 343, 345, 346, 389,
390, 403, 470, 486, 489
Artificial Sweeteners 364
ARVO Association for Research in
Vision and Ophthalmology
97, 460, 463
Ascorbic acid 314, 315, 368
Asopt (brimonidine) 132, 133,
146, 222
Aspartame (NutriSweet) 365, 366,
477
Aspirin 25, 46, 52, 134, 174, 187,
193, 289, 302, 314, 335,
347, 353, 383, 384, 390
Atenolol 126
Atherosclerosis 41, 50, 106, 284,
322, 326
Atropine 37, 94, 179, 272, 392
Atropisol. *See* Atropine
Autosomal Recessive 224
Axenfeld-Rieger Syndrome 226
Axons 11, 15, 16, 20, 21, 24, 217,
222, 223, 234, 235
Ayurveda 247, 280, 284

B

Baikal skullcap 280
Baltimore Eye Survey 27, 28
Banister, Richard 26
Barberry *(Berberis vulgaris)* 278
Bates, Dr.W.H. 258, 265
Beaver Dam Eye Study 28, 30, 64, 320, 356
Behcet's Syndrome 480
Belladonna 272
Bentyl 391. *See* Dicyclomine
Benzalkonium (BAK) 141, 480
Berberine 279
Berberis vulgaris *(barberry)* 278
Beta-Blockers 10, 11, 24, 65, 123, 124, 125, 126, 127, 134, 138, 142, 144, 174, 223, 480
Beta-carotene 221, 295, 314, 315, 318, 319, 322, 341, 350
Betagan 124, 142, 143, 220, 512. *See* Levobunolol
Betaxolol (Betoptic) 119, 124, 125, 156, 220
Betoptic 124, 142, 143, 156, 222, 512. *See* Betaxolol
Bilberry *(Vaccinum myrtillus)* 174, 193, 221, 273, 277, 278, 312, 313, 317, 371, 384
Biofeedback 246, 247, 270
Bioflavonoids 291, 311, 312, 316, 317, 473
Biotin 336
Bipolar cells 480
Birefringence 98
Birth control 334, 384
Bleb 93, 170, 173, 174, 175, 176, 177, 178, 179, 181, 183, 184, 186, 189, 190, 191, 192, 194, 209, 211, 480
Blepharitis 61, 134, 278, 304, 480

Blindness. *See* Vision loss
Blind spot 94, 108, 480
Blood cholesterol 332
Blood clotting herbs 193, 278, 279, 302, 331, 343, 384
Blood pressure 18, 23, 29, 30, 31, 32, 33, 34, 47, 48, 61, 74, 75, 80, 87, 103, 116, 123, 126, 128, 131, 132, 139, 147, 193, 219, 243, 248, 249, 252, 278, 289, 298, 302, 303, 323, 329, 332, 339, 347, 352, 381, 384, 385, 389, 391, 393, 394, 410, 459, 480, 498. *See* Hypertension
Blood shot eyes. *See* Conjunctival hyperemia
Blue Mountain Study 95, 284, 345
B-lymphocytes 287
Books on Tape 437, 510
Brachycardia 129, 143
Brain Derived Neurotropin Factor (BDNF) 217, 227
Bravewell Collaborative 240
Breathing 34, 50, 92, 94, 137, 219, 250, 251, 252, 253, 254, 259, 267, 310, 359, 374, 395, 462
Brimonidine (Alphagan) 129, 130, 138, 159, 220
Bromelain 280
Bruch's membrane 63, 165
Butylated hydroxyanisole (BHA) 368
Butylated hydroxytoluene (BHT) 368
B vitamins 295, 303, 313, 330, 331, 338

C

Café au lait spots 74
Caffeine 298, 384
Calcium 8, 125, 126, 133, 215, 218, 219, 220, 221, 222, 243, 289, 292, 295, 298, 304, 308, 312, 313, 316, 317, 329, 331, 337, 338, 371, 384, 474, 480
Calcium-channel blockers 126
Capsulotomy 154, 212, 462, 481
Carbacohl 10, 40, 90, 114, 131, 134, 144, 149, 166, 392
Carbon dioxide 51, 132, 133, 146, 153, 154, 252, 341, 365
Carbonic anhydrase inhibitors 11, 132, 138, 146, 174
Cardiac agents 391
Cardiovascular disease 23, 47, 310, 314, 318, 393
Carotenoids 107, 271, 286, 290, 295, 312, 313, 315, 318, 319, 320
Carotid arteries 46, 289
Carotid Artery Occlusive Disease 46
Catapres 143
Cataracts 5, 9, 18, 37, 41, 46, 74, 77, 80, 81, 82, 88, 114, 115, 135, 136, 137, 144, 181, 186, 194, 198, 199, 201, 202, 203, 204, 206, 208, 209, 245, 277, 284, 290, 309, 314, 315, 319, 320, 321, 322, 326, 327, 332, 333, 338, 343, 350, 357, 366, 393, 421, 474, 488
    Cortical 202, 203, 267, 314, 345, 357
    Nuclear 9, 198, 201, 202, 203, 288, 308, 312, 315, 320, 332, 357

Cataract surgery 19, 38, 43, 59, 101, 166, 189, 193, 203, 205, 207, 211, 213, 357, 468
    Posterior subcapsular 198, 202, 345
Central Retinal Vein 50, 51, 105, 140
Chandler's syndrome 52, 54
Chi 246, 251, 263, 269
Chloroquine 390
Chlorothiazide 391
Chlorthalidone 391
Cholesterol 87, 126, 143, 281, 282, 284, 289, 290, 297, 302, 304, 323, 326, 333, 342, 345, 348, 385, 393, 395, 463, 471
Choline 134, 326, 336, 479
Cholinergic agent 134
Choroid 4, 23, 43, 44, 50, 63, 74, 76, 88, 147, 148, 192, 193, 194, 296, 481, 484, 489, 490
Chromium 305, 316, 342, 343, 355, 371
Chromosome 31, 39, 69, 74, 78, 79, 225, 233, 335
Ciliary body 10
Ciliary muscle 12, 57, 88, 134, 135, 145, 227, 257, 489
Ciliary neurotropin factor (CNTF) 217
Ciliary processes 14, 481
Cinera martima. See silver ragwort
Circadian rhythm 17, 23, 481
Clonidine (Catapres) 391
Cocaine 391
Coenzyme Q10 323
Cogan-Reese Syndrome 54
Colace 187
Collaborative Initial Glaucoma Treatment Study 420, 472

Collaborative Normal-Tension
Treatment Study 119
Complementary therapies 239,
240, 242, 245, 246, 349,
387, 444
Computerized Axial Tomography
(CAT) 240
Computers 96, 199, 224, 257, 305,
311, 370, 430, 431, 433, 434
Eye protection 399
On line 278
Training 427
Cones 14, 15, 16, 17, 91, 108, 111,
116, 480, 486
Confocal Scanning Laser Ophthal-
mology (CSLO) 20, 100,
101
Congenital 21, 67, 68, 69, 70, 71,
72, 74, 79, 80, 83, 89, 156,
159, 183, 224, 225, 226,
231, 270, 466, 479, 487
Congenital glaucoma 67, 68, 69,
70, 71, 83, 89, 156, 183,
224, 225, 226, 270, 466
Microcornea 73, 83
Rubella 68, 80, 84
Conjunctival Buttonhole 191
Conjunctival hyperemia 61
Conjunctivitis 69, 71, 131, 137,
278, 279
Consumer Labs 273
Contact Lenses 5, 49, 58, 73, 89,
93, 132, 191, 235, 378, 406,
407, 459, 461, 502
Contrast sensitivity xvi, 15, 23, 88,
96, 207, 317, 400, 402, 410,
423, 424
Copaxone 24, 223
Copper 294, 302, 310, 316, 317,
327, 339, 340, 341, 350,
355, 358, 361, 370

Corgard 126. *See* Nadolol
Cornea 4, 5, 6, 7, 8, 9, 10, 11, 12,
14, 34, 38, 39, 42, 45, 53,
54, 55, 57, 60, 68, 69, 70,
71, 72, 73, 74, 84, 86, 89,
90, 91, 92, 101, 116, 120,
134, 141, 144, 147, 160,
162, 163, 169, 170, 173,
174, 180, 183, 185, 194,
195, 200, 201, 205, 208,
211, 225, 227, 231, 232,
321, 327, 343, 390, 421,
450, 458, 479, 480, 482,
483, 485, 488, 490
Cloudiness of 69, 89, 136, 212,
422
Corneal 6, 7, 29, 30, 34, 42, 52,
53, 54, 55, 60, 61, 72, 73,
74, 84, 86, 89, 91, 92, 99,
100, 116, 120, 127, 129,
131, 134, 140, 141, 160,
167, 169, 170, 174, 185,
186, 190, 194, 203, 205,
211, 231, 232, 321, 327,
333, 409, 449, 455, 457,
466, 468, 482, 484, 485,
486, 487
decompensation 42, 482
dellen 194
edema 482
ring segments 170
Corticosteroids 332, 333, 371
Cosmetics, use of 368, 407, 408,
409
Chemicals in 409
Cow's eye 482
COX-2 Inhibitor 25
Cryotherapy 162, 190
Crystalline lens 8, 481, 486, 488
Cupping 19, 23, 57, 68, 70, 270,
482

Cyclocryotherapy 70, 71, 482
Cyclopentolate (cyclogyl) 94, 392
Cyclophotocoagulation 71, 154,
    163, 193, 482
Cyclotherapy. *See* cyclophotocoagu-
    lation
Cycologyl. *See* cyclopentolate
CYPIBI gene 69, 226
Cysteine 168, 200, 218, 313, 324,
    325, 336, 484, 486
Cystoid macular edema 51, 462,
    482

D

Damato Campimeter 93
Daminozide 359
Daranide. *See* Dichlorphenamide
DARC (Detection of Apotosing
    retinal Cells) 102
Demecarium (Humersol) 136, 392
Descemet's membrane 52, 180,
    181, 482
Diabetes xv, 10, 18, 27, 31, 44,
    47, 48, 49, 73, 84, 87, 97,
    99, 103, 121, 164, 165, 199,
    202, 206, 216, 243, 284,
    293, 310, 318, 322, 326,
    329, 333, 341, 359, 364,
    394, 410, 449, 482, 497, 498
Diabetic Retinopathy xv, 19, 46,
    47, 48, 49, 80, 84, 99, 100,
    121, 139, 140, 153, 164,
    165, 183, 233, 243, 305,
    317, 331, 334, 342, 390,
    460, 482
Diamox 52, 132, 133, 194, 315,
    338, 386. *See* Acetazolamide
Diastolic pressure 32
Dichlorphenamide (Daranide, Ora-
    trol) 132. *See also* Carbonic
    Anhydrase Inhibitors

Dicyclomine (Bentyl) 391
Diet 17, 47, 49, 65, 203, 239, 243,
    246, 247, 268, 277, 280,
    281, 283, 284, 285, 286,
    288, 289, 290, 291, 292,
    293, 294, 295, 296, 301,
    302, 303, 304, 308, 312,
    313, 318, 320, 322, 327,
    331, 335, 337, 339, 342,
    343, 345, 347, 348, 350,
    361, 366, 367, 386, 394, 473
Diisopropyl fluorophosphate (DPF,
    or Floropryl) 392
Dimenhydrinate *(Dramamine)* 391
Diode laser 98, 100, 104, 154, 158
Dipivefrin 131, 157
Disopyramide (Norpace) 391
Docosahexaenoic acid (DHA) 128,
    297, 319, 346
Doctor-patient relationship 40,
    374, 375, 377, 378, 381,
    382, 383, 444
Donnagel 391. *See* Scopolamine
    (Donagel)
Doppler flow meter 29
Dorzolamide (Trusopt) 132, 133,
    343, 387
Down's syndrome 79, 83, 95
Dramamine 391. *See* Dimenhydri-
    nate
Driving 10, 38, 40, 82, 101, 135,
    195, 202, 394, 410, 411, 420
Drug interactions 383, 386, 395
Drusen 63, 77, 375, 482
Dry Eye Syndrome 66, 313, 365,
    476

E

Early Manifest Glaucoma Trial
    (EMGT) 28, 118, 156
Ecothiophate. *See* Phopholine Iodide

Edema 18, 19, 45, 49, 51, 52, 53,
    54, 55, 74, 89, 128, 136,
    140, 211, 333, 348, 462,
    482, 483
Elavil (Amitriptyline) 391
Electrodiathermy 162
Electrolytes 12, 303
Electronic Reading Enhancement
    Systems (CCTV) 429
Electrophysiology 105
Electroretinogram (ERG) 483
Endocyclophotocoagulation 163
Endogenous Endophthalmus 44,
    81, 128, 139, 285
Epidemiological 27, 30, 345
Epifrin (Epinephrine) 131
Epinal (Epinephrine) 131
Epinephrine 131, 132, 144, 340,
    365, 388, 392, 480, 481
Episcleral glaucoma 11, 56, 75, 76,
    84, 181, 483
Episcleral veins 11, 56, 181
Epithelium 6, 11, 46, 63, 226, 227,
    229, 232, 483
Epitrate (Epinephrine) 131
Eppy (Epinephrine) 131, 132, 144,
    340, 365, 392, 480, 481
Essential Fatty Acids 65, 313, 321,
    322, 345, 346, 348, 359
Ethacrynic acid 146
Exercise 47, 54, 61, 65, 93, 123,
    187, 210, 242, 243, 246,
    247, 248, 251, 253, 254,
    255, 260, 261, 262, 263,
    268, 269, 270, 289, 294,
    299, 305, 322, 383, 394,
    405, 415, 421, 449
Exfoliation syndrome 12, 13, 27,
    33, 38, 39, 40, 41, 43, 58,
    59, 78, 84, 119, 135, 157,

    197, 198, 206, 211, 213,
    216, 289, 397, 449, 483
Extraocular muscles 185, 483
Eye
Examination 18, 30, 33, 43, 69,
    87, 90
Pressure 357
Eyebright 278
Eye Drops 46, 53, 131, 187, 381,
    388, 422, 462
Eyeglasses 31, 153, 204, 257, 420,
    428
Eyes xv, 4, 7, 8, 9, 10, 12, 13, 15,
    17, 18, 20, 21, 23, 24, 27,
    28, 31, 34, 36, 39, 42, 43,
    44, 46, 47, 51, 54, 57, 58,
    62, 64, 65, 67, 68, 69, 71,
    72, 73, 74, 75, 77, 78, 80,
    81, 82, 83, 85, 87, 88, 89,
    91, 92, 93, 95, 96, 97, 98,
    100, 105, 108, 120, 121,
    123, 124, 125, 127, 128,
    129, 133, 135, 136, 137,
    145, 147, 148, 149, 161,
    165, 167, 168, 169, 174,
    175, 176, 179, 181, 185,
    187, 191, 192, 195, 200,
    201, 203, 204, 205, 206,
    214, 220, 222, 223, 226,
    227, 229, 230, 231, 241,
    243, 250, 254, 255, 257,
    258, 259, 260, 261, 262,
    263, 264, 265, 268, 275,
    278, 279, 284, 285, 286,
    287, 288, 303, 305, 310,
    312, 316, 318, 319, 323,
    327, 328, 329, 330, 332,
    333, 339, 341, 342, 344,
    345, 350, 358, 360, 361,
    367, 375, 385, 386, 390,
    396, 397, 399, 406, 408,

409, 411, 414, 415, 420,
423, 424, 425, 427, 429,
434, 435, 437, 442, 456,
462, 464, 465, 470, 474,
475, 481, 482, 484, 488,
489, 501, 502, 512, 513
Eye safety 399
Eye Vitamins xii, 11, 80, 193, 200,
201, 221, 246, 257, 286,
290, 291, 294, 295, 297,
300, 303, 304, 305, 311,
312, 313, 314, 315, 320,
324, 330, 331, 338, 341,
345, 349, 350, 351, 352,
362, 363, 366, 393, 395

F

Factor H 63
False Negative 99, 113
False Positive 99, 113
Fanconi syndrome 202
Fibulin 5,6 genes 226
Filtration surgery 61, 126, 149,
152, 155, 173, 193, 194,
195, 203, 381, 382, 452,
468, 490
5-fluorouracil 176
Flavonoids 271, 290, 291, 295,
302, 307, 316, 317, 473
Floaters 10, 43, 45, 50, 484
Floropryl 392. *See* Isoflurophate
Fluoride 153, 154, 222, 299, 300,
310, 361, 477
Fluoroscein angiography 48, 104
Fluphenazine (Prolixen) 391
Folic acid 302, 303, 313, 330, 332,
334, 335, 336
Food additives 283, 299, 300, 363,
364, 408
Food colorings 488
Forskolin 278

Fovea 18, 50, 62, 101, 116, 484
Framingham Eye Study 28, 198
Free radicals 48, 129, 168, 200,
221, 276, 277, 285, 290,
309, 310, 311, 313, 314,
317, 318, 319, 321, 322,
323, 324, 325, 327, 343,
357, 359, 476, 484
Frequency Doubling Technology
(FDT) 115, 483
Fructus ligustri lucidi (FLL) 279
Fuch's endothelial corneal dystrophy
54
Full thickness surgery 190
Functional Magnetic Resonance
Imagery (FMRI) 22

G

Galactosemia 202
Ganglion cells xii, 4, 11, 13, 15, 16,
17, 97, 105, 115, 117, 200,
201, 216, 217, 219, 220,
222, 226, 227, 232, 234,
236, 326, 464, 480
Genetically-Modified Foods 361
Genistein 177
Genomics 224
German measles 80
Ghost Cell Glaucoma. *See* Glaucoma ghost cell
Ghost cells 60, 84, 212
Ginkgo (Ginkgo biloba) 221, 222,
275, 276, 277, 278, 313,
347, 352, 353, 384, 385
Ginseng 281, 352, 384, 385
Glare 8, 88, 166, 170, 201, 202,
204, 207, 317, 410, 413,
414, 415, 423, 424, 425,
434, 435
Glasses. *See* See eyeglasses, safety
glasses, sun glasses

Glaucoma vii, ix, x, xi, xii, xiii, xiv,
     xv, xvi, 4, 5, 6, 7, 8, 9, 10,
     11, 12, 13, 14, 15, 16, 17,
     18, 19, 20, 21, 22, 23, 24,
     25, 26, 27, 28, 29, 30, 31,
     32, 33, 34, 35, 36, 37, 38,
     39, 40, 41, 42, 43, 44, 45,
     46, 47, 48, 49, 51, 52, 53,
     55, 56, 57, 58, 59, 60, 61,
     62, 64, 65, 66, 67, 68, 69,
     70, 71, 72, 73, 74, 75, 76,
     77, 78, 79, 80, 81, 82, 83,
     84, 85, 86, 87, 88, 89, 90,
     91, 93, 94, 95, 96, 97, 98,
     99, 101, 102, 103, 104, 105,
     106, 107, 108, 109, 111,
     113, 114, 115, 116, 117,
     118, 119, 120, 121, 122,
     123, 124, 125, 126, 127,
     130, 131, 134, 135, 136,
     137, 138, 141, 143, 144,
     145, 146, 147, 148, 150,
     152, 153, 155, 156, 157,
     158, 159, 160, 161, 164,
     165, 167, 168, 170, 171,
     172, 173, 174, 175, 179,
     181, 182, 183, 184, 185,
     186, 188, 189, 192, 194,
     195, 197, 198, 201, 203,
     204, 205, 206, 207, 209,
     210, 211, 212, 213, 214,
     215, 216, 217, 219, 220,
     221, 222, 223, 224, 225,
     226, 227, 228, 229, 231,
     232, 234, 235, 236, 241,
     242, 243, 245, 246, 247,
     248, 250, 256, 257, 260,
     263, 267, 268, 270, 271,
     272, 273, 274, 275, 276,
     277, 278, 279, 280, 281,
     284, 285, 287, 288, 289,
     299, 301, 304, 310, 312,
     314, 315, 316, 318, 320,
     322, 323, 324, 327, 331,
     334, 336, 338, 341, 342,
     343, 344, 346, 347, 356,
     357, 358, 360, 364, 371,
     372, 373, 374, 375, 376,
     377, 378, 379, 380, 381,
     382, 383, 384, 385, 386,
     387, 388, 389, 390, 391,
     392, 393, 396, 397, 399,
     400, 401, 404, 406, 407,
     410, 412, 414, 415, 417,
     419, 420, 421, 422, 423,
     424, 430, 433, 435, 437,
     443, 444, 445, 446, 447,
     448, 449, 450, 455, 456,
     457, 458, 459, 460, 461,
     462, 463, 464, 465, 466,
     467, 468, 469, 470, 471,
     472, 473, 474, 475, 479,
     480, 481, 482, 485, 486,
     487, 488, 489, 490, 491,
     492, 493, 494, 495, 496,
     497, 498, 499, 501, 503,
     510, 511
Acute angle closure 449
Angle closure 35, 449
Cataracts and 82, 88, 198, 201,
     203, 204, 474
Chronic angle-closure 38
Congenital 67, 70, 83, 89, 156,
     183, 224, 225, 226, 270, 466
Diet and 285
Effects on African-American 31,
     101
Effects on Asians 34, 35, 38, 294,
     295
Episcleral 56
Exfoliation 58
Ghost cell 60

In children 449
Infantile 68, 69, 70, 81
Laser treatment and 10, 76, 77, 161, 164, 194, 449
Malignant 192, 481, 486
Medically induced 59
Medication and xii, 9, 10, 25, 35, 42, 48, 49, 51, 58, 60, 62, 76, 79, 82, 85, 116, 117, 119, 120, 121, 122, 123, 124, 125, 126, 127, 128, 129, 130, 131, 133, 134, 137, 138, 139, 140, 141, 142, 143, 144, 145, 146, 147, 148, 149, 150, 151, 156, 158, 162, 164, 167, 172, 173, 174, 176, 178, 181, 183, 185, 186, 189, 211, 222, 223, 234, 235, 249, 250, 276, 315, 352, 356, 373, 376, 382, 383, 384, 385, 386, 387, 388, 389, 390, 394, 395, 396, 397, 411, 412, 416, 423, 424, 427, 440, 513
Narrow-angle 35, 39, 89, 101, 136, 160, 167, 168, 389, 390, 391, 392, 393
Neovascular 46, 47, 49, 51, 52, 59, 60, 106, 139, 179, 189, 211, 392
Normal-tension (NTG) 39, 103, 115, 118, 119, 128, 174, 226, 276, 338
Open angle 27, 222, 449
Pigmentery dispersion syndrome (PDS) 12, 27, 30, 39, 58, 63, 84, 85, 90, 102, 140, 146, 220, 229, 268, 296
Post-cataract 59
Primary infantile 70

Primary open-angle (POAG) 30, 84, 226
Retinal disorders and 58
Secondary infantile 81
Seconday 68
Steroid induced 19, 25, 45, 52, 58, 59, 61, 62, 159, 179, 184, 186, 190, 211, 482
Surgery and xii, 9, 18, 19, 28, 30, 38, 40, 41, 42, 43, 45, 46, 59, 60, 61, 70, 72, 73, 76, 82, 84, 85, 92, 101, 126, 135, 148, 149, 151, 152, 153, 154, 155, 156, 157, 159, 161, 164, 166, 167, 168, 169, 170, 171, 172, 173, 174, 175, 176, 178, 180, 182, 183, 184, 185, 186, 188, 189, 190, 191, 192, 193, 194, 195, 203, 205, 207, 208, 209, 210, 211, 213, 228, 235, 245, 247, 249, 257, 266, 280, 315, 340, 352, 357, 381, 382, 384, 385, 390, 397, 419, 427, 449, 468, 469, 481, 486, 489, 490, 498
Treatment of 19, 28, 66, 76, 118, 172, 242, 246
Wipe-out 194
Glaucon 131. See Epiniphrine
Glial cells 16
Glucose tolerance 322. See also Diabetes
Glutamate 16, 123, 146, 215, 216, 218, 219, 221, 223, 224, 276, 280, 285, 292, 331, 344, 363, 465, 478, 484. See Glutamic acid
Glutamate antagonists 331

Glutamic acid 168, 200, 313, 324, 325, 344, 363
Glutamine 285, 344, 473, 475
Glutathione 168, 200, 201, 218, 292, 298, 310, 313, 324, 325, 326, 332, 343, 474, 484
Glycine 168, 200, 313, 324, 325, 484
Glycosaminoglycans 62, 313
Golden Shunt 170
Goldmann tonometers 387
Goldmann visual field analysis 90, 91, 92, 93, 110, 113, 484
Goniolens 89, 484
Goniotomy 70, 73, 76, 81, 484
Groopman, Dr. Jerome 241, 470
Guggal 281

H

Headache 37, 50, 131, 219, 365
Heat shock proteins 219, 367
Heidelberg Retinal Tomography (HRT) 97
Hemorrhage 20, 21, 23, 34, 46, 51, 60, 76, 165, 193
Hepatocerebroretinall syndrome 83
Herbal medicine 272, 279
Herb-drug interactions 353
Herpes simplex virus 53, 228
Herpetic eye disease 129
Hippocampus 232, 243, 252
Holmium laser 169
Homatro 392. See Atrophine
Homocystinuria 41, 79, 80, 84
Hormones 13, 48, 123, 242, 244, 288, 300, 334, 337, 345, 352, 391
House plant detoxifiers 361
H. pylori bacter 457
Humorsol (Demecarium) 136, 138, 392

Humphrey Visual Field Analyzer 105, 106, 108, 110
Huperzine A 280
Hyaluronic acid 4, 10, 30, 344, 390, 484
Hydralazine (Apresoline) 391
Hydrobromide 392. See Artropine
Hydroxyamphetamine (Paredrine) 392
Hyoscine 392. See Scopolamine (Donagel)
Hyperopia 410, 484
Hyperpigmentation 129
Hypertension 23, 27, 28, 29, 30, 31, 32, 34, 41, 50, 91, 101, 103, 119, 120, 143, 147, 192, 243, 302, 328, 329, 346, 365, 375, 393, 449, 458, 459, 460, 463, 477, 496
Hypothyroidism 30, 299, 340
Hypotony Maculopathy 162, 176, 178, 180, 181, 184, 185, 190, 192, 194, 211, 475, 477, 485

I

ICE syndrome (Iridocorneal Enthothelium syndrome) 52, 53, 54
Immune privilege 7, 226
Incontinentia Pigmenti 77
Inderal 126, 385. See Propranolol
Indocyanine Green 65, 104
Infantile glaucoma 68, 69, 70, 81, 82, 83. See Glaucoma
Infection 19, 30, 32, 44, 47, 53, 66, 80, 81, 84, 140, 175, 179, 181, 185, 186, 189, 190, 191, 268, 282, 304, 367, 389, 406, 408, 482, 483, 484, 485, 486, 490

Infiniti 208, 209
Inflammation 8, 12, 19, 24, 25,
    33, 41, 43, 44, 45, 46, 50,
    51, 60, 61, 62, 63, 65, 68,
    69, 71, 76, 81, 85, 127, 129,
    134, 135, 137, 141, 144,
    159, 165, 167, 174, 179,
    186, 192, 193, 207, 211,
    216, 219, 228, 242, 278,
    280, 281, 285, 288, 293,
    295, 301, 313, 322, 327,
    328, 344, 345, 347, 348,
    366, 367, 391, 480, 483,
    484, 486, 487, 489, 490
Infrared Scanning Laser Tomogra-
    phy 104
Internal Sclerostomy 194, 461
Intracapsular cataract extraction
    485
Intraocular pressure xi, xii, 6, 11,
    12, 16, 17, 18, 19, 20, 25,
    26, 27, 29, 32, 33, 34, 40,
    42, 56, 58, 79, 86, 87, 88,
    90, 91, 93, 100, 108, 118,
    120, 121, 123, 125, 135,
    146, 152, 156, 162, 178,
    181, 215, 218, 222, 243,
    268, 275, 278, 279, 280,
    340, 357, 376, 381, 385,
    390, 391, 405, 449, 462,
    463, 478, 482, 485, 488, 490
Iopidine 129, 130, 143, 167.
    See Apraclonidine (Iopidine)
Iridectomy 67, 160, 161, 167, 173,
    185, 205, 211, 485
Iridocorneal enthothelium syn-
    drome. See ICE syndrome
Iridodesis 173

Iridotomy 37, 38, 39, 40, 59, 153,
    154, 160, 161, 162, 177,
    193, 206, 211, 485
Iris 4, 5, 7, 8, 11, 12, 14, 30, 35,
    36, 37, 38, 39, 40, 42, 43,
    45, 47, 52, 54, 55, 58, 67,
    68, 71, 72, 73, 74, 75, 78,
    79, 80, 81, 83, 84, 86, 89,
    90, 95, 101, 129, 136, 140,
    160, 161, 162, 163, 167,
    170, 173, 174, 177, 183,
    185, 193, 194, 206, 211,
    212, 227, 231, 344, 390,
    392, 479, 480, 481, 485,
    488, 490
Iritis 8, 43, 129, 137, 211, 279
Iron 222, 291, 294, 295, 298, 307,
    308, 310, 313, 318, 337,
    339, 340, 343, 370
Isoflurophate (Floropryl) 392

J

JAMA Journal of American Medical
    Association 66, 201, 459,
    476

K

Keraplasty 169
Ketamine 220, 390
Kinetic Perimetry 110
Kneist Gapo syndrome 83
Krukenberg spindles 38, 39, 90,
    485
Krupin shunt 184

L

Lacriminal glands 10, 149
Lamina cribosa 20, 21
Lane, Benjamin, OD xiv

Large-print 436, 437, 509, 510,
    513
Laser treatment 10, 45, 48, 58, 76,
    77, 89, 106, 118, 119, 120,
    121, 130, 140, 155, 156,
    157, 160, 161, 164, 168,
    170, 179, 193, 194, 310, 449
  exfoliative glaucoma and 118
Latanprost (Xalatan)
  side effects 124
Lazy eye 80, 479
L-Carnitine 326, 474
L-Carnosine 327
Leber's disease 229
Legal blindness xv, 73, 185, 413,
    423, 425, 426
Lens 4, 5, 6, 7, 8, 9, 10, 11, 36, 38,
    39, 40, 41, 42, 43, 45, 59,
    61, 65, 68, 72, 73, 78, 79,
    80, 81, 84, 88, 89, 90, 92,
    99, 101, 116, 129, 136, 137,
    140, 148, 157, 161, 162,
    163, 164, 166, 170, 188,
    191, 192, 193, 194, 197,
    198, 199, 200, 201, 202,
    203, 204, 205, 206, 207,
    208, 209, 210, 211, 212,
    233, 235, 257, 304, 310,
    313, 315, 324, 327, 330,
    332, 345, 390, 391, 392,
    397, 406, 428, 429, 443,
    458, 461, 468, 469, 471,
    479, 480, 481, 483, 484,
    485, 486, 488, 490, 502
Lens Epithelial cell derived Factor
    (ECDF) 140
Levobunolol (Betagan) 124
Lighting 15, 114, 115, 204, 379,
    400, 401, 413, 414, 415,
    417, 434, 435, 436, 444, 510
Light sensitivity 129

Linear scleroderma 83
Linoleic acid 345, 346, 347
Linolenic acid 313, 326, 346
Lipofuscin 140, 141
Lithium 153, 154, 223, 226, 476
Los Angeles Latino Eye Study 121,
    460
Lou Gehrig's disease 325
Louis-Bar Syndrome 74, 78
Lowe's syndrome 68
Low vision imaging xiii
Lucentis 139
Lutein 201, 247, 290, 295, 311,
    313, 319, 320, 350
Lycopene 291, 295, 319, 321

M

Macrocephaly 75, 486
Macula 17, 18, 19, 45, 49, 51, 62,
    77, 101, 102, 107, 108, 116,
    128, 140, 211, 277, 286,
    433, 481, 484, 486
Macular degeneration vii, xv, 17,
    23, 49, 62, 63, 64, 65, 77,
    106, 107, 109, 116, 139,
    141, 145, 154, 164, 165,
    200, 207, 218, 226, 227,
    233, 242, 247, 270, 284,
    286, 289, 296, 304, 310,
    312, 319, 320, 322, 325,
    330, 341, 345, 350, 356,
    390, 433, 442, 449, 462,
    467, 471, 482, 488, 495,
    502, 506
Mad cow disease 307, 324
Magnesium 220, 243, 294, 302,
    303, 305, 307, 312, 313,
    317, 337, 338, 352, 355, 371
Magnetic resonance imagery (MRI)
    240, 249
Magno cells 14, 115, 486

Manganese 303, 308, 318, 339, 341, 358
Map-dot fingerprint dystrophy 54
Marchesani's syndrome 79
Marfan syndrome 78
Marijuana 273, 274, 275, 463, 474
Marinol 275
Massage 178, 239, 245, 246, 247, 261, 263, 264, 265, 270, 471, 489
Medic Alert 404, 511
Medication 51, 62, 82, 85, 140, 156, 158, 387, 389. *See also* Individual medications
Charts 386
Driving 394
Meditation vii, 188, 240, 246, 247, 249, 250, 251, 253, 254, 265, 383, 449, 469
Melatonin 73, 313, 325, 326, 474, 486
Memantine 218, 463
Menstrual cycle 63
Mental retardation 76, 79, 80, 83, 365
Mercury 67, 296, 297, 308, 326, 328, 341, 343, 349, 358, 361, 408
Methazolamide (Neptazane) 132. *See* Carbibuc anhydrase inhibitor
Methylsulfonylmethane (MSM) 338
Metipranolol (Optipranolol) 124
Microprostheses 183
Mindful meditation 250, 251
Minerals 11, 153, 154, 246, 291, 294, 296, 303, 306, 308, 311, 312, 316, 336, 337, 338, 339, 341, 350, 355, 371

Mineral supplementation 201, 270, 310, 312, 314, 322, 324, 326, 330, 332, 342, 345, 349, 350, 351, 353, 382, 444
Miotics 40, 123, 134, 135, 136, 138, 144
Mitochondria 198, 215, 224, 241, 252, 288, 323, 326, 327, 334, 469
Mitomycin C 486
Mobility training 427, 441
Molds 367, 477
Molteno shunt 184
Molybdenum 317, 332, 342, 343
Monocytes 287
Monosodium glutamate (MSG) 363, 478
Morcher capsular tension ring 206
Muller cells 16, 227
Multifocal visually evoked potential (MFVEP) 105
Mydriacyl 392. *See* Tropicamide (Mydriacy)
Myocillan gene 225
Myopia 23, 27, 31, 34, 39, 58, 68, 69, 72, 74, 79, 83, 84, 87, 116, 135, 137, 169, 170, 257, 258, 285, 317, 390, 410, 422, 486

N

Nadolol (Corgard) 126
Nail partella syndrome 226
Nanophthalmos 102, 166, 390, 486
Nardil (Phenelzine) 391
Narrow angle glaucoma 36, 212
Drugs to avoid 390
National Eye Institute 32, 198, 218, 385, 433
Near-point accommodation 258

Nearsightedness (myopia) 70, 154, 471, 486
Needling 178, 189, 190
Neodymium yttrium aluminum Garnet laser (ND:YAG) 153, 154, 161, 193, 212, 462, 481
Neovascularization 51, 63, 64, 76, 105, 139, 140, 165, 211, 298, 475, 487
Neptazane (Methazolamide) 132, 133, 315, 338
Nerve fiber layer 20, 29, 97, 98, 100, 101, 215, 456, 487
Neurofibromatosis (von Recklng-hausen Disease) 74, 83
Neurological disorders 74, 219, 251, 293
Neurotropic deprivation 217
Neurotropins 223
Niacin 294, 326, 331, 332, 333, 336, 342
Niacinamide 332, 333
Nightshade 272, 281
Nirtric oxide synthase 200
Nitric acid 304
Nitroglycerine 222
Nitrous oxide 200, 221, 222, 390
n-mythl-d-aspartate (NMDA) 215, 218, 219, 220, 223
Norgesic 390. *See* Orphenadrine citrate (Norgesic)
Normal tension glaucoma 24, 33, 90, 91, 102, 462, 474
Norpace 391. *See* Disopyramide
NutraSweet 365, 366
Nystagmus 78, 95, 159, 167, 245, 459

O

Obesity 27, 84, 94, 202, 293, 294, 336
Occlusion 19, 41, 44, 46, 50, 51, 105, 138, 140, 149, 193, 458, 460, 464
Octopus Visual Field Test 484, 487
Ocular hypertension 23, 28, 29, 32, 34, 91, 119, 120, 375, 449, 459, 460
Ocular Hypertension Study 28, 29, 32
Olestra 363
Omega-3 essential fatty acids 27, 128, 297, 303, 345, 346
Omega-6 essential fatty acids 27
Open angle glaucioma. *See* Glau-coma
Ophthalmoscope 18, 88, 89, 95, 97, 99, 100, 104, 153, 466, 481, 487
Ophthalmoscopy 20, 154
Optical coherence tomography (OCT) 36, 100, 455, 456
Optic nerve xi, xii, 3, 5, 12, 16, 17, 19, 20, 21, 24, 26, 27, 29, 32, 33, 34, 37, 43, 45, 47, 50, 57, 65, 68, 70, 73, 74, 75, 76, 86, 89, 90, 91, 94, 95, 97, 98, 100, 101, 102, 103, 106, 107, 108, 109, 115, 116, 118, 119, 130, 132, 137, 145, 146, 182, 186, 193, 197, 201, 204, 206, 214, 216, 217, 218, 220, 221, 222, 225, 226, 232, 234, 236, 246, 247, 259, 273, 276, 279, 330, 331, 356, 381, 389, 449,

455, 456, 463, 465, 480,
482, 484, 485, 487, 488
Optic neuritis 21, 365
Optipranolol 124. *See* Metapranolol
Oral contraceptives 330, 334
Organic foods 285, 306, 307, 308,
309, 362
Orphenadrine citrate (Norgesic)
390
Osteoporosis 80, 298, 299, 329,
335
Oxidation 141, 221, 268, 290,
302, 309, 310, 319, 320,
321, 346, 351, 368, 388,
479, 487

P

PABA 336. *See* Para-aminobenzole
zcid
Pachymetry 90
Pallor 20, 95, 103, 104, 487
Palming 245, 265
Para-aminobenzoic acid (PABA)
336
Paradrine I. *See* hydroxy amphet-
amine
Parasympatholytic agents 392
Parasympathomimetic agents 392
Parnate 143, 391. *See* Tranylcy-
promine (Parnate)
Partial thickness surgery 176
Parvo cells 14, 487
Pasque flower *(Anemone Pulsitilla)*
278
Pedigree 224
Penetrating Keratoplasty 60
Perception, stimulation 84, 105,
135, 140, 158, 235, 263,
267, 488
Peripheral ischemia 143

Peripheral nerves 326
Peripheral vision 49, 63, 64, 93,
165, 261, 313, 400, 406,
410, 417, 420, 421, 442
Perphenazine (Triafon) 391
Perri, Dolores xiv, 316
Pesticides 199, 283, 285, 295, 300,
306, 307, 308, 309, 326,
348, 357, 359, 361, 476, 477
Peter's Anomaly 71, 72, 73
Phacoemulsification 205, 206, 207,
208, 488
Phagocyte cells 242
Phenelzine (Nardil) 391
Phenotype 224
Phospholine Iodide (Echothiophate)
136, 174, 392
Photocoagulation 140, 153, 154,
163, 164, 165, 488. *See* laser
surgery
Photodynamic therapy 106, 139,
140, 153, 488
Photoreceptors 4, 63, 232, 325,
330, 457, 477
Physostigmine 272
Phytochemicals 291, 295, 307, 352
Pigmentary Dispersion Syndrome
8, 30, 38, 58, 84, 102, 162,
449, 485. *See* Glaucoma
Pigment epithelial derived factor
(PEDF) 487
Pilocarpine 40, 82, 90, 114, 131,
134, 135, 136, 144, 157,
162, 166, 272, 392
Plaque 12, 50, 216, 268, 298, 301,
327, 336, 359
Plateau *iris* 38, 102, 161, 488
Pneumotonometer 92, 93, 488
Polarimetry 20, 97, 98, 461, 489
Pollutants 199, 324, 337, 360, 476

Polymorphous dystrophy 54, 55, 84
Polypharmacy 389
Polyphenols 290, 298, 311, 316, 318
Post-Cataract Glaucoma 59
Potassium 133, 202, 216, 243, 291, 295, 308, 312, 337, 338, 339, 364, 368, 371, 386
Potential acuity meter (PAM) 487, 488
Preservatives 122, 141, 142, 289, 304, 305, 361, 407, 409, 464
Prevent Blindness America 93, 399, 424, 446, 504
Primary infantile glaucoma 70, 82
Pro-Banthine 391. *See* Propantheline (Pro-Bantine)
Progressive iris atrophy 52, 54
Prolixin 391. *See* Fluphenazine
Propanolol (Inderal) 126, 385
Propantheline (Pro-Bantine) 391
Prophylactive, use of 382
Propine 131, 512
Prostaglandins 28, 31, 40, 46, 81, 123, 124, 127, 128, 129, 130, 138, 347
Proview 93
Pseudoexfoliation xi, 457, 461, 488
Puncta 485
Pupillary block 35, 39, 41, 79, 80, 81, 161, 162, 174, 193, 205, 392
Pupils 42, 88, 99, 131, 198, 391, 393
Pyridoxine. *See* Vitamin B

Q

Quercetin 219, 317, 474

R

Raman Spectroscope 107
Reactive oxygen species (ROS) 199, 200, 330
Relaxation 242, 246, 253, 254, 338, 449
Rescula 127, 128, 129, 142
Research in Vision and 51, 470, 471, 472, 474, 475, 478
RESTOR lens 207
Rhodopsin 3, 200, 221, 277, 318, 319, 487
Ribonucleic acid 218
Ribonucleic acid (RNA) 218
Rieger's Anomaly 71, 72
Ritch, Dr, Robert xiii, xiv, 39, 268, 269, 457, 461, 475, 495, 497
Rods 14, 16, 111, 277, 318, 480, 486, 489
Rubella
  Congenital 68
Rubinstein-taybi syndrome 83
Rutin 317

S

Saccharin 366
Safety glasses 399, 400
Scanning laser acuity potential (PAM) 203
Schepens Eye Institute 390
Schlemm's canal 5, 11, 12, 13, 42, 56, 70, 176, 180, 181, 182, 183, 185, 189, 464, 485, 489
Schwartz, Dr. Michal 24, 58, 223, 287, 466, 472
Sclera 4, 6, 11, 14, 21, 27, 58, 70, 76, 89, 131, 148, 163, 173, 176, 180, 181, 191, 192, 343, 344, 483, 489
Scleral flap disinsertion 191
Scopolamine (Donagel) 94, 391, 392

Seizures 75, 76, 77, 219
Select laser 155
Selenium 291, 303, 307, 308, 312,
   313, 317, 322, 332, 343
Self-healing 242, 245, 246, 247,
   252
Senecio cineraria. *See* silver ragwort
Seton implant 184
Shiatsu 262, 264, 489
SHORT syndrome 83
Short wave length automated perim-
   etry (SWAP) 489
Sickle cell disease 50, 66, 315
Siegel, Dr. Bernie 242, 472
Simmons shell 178, 190
Simplesse 363
Sjogren's syndrome (dry eye) 9, 44,
   345, 489
Skeletal deformation 75
Slit lamp 88, 89, 90, 100, 489
Snellen chart 87, 89, 197, 421,
   479, 489
Soap 361
  kosher 361
Sodium 53, 103, 132, 133, 134,
   141, 142, 192, 202, 218,
   220, 243, 298, 337, 339,
   363, 368, 390, 409, 472, 473
Sodium chondroitin sulfate 221
Sodium lauryl sulfate 409
SOLX Titanium Sapphire Laser
   170
Spaeth, Dr. George 375, 458
Spherophakia. *See* Marchesani's syn-
   drome
Sphincterotomy 166
Spiral computed tomography 106
Spironolactone 391
Stabilized oxychloro complex (SOC)
   141
Staphylococcus 191

Static perimetry 110, 111
Steroids 12, 25, 45, 49, 52, 58, 61,
   62, 82, 139, 186, 190, 191,
   193, 194, 198, 199, 206,
   210, 347, 410
Strabismus 73, 78
Streptococcus 191, 305
Stress 29, 37, 41, 43, 63, 65, 123,
   146, 165, 200, 208, 219,
   220, 243, 244, 245, 248,
   250, 252, 266, 267, 270,
   280, 281, 288, 291, 292,
   310, 324, 326, 336, 347,
   376, 379, 381, 411, 415,
   417, 469, 471, 476, 477
Sturge-Weber syndrome 68, 74, 75,
   83
Succinylcholine 390
Sulfur 132, 133, 291, 303, 317,
   336, 337, 338, 343, 368, 463
Sunglasses 7, 10, 64, 140, 148,
   166, 187, 201, 330, 401,
   406, 410, 411, 412, 424, 425
Superciliary Effusion 194
Superior oblique muscle 4, 489
Superoxide dismutase 221, 291,
   292, 310, 328, 341, 489
Support groups xi, xii, 497, 506
Support services vii, 426, 497, 501
Surgery xii, 9, 18, 19, 28, 30, 38,
   40, 41, 42, 43, 45, 59, 60,
   61, 70, 72, 73, 75, 76, 81,
   82, 84, 85, 92, 101, 126,
   135, 141, 148, 149, 151,
   152, 153, 154, 155, 156,
   157, 159, 161, 164, 166,
   167, 168, 169, 171, 172,
   173, 174, 175, 176, 178,
   179, 180, 182, 183, 184,
   185, 186, 188, 189, 190,
   191, 192, 193, 194, 195,

203, 204, 205, 207, 208,
209, 210, 211, 213, 228,
235, 245, 247, 249, 257,
266, 280, 315, 340, 352,
357, 381, 382, 384, 385,
390, 396, 397, 419, 427,
449, 456, 459, 462, 467,
468, 469, 481, 486, 489,
490, 498
Sweeteners 302, 364, 366
Sympathomimetic agents 392
systemic lupus erythematosus 44

T

Tears 9, 62, 116, 135, 142, 154,
164, 189, 243, 263, 483,
485, 486
Telemedicine 195, 455
Telescopes 410, 420, 428, 429
Television and movie access 438
Tenormin (Atenolol) 126
The Glaucoma Foundation x, 447,
457, 464, 465, 495, 496, 503
The Glaucoma Research Foundation
143, 433, 465
Thyroid 30, 56, 278, 287, 288,
299, 342, 343, 345, 348,
352, 359, 391, 470, 472,
477, 498
TIGR (gene) 13, 30, 31, 62, 84
Timolol (Timoptic) 123, 124, 127,
134, 138, 157, 275, 324,
387, 512
T-lymphocytes 287
Tobacco 301, 310, 357, 392
Toric lens 207
Toxoplasmosis 44, 490
Trabectome 155, 183, 227, 467,
490
Trabecular meshwork 5, 11, 12, 13,
25, 30, 32, 38, 40, 42, 45,

47, 48, 51, 56, 57, 58, 59,
60, 62, 67, 68, 70, 71, 73,
75, 76, 77, 78, 81, 82, 83,
84, 123, 134, 135, 145, 146,
155, 156, 157, 158, 167,
170, 176, 180, 181, 183,
200, 207, 215, 225, 226,
227, 231, 232, 234, 236,
241, 268, 313, 314, 344,
390, 461, 480, 485, 488, 490
Trabeculectomy 36, 53, 56, 68, 76,
81, 82, 120, 122, 138, 156,
159, 161, 162, 173, 175,
176, 177, 178, 179, 180,
181, 182, 183, 184, 185,
192, 209, 211, 228, 449,
468, 490
Trabeculoplasty 32, 40, 119, 130,
138, 151, 152, 153, 154,
155, 157, 159, 160, 167,
173, 398, 449, 461, 462,
464, 468, 490
Trabeculotomy 70, 73, 76
Trace elements 308, 342. *See* Minerals
Transderm scop. *See* scopolamine
Transillumination 38, 90
Tranylcypromine (Parnate) 391
Trauma 6, 43, 50, 56, 57, 68, 81,
82, 84, 179, 186, 215, 244,
266
Treatment Study 33, 34, 91, 119,
156, 420, 459
Trental. *See* Pentoxifylline
Triamcinolone (Kenalog) 46, 52
Trichlormethiazide 391
Trichloroacetic acid 190
Trihexyphenidyl(Artane) 391
Trilafon 391. *See* Perphenazine
(Triafon)
Trisomy 79, 83

Tropicamide (Mydriacy) 94, 392
Trusopt 11, 132, 133, 134, 142, 146, 222, 387
Tuberous sclerosis (Bourneville Disease) 74, 76
Tumors 56, 58, 68, 74, 75, 76, 77, 81, 84, 102, 291, 360, 364
Tylenol 187, 324, 385. *See* Acetaminophen
Tyrosinase 39, 129

U

Ubiquinone (CoQ10) 323
UK 99, 145, 494, 497
Ultrasound biomicroscopy 34, 90, 101, 488
Ultraviolet rays 7, 9, 148, 235, 305
Uvea 4, 34, 43, 61, 179, 211, 484, 490
Uveitis 8, 19, 24, 27, 30, 43, 44, 45, 46, 56, 62, 78, 81, 129, 137, 156, 167, 174, 179, 185, 189, 206, 207, 211, 216, 242, 392, 455, 458, 459, 460, 461, 484, 495

V

Vaccinium myrtillus. *See* Bilberry (Vaccinum myrtillus)
Vanadium 317, 342
Vascular endothelial growth factor (VEGF) 49, 139, 490
Vasodilation 252
Viramin B1 (thiamine) 294, 326, 331, 333
Viscoelastic 181, 205, 206, 344, 464
Vision, color 96, 116
Vision loss xv, 15, 26, 29, 32, 34, 48, 51, 63, 90, 91, 98, 99, 100, 101, 109, 115, 119, 120, 141, 156, 165, 168, 188, 223, 228, 288, 373, 377, 444, 456, 474, 476
Visual aids 402, 420, 428, 449, 506
Visual-evoked potential (VEP) 105
Visual field xi, xii, 17, 30, 32, 33, 34, 37, 41, 51, 57, 86, 93, 96, 98, 99, 101, 105, 106, 107, 108, 109, 110, 111, 113, 114, 118, 120, 123, 130, 138, 167, 172, 174, 186, 204, 222, 225, 270, 276, 279, 326, 338, 356, 365, 377, 381, 410, 420, 423, 425, 449, 455, 456, 457, 472, 477, 480, 483, 484, 487, 489, 490
Visudyne 106, 140, 165, 166
Vitamin A 66, 318, 329, 351, 355, 474, 476
Vitamin B2 (riboflavin) 332
Vitamin B3 (niacin, niacinamide) 332
Vitamin B6 (pyridoxine) 334
Vitamin B12 (methylcobalimin) 334
Vitamin C (ascorbic acid) 294, 312, 313, 314, 315, 316, 331, 332
Vitamin D 328, 329, 474
Vitamin E 314, 321, 322
Vitamin K 331
Vitamins xii, 11, 80, 193, 200, 201, 221, 246, 257, 273, 286, 290, 291, 294, 295, 297, 300, 303, 304, 305, 311, 312, 313, 314, 315, 319, 320, 324, 328, 330, 331, 338, 341, 345, 349,

350, 351, 352, 355, 362, 363, 366, 393, 395

Vitamin supplementation 201, 350, 444

Vitreous body 5, 10, 60, 490

Vitreous humor 4, 488, 490

Vogt-Koyanagi Harado Syndrome 44

Von Hippel-Lindau Disease 77

Von Recklinghausen's Disease 74

W

Water 4, 10, 14, 44, 61, 67, 102, 133, 146, 149, 166, 199, 201, 208, 220, 241, 242, 243, 255, 260, 269, 274, 278, 279, 281, 283, 284, 290, 295, 297, 299, 300, 303, 304, 307, 310, 324, 326, 327, 337, 339, 340, 344, 346, 348, 351, 353, 359, 360, 361, 369, 370, 371, 408, 439, 476, 482

Weill-Marchesani Syndrome 79

Whipple's Disease 44, 490

X

Xalatan (Latanoprost) 40, 56, 124, 127, 128, 129, 142, 223, 387, 388, 512

Xanthogranuloma 81, 84

Y

Yoga 188, 246, 247, 248, 250, 253, 255, 261, 265, 268, 269, 382, 400, 405, 444, 449

Yogurt 294, 304, 305, 331, 332, 336, 364, 367

Z

Zinc 227, 243, 246, 291, 294, 303, 308, 312, 313, 318, 325, 332, 337, 339, 341, 342, 350, 355, 358, 361, 371, 475

Zonular fibers 11, 490

Zonules 8, 38, 40, 42, 59, 88, 197, 198, 205, 206, 390, 481

LaVergne, TN USA
01 July 2010
188112LV00007B/77/P